Diagnosis and
Treatment Planning Skills for
MENTAL HEALTH
PROFESSIONALS

Diagnosis and Treatment Planning Skills for MENTAL HEALTH PROFESSIONALS

A Popular Culture Casebook Approach

Alan M. Schwitzer ▪ **Lawrence C. Rubin**

Old Dominion University

St. Thomas University

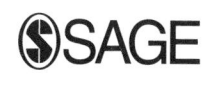

Los Angeles | London | New Delhi
Singapore | Washington DC

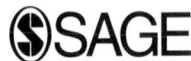

Los Angeles | London | New Delhi
Singapore | Washington DC

FOR INFORMATION:

SAGE Publications, Inc.
2455 Teller Road
Thousand Oaks, California 91320
E-mail: order@sagepub.com

SAGE Publications Ltd.
1 Oliver's Yard
55 City Road
London EC1Y 1SP
United Kingdom

SAGE Publications India Pvt. Ltd.
B 1/I 1 Mohan Cooperative Industrial Area
Mathura Road, New Delhi 110 044
India

SAGE Publications Asia-Pacific Pte. Ltd.
33 Pekin Street #02-01
Far East Square
Singapore 048763

Acquisitions Editor: Kassie Graves
Editorial Assistant: Courtney Munz
Production Editor: Karen Wiley
Copy Editor: Amy Rosenstein
Typesetter: C&M Digitals (P) Ltd.
Proofreader: Kristin Bergstad
Indexer: Sheila Bodell
Cover Designer: Scott Van Atta
Marketing Manager: Katie Winters
Permissions Editor: Adele Hutchinson

Printed in the United States of America

Library of Congress Cataloging-in-Publication Data

Schwitzer, Alan M.

Diagnosis and treatment planning skills for mental health professionals: a popular culture casebook approach / Alan M. Schwitzer, Lawrence Rubin.

p. cm.
Includes bibliographical references and index.

ISBN 978-1-4129-8882-7 (pbk. : acid-free paper)

1. Counseling—Methodology. 2. Counseling—Case studies. 3. Popular culture—United States—Case studies. 4. Managed mental health care—Case studies. I. Rubin, Lawrence C., 1955- II. Title.

BF636.6.S39 2012
362.196′89—dc23   2011037033

This book is printed on acid-free paper.

11 12 13 14 15 10 9 8 7 6 5 4 3 2 1

CONTENTS

LIST OF TABLES AND FIGURES

TABLES

FIGURES

ACKNOWLEDGMENTS

First and foremost, it has been a pleasure to complete such a successful collaboration with Lawrence Rubin. Larry's mastery of popular culture and psychology, energy for writing and educating, and clinical expertise have made this project a truly rewarding one. Working with Larry "made it so." Thanks next to my wife. Lisa is forever young and helped me keep the good times rolling even during the long hours and the pressures of writing this text. Buddy, Mae, and Rex provided psychosocial support and always reminded me when it was time to play, walk, or go to my pillow. My Department Chair Danica Hays, Dean Linda Irwin-Devitis, and Provost Carol Simpson all have been supportive. The concepts I brought to this project have been in development for many years. I am grateful to my early mentors at Virginia Commonwealth University (VCU) and The University of Texas at Austin (UT), and to the hundreds of clients, students, and colleagues at VCU, UT, Tulane, James Madison University (JMU), and Old Dominion University who have influenced my clinical thinking over the years. Finally, thanks to Acquisitions Editor Kassie Graves and SAGE Publications. Kassie and SAGE are amazing publication partners and are much appreciated.

—*AMS*

Fortunately, there were no marriages or parent-child relationships that were harmed or sacrificed in the making of this volume. The only casualty was my sleep. But it was well worth it. I am so proud to have collaborated with intellectual and clinical powerhouse Alan "Woody" Schwitzer in the creation of this book and truly believe that we offer a unique, powerful, and enjoyable teaching tool for therapists and counselors everywhere. Hey howdy hey, Woody! My wife Randi, as always, but even more so in this volume, supported and nurtured both me and my passion for popular culture by spending endless hours on the couch and in the theaters drinking in all of these fascinating characters with me. My son Zach, now 17, brought his own unique blend of pop culture appreciation into my consciousness, while my daughter Rebecca gave me an appreciation for a whole new generation of popular culture characters. I am ever grateful to my Energizer Bunny parents Esther and Herb, whom I know will be so very proud of me for once again adding to the Larry Rubin wing of their private library. I love you. And finally, I wish to thank the students of my PSY 495 class (Popular Culture and Psychology) at St. Thomas University in Miami, Florida, who helped me to better understand the characters in this book. These students are: Lisandra Abraham, Ernie Fernandez, Diamond Howard, Nathali Geitan, Ronise Labrando, Monica Lobos, Stephanie Maldonado, Roxanne Madrid, Madeline Marquiz, Keira Peralta, Stephanie Rodriguez, Kizzy Rose, and Melissa Wolozny. And lastly, thanks to Kassie Graves, Acquisitions Editor at SAGE, who has been as excited about this project as we have been.

—*LCR*

PART I

INTRODUCTION AND OVERVIEW

*Developing Diagnosis, Case Conceptualization,
and Treatment Planning Skills:
A Popular Culture Casebook Approach*

1

OVERVIEW OF THE BOOK

INTRODUCTION TO THE BOOK AND ITS APPROACH

Welcome to the first edition of *Diagnosis and Treatment Planning Skills for Mental Health Professionals: A Popular Culture Casebook.* We hope that students and new professionals—as well as their classroom instructors, faculty, and clinical supervisors—will find this book to be an exceptionally effective learning tool for developing the clinical thinking skills needed in today's world of professional counseling. Clinicians at all levels of education, training, and experience—from those currently in graduate and professional programs, to those currently in residence or preparing for licensure, to those who are seasoned professionals—and in all counseling and mental health disciplines—including professional counselors specializing in community, mental health, school, and college counseling; psychotherapists and marriage and family therapists; clinical social workers; psychologists; psychiatrists; and others in the allied mental health fields—rely on a core set of clinical thinking skills and tools to guide their effective intervention in the lives of their clients. These include: (a) *diagnosis,* which allows the counselor to describe and communicate about client presentations by matching his or her observations and the client's report of symptoms with the criteria for the various disorders found in *Diagnostic and Statistical Manual of Mental Disorders, Fourth Edition, Text Revision (DSM-IV-TR),* (b) *case conceptualization,* which provides the professional with a rationale and framework for working with clients by integrating clients' presenting thoughts, feelings, and behaviors into meaningful patterns, and (c) *treatment planning,* which integrates the information from the diagnosis and case conceptualization into a coherent therapeutic plan of action. This text fully addresses and illustrates the skills needed in all three of these areas.

Extensive Coverage of Core Clinical Thinking Skills

Historically, most textbooks have focused heavily on the development of just one or two of the core clinical thinking skills we present in this text. They might fully cover use of the *DSM-IV-TR* to make a diagnosis, methods of moving from theory to practice via a case conceptualization, or the steps needed to design a treatment plan—but usually not all of these. By comparison, this text begins with all of the details associated with multiaxial mental health diagnosis, moves on to a full review of case conceptualization specially written for new counselors, and wraps up with the important components of treatment planning. We worked hard to bring all three skills together and show how they are used in connection with one another in actual, everyday practice—and to write each chapter with students and new counselors in mind.

Detailed Case Illustrations

Further, traditionally, typical counseling and psychotherapy clinical textbooks have offered only snippets of case illustrations, rather than walking you through case development, step by step, from beginning to end. Often these are partial or whole cases that are amalgams of various cases from the author's own caseload or are fictitious cases designed to show some aspect of diagnosis, case conceptualization, or treatment planning. In contrast, our textbook provides 30 fully prepared case illustrations— each of which introduces you to the client, shows a professional intake summary, presents and explains a case conceptualization, and develops a fully prepared treatment plan. Most interestingly, the cases from which you will learn and practice using this text are drawn directly from popular culture (i.e., television, movies, literature, advertising, the musical stage, song lyrics, comics, and even video games). We have chosen 30 characters who become fascinating clients, most of whom will be either somewhat or very familiar to you. Together they represent a wide range of individual differences, including various ages, ethnic identities, cultures, socioeconomic statuses, and sexual identities. In addition, they illustrate a wide range of presenting concerns, different types of client needs and issues, and various forms and levels of diagnosable disorders. For many of these clients, we also provide recommended links to video portrayals of characters, which further brings them to life for you.

The characters you will meet and analyze in this book include:

- *Children's Characters and Video Game Characters:* The Muppets' Miss Piggy, Mario of video game fame, Gretel, anime superstar Naruto Uzumaki, and Snoopy
- *Troubled Youth in Film and on Stage: Twilight's* Edward Cullen, Jamal Malik from *Slumdog Millionaire, Juno's* Juno MacGuff, Claire from *The Breakfast Club,* and *Wicked's* Elphaba Thropp
- *Animated Characters:* Cartoon character Cleveland Brown, Jessie the Yodeling Cowgirl, Tinkerbell, *The Simpsons'* Waylon Smithers, and *Beauty and the Beast's* Belle
- *Adults in Television Sitcoms and Drama:* TV drama star Jack Bauer, *Golden Girls'* Sophia Petrillo, George Lopez, *Star Trek's* Lieutenant Commander Data, and Jack McFarland from *Will and Grace*
- *Characters in Music, Musicals, and Advertising:* Dunkin' Donuts' Fred the Baker, *West Side Story's* Maria, Billie Jean from the Michael Jackson song of the same name, the Beatles' Eleanor Rigby, and the Geico Caveman
- *Characters in Literature and Comics: Misery's* Annie Wilkes, *The Color Purple's* Miss Celie, Chief Bromden from *One Flew Over the Cuckoo's Nest,* Peter Parker, aka Spider-Man, and A. A. Milne's Christopher Robin

Rather than offering snippets of these cases, we take you from start to finish—from intake through treatment planning—so that you can develop a full understanding and appreciation of how diagnosis, case conceptualization, and treatment planning skills are applied to rich, complex, and engaging clinical cases. Further, within the discussion of each of these 30 cases, we provide extensive, step-by-step, empirically supported guidelines to help you to develop each of the three critical clinical thinking skills.

HOW TO USE PART I OF THE BOOK

This book is divided into four parts. In Part I, Introduction and Overview, we provide a rationale for using popular culture cases in the development of your case conceptualization, diagnosis, and treatment planning skills. The current chapter provides readers with an overview of the book's approach to the learning. Then, in Chapter 2: Popular Culture as a Learning Tool in Counseling and Psychotherapy, we discuss the role of popular culture in our everyday lives, the debate over the effects of popular culture on our lives, the importance of assessing your Popular Culture IQ (PCIQ), the value of using popular culture clients to build a clinical caseload, and how popular culture can be a resource for counselor development and growth. We include the professional perspectives of practicing counselors and real-life client examples. This part of the book sets the stage for the learning that will follow, so to make the best use of Part I, you will want to read the chapters and complete an exercise in Chapter 2 that asks you to begin exploring the 30 case illustrations we will be using later on.

HOW TO USE PART II OF THE BOOK

In Part II, Diagnosis, Case Conceptualization, and Treatment Planning, we provide extensive, didactic coverage of the knowledge, information, and skills you will need to perform diagnosis, case conceptualization, and treatment planning. First, Chapter 3, Clinical Thinking Skills: Diagnosis, Case Conceptualization, and Treatment Planning, introduces and defines the three clinical thinking tools. This chapter was written to show how the different skills are used together in counseling practice and to highlight how students and new professionals can best approach learning and skill development in these areas.

Next, in Chapter 4, Diagnosis: Understanding and Using the *DSM-IV-TR,* we offer a comprehensive discussion of the *DSM-IV-TR,* including diagnosis in the context of professional counseling, the benefits and limitations of diagnosis, and an in-depth analysis of the complete multiaxial system. Then, in Chapter 5, Case Conceptualization: Making Sense of the Client's Concerns, we provide a rich discussion of the importance of case conceptualization—and present a detailed discussion of case conceptualization for students

and new professionals using our four-step Inverted Pyramid Method (the process includes problem identification, thematic groupings, theoretical inferences, and narrowed inferences). Finally, Chapter 6, Treatment Planning: Designing a Plan for Change, provides a comprehensive discussion of the process of treatment planning, in which we build on the information derived from the diagnosis and case conceptualization in order to create a logical plan of action. We use a four-step approach to the treatment plan includes establishing a behavioral definition of the problem(s), identifying and articulating goals for change, describing the therapeutic intervention(s), and providing outcome measures of change.

Each of these chapters gives readers an introduction, sets the professional counseling context, offers step-by-step instructions regarding each aspect of the skill covered, and then presents a "Pulling It All Together" section. Each chapter provides professional viewpoints and several also provide clinical snapshots drawn from practice, they all suggest ample skill-building and learning exercises, and give clear learning goals. In addition, the chapters include as many helpful tables and figures as possible. To most effectively use Part II, you will want to read the chapters in sequence, keep track of your learning goals, complete as many of the exercises as possible, continue exploring the 30 case illustrations, and follow the various suggestions for practice and application.

SPECIAL FEATURES IN PARTS I AND II

As we have indicated, at selected points in the text, you will find several special features. These include:

- Snapshots: Professional Perspectives
- Clinical Spotlights
- Skill and Learning Exercises

You will find each of these features set off in highlighted boxes. The *Snapshots: Professional Perspectives* share the impressions of practitioners

Figure 1.1 Special Features Found in Highlight Boxes

Snapshots: Professional Perspectives	Present selected impressions of practicing counselors
Clinical Spotlights	Present selected themes from real-life client experiences
Skill and Learning Exercises	Present suggested activities for integrating chapter material

as they relate to the material covered. The *Clinical Spotlights* add to the learning by sharing a few, selected real-life client experiences. The *Skill and Learning Exercises* suggest activities you can use to integrate the material covered, most often by referring to and using this text's popular culture case illustrations. We hope you will read all of the snapshots and spotlights, and engage in the learning activities, when you come to them in your reading. These can be approached on your own, working with a partner, or as group exercises during class meetings.

HOW TO USE PART III OF THE BOOK

Building on the information and knowledge covered in Chapters 3 through 6, in Part III: Diagnosis, Case Conceptualization, and Treatment Planning: 30 Case Illustrations, we go on to illustrate the clinical thinking tools using our case examples. In this part of the book, we take you from start to finish in the analysis of each of the 30 popular culture–based cases—moving from intake to assessment and case conceptualization to diagnosis and finally to treatment planning. Each case can be read all on its own. We explain what was done to complete the intake, the counselor's decision-making during

diagnosis, the clinician's thought process during case conceptualization, and the method followed to build the treatment plan.

We have attempted to make our 30-client "case-load" as illustrative as possible. As you will see in Table 1.1, by reviewing all 30 case illustrations, you will find examples covering nearly every class of diagnosable disorders and other conditions found in the *DSM-IV-TR*. Somewhere among the cases you should be able to find the presenting concerns and client needs that are of most interest to you, are most relevant to your professional interests, and most salient to your educational and training focus. Further, you can widen your knowledge base by examining all of the cases in detail in order to see how concerns drawn from every corner of diagnosis are addressed.

We also have attempted to present a wide range of theoretical and practice approaches when forming our case conceptualizations and designing our treatment plans. As you will see in Table 1.2, by reviewing all 30 case illustrations, you will find examples covering nearly all of the major theoretical approaches commonly used in practice, extensive examples using psychotherapeutic integrations that combine multiple approaches, and further examples using eclectic and solution-focused methods. Here again, you are likely to find illustrations using many of the approaches that will be most important in your own education and clinical training, and in real-life practice. Wherever possible, we have emphasized evidence-based practices; elsewhere, we explain the practical rationale for the counseling method selected.

Further, along with showcasing a broad range of presenting concerns and a mixture of treatment approaches, we have worked to build a caseload that emphasizes and illustrates the individual differences typically seen among clients. As Table 1.3 shows, our 30 cases are relatively diverse. Throughout Part III, we identify the significant demographic features that differentiate our clients according to age, ethnicity, culture, American or international residence, socioeconomic status, sexual/gender identity, and additional

(Continued)

Table 1.1 Our Popular Culture Caseload: *DSM-IV-TR* Diagnoses and Presenting Concerns

Client	Page	Diagnoses and Presenting Problems Illustrated	
		DSM-IV-TR **Section**	*DSM-IV-TR* **Axis I and Axis II Diagnoses**
Miss Piggy	130	Personality Disorders	Borderline Personality Disorder
Mario	142	Substance-Related Disorders	Cocaine Dependence, Alcohol Abuse
		Sleep Disorder	Substance-Induced Sleep Disorder
Gretel	156	Disorders Usually First Diagnosed in Infancy, Childhood, or Adolescence	Oppositional Defiant Disorder
Naruto	167	Disorders Usually First Diagnosed in Infancy, Childhood, or Adolescence	Attention-Deficit/Hyperactivity Disorder Conduct Disorder
Snoopy	185	Disorders Usually First Diagnosed in Infancy, Childhood, or Adolescence	Autistic Disorder
Edward Cullen	202	Mood Disorders	Major Depressive Disorder
Jamal Malik	215	Anxiety Disorders	Acute Stress Disorder
Juno	225	Other Conditions That May Be a Focus of Clinical Attention	Parent-Child Problem
Claire	237	Eating Disorders	Eating Disorder Not Otherwise Specified
		Substance-Related Disorders	Cannabis Abuse
		Impulse Control Disorders Not Classified Elsewhere	Trichotillomania
Elphaba	249	Somatoform Disorder	Body Dysmorphic Disorder
		Personality Disorder	Antisocial Personality Disorder Features
Cleveland Brown	266	Substance-Related Disorder	Alcohol Abuse
		Mood Disorder	Dysthymic Disorder
		Sexual and Gender Identity Disorders	Erectile Dysfunction
		Other Conditions That May Be a Focus of Clinical Attention	Relational Problem Not Otherwise Specified
Jessie	282	Disorders Usually First Diagnosed in Infancy, Childhood, or Adolescence	Reactive Attachment Disorder

(Continued)

Table 1.1 (Continued)

Client	Page	Diagnoses and Presenting Problems Illustrated	
		DSM-IV-TR Section	*DSM-IV-TR* Axis I and Axis II Diagnoses
Tinkerbell	292	Schizophrenia and Other Psychotic Disorders	Schizoaffective Disorder
		Personality Disorders	Borderline Personality Disorder Features
Waylon Smithers	306	Other Conditions That May Be a Focus of Clinical Attention	Identity Problem
The Beast's Belle	318	Anxiety Disorder	Social Phobia
		Personality Disorder	Avoidant Features
Jack Bauer	335	Anxiety Disorder	Posttraumatic Stress Disorder
		Other Conditions That May Be a Focus of Clinical Attention	Bereavement
		Personality Disorder	Antisocial Personality Disorder Features
Sophia	347	Delirium, Dementia, Amnestic, and Other Cognitive Disorders	Dementia of the Alzheimer's Type
George Lopez	359	Adjustment Disorders	Adjustment Disorder With Mixed Mood
		Other Conditions That May Be a Focus of Clinical Attention	Acculturation Problem
Lieutenant Commander Data	373	Mood Disorders	Major Depressive Disorder
		Mental Disorders Due to a General Medical Condition	Amnestic Disorder Due to a General Medical Disorder
		Other Conditions That May Be a Focus of Clinical Attention	Identity Problem
			Religious or Spiritual Problem
Jack McFarland	388	Disorders Usually First Diagnosed in Infancy, Childhood, or Adolescence	Attention-Deficit/Hyperactivity Disorder
		Mood Disorders	Major Depressive Disorder
		Personality Disorder	Histrionic Personality Disorder Features
Fred the Baker	410	Adjustment Disorders	Adjustment Disorder With Depressed Mood
Maria	423	Anxiety Disorders	Acute Stress Disorder
		Other Conditions That May Be a Focus of Clinical Attention	Bereavement

Client	Page	Diagnoses and Presenting Problems Illustrated	
		DSM-IV-TR Section	*DSM-IV-TR* Axis I and Axis II Diagnoses
Billie Jean	434	Schizophrenia and Other Psychotic Disorders	Delusional Disorder
Eleanor Rigby	447	Disorders Usually First Diagnosed in Infancy, Childhood, or Adolescence	Mental Retardation
		Mental Disorders Due to a General Medical Condition	Mood Disorder Due to a General Medical Condition
Geico Caveman	458	Adjustment Disorders	Adjustment Disorder With Depressed Mood
		Other Conditions That May Be a Focus of Clinical Attention	Identity Problem, Acculturation Problem
Annie Wilkes	474	Mood Disorders	Bipolar Disorder
		Personality Disorders	Antisocial Personality Disorder
Miss Celie	488	Mood Disorders	Dysthymic Disorder
		Anxiety Disorders	Posttraumatic Stress Disorder
Chief Bromden	503	Schizophrenia and Other Psychotic Disorders	Schizophrenia
Peter Parker	517	Mood Disorders	Major Depressive Disorder
		Mental Disorder due to a General Medical Condition	Personality Change due to a General Medical Condition
Christopher Robin	532	Disorders Usually First Diagnosed in Infancy, Childhood, or Adolescence	Asperger's Disorder

contextual features such as educational status; factors of religion, spirituality, or faith; and involvement in occupational settings, school systems, or the legal system. Wherever relevant, you will find case information illustrating the thought processes needed to form diagnoses, case conceptualizations, and treatment plans that are responsive to individual differences.

Taken together, the 30 cases found in the six chapters comprising Part III of the book present a wide range of examples of clinical thinking as it is applied to child, adolescent, and adult clients representing a diverse set of populations, presenting a wide range of concerns and needs, and for whom a variety counseling approaches are used. You can make the most of the cases in Part III by following all of the learning and skill building exercise found in the earlier chapters, most of which refer to our case illustrations; reading through, comparing and contrasting, and

(Continued)

Table 1.2   Our Popular Culture Caseload: Theoretical Approaches to Case Conceptualization and Treatment Planning

Client	Page	Theoretical and Treatment Approaches Represented	
		Individual Counseling and Psychotherapy	Additional Treatment Modalities
Miss Piggy	130	Dialectical Behavior Therapy	Case Management
Mario	142	Integrative: Multicomponent Psychosocial Intervention Approach Motivational Interviewing	Inpatient Treatment Narcotics Anonymous (NA)
Gretel	156	Integrative: Client-Centered Play Therapy Cognitive Behavioral Play Therapy	Family Play Therapy
Naruto	167	Multicomponent Psychosocial Intervention Approach	Psychopharmacology Consultation Family Counseling Parent Support Group
Snoopy	185	Eclectic: DIR (Floor Time) Therapy Behavior Therapy Expressive Creative Arts Play Therapy	Family Counseling and Psychoeducation Social Skills Psychoeducational Group
Edward Cullen	202	Integrative: Cognitive Behavior Therapy Interpersonal Psychotherapy	Psychopharmacology Consultation Family Counseling
Jamal Malik	215	Brief Solution-Focused Counseling Emphasizing Cognitive Behavioral Interventions With Adolescents	Psychopharmacology Consultation Relaxation Training
Juno	225	Client-Centered Counseling	Family Counseling Support Group
Claire	237	Brief Contemporary Psychodynamic Psychotherapy	Group Counseling
Elphaba	249	Cognitive Behavior Therapy	Gestalt-Oriented Group Counseling

Client	Page	Theoretical and Treatment Approaches Represented	
		Individual Counseling and Psychotherapy	Additional Treatment Modalities
Cleveland Brown	266	Integrative: Schema Focused Cognitive Therapy Interpersonal Psychotherapy	Couples Counseling Family Counseling
Jessie	282	Theraplay	Dyadic Family Therapy
Tinkerbell	292	Solution-Focused Counseling Emphasizing Cognitive Interventions and Dialectical Behavioral Interventions	Inpatient Hospitalization Psychopharmacology Consultation
Waylon Smithers	306	Person-Centered Counseling	
The Beast's Belle	318	Cognitive Behavior Therapy	
Jack Bauer	335	Cognitive Behavior Therapy	Eye Movement Desensitization and Reprocessing and Exposure Relaxation Training
Sophia	347	Integrative: Behavior Therapy Cognitive Stimulation Therapy	Family Counseling and Psychoeducation
George Lopez	359	Reality Therapy	
Lieutenant Commander Data	373	Integrative: Cognitive Behavior Therapy Existential Counseling	Group Counseling
Jack McFarland	388	Integrative: Brief Psychodynamic Psychotherapy Cognitive Behavior Therapy	Career Planning Relaxation Training
Fred the Baker	410	Person-Centered Counseling	
Maria	423	Cognitive Behavior Therapy	Bereavement Support Group
Billie Jean	434	Brief Solution-Focused Counseling Emphasizing Cognitive Interventions With Adolescents	Psychopharmacology Consultation Family Counseling Day Treatment With Group and Psychoeducational Group Counseling

(Continued)

Table 1.2 (Continued)

Client	Page	Theoretical and Treatment Approaches Represented	
		Individual Counseling and Psychotherapy	Additional Treatment Modalities
Eleanor Rigby	447	Brief Solution-Focused Counseling	General Medical Pharmacology Referral Support Group
Geico Caveman	458	Adlerian Therapy	
Annie Wilkes	474	Cognitive Behavior Therapy	Inpatient Hospitalization Psychopharmacology Consultation Psychoeducational Group Counseling
Miss Celie	488	Integrative: Schema-Focused Cognitive Therapy Feminist Therapy	Support Group
Chief Bromden	503	Integrative: Cognitive Behavior Therapy Cognitive Remediation	Psychopharmacology Consultation Day Treatment With Group and Individual Counseling Psychoeducational Group Counseling
Peter Parker	517	Integrative: Cognitive Behavior Therapy Reality Therapy	Stress Management Training
Christopher Robin	532	Expressive Creative Arts Play Therapy	Parent Consultation Teacher Consultation

Note: As we have written the case scenarios in this book, many of our characters are experiencing complex situations that can be characterized as diagnosable mental health concerns. In addition, as often occurs in your real-life work as counselors and psychotherapists, you will find that many of these characters are experiencing more than one concern. These types of diagnosable and co-occurring client situations sometimes require, or suggest the need for, multiple forms of counseling and other interventions. The counseling approaches and interventions you will find presented in this table and in our 30 case conceptualizations and treatment plans were selected from among the most important approaches taught in counseling theories classes, from today's documented best mental health practices, and from evidence-based counseling recommendations derived mostly from large-scale treatment outcome studies and meta-analyses of treatment outcome research. They are a starting point for clinical conversation!

Table 1.3 Our Popular Culture Caseload: Client Populations and Individual Differences

Client	Page	Populations and Characteristics Illustrated				
		Lifespan	Age	Gender	Ethnicity/Culture	Sexual Orientation	Additional Contextual Information
Miss Piggy	130	Adult	32	Female	White	Heterosexual	French–American heritage
Mario	142	Adult	44	Male	White	Heterosexual	Italian-American heritage
Gretel	156	Child	10	Female	Austrian, White	Heterosexual	International client
Naruto	167	Child	09	Male	Japanese	Heterosexual	International client
Snoopy	185	Child	12	Male	White	Heterosexual	Middle school student
Edward Cullen	202	Adolescent	17	Male	White	Heterosexual	High school student Adopted family
Jamal Malik	215	Adolescent	17	Male	Indian	Heterosexual	International client Muslim faith Impoverished
Juno	225	Adolescent	16	Female	White	Heterosexual	High school student
Claire	237	Adolescent	17	Female	White	Heterosexual	Affluent suburban context
Elphaba	249	Young adult	22	Female	Of color (Green)	Heterosexual	College student
Cleveland Brown	266	Adult	42	Male	African American	Heterosexual	Stepfamily
Jessie	282	Child	11	Female	White	Heterosexual	Foster care
Tinkerbell	292	Adult	45	Female	Of color (Pink)	Heterosexual	Workplace-referred client
Waylon Smithers	306	Adult	38	Male	White	Homosexual	Mandated client
The Beast's Belle	318	Adult	31	Female	British, White	Heterosexual	International client

(Continued)

Table 1.3 (Continued)

Client	Page							
		Populations and Characteristics Illustrated						
		Lifespan	Age	Gender	Ethnicity/Culture	Sexual Orientation	Additional Contextual Information	
Jack Bauer	355	Adult	43	Male	White	Heterosexual	Mandated client	
Sophia	347	Adult	85	Female	White	Heterosexual	Older adult client	
George Lopez	359	Adult	48	Male	Hispanic	Heterosexual	Mexican American heritage Catholic faith	
Lieutenant Commander Data	373	Adult	25	Male	Other (Android)	Heterosexual	Workplace-referred client	
Jack McFarland	388	Adult	34	Male	White	Homosexual	Large city context	
Fred the Baker	410	Adult	72	Male	White	Heterosexual	Older adult client	
Maria	423	Young adult	18	Female	Hispanic	Heterosexual	Puerto Rican–American heritage Catholic faith	
Billie Jean	434	Adolescent	15	Female	African American	Heterosexual	Impoverished background Large city context	
Eleanor Rigby	447	Adult	62	Female	British, White	Heterosexual Anglican faith	International client	
Geico Caveman	458	Adult	31	Male	German, White	Heterosexual	International client	
Annie Wilkes	474	Adult	42	Female	White	Heterosexual	Rural geographic context	
Miss Celie	488	Adult	51	Female	African American	Bisexual	Rural geographic context	
Chief Bromden	503	Adult	37	Male	Native American	Heterosexual	Inpatient treatment context	
Peter Parker	517	Adolescent	17	Male	White	Heterosexual	High school student client	
Christopher Robin	532	Child	6	Male	White	Heterosexual	Elementary school client	

(Continued)

forming your own impressions and critiques of, the entire group of cases; and/or by focusing especially closely on a few clients you find most useful or salient and studying these in greater detail.

HOW TO USE PART IV OF THE BOOK

Part IV wraps up the textbook with two final chapters: Chapter 13, Epilogue, and Chapter 14, Getting to Know the Clients Through Internet Sources, Published Literature, and Film. In Chapter 13, Epilogue, we bring it all together for you by summarizing what we have attempted to accomplish in the book, that is, teaching you how to implement diagnosis, case conceptualization, and treatment planning skills in the context of analyzing 30 cases drawn from the personages in popular culture. We then offer a number of caveats regarding popular culture and clinical work that will further guide you in the development of these skills. We also try to make the case for incorporating the intriguing lives of popular culture characters, when useful, in your professional world—whether it be in the counseling office, classroom, or supervisory relationship. Chapter 13 concludes by offering a number of "next learning steps" through which you can continue developing your clinical thinking skills.

Bringing the book to a close, Chapter 14, Getting to Know the Clients Through Internet Sources, Published Literature, and Film, then provides readers with a variety of web links leading to audio and video portrayals, further background and life span information, and more historical context that we think will allow you to get to know our clients even more personally and in even greater detail. You can use these websites to bring alive our illustration caseload.

We believe it is important for you to read and understand the caveats and limitations we have

outlined pertaining to the popular culture characters we the selected, the methods we used to transform them into counseling clients, and the clinical choices we made. This will help you develop your own critical counseling insights about clinical thinking. Likewise, because use of this text is just the beginning of your skill development, we hope you will make note of the next learning steps we recommend. Being able to see, hear, and learn more about the characters will enable to you to more fully engage in the clinical thinking process as you learn from our case write-ups. Naturally, we also hope that you will consider the value of popular culture in professional counseling education, training, and practice!

CHAPTER SUMMARY AND WRAP-UP

Part I of our text sets the stage for the learning to follow. In it, Chapter 1 has given an overview of the book's organization and contents, and Chapter 2 will orient readers to the use of popular culture in the learning process. In the first chapter, we outlined the critical contents to be found in Part II of the book—where Chapters 3, 4, 5, and 6 fully cover all of the details needed to begin practicing diagnosis, case conceptualization, and treatment planning. The chapter also previewed the 30 separate, start-to-finish case examples you will find in Part III of the text. The three tables in Chapter 1 presented easy-to-use summaries of the characters, divided according to presenting concerns and needs, counseling and psychotherapeutic approaches used in the cases, and individual differences. You are likely to refer back to these tables throughout the learning when searching for specific types of case illustrations. Our hope is that the book will be exceptionally valuable to you in your development as a counseling professional.

2

Popular Culture as a Learning Tool in Counseling and Psychotherapy

Introducing Chapter 2: Reader Highlights and Learning Goals

Popular culture comprises all of the various and varied mediums through which information and entertainment reaches us in the course of our daily lives. These include television, movies, music, literature, advertising, and video games. Whether a song, sitcom, superhero comic, or Broadway musical, each of these, in one way or another, tells a story about a person. The lives of these people may be of particular interest to counselors who are in the process of learning skills with which to help people.

In this chapter, we introduce the field of popular culture as a source for deepening your understanding of people. First, we will explore the role of popular culture in our everyday lives, followed by a review of the debate over its value as both a field of study and its potential role for counselors. Next, we will encourage you to develop your PCIQ (Popular Culture IQ) by becoming more intimately familiar with some of its more popular characters. We will then describe the ways in which a systematic exploration of popular culture characters can provide a useful alternative to traditional training models. In so doing, we will lay the groundwork from which you will build and then strengthen your clinical skills in the areas of case conceptualization, diagnosis, and treatment planning.

At the end of this chapter, you should be able to:

- Discuss the meaning and importance of popular culture, particularly as it relates to characters in film, television, music, literature, advertising, and video games.
- Develop an opinion as to the relative merits of familiarizing yourself with popular culture.
- Appreciate the importance of building your PCIQ as a potential vehicle for relating to clients.
- Evaluate the merits of incorporating stories drawn from the lives of popular culture characters into your counseling tool bag, particularly as a means of building case conceptualization, diagnosis, and treatment planning skills.

THE ROLE OF POPULAR CULTURE IN OUR EVERYDAY LIVES

Have you ever had the experience of watching a movie, a cartoon or television show, or reading a book in which one or several of the characters was so intriguing that you thought about him or her for days? Or perhaps you have heard a song that told such a poignant story, that for a moment you were transported into the lyrics and the very life of the person in that song. What about television commercials? We know that they are designed solely for the purpose of selling us something; but sometimes commercials and advertisements capitalize on a story about a person just like you and me, and for that reason, their story becomes interesting.

If the answer to one or several of these questions is "yes," then you appreciate, perhaps without even realizing it, the power of popular culture as mythologist Joseph Campbell said, "to grab us" (Konner & Perlmutter, 1988). Although Campbell was talking more specifically about the power of mythology to resonate with us, he believed, as do we, that the tales and stories of everyday people, whether true or fictionalized— as they are in popular culture, are fascinating (Campbell, 1968).

Throughout history, whether in word, picture, or, more recently, in electronic or digital form, people have told stories—it is in our nature to understand and share our experiences. Sometimes the stories we tell are of people who lead exemplary lives replete with success and fortune. These stories may inspire us to do great things in our own lives. Other times, we are powerfully moved by the stories of people who confront and overcome great obstacles and challenges, both inner and outer. Most fascinating perhaps, are the stories of people who struggle in their day-to-day lives to cope with adversities both great and small. These adversities may include but are certainly in no way limited to loss of a loved one, physical or mental deterioration, abuse and trauma, or the effects of drugs and alcohol. It is to these particular stories that you as future mental health practitioners will be drawn in attempts to understand and help.

The storied lives of those people who will be your clients will not be fantasy tales of good overcoming evil, nor will they take place in distant lands populated by fantastical beings. Their stories will, in some ways, be similar to your own and contain elements, individuals, and events that may seem familiar.

We have chosen to structure this book around the lives of 30 fascinating characters who, although not real per se, are in many ways fashioned after the stories of real people. You may know them through your experience as consumers of popular culture, for they have, either directly or indirectly, been a part of your life, whether or not you realize it. These characters of movie, television, music, and musicals as well as animation, literature, advertisement, and even Broadway, are each, in their own way, fascinating people, albeit fictional, or should we say, fictionalized.

You may very well wonder, "What can I possibly learn from studying the lives of fictional characters?" And once this question is asked, others must invariably follow. These include: "What role can popular culture play in the training of mental health professionals, and in particular, those studying to become counselors and psychotherapists?" "Is popular culture, which has been maligned for its potential detrimental effects on our sensibilities, a potential source for learning and professional growth?" "Can the various mediums of today's popular culture, including but not limited to television, film, literature, advertising, video games, and music, play an integral role in this training and growth, and if so, how?"

THE DEBATE OVER THE EFFECTS OF POPULAR CULTURE ON OUR LIVES

Most important, the popular culture of a country is the voice of the people—their likes and dislikes, the lifeblood of daily experience, their way of life . . . [it is] all aspects of the world we inhabit: the way of life we inherit, practice and pass on to our descendants . . . it is the everyday world around us: the mass media, entertainments, diversions, heroes, icons, rituals, psychology, religion—our total life picture. (Browne, 1984, p. 1)

As the above quote from Ray Browne, cofounder, along with Marshall Fishwick of the Popular Culture Association, suggests popular culture is a *lingua franca*—a primary voice of the people, by the people, and for the people. Its study comes not from the fields of counseling and psychotherapy as the title of this book might suggest, and not even from their parent discipline of psychology. Instead, it derives from the humanities, the same scholarly discipline and domain of lived experience that has given us art, music, and literature.

When you hear the term *popular culture,* what comes to mind? Do you think of a Puccini opera or a Marilyn Manson concert, a Picasso painting or a Hannah Montana lunchbox, a Hemmingway novel or a Superman comic, a movie like *Gone With the Wind* or the latest installment in Stephanie Meyer's *Twilight* vampire saga? In actuality, popular culture is not any one thing, nor is it any one genre of media. It is the sum total of the all of the products, ideas, and people that are known to the majority of society at a given point in time. It is both classical music and underground death metal, haute cuisine and fast food, revered politicians and reviled pop stars, pornography and Internet porn sites, disposable flip phones and global social networking sites, C-movies and Academy Award winners, television toy commercials and world-changing documentaries. Popular culture is timely and timeless, fleeting and fundamental, highbrow and lowbrow, and everything in between.

For some, popular culture is synonymous with terms such as *formulaic, fleeting,* and *foolish*—those things and experiences that are mass-produced for the sole purpose of mass consumption (Macdonald, 1998). Perhaps "mass" is the key word here, as it implies large, anonymous, and artificial. The success of popular culture depends on mass-production and mass-consumption. Since, according to Karen Brooks, "Young people are concurrently constructed as both product and market" (2006, p. 10), the glamorization of sex, drugs, and violence becomes an integral selling point for all things popular. Movies, television shows, Internet sites, and video games, instead of being solely a form of entertainment, become seductive gateways to potentially destructive belief systems, behaviors, and relationships.

Brooks continues by suggesting that

when people, young and not-so-young, are continually inundated with images of [others] being reckless, experimenting with drugs and alcohol, adorning themselves in particular clothes and accoutrements, inscribing their bodies and ritualizing their appearance, it starts to be regarded as normal . . . that is, a mindset develops that responds to the manufactured images [of popular culture] as "truth" and as representing all people. (p. 10)

Given the ubiquity of popular culture, it is easy to appreciate Brooks's concern. Hers is not a lone voice. Ever since mass media was ushered in with radio in the 1920s, there has been concern for the dehumanizing and demoralizing effects of capitalism, violence, and sexuality on our most vulnerable and impressionable citizens. These concerns culminated in the comics code of the 1950s, the national Television Violence Study of the 1970s, and the more recent work of researchers like Dorothy and Jerome Singer (2007) who have demonstrated that violence, particularly in video games, contributes, in many ways, to potentially violent behavior.

On the other side of the argument as to whether popular culture helps or hurts, Marshall Fishwick noted that "culture has always been popular, thriving on formula, archetypes and stereotypes . . . cyclic, repetitive and powerful" (2002, p. 3). Those such as Fishwick believe that the distinctions between elite and popular, as well as between highbrow and lowbrow, are little more than meaningless and divisive class distinctions that seek to trivialize and marginalize people. Popular culture is a medium for expression without prerequisites. It is a democratizing force, one in which all can partake.

Along similar lines, and arguing in part from the vantage point of neuroscience, Steven Johnson in *Everything Bad Is Good for You* (2006) suggested that in contrast to the popularly held belief that mass culture follows a steadily declining path, popular video games, violent television dramas, and even juvenile sitcoms challenge their audiences to think and problem-solve. He was referring to the many ways in which the plots of today's television shows, and by association movies, stimulate and challenge us.

SKILL AND LEARNING EXERCISE 2.1

How in Tune Are You With Today's Popular Culture?

Think for a moment! What is the most popular reality show on television? What is the hottest gadget that people are using today? What is the difference between metal and gangsta rap? What is the most popular sneaker that kids are wearing? Which social networking Internet site is drawing the most attention? What poplar book has most recently been reincarnated on the silver screen? As you answer these questions, ask yourself, "Are they necessarily good or bad" and "How can each one of these cultural artifacts be of value to society?"

ASSESSING AND ENHANCING THE COUNSELOR'S PCIQ (POPULAR CULTURE IQ)

> Today's 10 year-old is capable of following dozens of professional sports teams, shifting effortlessly from phone to IM [instant messaging] to e-mail in communicating with friends and telescoping through immense virtual worlds [and] adapting and trouble-shooting new media technologies without flinching. (Taffel, 2005, p. 144)

Just how tuned-in should a therapist be to popular culture? If, as some suggest, movies, television, the Internet, games, and comic books are at best entertainment, and at worst potentially dangerous distractions, then is it not a waste of time for clinicians to bother themselves with these passing fads? And do we really serve clients by buying into the chit-chat and chatter of popular culture? Perhaps, but consider that a recent Kaiser Family Foundation survey titled "Talking with Kids About Tough Issues" (2001) found that children and teens are turning to sources other than their parents, including television,

movies, and the Internet, for information about complicated topics such as alcohol, drugs, sex, and violence. Each of these facets of popular culture is a potential resource for our clients, particularly children and teens who may be more readily influenced by their popular culture.

We are not advocating that clinicians become experts on all things popular. However, we are suggesting that whether you work, or plan to work with children, adolescents, or adults in private practice, community mental health settings, school or college counseling centers, or even hospitals, that you appreciate that popular culture is like oxygen. It is everywhere, and influences everyone—some more than others. So, what is your PCIQ? How familiar are you with the current fashion trends, music genres, animated films, and television dramas? If an extraterrestrial stopped you on the street and asked you to describe what people are watching, buying, and eating in your immediate world, what would you say? How prepared are you to engage clients in conversations about what may seem quite trivial and superficial to you, but very important to them?

SNAPSHOT: PROFESSIONAL PERSPECTIVE 2.1

Breaking Through to Teens

In his *Breaking Through to Teens: A New Psychotherapy for the New Adolescence* (2005), master therapist Ron Taffel advocates that the therapist working with today's teen must become familiar with the sights and sounds of the world of the adolescent. This includes a familiarity with movies, television shows, and music icons.

Using Popular Culture Clients to Build a Caseload for Learning

> The various mediums through which popular culture flows, including movies, board games, music, literature, television and the Net, move from the realm of commodity to that of therapeutic resource, and can be referred to as popular culture intervention. (Rubin, 2008, p. xxxiv)

It was indeed conversations between the authors around popular culture that were the impetus for this book. Schwitzer's ongoing work in both the clinic and classroom using historical and popular culture characters to teach assessment and intervention skills was highly useful to students. My (Rubin) volume *Popular Culture in Counseling, Psychotherapy and Play-Based Interventions* (Rubin, 2008) brought my own clinical experience together with that of other clinicians who had successfully used the various facets of popular culture in their clinical work with children, adolescents, adults, and the elderly. Examples included using:

- Popular music with the elderly to consolidate life stories.
- The characters and plots from fantasy films to help adolescents problem solve.
- Animated film and television characters in the treatment of childhood abuse.
- Board and video games to build solidarity among disenfranchised youth.
- Sport metaphors in the service of emotional regulation.
- Cutting-edge technology and social networking to mend family and social ties.

Research leading up to our collaboration had clearly demonstrated that the ubiquity and influence of popular culture in our lives was significant. As such, it made good sense to draw from that source for clinical and pedagogical possibilities. Mattingly's therapeutic use of popular culture narratives with inner-city youth (2006), Moni and Jobling's incorporation of popular culture characters into the literacy education of adults with Down syndrome (2008), Beres's reliance on popular romance literature to re-educate victims of domestic abuse (2002), and Ashcraft's application of popular movie themes into sex education (2003) all affirmed our conviction in the belief that popular culture can be a valuable therapeutic resource.

SNAPSHOT: PROFESSIONAL PERSPECTIVE 2.2

Popular Culture Offers a Wealth of Fascinating Individuals

Aside from the obvious multisensory appeal of all things popular, our favorite television shows, movies, video games, comics, and songs are inhabited by a population of fascinating characters and personalities that range from the deeply mysterious to the unfathomably complex. I (Rubin) often utilize my client's interests in superheroes (Superman and Spider-Man) to address deeply personal and meaningful issues in their own lives. Similarly, Schwitzer has incorporated the stories of John Basil Henderson and Gollum into both his college counseling practice and pedagogy to help students hone their case conceptualization skills.

Popular Culture as a Resource for Counselor Development and Growth

In the final analysis, popular culture, for us, is about people! It is not about how many video games feature Mario the plumber, how many tickets *Toy Story 3* sold in its first week in the theaters, or even whether Jack Bauer is a criminal. It is about the unlimited ways in which the backstories of these popular characters can be used in the service of clinical training, both in the classroom and in the field that is of interest to us.

In 2005, the USA cable television network launched its "Characters Welcome" advertising campaign. It was designed to, and was successful at drawing viewers' attention to their unique and out-of-the-box offerings such as *Monk; House MD; Becker; Psych; and Walker, Texas Ranger.* Each of these highly popular shows, which ran the gamut from serious drama to intelligent comedy, featured a main character that was, by all standards, both psychiatric and non, powerfully engaging, intriguing, and psychologically complex. America was fascinated by the obsessive-compulsive detective Adrian Monk and the sardonic and depressed, yet brilliant physician Gregory House.

The USA logo very nicely captures our intent in creating this book. We welcome characters from all facets of popular culture, not only television shows, but from movies, board and video games, literature and comics, advertising, and music. Other volumes on case conceptualization, diagnosis, and treatment planning, construct their clinical vignettes from either amalgams, that is, those constructed (and embellished) from bits and pieces of real clinical cases, or those drawn directly from the authors' own caseloads.

In contrast, the training cases in this book will draw directly from the fascinating personages of popular culture—our shared *lingua franca*. It is our contention, as Schwitzer et al. have previously noted (Schwitzer, Boyce, Cody, Holman, & Stein, 2006), that "the use of cases drawn from historical figures and popular characters to practice and demonstrate case-formulation skills is well established" (p. 60). In addition to reducing practitioner (and trainee) discomfort, increasing familiarity and comprehension, providing immediate experience for skill development and enhancing confidence, the use of fictional characters from popular culture can, according to Schwitzer et al.:

- Help clinicians avoid the difficulties involved in obtaining sufficient caseloads with which to practice skill development.
- Mitigate for new clinicians the ethical problem of working within the limits of their existing competencies, such as worrying about harming real clients.
- Allow new clinicians to freely explore their own attitudes regarding the role of assessment, diagnosis, and treatment planning in their work, without concerns over the impact of their own self-explorations on the provision of services to clients.
- Circumvent ethical and legal issues related to confidentiality.
- Assist the clinician in collecting large amounts of client-related information that might not otherwise be available until later on in therapy, due to the absence of collateral sources of data or because of the client's discomfort sharing it.

CLINICAL SPOTLIGHT 2.1: The Popular Culture Case of Roberto and Superman

Roberto was 5 years old when his mother first shared with him the story of Superman. He recalled with great fondness Superman's incredible adventures and how he and his mother would eagerly await each week's newest installment. Of even greater significance to young Roberto, was the adoption narrative that formed the foundation of Superman's story . . . and his own. Roberto was adopted at birth. His mother, who had learned to speak English by reading Superman comics with her own mother, decided early on that she would teach her son about his adoption by sharing with him the story of Superman, who was adopted by Jonathan and Martha Kent after being jettisoned to Earth by his Kryptonian parents Jor-el and Lara. Although Roberto struggled over the years to integrate adoption into his own life story, Superman was always there to lend a hand. When I (Rubin) had the opportunity to meet with Roberto in a nonclinical context, his story was inspirational, and reaffirmed the important role that popular culture can play in the people's lives and its potential therapeutic value.

CLINICAL SPOTLIGHT 2.2: The Popular Culture Case of Alex and Luke Skywalker

When Alex first came to counseling at 11 years old, he was sad, angry, and confused. He and his family had just returned from another summer vacation with extended family. While these gatherings were large and loving, they were continual reminders to Alex that he was adopted because he was of Central American descent and his adopted family was Scandinavian. In counseling, Alex was intrigued by *Star Wars,* and in particular, by the relationship between Darth Vader and his son Luke Skywalker (both characters were adopted). Over the course of therapy, Alex's play themes in the both the sandtray and storytelling centered on Luke's adventures. Together with the therapist, Alex wrote the outline for a script to a new *Star Wars* adventure that highlighted adoption, and how its effects, both good and bad, affected all the characters. His love, and the therapist's appreciation for and willingness to use the *Star Wars* story, were significant in the resolution of Alex's conflicts with regard to adoption.

SKILL AND LEARNING EXERCISE 2.2

Popular Culture Characters on the Couch

When you think of some of the following characters, what type of developmental challenges, psychological issues, and possible counseling needs come to mind? These are some of the fascinating individuals who will form the foundation of our work ahead in this book:

- Chief Bromden (Chapter 12), the oppressed Indian star of *One Flew Over the Cuckoo's Nest*
- Eleanor Rigby (Chapter 11), the lonely church-keep from the Beatles' song of the same name
- Tinkerbell (Chapter 9), the feisty and vindictive sprite from the Disney classic *Peter Pan*
- Elphaba Thropp (Chapter 8), the green-skinned heroine in the Broadway musical *Wicked*
- Sophia Petrillo (Chapter 10), the wisecracking octogenarian from television's *The Golden Girls*
- Fred Wozniak (Chapter 11), the perennially fatigued baker from the Dunkin' Donuts commercials
- Mario (Chapter 7), brother of Luigi, the indefatigable hero of Nintendo video game fame

CHAPTER SUMMARY AND WRAP-UP

This chapter introduced you to popular culture by highlighting its many constituent parts, including television, film, music, literature, and the Internet. First, we discussed the role of popular culture in our everyday lives, briefly tying its study to mythology and then suggesting that both fields are most interested in people and the stories of their lives. We then discussed the long-running debate over whether popular culture, with its focus on consumerism, fads, and trends, was in some way detrimental, particularly to children and teens who are highly impressionable. This argument was countered with research suggesting that popular culture can stimulate problem-solving and challenge us intellectually and emotionally. Next, we addressed the concept of PCIQ by discussing how influential the media of popular culture can be to young people as a resource for information and discussion on topics of relevance to them. The implication is that the more clinicians know about popular culture, the more intimately they may be able to appreciate the concerns of their clients, both young and old.

In order to bring this discussion to life, we provided examples of ways in which each of us has brought the plots and characters of popular culture into our roles as counselors and counseling educators and then highlighted supportive research. As the chapter progressed, we identified specific and fascinating popular culture characters, each of whom provides poignant insights into the human condition. We suggested that each of these characters, and the many more we will highlight in the chapters to follow, provide both counseling students and seasoned therapists with the opportunity to hone their case conceptualization, diagnostic, and treatment planning skills. We demonstrated that the use of characters drawn from popular culture (as opposed to real clients) can help clinicians avoid certain professional and ethical challenges—all the while deepening the learning experience. We concluded the chapter by discussing actual cases drawn from our clinical caseloads in which popular culture characters such as Superman and Luke Skywalker were effectively used. The chapter prepared you for subsequent discussions about the theoretical bases and mechanics of case conceptualization, diagnosis, and clinical treatment planning, which will, in turn, lay the foundation for enjoyable and highly useful analyses of characters drawn from all corners of popular culture.

PART II

DIAGNOSIS, CASE CONCEPTUALIZATION, AND TREATMENT PLANNING

3

CLINICAL THINKING SKILLS

*Diagnosis, Case Conceptualization,
and Treatment Planning*

INTRODUCING CHAPTER 3: READER HIGHLIGHTS AND LEARNING GOALS

Individuals who choose careers as mental health professionals—including counselors, psychotherapists, social workers, counseling and clinical psychologists, psychiatrists, and those in similar career paths—often enter the counseling field because earlier in their lives, in their families of origin, in their schools and neighborhoods, and among their friends and peers, they previously found themselves in the role of good listener, intelligent analyzer, or effective problem-solver when those around them encountered life's difficulties (Neukrug & Schwitzer, 2006). In other words, many people already are "natural helpers" when they decide to become professionals (Neukrug & Schwitzer, 2006, p. 5). As natural helpers for friends and family, they have relied on their intuition, personal opinions, and natural inclinations as they spontaneously listen, support, analyze, encourage, push, or make hopeful suggestions.

However, the demands of professional counseling work go beyond the qualities needed by natural helpers. Compared with the spontaneous nature of natural helping, professional counseling requires us to rely on purposeful skills and to systematically guide the counseling relationship through a sequence of organized stages, intentionally aiming to achieve specific client outcome goals (Neukrug & Schwitzer). That is, professional counseling requires us to become competent at using clinical thinking skills "to facilitate [the] provision of mental health treatment" (Seligman, 1996, p. 23). These skills include diagnosis, case conceptualization, and treatment planning. The goal of our textbook is to help you understand and become competent at these three important clinical thinking skills. Part II of the text explores each skill in detail. In Chapter 3 we introduce all of the key concepts and then in Chapters 4, 5, and 6 we discuss them more fully.

(Continued)

(Continued)

In the current chapter, first we discuss the role that clinical thinking skills play in counseling and psychotherapy. Next, we define *diagnosis, case conceptualization,* and *treatment planning.* Following our definitions, we relate these skills to caseload management, and explain how they fit into the stages of the professional counseling process, and summarize. We then will be ready to explore each skill more fully in the separate chapters that follow.

At the end of this chapter, you should be able to:

- Discuss the role of clinical thinking skills in counseling and psychotherapy as they are practiced in today's professional mental health world
- Define diagnosis, case conceptualization, and treatment planning
- Distinguish among these skills and caseload management
- Summarize the stages of the professional counseling relationship and discuss where diagnosis, case conceptualization, and treatment planning fit into the process
- Be ready to move on to the three specific chapters that follow, dealing in detail with diagnosis, case conceptualization, and treatment planning

THE USE OF CLINICAL THINKING SKILLS IN COUNSELING AND PSYCHOTHERAPY

The transition from natural helper to professional counselor can be a daunting one. We become aware that a client's decision to seek counseling is an important "investment in time, money, and energy" (Vaughn, 1997, p. 181). We realize that when clients choose us as professional consultants for their therapeutic "journey," it takes substantial determination for them to stay the course with us "when the going gets tough" (p. 181). We learn that counselors are responsible for helping the individual understand his or her own view of himself or herself and his or her life, discover new choices, create a new view of himself or herself, and bring about his or her own changes (Weinberg, 1996). We recognize that when counseling succeeds, our clients should be better able to form their own insights and apply the benefits of psychotherapy to new life situations when they arise (Vaughn, 2007). To accomplish these tasks, we make judgments about our clients, decide what goals seem reasonable and feasible, consider how we will communicate with our clients, and determine how to implement the change process (Basch, 1980). Further, we must pay attention to what we know about empirically supported

practice, evidence-based practice, and other best practice information (Wampold, 2001). Basch (1980) referred to all of this as "listening like a psychotherapist" (p. 3). It means a lot of decision-making responsibility rests on our shoulders.

Correspondingly, to accomplish the shift from natural helper—giving advice at the dinner table or comforting a coworker who is upset—to counseling professional—meeting in a therapeutic setting with child, adolescent, young adult, adult, couple, family, or group clients who are in need—a set of tools is required with which to describe the client's functioning, gain an understanding of the person's situation and needs, identify goals for change, and decide on the most effective interventions for reaching these goals. Specifically, diagnosis is a tool for *describing* client needs, case conceptualization is a tool for *understanding* these needs, and treatment planning is a tool for *addressing* these needs to bring about change. When employed by counseling professionals, the treatment plan follows directly from the case conceptualization, which builds on the diagnostic impressions. All three of these clinical thinking skills are required competencies for today's counseling and psychotherapy professionals (Seligman, 1996, 2004).

Figure 3.1   Clinical Thinking Skills

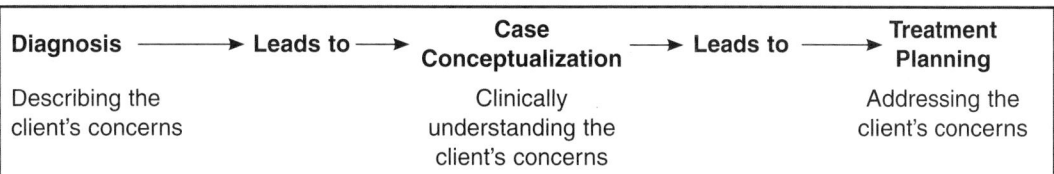

Diagnosis ——→ Leads to ——→ Case Conceptualization ——→ Leads to ——→ Treatment Planning

Describing the client's concerns — Clinically understanding the client's concerns — Addressing the client's concerns

DEFINING DIAGNOSIS

In today's professional counseling world, diagnosis refers to the use of the *Diagnostic and Statistical Manual of Mental Disorders, Fourth Edition, Text Revision (DSM-IV-TR)* (American Psychiatric Association [APA], 2000a) to identify and describe the clinically significant patterns associated with our clients' distress or impairment or risk. Certainly there are other mental health diagnostic systems besides the *DSM-IV-TR*. The World Health Organization's (WHO) *International Classification of Diseases, Tenth Edition (ICD-10)* is an important example. Further, some fields of counseling and psychotherapy maintain their own systems of diagnostic formulation; for instance, there are psychoanalytic systems for diagnosing client personality structures (McWilliams, 1994, 1999). However, it is the *DSM-IV-TR* that is the widely accepted, official nomenclature for making a mental health diagnosis in today's clinical practice. It is used throughout the United States and, increasingly, around the world. The *DSM-IV-TR* has been translated into more than 14 languages. As mental health professionals who work with multiple constituencies and colleagues of various disciplines, mastering the *DSM-IV-TR* is a professional survival skill for counselors and psychotherapists in all settings and contexts.

Specifically, the *DSM-IV-TR* is a classification system that divides client presentations into mental disorders based on sets of criteria that are made up of observable features. In other words, diagnoses of mental disorders in the *DSM-IV-TR* are *criterion-referenced.* This categorical approach stems from the traditional scientific/medical

method of organizing, naming, and communicating information in as objective a fashion as possible. The job of the counselor is to find the best match between what the clinician observes the client to be experiencing and the various criteria for the different clinically significant patterns found in the *DSM.* This type of diagnosis can help us determine the primary focus of counseling. For example, a focus on a mood problem might need different counseling responses than a focus on anxiety complaints, and a focus on an adjustment problem would be addressed differently than a focus on long-term life problems like personality disorders.

The *DSM-IV-TR* provides about 300 separate diagnoses. It includes disorders of infancy, childhood, adolescence, and adulthood; describes both short-term client concerns, such as adjustment disorders, and longer-standing problems, such as mental retardation and personality disorders; covers a wide range of behavior, from substance abuse to sleep disorders to bereavement; and pays attention to characteristics of thought, mood, behavior, and physiology. A fully prepared, start-to-finish *DSM* diagnosis requires five different types of information, each of which helps the counselor to describe what the client is experiencing or presenting. Each of the five types of information is called an *Axis,* and taken together, the system is described as *Multiaxial.* The five types of information include clinical disorders of children and adults and other conditions that may be a focus of counseling (comprising Axis I and Axis II of the multiple-axis system); medical conditions (Axis III); psychosocial and environmental problems encountered by the client (Axis IV); and the counselor's numerical estimate of the person's overall everyday function on a quantitative scale (Global Assessment of Functioning [GAF], Axis V). Further, the criteria—or requirements—for each clinical diagnosis appearing on Axis I or Axis II has four parts: (a) client behaviors, thoughts, mood, and physiological symptoms; (b) the frequency and duration of the person's concerns; (c) the severity of the distress or life dysfunction the person encounters as a result of his or her concerns; and (d) the ruling out of other possible conditions that might account for the person's needs. As an illustration, the criteria that must be met for a diagnosis of Generalized Anxiety Disorder include excessive anxiety, worry, and physical stress (thought, behavior, mood, and physiological features) present at least 6 months (duration) that are interfering with daily functioning (severity) and are not due to substance use or a medical problem (ruling out differential diagnoses). In addition, the system has severity specifiers, course specifiers, and subtypes that are used to describe individual client variations within a diagnosis.

SKILL AND LEARNING EXERCISE 3.1

Taking a Look at a Multiaxial Diagnosis

Find the case of Jamal Malik appearing in Chapter 8, Troubled Youth in Film and on Stage, located later in this text. Find the fully completed multiaxial *DSM-IV-TR* diagnosis describing Jamal's presenting concerns. Working alone or with a partner, refer to your copy of the *DSM*. What thoughts, feelings, behaviors, or physiological symptoms must Jamal be experiencing to suggest a diagnosis of Acute Stress Disorder on Axis I? Have any medical problems or environmental problems been identified on Axis III and Axis IV? What did the counselor mean when he estimated a GAF = 51 on Axis V?

The primary purpose for making a *DSM-IV-TR* diagnosis is to describe and communicate with other professionals who are familiar with the system. Having all mental health professionals using the same diagnostic system is intended to enhance agreement among clinicians about the client picture they are seeing and should improve the sharing of information about client presentations and client needs. By itself, a diagnosis does not reflect any specific theoretical perspective (such as person-centered counseling or cognitive-behavioral therapy) or indicate any specific mental health field (professional counseling, psychology, etc.); rather, the *DSM-IV-TR* diagnoses are theory-neutral and do not reflect any one orientation. As a result, using *DSM-IV-TR* categories and descriptions allows clinicians to describe client needs and communicate with mental health colleagues across disciplines—and then later apply their own professional viewpoint and theoretical approach during case conceptualization and treatment planning.

DEFINING CASE CONCEPTUALIZATION

Following diagnosis, which provides a method for describing and communicating about client presentations, effective treatment in today's mental health world next requires that we use case conceptualization to evaluate and make sense of the client's needs (Hinkle, 1994; Seligman, 2004). Conceptualization skills provide the counselor with a rationale and a framework for his or her work with clients—and with today's emphasis on briefer counseling approaches, extensive use of integrated and eclectic psychotherapy models, and greater focus on evidence-based best practices, efficient case conceptualization has become essential (Budman

& Gurman, 1983; Mahalick, 1990; Neukrug, 2001; Wampold, 2001). Specifically, case conceptualization is a tool for observing, understanding, and conceptually integrating client behaviors, thoughts, feelings, and physiology from a clinical perspective (Neukrug & Schwitzer, 2006).

Case conceptualization involves three steps (Neukrug & Schwitzer, 2006): First, the counselor thoroughly *evaluates* the client's concerns by observing, assessing, and measuring his or her behaviors. Second, the clinician *organizes* these observations, assessments, and measures to his or her *patterns and themes* among the client's concerns. Third, the therapist selects a *theoretical orientation* to interpret, explain, or make clinical judgments about what the client is experiencing. When the case conceptualization is completed, the counselor should have a picture of what he or she believes has led to the client's concerns (etiology) and what features are maintaining or perpetuating the problem (sustaining factors). Understanding the etiology and sustaining factors will then lead to treatment planning, which uses the case conceptualization to decide how to best address, reduce, manage, or resolve the client's issues.

Naturally, the first component of case conceptualization is assessment, measurement, or appraisal of the client's presenting problems or reasons for referral. As mentioned above, behavioral, cognitive, affective, and physiological components all are taken into account. For instance, while the experience of a depressive disorder is most clearly associated with low mood and feeling sad or "down," it is typical for clients with depressive disorder to simultaneously experience cognitive symptoms of depression like hopeless or helpless pessimistic thinking, physical symptoms like sleep or appetite difficulties, and behavioral problems such as losing interest in everyday activities. All of these components of the presenting problem contribute to the case conceptualization.

However, in order to form a full case conceptualization, effective clinicians also go beyond the presenting concerns or reason for referral. They evaluate additional issues with work, school, or other major life roles and with social and personal-emotional adjustment; they examine developmental and family history such as current and past family and parental relationships, previous school and work experiences, and previous peer and social experiences; they make in-session observations; they make clinical inquiries about present and past medical, psychiatric, substance use, and suicidal experiences; and they collect formal psychological assessment data, that is, psychological tests.

Once the clinician has collected as much information as possible, his or her second step in the case conceptualization process is to begin organizing the various client data. The counselor uses his or her conceptual skills to weave together the different pieces of information about the client's adjustment, development, distress, or dysfunction into logical groupings that elucidate the person's larger clinical concerns, the problematic themes underlying the person's difficulties with life situations or life roles, or critical problems found in the person's intrapsychic or interpersonal approach to his or her world. Later on, these themes help form the targets for change that will be addressed by treatment planning.

After organizing themes that meaningfully sort together the different pieces of client information that have been collected, the counselor's third step is to apply a theoretical approach to infer, explain, or interpret the identified themes. Today's clinicians are expected to match the best counseling approach for addressing the client's needs (Wampold, 2001). This means that when forming a case conceptualization, today's counselors might apply to their understanding of the client's themes and patterns one of the many well-documented purist theoretical approaches (such as Cognitive Behavior Therapy, person-centered counseling, or Reality Therapy), an integration of two or more theories, an eclectic mix of theories, or a brief solution-focused approach (Corey, 2009; Dattilo & Norcross, 2006; de Shazer & Dolan, 2007; Norcross & Beutler, 2008; Wampold, 2001). In other words, part of the counselor's job is to decide which theoretical approach is a good fit with the client's needs, and then use that approach to finish the case conceptualization.

Comparing Theoretical Approaches to Case Conceptualization

Find the cases of Snoopy (appearing in Chapter 7, Children's Characters and Video Game Characters), George Lopez and Lieutenant Commander Data (appearing in Chapter 10, Adults in Television Sitcoms and Drama), and Eleanor Rigby (appearing in Chapter 11, Characters in Music, Musicals, and Advertising) located later in this text. Find the section of each case discussing case conceptualization. Working alone or with a partner, consider the following: What theoretical approach did the counselor select to explain Snoopy's, George's, Data's, and Eleanor's concerns? Did the counselor select a purist theory, integration of two or more theories, eclectic mix of theories, or brief solution-focused approach? What was the counselor's rationale for his or her selection?

Inverted Pyramid Method of Case Conceptualization

Taken together, a start-to-finish case conceptualization begins with learning about the client's concerns (first step), moves on to meaningfully organizing this information into patterns and themes (second step), and finishes by explaining the patterns and themes using our choice of theory or theories (third step). As with learning diagnostic skills, learning to form this type of case conceptualization can be overwhelming for beginning counselors and trainees (Neukrug & Schwitzer, 2006). Beginning clinicians often experience ambiguity and feel confused when they start the process of forming reliable, accurate case conceptualizations for each new client they encounter (Loganbill, Hardy, & Delworth, 1982; Martin, Slemon, Hiebert, Halberg, & Cummings, 1989). In fact, over the years, students in training sites (Robbins & Zinni, 1988) as well as newly employed therapists and counselors (Glidewell & Livert, 1992; Hays, McLeod, & Prosek, 2010) consistently have reported lacking confidence in their case conceptualization skills. By comparison, more experienced therapists are able to systematically apply a consistent set of clinical thinking skills to the different problems presented by each new client.

In turn, to help you more easily develop case conceptualization skills and become more confident in your abilities, in this textbook we use a step-by-step method specifically designed to assist new counselors in becoming consistent, accurate, case conceptualizers. This method, known as the *inverted pyramid* (Neukrug & Schwitzer, 2006; Schwitzer, 1996, 1997), gives you a specific way to form your conceptualizations of clients. The inverted pyramid method is presented later in the text and is illustrated in all 30 case examples.

DEFINING TREATMENT PLANNING

Once our earlier clinical thinking is completed, a treatment plan is built that integrates the information from the diagnosis and case conceptualization into a coherent plan of action. Treatment planning is a vital aspect of today's mental healthcare delivery (Jongsma & Peterson, 2006; Jongsma, Peterson, & McInnis, 2003a, 2003b; Seligman, 1993, 1996, 2004), and competent clinicians are expected to be able to move methodically from conceptualization to the formulation and implementation of the treatment plan (Jongsma & Peterson, 2006; Schwitzer & Everett, 1997). Whereas natural helpers typically "shoot from the hip," counseling professionals are expected to carefully select achievable goals, determine what intervention approach will be used, and establish how change will be measured (Neukrug & Schwitzer, 2006, p. 224). A widely accepted definition of treatment planning is as follows:

[Treatment planning is] plotting out the counseling process so that both counselor and client have a road map that delineates how they will proceed from their point of origin (the client's presenting concerns and underlying difficulties) to their destination, alleviation of troubling and dysfunctional symptoms and patterns, and establishment of improved coping. (Seligman, 1993, p. 288; 1996, p. 157)

As Seligman indicated, the treatment plan maps out a logical and goal-oriented strategy for making positive changes in the client's life. It is a blueprint for the counseling process that is based on the clinical themes identified, and the theoretical approach used, in the case conceptualization.

A basic treatment plan comprises four steps (Neukrug & Schwitzer, 2006). First, the clinician *behaviorally defines* the counseling problems to be addressed. Second, *achievable goals* are selected. Third, the modes of treatment and *methods of intervention* are determined. Fourth, the counselor explains *how change will be measured* and how outcomes will be demonstrated.

More specifically, the behavioral definition of the problem consolidates the case conceptualization into a concise hierarchical list of issues and concerns that will be the focus of treatment. Achievable goals are selected by assessing and prioritizing the client's needs into a hierarchy of urgency that also takes into account such factors as the level of dysfunction the person is experiencing, the client's motivation for change, and real-world influences on the client's needs. Urgency typically increases for issues of suicidality,

potential for harm to self or others, certain diagnostic red flags, substance use concerns, and other issues causing substantial distress or impairment in daily functioning. At the same time, the client's own motivations and ability to engage in the therapeutic process influence the goals that are agreed on, as do real-world factors such as the client's availability to attend counseling, session limits, and the like. Treatment modes and methods of intervention are selected by taking into account the client's particular dynamics and then applying the specific theoretical orientation or clinical approach that is to be employed. Decisions about treatment modes often center on: who the service provider will be, including what type of counseling professional will provide services and who specifically will be the clinician; what type of outclient or inpatient setting the client will visit, and what types of individual counseling or group psychotherapy formats the person will attend. Methods of intervention are derived from the specific theoretical approach, integration of two or more theoretical approaches, eclectic mix of theories, or solution-focused intervention approach we endorse for our work with the client; these decisions should be made based on our knowledge of best practices, evidence about treatment efficacy, and other professional knowledge. *Changes and outcomes* that are achieved can be demonstrated using various sources of information such as client report, counselor observation, pre-post treatment comparisons, and other means of documenting the results of our counseling work.

SKILL AND LEARNING EXERCISE 3.3

Taking a Look at a Basic Treatment Plan

Find the case of *The Color Purple's* Miss Celie appearing in Chapter 12, Characters in Literature and Comics, located later in this text. Find the fully completed treatment plan and the treatment plan summary table. Working alone or with a partner, consider the following: What are the goals for treatment listed for each clinical concern? Are they behaviorally defined? What are the modes of treatment and methods of intervention? These come from an integration of which two theoretical approaches? Do the outcome measures seem appropriate? Are they likely to show the counselor and Miss Celie whether progress has been made toward her goals? Overall, how successful is the treatment plan at providing the counselor with structure and direction for her work with the client?

The use of a treatment plan that selects the goals for change, determines the counseling methods for achieving change, and presents ways of measuring the changes that are produced provides structure and direction to the counseling process. It helps the counselor and the client track their progress and determine the degree to which goals are being met, and allows the counseling professional to demonstrate accountability and effectiveness (Seligman, 1996). When the treatment plan is completed, the counselor should have a clear picture of what the goals are, how to reach the goals, and how to know when they have been reached.

CLINICAL THINKING SKILLS AND CASELOAD MANAGEMENT

So far in this chapter we have introduced and defined the three clinical thinking skills that are the focus of our text. Along with diagnosis, case conceptualization, and treatment planning, students and new professionals also often are exposed to another term that also is important to the practice of professional counseling and is related to these clinical tools: *caseload management*. In this brief section of the chapter, we want to explain what comprises caseload management and how the three clinical thinking skills fit in. Caseload management "encompasses the knowledge, skills, and activities involved in managing an entire [client] caseload" (Woodside & McClam, 1998, p. 4). Being skilled at managing our overall load of clients includes using all of the tools needed to move the individuals with whom we are working "through the service delivery process from intake to closure" (Woodside & McClam, 1998, p. 3). Novice counselors who are new to their professional work settings report having discovered that caseload management involves "the paperwork and documentation for each client on your caseload" and "handling the records, files, communications, supervision, working with other staff on a case, and everything else you do in the office besides sit down with the client himself or herself" (Woodside

& McClam, 1998, p. 3). In sum, new counselors have commented that caseload management "isn't just filling out paperwork—it's how you handle every phone call, insurance form, scheduling, information request, follow-up, time management, and giving good client service" (Neukrug & Schwitzer, 2006, p. 257). More specifically, caseload management comprises each of the following elements (Neukrug & Schwitzer, 2006):

- Documentation
- Supervision, consultation, and collaboration
- Communication with stakeholders
- Business-related activities
- Time management, schedule management, and caseload tracking

Several of these elements of caseload management fit together closely with the use of our clinical thinking tools.

First, *documentation* involves all of the record-keeping involved in professional counseling work. This includes our note-taking, monitoring, and documenting of all client information, and storing of records. Included are pre-interview and intake materials, case notes, termination materials, testing data, billing and payment-related materials, including insurance forms, and other materials. Naturally, our diagnostic impressions, case conceptualization notes, and written treatment plans are part of documentation. These clinical thinking products all are components of the client's or patient's record—and accurately recording and keeping these records is extremely important in today's professional mental health world (Kleinke, 1994; Reynolds, Mair, & Fischer, 1995). Although often we refer to professional documentation as being "the client's record" or "belonging to the client," in actuality all of the clinical documents in the caseload file are clinical tools used by the clinician and are the property of the agency or counseling setting in which the therapist is working. Therefore, diagnosis, case conceptualization, and treatment notes all must be prepared carefully and professionally, with an awareness that they will contribute to the client's record and may be used by a variety of people for a wide range of professional purposes (Reynolds et al., 1995). Further, clinicians must prepare their clinical thinking documents to adhere to agency rules, ethical guidelines, and legal statutes, including Health Insurance Portability and Accountability Act (HIPAA)-related materials.

Second, clinicians rely on *supervision, consultation, and collaboration with other professionals* as they manage their caseloads in an effort to provide effective client services. Ethical codes for essentially all of the mental health professions as well as state statutes and other regulations require that clinicians practice within the limits of their competence. In turn, much of our work occurs with the support of others.

Among these supportive professional relationships, counseling *supervision* is most prominent. Counseling supervision is an intensive, interpersonally focused relationship in which one person is designated to facilitate the professional competence of one or more other persons (Loganbill et al., 1982). Students rely on supervision for intensive support and extensive expert advice as they begin learning to be a counselor;

interns and licensure residents rely on supervision to provide moderate support and solid expertise as they continue building their skills; and even licensed and experienced clinicians rely on supervision for expert guidance, to learn new approaches, and for help with special client challenges. Regarding clinical thinking, earlier in their training, students, trainees, and novice counselors tend to rely extensively on their supervisors for help and advice making diagnostic decisions, moving through the steps of case conceptualization, and formulating and writing out a treatment plan. Often, the novice's supervisor provides expert advice about which theoretical perspective, evidence-based approach, or best practice to match with the client's needs. Correspondingly, clinical thinking often is a major component of early counseling supervision (Bernard & Goodyear, 2004). Later, over the course of one's professional development, the responsibility for diagnosis, case conceptualization, and treatment planning gradually shifts from supervisor to supervisee (Bernard & Goodyear, 2004; Loganbill et al., 1982).

SNAPSHOT: PROFESSIONAL PERSPECTIVE 3.1

Using Counseling Supervision

Supervision can be useful throughout our professional lives. One of the authors (Schwitzer) has returned to supervision on more than one occasion to update his skills. He sought supervision at one time for specialized support understanding and conceptualizing Mexican and Mexican American family dynamics when he relocated to the state of Texas and found that Hispanic clients comprised an important portion of his caseload. He later returned to supervision when he was interested in adding elements of clinical hypnosis to his counseling repertoire and required an expert in hypnosis to help him learn the needed skills and make decisions about when to include them in the treatment plan. The other author (Rubin) has become interested in the use of Narrative Therapy with child, adolescent, and adult clients, toward which end he has attended numerous workshops on the topic and sought out individualized supervision with an clinician who is highly experienced in this modality.

Compared with supervision, which is an intensive, ongoing professional relationship, *consultation* is a time-limited relationship through which the counselor seeks the advice,

expert opinion, or professional support of another professional about the needs of a specific client. Very often, consultation provides us with needed guidance pertaining to our clinical thinking about a client situation. The counselor sometimes meets directly with the consultant to discuss a case situation—or, alternatively, refers the client to meet with the consulting professional, who then provides his or her diagnostic, conceptual, or treatment impressions. Commonly used consultants include: (a) another, more expert or more specialized mental health professional who can add to our exploration, understanding, and formulation of the client's dynamics and needs; (b) a medical consultant such as a physician (or another medical practitioner like a nutritionist) who can conduct physical exams or medical evaluations and provide us with information useful to our diagnostic, conceptual, or treatment decisions; and (c) specific discussions with or referral to a psychiatrist in order to rule out certain diagnoses or evaluate for psychiatric medication as a component of the treatment plan. Effective caseload management includes recognizing when consultation would be beneficial to our clinical thinking—outside opinion about a diagnosis, input regarding etiology and underlying causes of a conceptualized concern, advice about the interventions that will form the treatment plan—and to the provision of counseling that results from our clinical thinking.

In addition to supervision and consultation, through which we rely on third-party professionals for guidance, caseload management also sometimes involves direct *collaboration* with a colleague. Common collaborations include: cotherapy, in which two or more clinicians work together directly with the same client for example, providing play therapy, group coleadership, couples or family cotherapy, and other roles such as coleading a workshop. When these formats are used, the colleagues must agree on their clinical thinking as it pertains to the client, coming to a collaborative understanding of the diagnosis, conceptualization, and plan for treatment. The various modes of collaborative counseling in which the client will participate also must be documented in the treatment plan.

Third, when counseling professionals *communicate with stakeholders* besides the client or *conduct business matters,* they often confront questions about, and staked interest in, their clinical thinking. Common stakeholders are parents and legal guardians, spouses, and other family members; referral sources such as teachers and other school personnel, or employers and other workplace personnel; courts and other criminal justice personnel; and individuals making inquiries pertaining to employment checks and background investigations. Common business situations include interactions with third-party payers such as insurance company representatives, health maintenance organization (HMO) staff, and governmental agency personnel. Counseling generally operates confidentially; however, when it is ethically suitable, or when legally required to do so, counseling professionals might find themselves communicating verbally or in writing about a client with any of these stakeholders. In fact, those interested in the client's well-being often place a lot of pressure on us as professionals to discuss private information about the client. Further, generally speaking, parents and legal guardians have easy access to their minor children's records, and some counselors, such as those working in military settings with service members, do not have the same confidentiality protections as in other settings. Such communications with stakeholders and business representatives sometimes include sharing the written materials that are a part of the client's agency records. In turn, we must carefully and thoughtfully prepare, and professionally word, all of our written clinical thinking materials—and be cognizant that any diagnostic notes, conceptualizations, or treatment plans we prepare could potentially be seen by individuals outside our office, who may or may not be other mental health professionals, and may or may not have the same client interests as we do. As a result, for new counselors, documentation, communication with stakeholders, and the conducting of business matters often become another important focus of clinical supervision, as we begin learning how to carefully but accurately communicate our clinical impressions of clients (Bernard & Goodyear, 2004; Hall & Sutton, 2004).

Time management, schedule management, and caseload tracking round out this chapter's brief discussion of caseload management as it relates to clinical thinking. It is sufficient here to mention the following points: Time and schedule management includes the timely completion of all record-keeping. In turn, intake materials for clinical use and business purposes, such as diagnostic impressions, case conceptualizations, and treatment plans when any of these are required, should be completed in time to be useful as guides to the implementation of counseling. Further, the counselor's case notes, including the treatment plan and subsequent documentation of counseling outcomes and measure of progress and change, should be prepared so that they are easily usable for caseload tracking—including describing front-end diagnostic and conceptual impressions, measures of progress throughout the counseling process, and evidence of outcomes and final impressions at the conclusion of the psychotherapy relationship. A clinician's collection of case materials should provide a clear, ongoing snapshot of his or her current caseload.

This final aspect of caseload management also means paying attention to our ability to manage our various workplace demands. For example, we must be able to recognize when our caseloads might be too large, become too emotionally demanding, require too many weekly contacts, or involve too many competing roles. Ideally, we can use our clinical thinking—the diagnostic impressions, theoretical conceptualizations, and plans for treatment pertaining to our caseload—to help us monitor and track the nature, content, and strenuousness of the work we are doing. The bottom line is that our clinical thinking tools should be helpful for caseload management. That is, effective clinical thinking practices should help us more carefully track and manage our clinical efforts, professional responsibilities, and office practices, and more closely follow the needs and progress of our individual clients.

CLINICAL THINKING SKILLS AND STAGES OF THE CHANGE PROCESS

This chapter has so far focused on the role of the three most important clinical thinking tools in professional counseling practice. The final point to be made is that for counseling and mental health practitioners, diagnosis, case conceptualization, and treatment planning occur in the context of an unfolding, more-or-less sequential professional counseling process. Generally speaking, the prototypical counseling experience follows several logical stages, as follows (Neukrug, 2002, 2003): The earliest steps include pre-interview preparation, first contacts with the client or referral sources, and initial meetings with the client. The next early steps include a period of rapport and trust-building, and problem identification. This typically is followed by another early period of deepening understanding of the client's needs and goal-setting. At this point, often referred to as the work stage, the counseling interventions or treatment approach is fully implemented. Finally, the later steps include closure or termination, which is the ending and consolidating phase of the counseling relationship, and then follow-up or other office practices that finish up and close out the process.

In today's mental-health world, counselors are expected to work quickly and efficiently to form initial diagnostic impressions, formulate useful case conceptualizations, and build effective treatment plans early on in the process; monitor and revise their diagnostic impressions and conceptualizations as needed, and provide intermediate measures of counseling effectiveness, during treatment implementation; and reevaluate diagnoses and revisit case conceptualizations and provide evidence of the outcomes achieved at the point of termination and closeout of a case (Budman & Gurman, 1983; Jongsma & Peterson, 2006; Mahalick, 1990; Neukrug, 2002, 2003; Neukrug & Schwitzer, 2006). Figure 3.2 provides a generic summary of the prototypical counseling process

Figure 3.2   Generic Summary of the Professional Change Process: Clinical Thinking Tools in Context

Stage of Counseling Process	Counseling Relationship Tasks	Primary Clinical Thinking Tasks
Very Earliest Stages	Pre-interview preparation First contact with client or referral source Initial meetings with client Rapport and trust-building Problem identification	Conduct assessment and evaluation Facilitate intake and screening
Moderately Early Stages	Continued relationship-building Deepening understanding of client needs Goal-setting	Form initial diagnostic impressions Develop case conceptualization Prepare treatment planning
Work Stage	Implementation of treatment plan Planful counseling intervention	Monitor, update, or revise diagnosis Provide ongoing measures of change Update case conceptualization Adjust treatment plan
Later Stages	Closure Consolidation of change Relationship termination Follow-up or other office wrap-up	Reevaluate diagnosis at termination Revisit case conceptualization Demonstrate outcomes achieved

as it is usually described by today's authors and clinicians.

As can be seen, although the professional counseling relationship is somewhat front-loaded with diagnosis, case conceptualization, and treatment planning tasks, these tools are used throughout the process. During the middle working period, we are expected to monitor, revise, and update our formulations as needed as we come to better understand and evaluate our client's experiences and presentations. We also assess our progress, as operationalized by the treatment plan, throughout the process. We then heavily rely on our diagnostic skills, and our treatment plan measures, again as we terminate and wrap-up. In sum, being skilled at diagnosis, case conceptualization, and treatment planning will be of benefit from start to finish in the transition from natural helper to counseling professional.

Diagnosis, Case Conceptualization, and
Treatment Planning in a Professional Setting

Select a professional counseling setting in which you are interested, such as a community mental health agency, independent psychological practice, school counseling office, college or university counseling center, inpatient hospital or residential treatment center, or another setting. Interview a staff member to find out what roles diagnosis, case conceptualization, and treatment planning play in his or her daily work. What is expected or beneficial during initial client contacts and early in counseling relationship in the setting? What documents are required? What is expected or beneficial during the working stage when counseling is implemented? How is progress measured? What is expected or beneficial during the final stages, at closure and during follow-up or wrap-up? What final documents are included in the client record at termination? Which diagnostic, case conceptualization, and treatment planning skills are most important or most essential in this setting at the beginning, middle, and end of the counseling relationship? You may want to share your findings in class or discuss your findings during clinical supervision.

CHAPTER SUMMARY AND WRAP-UP

This chapter began Part II of our text: Diagnosis, Case Conceptualization, and Treatment Planning. In the chapter, we introduced the primary skills and tools that are the focus of our text: mental health diagnosis, counseling case conceptualization, and psychotherapeutic treatment planning. Each of these skills will be addressed more fully in the remaining three chapters of this section.

First, we introduced the perspective that, for many learners, education and training in the fields associated with professional counseling can be characterized as a transition from one's background experiences as a successful natural helper in one's everyday interpersonal relationships, to a formal career in today's world of professional practice. We believe that mastering the tools that are the focus of this text is critical to the transition.

Next, we defined each of the three tools. We approached diagnosis as a tool for describing client needs, case conceptualization as a tool for understanding client needs, and treatment planning as a tool for addressing client needs—and summarized their interrelationship in Figure 3.1. Looking first at diagnosis, we indicated that clinical diagnosis in the mental health fields

refers to using the *DSM-IV-TR,* which is a criterion-referenced classification system for organizing and naming what we see and hear our clients experiencing, to form multicomponent diagnoses (with each component of diagnostic information called an axis). We introduced each axis, including: Axis I for almost all of diagnosable mental disorders and other conditions that might be a focus of counseling; Axis II, which is reserved exclusively for diagnoses of mental retardation and personality disorders; Axis III, which presents medical conditions; Axis IV, which lists environmental problems and psychosocial stressors; and Axis V, which provides an estimate of client functioning called the GAF. As we indicated, the primary purpose of such a diagnosis is to describe client concerns and communicate about them with other clinicians.

Looking next at case conceptualization, we indicated that case conceptualization in professional counseling refers to a process of evaluating client behaviors, organizing these presentations into patterns and themes, and then applying a selected theoretical orientation to interpret, explain, or make sense of the etiological factors (features leading to or causing the client's concerns) and sustaining factors (features maintaining the concerns, that is, keeping them going). As we discussed, via case conceptualization, contemporary clinicians select one of the pure counseling theories, a psychotherapeutic integration of two or more theories, an eclectic mix, or a brief solution-focused approach. We will use these distinctions throughout the text when we discuss and illustrate case conceptualization. As we mentioned at the beginning of the book, throughout our text we will be applying the Inverted Pyramid Method, which was developed especially for use by new trainees and emerging professionals.

Looking then at treatment planning, we indicated that psychotherapeutic treatment planning involves plotting out a road map for the counseling process to be undertaken by the counselor and client. It gives a picture of the strategy to be used to facilitate change. We summarized treatment planning to include four steps: behaviorally defining counseling problems or targets, setting achievable goals, selecting the methods of intervention to be employed, and identifying how outcomes change will be shown. We explained some of the many factors that contribute to the selection of goals and determination of modes of intervention, and we emphasized that the client themes and patterns that are derived and the theoretical perspective that is selected during case conceptualization form the basis for developing the treatment plan. We offered three skill-building and learning exercises to further familiarize readers with the three tools and the text's case illustrations.

Finally, we offered some context: We discussed the relationships among diagnosis, case conceptualization, and treatment planning and several aspects of caseload management as it is practiced in professional settings. These included how the clinical thinking tools contribute to documentation; the reasons the tools are the focus of clinical supervision and consultation, and a point of discussion during professional collaborations; the ways in which the tools become topics of communication with stakeholders and when taking care of business activities that are auxiliary to our actual time spent in the counseling session; and how they are associated with daily management of our client workloads. Likewise, we briefly discussed where the tools fit into the start-to-finish stages of the counseling relationship. Figure 3.2 provided a summary of the stages and where the tools are used most heavily. This should help you understand how diagnosis, case conceptualization, and treatment planning connect to the overall counseling process with which you are becoming familiar. We now are ready to examine each tool in detail!

4

DIAGNOSIS

Understanding and Using the DSM-IV-TR

INTRODUCING CHAPTER 4: READER HIGHLIGHTS AND LEARNING GOALS

In comparison with everyday natural helpers, and in comparison with other professional service providers in the human services and related fields, being able to form diagnostic impressions using the *Diagnostic and Statistical Manual, Fourth Edition, Text Revision (DSM-IV-TR);* American Psychiatric Association [APA], 2000a) is an essential skill in today's mental health workplace. Practitioners, including professional counselors and psychotherapists, clinical social workers and psychologists, and psychiatrists are all expected to be proficient using the *DSM-IV-TR* classification system. Depending on the type of practitioner and setting, these professionals are ethically obligated and sometimes legally required to provide responsible diagnoses that set the stage for counseling and treatment (Robinson, 2003; Rosenberg & Kosslyn, 2011; Seligman, 1996). Even counseling professionals who do not actively make diagnoses on a daily basis—such as school counselors in typical school systems—must become conversant in the diagnostic language of the *DSM-IV-TR* in order to be effective in the multidisciplinary settings in which they work. As we indicated in the previous chapter, effective assessment and diagnosis leads to case conceptualization, subsequent treatment planning, and, in turn, the important work that occurs when we sit down with our clients with the goal of bringing about positive changes in their lives.

At the same time, learning to manage the *DSM-IV-TR* diagnostic classification system can seem especially daunting for new counselors: After all, the text comprises more than 900 pages, contains hundreds of diagnoses, and weighs about 4 pounds! Correspondingly, Chapter 4 provides the information you will need to start the learning process. In this chapter, first we introduce mental health diagnosis as it is practiced today, and define *diagnosable mental disorder*. We include an explanation of the term *criterion-referenced*. We discuss the purposes and benefits, as well as the limits, of making a diagnosis; and we identify some of the most common reservations counseling professionals have raised about *DSM-IV-TR* classifications.

(Continued)

(Continued)

Next, we present the *DSM-IV-TR's* multiaxial system and explain how to successfully use the system. Then, one by one, we take a more detailed look at each of the five individual axes comprising a diagnosis. Finally, we pull it all together, demonstrate how to make a start-to-finish diagnosis, and summarize what we have covered. Throughout the chapter, we offer learning activities and professional and clinical snapshots and refer to our 30 clinical cases in order to illustrate our main points about understanding and using the *DSM-IV-TR*.

At the end of the chapter, you should be able to:

- Discuss the role of diagnosis in today's professional counseling settings
- Describe the use of the *DSM-IV-TR* classification system in contemporary mental health diagnosis
- Discuss the purposes, benefits, and limited role of a diagnosis
- Identify and discuss the most important counselor reservations about diagnosis using the *DSM-IV-TR*
- Define each of the following: diagnosable psychological disorder, criterion referenced, and multiaxial
- Identify, explain, and demonstrate the use of each of system's five axes
- Demonstrate how to read and understand a fully prepared, multiaxial *DSM-IV-TR* diagnosis
- Demonstrate the ability to fully prepare start-to-finish, multiaxial diagnostic impressions using the *DSM-IV-TR* text in learning, skill-building, and supervised training contexts that are within the ethical domain of your competency and experience levels

DIAGNOSIS IN THE PROFESSIONAL COUNSELING CONTEXT: *DSM-IV-TR* CLASSIFICATION SYSTEM

The earliest European and North American mental health diagnostic systems referred to various forms of "madness" (Rosenberg & Kosslyn, 2011), and the earliest system of diagnosis formally used in the United States included only two classifications: "idiocy" and "lunacy" (APA, 2000a). Today, nearly all mental health professionals in the United States rely on the *DSM-IV-TR* as the primary system for making clinical diagnoses, and the system is used increasingly internationally. The *DSM* was introduced in 1952 by the American Psychiatric Association in collaboration with other mental health professional groups and underwent revisions in 1964 *(DSM-II)*, 1980 *(DSM-III)*, 1987 *(DSM-III-R)*, and 2000 *(DSM-IV-TR)*. The system is intended to be an official nomenclature, applicable to a wide range of clinical settings and contexts. It is

used by practitioners of many different clinical orientations; is used by "psychiatrists, other physicians, psychologists, social workers, nurses, occupational and rehabilitation therapists, counselors, and other health and mental health professionals"; and is used across settings that include "inpatient, outpatient [or outclient], partial hospital, consultation-liaison, clinic, private practice, and primary care, and with community populations [among others such as school settings and college and university health and mental health]" (APA, 2000a, p. xxiii).

The *DSM* provides a single, comprehensive system of diagnosis that covers all of the main concerns seen in infancy, childhood, and adolescence; and young adulthood, middle adulthood, and later adulthood. This means, for example, that concerns ranging from autistic disorder identified in childhood, through anxiety and mood disorders experienced in adulthood, to the later life onset of dementia of the Alzheimer's type, all appear together in the *DSM-IV-TR's* pages. This is illustrated in our group of popular culture cases found in Part III, where, for instance, Gretel (Chapter 7) presents the childhood and adolescent problem of Oppositional Defiant Disorder, Jack Bauer (Chapter 10) presents an adult occurrence of Posttraumatic Stress Disorder, and Sophia (Chapter 10) presents late life onset of Dementia, Alzheimer's Type.

The DSM-IV-TR is designed to cover client concerns in all four domains of client experience: mood, cognitions, behavior, and physiology. This means, for example, that concerns ranging from the mood problem of Major Depression, to the thought problem of Delusional Disorder, to the behavioral problem of Kleptomania, to physiological problems such as Personality Change Due to a General Medical Condition, all appear within the system. In our case illustrations, you will find diagnoses centering on problems of mood, such as Peter Parker's Major Depressive Disorder (Chapter 12), on problems of thinking, such as Elphaba's Body Dysmorphic Disorder (Chapter 8), and on problems with multiple facets, such as Tinkerbell's Schizoaffective Disorder (Chapter 9).

The system was built to include immediate, short-term, and time-limited problems; more long-standing concerns that follow the client over a greater time period; as well as entrenched lifelong difficulties. This means, for example, that shorter-term Adjustment Disorders, more longstanding Alcohol Dependence, and the lifelong problems of Mental Retardation and Personality Disorders all are contained within the *DSM's* covers. Among our pop culture illustrations, for instance, Mario's cocaine dependence (Chapter 7), Claire's eating disorder (Chapter 8), and Miss Piggy's Borderline Personality Disorder (Chapter 7) each are covered.

SKILL AND LEARNING EXERCISE 4.1

Searching the *DSM-IV-TR*

Refer to Table 1.1 in this text. Working alone or with a partner, select three different popular culture characters that are of special interest to you. Find their case illustrations in Part III of our book (Chapters 7–12), and review the diagnostic impressions provided for each case. Now, using your own copy of the *DSM-IV-TR,* locate the page on which the primary diagnosis or diagnoses used to describe each of the three client's concerns is found. Answer the following: In which diagnostic classes or chapters do the diagnoses appear? Are they primarily diagnoses first made in childhood or in another phase of life? What are the time frames of the diagnoses (short-term, midrange, lifelong)? What are main domains affected (feelings, thoughts, behavior, physiology)?

At the same time, although the *DSM-IV-TR* system is extensive, it also is designed to have limits and boundaries. Two important aspects of the system that are critical to our understanding of the *DSM* pertain to these limits and boundaries. They are the system's limited scope and its limited purpose.

Limited Scope: Definition of a Diagnosable Disorder

One common misperception about clinical diagnosis is that human experience is interpreted exclusively from a pathological point of view— that making a diagnosis leads to a pathological view of all of client concerns. In contrast to this misperception, the *DSM* is designed only to cover a small portion of human behavior or client experience, namely, conditions that meet the definition of *mental disorder,* also known as *psychological disorder* (we will use these two terms interchangeably in our text). According to the *DSM, each diagnosable psychological disorder is a distinct pattern of thoughts, feelings, behaviors, or physiological symptoms that occurs in an individual and causes clinically significant personal distress, clinically significant impairment in one or more important areas of daily functioning, and/or significantly increased risk of harm (where risk of harm includes increased risk of pain or disability, loss of important freedoms, or death).* Every *DSM-IV-TR* diagnosis includes a requirement that the client's experiences of distress, impaired functioning, or risk of harm are clinically significant—meaning that they are having a substantial negative effect on the person's life. In addition, these clinically significant symptoms must be unusual for their context—so that client experiences that are considered to be normally expectable reactions or culturally appropriate reactions to life events are not diagnosable as psychological disorders.

Given this limited definition of a diagnosable mental disorder, it follows that from a diagnostic standpoint that most human behavior or experience is considered functional, normal, and ordered, rather than dysfunctional, abnormal, or disordered. Further, there are several specific types of client experiences that do not fall into the diagnosable category: These include normally expected, culturally appropriate, and life-phase appropriate experiences, and a few other types of nondiagnosable behavior.

Normally Expected, Culturally Appropriate, and Developmentally Appropriate Experiences. Client experiences that we believe are normally expectable responses and culturally appropriate reactions to life events or situations are not diagnosable as psychological disorders, even when they cause the person some distress or difficulty in daily living. For example, although grief following the death of a loved one may be a focus of counseling, a diagnosis of Major Depressive Disorder is not made even when the person experiences major depressive criteria like extreme sadness, loss of interest in everyday activities, insomnia, or poor concentration during the first 2 months following the loss. Likewise, a diagnosis of a psychotic reaction usually is not made even when the client reports seeing, hearing, and talking to his or her loved one immediately following a loss when his

or her culture finds this behavior appropriate. Even substantial changes in mood and functioning are normally expected and culturally appropriate during the bereavement process and therefore are not diagnosable psychological disorders. In our text's popular culture caseload, for example, Jack Bauer and *West Side Story's* Maria both deal with Bereavement.

Similarly, client behavior that we view as normally expectable phase-appropriate life-developmental experiences are not diagnosable as psychological disorders even though they cause distress or some difficulty with functioning. For instance, identity confusion in adolescence, which often is associated with distress about long-term life plans, relationships, and other decisions, is not diagnosable because it is considered a phase-appropriate developmental occurrence. Moderate changes in mood and functioning following a job lay-off, divorce, or retirement generally fall into this area as well. In our text's pop culture caseload, for instance, the Geico Caveman presents an Acculturation Problem (Chapter 11), and Lieutenant Commander Data presents a Religious or Spiritual Problem (Chapter 10), which are to be a focus on counseling but are not diagnosable psychological disorders.

Other Nondiagnosable Behavior. A few other conditions that are not diagnosable also should be noted. One is behavior that is considered by nonclinicians to be "deviant." The *DSM-IV-TR* does not address conflicts between an individual and society—such as political, religious, or sexual deviations from societal norms—unless these are the result of a diagnosable mental disorder. Likewise, because a client's negative experiences meet the legal or other nonclinical criteria for mental disorder or mental disability does not necessarily mean that the *DSM-IV-TR* criteria for a diagnosable psychological disorder has been met. In addition, there are psychological patterns that, although commonly used colloquially by nonprofessionals or even by professionals in their everyday conversations, are not diagnosable disorders because they do not appear in the classification system. For example, although *codependence* is a commonly used term in contemporary culture, it is not among the *DSM-IV-TR's* diagnosable disorders.

Specific Purpose: Benefits of a Diagnosis

So far we have described the *DSM* diagnostic system's limited scope. It also was designed with a narrowly defined primary purpose: to assist clinicians in describing client concerns in order to communicate their view of the client's needs. In other words, diagnosis is a *descriptive tool.* It provides an agreed-upon language for characterizing a client's behavior, thoughts, feelings, and other aspects of distress, impairment, or risk. It should help enhance agreement and improve the sharing of information among clinicians about the "client picture they are observing" (Neukrug & Schwitzer, 2006, p. 168). For example, when it is indicated by a previous counselor that our new client has been experiencing a Major Depressive Disorder, we are provided a great deal of information about the nature of the person's concerns. We know about the primary symptoms (low mood, loss of pleasure), associated symptoms (disruptions in sleep, appetite, concentration, etc.), minimum duration (at least 2 weeks), and severity of the distress, and that his or her mood problems are not due to substance use—all because we are familiar with the Major Depressive Disorder diagnosis. You will see a good example of this by reading the case notes and diagnostic impressions we present in Edward Cullen's case illustration in Chapter 8 of our text.

Importantly, *DSM-IV-TR* diagnoses are theory-neutral categorizations. Using the system to describe client experiences does not reflect any specific theoretical interpretation, disciplinary viewpoint, or causal inference. Instead, the system relies on the traditional medical/scientific approach of naming and organizing our client information in as objective a fashion as possible. The classification system divides client presentations into psychological disorders based on sets of criteria that are made up of observable features. In other words, *diagnoses in the DSM-IV-TR are criterion-referenced, and our job is to match up client information with the sets of criteria the DSM provides for the various diagnoses.* Being objective and theory-neutral means that in and of themselves, diagnoses do not identify the etiology of the person's concerns, apply a theory to infer the causes or sustaining factors contributing to the situation, or offer a plan for intervention. For instance, the system does not use terms such as *neurosis* and *psychosis* that might indicate a psychoanalytic theoretical viewpoint, or terms such as *organic* and *inorganic* that might favor the biopsychiatric discipline. It is built with multidisciplinary users in mind.

However, the diagnoses *do* provide our starting point for moving on to the next steps of case conceptualization and treatment planning—where we apply our preferred theoretical viewpoint and counseling approach on the basis of our own clinical decision making. The diagnosis provides our foundation for determining what the primary focus of counseling should be—for example, mood problems versus somatic symptoms, or solution focus versus life patterns such as a personality disorder. It helps us see what our treatment goals might be in the form of reducing or eliminating specific symptoms that are part of the diagnostic criteria set. It can help sort out the need for physiological interventions such as medical treatment; counseling interventions such individual or group interventions; and social interventions such as environmental adaptations in the community, school, or family. You will find good illustrations of this by reading the diagnostic impressions, case conceptualizations, and treatment plans we present in both Naruto's and Snoopy's case illustrations in Chapter 7 of the text.

In addition, when the information is known, the *DSM* provides data for each diagnosis pertaining to primary features, associated features, subtypes, and variations in client presentations; typical pattern, course, or progression of symptoms; and how to differentiate the diagnosis from other, similar ones. It also provides research findings about predisposing factors, complications, and associated medical conditions when they are known. All of these elements are benefits of making the diagnosis.

Figure 4.1 The *DSM-IV-TR* in Context

Limited Scope	
What the Diagnostic System Covers	**What the Diagnosis System Does Not Cover**
Diagnosable psychological disorders defined as distinct patterns of thoughts, feelings, behaviors, and/or physiological symptoms that cause an individual clinically significant distress, impairment in functioning, and/or increased risk of harm	Normally expectable reactions to life events or situations
	Culturally appropriate reactions to events or situations
	Life-phase appropriate developmental patterns
Unusual for their situational and cultural context	Conflicts between individual and society (Deviance) that are not due to another diagnosable disorder
	Patterns meeting legal or other professional definitions but not meeting *DSM-IV-TR* criteria
	Patterns described by colloquial definitions but not meeting any specific *DSM-IV-TR* criteria

Specific Purpose	
What the Diagnostic System Does	**What the Diagnostic System Does Not Do**
Provides an agreed-upon language for describing client concerns	Reflect any specific theoretical orientation
Enhances agreement and improves sharing of information about client situations	Reflect any specific disciplinary viewpoint
Provides criterion-referenced, theory-neutral descriptions that assist with determination of primary focus of counseling	Infer etiology, sustaining factors, or other conceptual interpretations (other than indicating a medical cause)
Sets the stage for case conceptualization and treatment planning	Determine the course of treatment

Counselor Reservations About Diagnosis

Along with the benefits of diagnosis, important counselor reservations have been raised about use of the *DSM-IV-TR* classification system. These reservations take the form of apprehensions, cautions, critiques, and criticisms. We believe it is essential for effectively functioning clinicians to understand the reservations that sometimes are raised about the system along with its benefits. We already have addressed the misperception that the system views human behavior from an exclusively pathological viewpoint by discussing the *DSM-IV-TR*'s limit of scope. We also have addressed the misperception that the system determines the theoretical or disciplinary approach of the case conceptualization and treatment plan by discussing the *DSM-IV-TR*'s limit of purpose. Other counselor reservations have to do with social-cultural cautions as well as clinical criticisms. We want to describe a few of the reservations we hear most commonly expressed by students and new counselors and suggest the ways in which the *DSM* system attempts to address these issues. They include: potential for diagnostic bias, potential for stigmatization and labeling, underresponsiveness to social change, and overresponsiveness to payment pressures.

Potential for Diagnostic Bias. This counselor reservation relates to the potential for diagnostic bias, whereby clinicians might routinely overdiagnose, underdiagnose, or misdiagnose clients populating specific demographic groups, such as on the basis of ethnicity, gender, age, or socioeconomic status (Kunen, Niederhauser, Smith, Morris, & Marx, 2005; Meehl, 1960). As examples, researchers have reported that African American clients with mood disorders are likely to be misdiagnosed with schizophrenic disorders (Neighbors, Trierweiler, Ford, & Muroff, 2003; Trierweiler, Muroff, Jackson, Neighbors, & Munday, 2005), while Latina/o clients may tend to have their presenting concerns underdiagnosed by their counselors (LaBruzza & Mendez-Villarrubia, 1994; Schmaling & Hernandez, 2005).

The *DSM's* authors attempt to address issues of gender and multiculturalism in several ways. Each diagnosis includes contextual information, when it is known, under the separate heading, "Specific Culture, Age, and Gender Features." For instance, cultural variations in presenting complaints (somatic complaints such as headaches among Latino cultures; complaints of fatigue or weakness among Asian cultures) are described along with the main criteria for the Major Depressive Disorder diagnosis. Age differences in the prominent features of many diagnoses are presented. For instance, variations in prominent Major Depression features include withdrawal among children, hypersomnia among adolescents, and cognitive symptoms like memory loss among older adults. Differences in prevalence according to socioeconomic status are described for some diagnoses, such as Conversion Disorder.

The *DSM-IV-TR* text also notes when the diagnosis of certain disorders among certain ethnic or age groups should raise questions for us (e.g., the *DSM* alerts us that it is known that clinicians may tend to inappropriately diagnose Schizophrenia instead of Bipolar Disorder among nonwhite ethnic groups and younger clients). Prevalence according to gender is indicated (e.g., Bipolar Disorders are equally common among women and men, unlike Major Depression, which is diagnosed more commonly among women, or Obsessive-Compulsive Disorder, which is diagnosed more commonly among men in the United States). Gender-specific information is provided. For instance, among people diagnosed with Histrionic Personality Disorder, women are more likely to present problems centering on the feminine relationship role, while men are more likely to present problems centering on machismo. As counseling professionals, we must remain up to date on the growing clinical research literature about diagnostic bias and carefully read the information already available inside the *DSM.*

In Part III of our text, you will find that we considered these issues when forming diagnostic impressions for a variety of our cases; as an illustration, see our case notes and the diagnostic discussion for case of Maria (Chapter 11).

Potential for Stigmatization and Labeling. Another commonly expressed reservation among counselors is that diagnosis can become a stigmatizing label, and therefore negatively affect how an individual views himself or herself, how others in the person's life react to him or her, or how the person accesses services and is responded to in his or her community (Eriksen & Kress, 2005; McAuliffe & Associates, 2008). To address this, counselors must be vigilant in correcting the common misperception that clinical diagnosis classifies or labels people; instead, the *DSM* really classifies the psychological disorders people are experiencing. To promote this, the *DSM-IV-TR* carefully uses phrases such as "an individual with Schizophrenia" and "an individual with Alcohol Dependence" rather than terms like "a schizophrenic" or "an alcoholic" throughout the text (APA, 2000a, p. xxxi). As counseling professionals, we must use the same vigilance in our own communications about our clients and our diagnosis of their concerns. In our case illustrations, for example, we are careful to use this language when describing Chief Bromden (Chapter 12) as a person with Schizophrenia rather than a schizophrenic.

Underresponsiveness to Social Change. One more type of social-cultural reservation expressed by counseling professionals is that diagnosis is too unresponsive to social change. However, the authors of the *DSM* attempt to address this through the rigor of the revision process used to update the system. This constant updating process includes expert participation in literature reviews, data analyses and re-analyses, and field trials that employ careful thresholds for revision. The *DSM's* historical management of the issue of homosexuality provides one example of the *DSM's* responsiveness to changing societal and professional viewpoints. "Homosexuality" was classified as a mental disorder in the *DSM-II,* in keeping with professional standards of the time. Based on a change in expert consensus viewpoint, the disorder was replaced by "Sexual Orientation Disorder" in later printings of the *DSM-II* and then by "Ego-dystonic Homosexuality" in *DSM-III.* Both of these refer only to the situation in which an individual experiences clinically significant distress or impairment related to his or her thoughts, feelings, or behaviors pertaining to a gay, lesbian, bisexual, or transgendered (GLBT) sexual orientation. The change in viewpoint was based on the corrected finding that having a nonheterosexual sexual identity per se did not meet the criteria for a diagnosis. Subsequently this disorder was removed from *DSM-III-Revised,* and did not appear at all in *DSM-IV.* Instead, "persistent and marked distress about sexual orientation" is provided in the *DSM-IV-TR* as one of several examples of a situation in which the diagnosis "Sexual Disorder Not Otherwise Specified" (APA, 2000a, p. 582) might be used to best describe a client's primary

concerns. Alternatively, today's clinicians simply indicate there is no diagnosable mental disorder, but that the client is dealing with a troubling "Identity Problem" that will be the focus of counseling. You will find that we employed this approach in our diagnostic impressions for text's popular culture client, Waylon Smithers (Chapter 9).

Overresponsiveness to Payment Pressures. Eriksen and Kress (2005) raised the concern that revisions, additions, and expansions to the *DSM* classification system sometimes may occur for reasons of payment pressure rather than clinical evidence or in response to professional advances. These authors suggested that because the mental health-care industry requires that a client or patient be experiencing an accepted diagnosable mental disorder in order to be reimbursed by health insurance companies or other third-party payers, some of the additions, expansions, or criteria changes in the *DSM* may sometimes occur to help clinicians gain coverage rather than for reasons based on clinical evidence. According to this line of thinking, having more diagnoses, or more payment-sensitive diagnoses from which to choose, might increase the chances of receiving payment. Naturally, this raises critical issues about how we go about our professional practices. Although the question of payment pressures is not addressed directly in the *DSM,* the text's introductory cautionary statement reminds counseling professionals that the purpose of the system is to "provide clear descriptions of diagnostic categories in order to enable clinicians and investigators to diagnose, communicate about, study, and treat people with various mental disorders" (APA, 2000a, p. xxxvii). It implies that diagnoses are designed for clinical and research purposes—rather than for other purposes. In this text and in our case illustrations, we take the traditional, orthodox view that the diagnosis is for the purpose of accurate clinical description and should not be influenced by any nonclinical factors such as payment pressures. However, this counselor criticism is one that raises questions we believe you will need to carefully consider and understand, discuss in classes and with your colleagues, and raise with your experienced clinical supervisors as you make the transition to professional mental health practice.

Additional Thoughts. We now have introduced the *DSM-IV-TR* diagnostic system in the professional counseling context, explained what is meant by a diagnosable mental disorder and what is and is not covered by the system, explained the purposes and benefits of making a diagnosis, and also explained some of the hesitations counselors express about diagnosis. Other reservations exist, of course, and many of these pertain to how the system itself operates, such as how the system handles medical illnesses that overlap psychological disorders, how the system handles commonly co-occurring problems such as coexisting depressive and anxiety disorders, the system's use of categorical criteria instead of criteria on a continuum, and so on. Later on, after you have developed a basic understanding of the *DSM* and basic diagnostic competencies, you may want to further investigate what the counseling research and professional literature have to say about these more advanced clinical criticisms. In the remaining portion of Chapter 4, we will turn to the nuts-and-bolts details of making a mental health diagnosis.

SKILL AND LEARNING EXERCISE 4.2

Analyzing Diagnostic Impressions

Refer to the case of *West Side Story's* Maria appearing in Chapter 11, Characters in Music, Musicals, and Advertising, located later in this text. Read the intake summary, diagnostic impressions, and discussion of the diagnosis. You may also want to have your copy of the *DSM-IV-TR* available. Working alone or with a partner, consider the following:

So far in this chapter we have discussed the limited scope of a mental health diagnosis. You will see that a diagnosis of Acute Stress Disorder was decided upon to describe Maria's presentation. What characteristics of Maria's presenting concerns fall within the scope of the *DSM* and allow the diagnosis of a psychological disorder? What specific criteria were needed for the diagnosis of Acute Stress Disorder? Why do the characteristics of Maria's presenting concerns pertaining to her grief about the loss of her boyfriend fall outside the scope of a mental disorder diagnosis? How did the counselor indicate that grief and loss was not diagnosable, but still would be focus of counseling?

In this chapter we discussed the specific descriptive purpose of a mental health diagnosis. What would it mean to you as a counselor to learn that Maria's symptoms were described by Acute Stress Disorder? What would you know about the types of symptoms she was experiencing? The types of life events she had experienced? About the time frame of her difficulties?

In this chapter we discussed common counselor reservations about *DSM* diagnoses, including criticisms related to social-cultural considerations. How are they relevant to Maria's situation? How did Maria's intake counselor address these considerations?

Considering the benefits, limitations, and reservations about making a diagnosis, what do you believe are the advantages of having diagnostic impressions to guide the focus of counseling, case conceptualization, and treatment planning for our work with Maria? Do you believe there are disadvantages, and if so, what are they?

Finally, if you were Maria's intake counselor, how comfortable would you be with the diagnostic impressions found in this case illustration?

MULTIAXIAL SYSTEM

We said in Chapter 3 of our text that a *DSM-IV-TR* diagnosis is *multiaxial*. We realize the term *multiaxial* can cause some confusion and even intimidation for students and clinicians who are new to diagnosis. Simply stated, each of the five "axes" that contributes to a fully prepared diagnosis gives us a different piece of information about the client with whom we are working. Having several mechanisms for describing *five different aspects* of a client's or patient's presentation gives the counseling professional more room to fully characterize and record what the person is experiencing. It allows us to describe our clients' experiences holistically, from several different points of view (Seligman, 2004)—including our view of their primary psychological concerns, related medical problems, life stressors, and overall levels of distress or functioning. For quick and convenient reference, instructions for using each axis of the multiaxial system are provided to us right in the *DSM-IV-TR* text itself, on pages 27–37, so that as long as you have your copy of the *DSM* with you, you have the support you need as a beginning diagnostician. The axes are summarized in Figure 4.2.

Figure 4.2   Multiaxial Assessment

Axis I.	Clinical Disorders
	Other Conditions That May Be a Focus of Clinical Attention
Axis II.	Personality Disorders
	Mental Retardation
Axis III.	General Medical Problems
Axis IV.	Psychosocial and Environmental Problems
Axis V.	Global Assessment of Functioning (GAF)

Axis I. Clinical Disorders and Other Conditions That May Be a Focus of Clinical Attention. Axis I probably is seen as the most salient and important part of the multiaxial assessment. It is on Axis I that we record almost all of the diagnosable psychological disorders of infancy, childhood, adolescence, and adulthood found throughout the entire *DSM-IV-TR*. There are only two exceptions: the diagnosis of Mental Retardation, and diagnosis of any of the Personality Disorders. Therefore, if we determine that our client is experiencing any diagnosable mental disorders at all (except Mental Retardation or a Personality Disorder), we record these on Axis I. Further, in addition to all of the diagnosable psychological disorders (except Mental Retardation or a Personality Disorder), we also record all of the client's nondiagnosable problem areas and counseling themes on Axis I. Using *DSM* language, these nondiagnosable issues are referred to as Other Conditions That May Be a Focus of Clinical Attention.

Axis II. Personality Disorders and Mental Retardation. Axis II is set aside for recording two specific types of diagnoses: Personality Disorders and Mental Retardation. Both of these are viewed as long-standing, entrenched, and, typically, lifelong conditions. Having a separate axis for these typically lifelong conditions reminds clinicians of their diagnostic importance.

Axis III. General Medical Conditions. Axis III gives us a place in the mental health diagnosis to list any medical problems and physical complaints that might be present in the client, especially when a medical or physical problem might be associated with the person's presenting psychological and counseling concerns.

Axis IV. Psychosocial and Environmental Problems. Axis IV gives us a separate place in the diagnosis to record any psychosocial, social, relational, social-environmental, or other life stressors or pressures the client might be experiencing, especially when these stresses might be associated with the individual's presenting psychological concerns and counseling issues.

Axis V. On Axis V, clinicians provide a one-shot estimate of the client's level of distress, the impact of the symptoms he or she is experiencing, and how well the person is functioning in his or her various life roles. This estimate is made using a

psychometric scale, the Global Assessment of Functioning (GAF), which appears in the *DSM-IV-TR* on page 34. Scores reflect a continuum ranging from a low of 1 (poorest functioning) to a high of 100 (maximum functioning).

SKILL AND LEARNING EXERCISE 4.3

Understanding Multiaxial Diagnosis

By now you have reviewed several of our case illustrations as you have completed our Skill and Learning Exercises, and probably thumbed through others you found interesting. All of the cases provide examples of multiaxial diagnoses. At this point in your reading, refer to the case of Eleanor Rigby of the Beatles' *Revolver Album,* appearing in Chapter 11, Characters in Music, Musicals, and Advertising. In this case, you will find an example of a fully prepared multiaxial assessment, based on our own unique version of Eleanor Rigby's situation.

Examining Axis I, you will see we recorded Eleanor Rigby's mood problem on Axis I because this is where the *DSM-IV-TR's* diagnosable psychological disorders (except Mental Retardation and Personality Disorders) are presented. Next you will see we recorded the Mental Retardation we described her as experiencing in this case on Axis II, since Axis II is the location for diagnoses of Mental Retardation and Personality Disorders (read through the case to for our unique take on Eleanor Rigby). On Axis III we listed Hypothyroidism, since her thyroid condition is directly related to her low mood symptoms (read through the case illustration for more details). On Axis IV, we listed the social and psychosocial problems that Eleanor Rigby confronts, which are related to living by herself since the loss of her husband, and her need for some supervised support. Finally, on Axis V, you will see that Eleanor Rigby's counselor used the GAF scale to estimate the client's current functioning. The estimate of GAF = 61 indicates Eleanor Rigby is experiencing some mild symptoms but generally is functioning pretty well.

Altogether, the five-axis diagnosis gives us a complete, holistic description of the client's current clinical situation. Now let us explore each of the axes in more detail.

A CLOSER LOOK AT AXIS I: CLINICAL DISORDERS AND OTHER CONDITIONS THAT MAY BE A FOCUS OF CLINICAL ATTENTION

Axis I and Axis II are the key components of the *DSM-IV-TR* multiaxial diagnostic system. Axis I is used to record nearly all of the 340 diagnosable disorders appearing in the system, and all of the other issues that might be a focus of counseling. On Axis I, counseling professionals answer the questions:

"Does the client show signs and symptoms of any of the fifteen major classes of Axis I mental disorders?," "Are there conditions other than [diagnosable psychological disorders] that should be a focus of clinical attention?," and "Which is the principal diagnosis and reason for today's visit?" (LaBruzza & Mendez-Villarrubia, 1994, p. 86)

Axis I is used to indicate when the counselor is uncertain or undecided about a diagnosis, when the diagnosis will be deferred until later assessment, when no Axis I diagnosis at all is indicated, and, alternatively, when multiple diagnoses are needed to characterize the client's presentation.

To become successful using Axis I, it is necessary to learn about two aspects of the *DSM* text: Interchapter organization and intrachapter organization.

Interchapter Organization

The long list of Axis I disorders is divided into 15 separate categories, called *classes of disorders.* Each class of disorders has its own chapter. Each of the diagnostic classes, or chapters, brings together various diagnosable psychological disorders that share common denominators—that is, each class or chapter of diagnoses in the DSM brings together various diagnoses that have natural similarities. For example, all of the diagnosable client problems related to substance use (e.g., alcohol dependence, cocaine abuse, withdrawal symptoms) are in the same class or chapter of disorders; all of the client concerns with mood (major depression, bipolar disorder, etc.) are in the same class or chapter of disorders, and all of the clinically significant client difficulties reacting to life stressors (adjustment disorder with depressed mood, adjustment disorder with anxiety) are in the same class or chapter.

A typical starting point for formulating an Axis I diagnosis is to first decide which diagnostic class, or chapter, seems to hold the best tentative match with the client's presentation. For example, a typical starting point is to think about whether the person's symptoms—her thoughts, feelings, behaviors, or physiological signs—seem primarily suggestive of panic, a phobia, or traumatic reaction (found in the Anxiety Disorders), troubles with falling asleep, maintaining sleep, and being rested (found in the Sleep Disorders), or possibly sexual desire or performance (the Sexual and Gender Disorders). In other words, using the *criterion-referenced approach,* the counselor might first ask, "Can I narrow down the client's presenting concerns from all of the various diagnosable disorders in all of the fifteen diagnostic classes (or chapters) to just a few possibilities?"

Further, the *DSM-IV-TR* text is organized from front cover to back cover in a way that is intended to help us answer this question. The chapters appear in a specific, useful order that helps us with our Axis I diagnostic decision making. They are ordered in a way that can guide our diagnostic thought process. You can see the order by thumbing through pages 13–26 of the *DSM.* What makes the order of the chapters useful to us? It presents the different types of disorders in the order of their critical nature to the client's well-being. Take another look at the order of the classes of disorders appearing on pages 13–26 of the *DSM.* You will notice the following contents:

Disorders Usually First Diagnosed in Infancy, Childhood, or Adolescence

As you will see, the Disorders Usually First Diagnosed in Infancy, Childhood, or Adolescence appear first, simply because they occur first in the lifespan. When the client is an infant, child, or adolescent, this is a natural starting point. Included are 10 different categories: Mental Retardation (recorded on Axis II), Learning Disorders, Motor Skills Disorders, Communication Disorders, Pervasive Developmental Disorders, Feeding and Eating Disorders of Infancy and Early Childhood, Tic Disorders, Elimination.

Child therapists, family clinicians, school counselors, and others who work extensively with individuals under age 18 years rely heavily on this chapter. Of particular note, school counselors and their clinical colleagues with child and adolescent caseloads often find the Learning Disorders (Mathematics, Reading, Written Expression), the Pervasive Developmental

Disorders (especially Autistic Disorder and Asperger's Disorder), Attention-Deficit Disorders and other Disruptive Behavior Disorders (especially Conduct Disorder and Oppositional Defiant Disorder) to be especially important to their diagnostic work.

Becoming Familiar With Disorders Usually First Diagnosed in Infancy, Childhood, or Adolescence

The childhood disorders are well represented in our popular culture caseload. We recommend that you closely read these this chapter in its entirety, and then turn to our case illustrations. Remember that you are gaining an initial familiarity at this point, not detailed expertise.

To increase your understanding of diagnostic decision-making with *Disorders Usually First Diagnosed in Infancy, Childhood, or Adolescence,* take time now to closely read or reread the intake summary, diagnostic impressions, and diagnostic discussion found in the following case illustrations: Gretel (Chapter 7), Naruto (Chapter 7), Snoopy (Chapter 7), and Christopher Robin (Chapter 12). It will be helpful to have your copy of the *DSM-IV-TR* available as you study the diagnostic aspects of these case illustrations.

At the same time, as the chapter's title indicates, these disorders are *usually but not always first identified in children.* When a counselor can trace an adult client's problematic symptoms back to an early life phase with relative certainty, diagnoses found in this chapter may be used. For example, an adult might first be identified with Attention-Deficit/Hyperactivity Disorder (one of the diagnoses in this chapter) during college, providing all of the criteria for onset and the other criteria can be determined.

Four Red Flags

Next come four *red flag* chapters. We refer to these as *red flags* because clinicians commonly believe that if any of these disorders are present, typically they must be identified, acknowledged, addressed, responded to, or treated first or very early on—that is, when a client or patient is experiencing any of the concerns found in these chapters, commonly it is assumed that this condition will take priority in treatment planning. The red flags include:

Delirium, Dementia, and Amnestic, and Other Cognitive Disorders. This class of disorders refers to prominent clinical disturbances. Further, these disturbances must be due to (a) a specific, physiological/medical condition for which there is evidence from medical history, physical examination, or laboratory findings; (b) the effects of a substance, including a drug of abuse, medication, or exposure to a toxin; or (c) a combination of these. Effects of a medical condition in the form of a *delirium* means that the client or patient is experiencing a disturbance in his or her conscious awareness of self and orientation to the world around him or her. *Dementia* indicates the client is experiencing memory problems as well as other cognitive deficits. *Amnesia* indicates memory impairment without the other cognitive deficits characteristic of dementia. Head trauma, vascular disease, prolonged substance use, human immunodeficiency virus

(HIV) disease, and Parkinson's and Huntington's diseases are commonly cited examples of conditions leading to these disorders.

Clinicians and counseling professionals in inpatient, medical, psychiatric, and alcohol and other drug treatment settings may rely more heavily on this chapter. Further, those working closely with older populations and in geriatric settings are especially familiar with Dementia of the Alzheimer's Type found here. A summary appears on *DSM-IV-TR* pages 135–136.

Mental Disorders Due to a General Medical Condition. These are psychological disorders that are "judged to be the direct physiological consequence of a general medical condition" (APA, 2000a, p. 181). Mood Disorders, Anxiety Disorders, Sexual Dysfunctions, Sleep Disorders, Personality Change, and various other mental disorders can have their origins in physiological medical conditions. These are outlined in this chapter and referred to again throughout the diagnostic system. Clinicians in medical and psychiatric settings may be especially expert with this red flag chapter. A summary appears on *DSM-IV-TR* pages 181–182.

Substance-Related Disorders. All of the disorders associated with clinically problematic *substance use* (including substance abuse and dependence) and with clinically significant problems that are *substance induced* are included in this extensive chapter. Included are intoxication and withdrawal; substance-induced delirium, persisting dementia, persisting amnesia, and persisting psychotic disorders; substance-induced mood and anxiety disorders, sexual dysfunctions, and sleep disorders. Further, for the purposes of diagnosis, all the various substances are referred to by this chapter, including alcohol, drugs of abuse (such as cocaine), medications

(prescription or nonprescription, including psychiatric medications), and exposure to toxins (such as lead paint). Readers will note that this chapter first presents the criteria for the various disorders, and then matches them with various substances. For example, the chapter defines diagnostic sets such as abuse and dependence, withdrawal, and substance-induced problems, and then goes on to connect each of these, one after another, to alcohol and other classes of substances. Naturally, professionals working in settings for which substance-use and substance-induced problems are especially prominent will need to become masters of this chapter. You will find a helpful one-page summary of the whole Substance-Related Disorders chapter on *DSM-IV-TR* page 193.

Schizophrenia and Other Psychotic Disorders. This chapter contains diagnoses for Schizophrenia, which is a mixture of psychotic symptoms (delusions, hallucinations) and other characteristically disturbing symptoms (disorganized speech or behavior, disturbed affect, volition, etc.) present intensely for a month and with residual symptoms present for 6 months, causing disturbances in the person's life and not due to another medical condition or other cause; and related problems such as Schizoaffective Disorder, in which the symptoms of both Schizophrenia and a Mood Disorder are troubling the client or patient. The chapter also contains diagnoses for other disturbing psychotic and delusional problems, including Delusional Disorder, in which the client vehemently holds nonbizarre but untrue beliefs in areas of romance, grandiosity, jealously, persecution, and so on; and Brief Psychotic Disorders and Shared Delusions. Clinicians in medical, psychiatric, and other settings in which these types of symptoms appear may be especially expert with this red flag chapter. A summary appears on *DSM-IV-TR* pages 297–298.

CLINICAL SPOTLIGHT 4.1: A Career Counseling Client Presenting Psychotic Symptoms?

Why are the red flag chapters so important to the typical counseling professional? We indicated above that certain types of clinicians in specific types of settings might be most likely to use diagnoses for these psychological problems. Often these are medical and psychiatric settings. However, our view is that all counseling professionals must be aware of the red flag disorders and be vigilant about evaluating for them among our client caseload. For instance, if our client presents all of the symptoms of a depressive disorder, but those symptoms are directly due to hypothyroidism, the effects of diabetes, or another medical cause, we must be able to identify this possibility and refer our client for adequate medical examination in order to determine what treatment (medical, counseling, or both) is needed. Therefore, we all must pay attention to the red flags.

As an example, one of the authors (Schwitzer) recalls conducting an intake interview with a college student who came into the university mental health center for career counseling. During the first few sessions, the client reported that he had been having conversations with his deceased grandmother, who was providing consultation and sage advice. He described being able to clearly hear her talking to him. The client came from a Mexican cultural background in which consultation with family ancestors was a normally expected practice. Therefore, as a counselor, there was a diagnostic question as to whether this client was presenting nondiagnosable information about his helpful use of culturally appropriate practices, or, alternatively, whether he was reporting the "red flag" symptoms of a possible psychotic or schizophrenic disorder.

The author followed the diagnostic path suggested by the *DSM*. Further mental status evaluation indicated that, in addition to the auditory experiences (hearing his grandmother), this student also was experiencing the tactile hallucination of feeling as though when he walked, he was stepping several inches above the earth rather than touching the ground with his feet. Follow-up evaluation and psychiatric consultation and referral did, in fact uncover that the student was experiencing a first incidence of Schizophrenia. Had Schwitzer not begun diagnostically with the red flags—with this career counseling client—he might have missed the correct diagnosis and therefore the needed treatment.

SKILL AND LEARNING EXERCISE 4.5

Becoming Familiar With Red Flag Classes of Diagnosis

All four red flag classes of disorders are represented in our popular culture caseload. We recommend that you closely read these chapters in their entirety, and then turn to our case illustrations. Remember that you are gaining an initial familiarity at this point, not detailed expertise.

To increase your understanding of diagnostic decision-making with *Delirium, Dementia, and Amnestic, and Other Cognitive Disorders,* take time now to closely read or reread the intake summary, diagnostic impressions, and diagnostic discussion found in the case illustration of Sophia (Chapter 10).

To increase your understanding of diagnostic decision-making with *Mental Disorders Due to a General Medical Condition,* take time now to closely read or reread the intake summary, diagnostic impressions, and diagnostic discussion found in the case illustrations of Lieutenant Commander Data (Chapter 10) and Eleanor Rigby (Chapter 11).

(Continued)

(Continued)

To increase your understanding of diagnostic decision-making with *Substance-Related Disorders,* take time now to closely read or reread the intake summary, diagnostic impressions, and diagnostic discussion found in the case illustrations of Mario (Chapter 1) and Cleveland Brown (Chapter 9).

To increase your understanding of diagnostic decision-making with *Schizophrenia and Other Psychotic Disorders,* take time now to closely read or reread the intake summary, diagnostic impressions, and diagnostic discussion found in the case illustrations of Billie Jean (Chapter 11) and Chief Bromden (Chapter 12).

It will be helpful to have your copy of the *DSM-IV-TR* available as you study the diagnostic aspects of these case illustrations.

Two Frequently Diagnosed Classes of Disorders

Next to appear in the *DSM-IV-TR* are two classes of disorders containing arguably the most frequently used sets of diagnoses among contemporary mental health populations: the Mood Disorders and Anxiety Disorders (Kessler et al., 1994; Seligman, 2004). It should make sense to us that after considering the red flags, next we would turn to frequently presented disorders as we move through our diagnostic decision-making process of comparing the client's presentation to all of the different *DSM* diagnosis criteria sets (as a note, Substance-Related Disorders also are common [APA, 2000a; Kessler et al, 1994; Munson, 2001], but of course we already have considered this by first carefully evaluating for the presence of red flag concerns).

Mood Disorders. This important chapter extensively covers diagnosable syndromes characterized by depressed, elevated, or irritable mood (Frances, First, & Pincus, 1995), where mood is defined as "a pervasive and sustained emotion that colors the person's perception of world" (APA, 2000a, p. 825). Two categories of disorders are covered: Depressive Disorders and Bipolar Disorders. Inside the chapter, the criteria sets first are explained for Major Depressive Episode, Manic Episode, and Hypomanic Episode. The chapter then uses these criteria sets as building blocks to form the diagnosable disorders. The mood disorder criteria sets include primary symptoms and associated symptoms pertaining to feelings as well as thoughts, behaviors, and physiological symptoms; minimum duration and timelines; and severity indicators.

The diagnosable disorders include Major Depressive Disorder, Single Episode; Major Depressive Disorder, Recurrent; Dysthymia; Bipolar I Disorder, Single Manic Episode; Bipolar I Disorder, Most Recent Episode Hypomanic; Bipolar I Disorder, Most Recent Episode Manic; Bipolar I Disorder, Most Recent Episode, Mixed; Bipolar II Disorder (Recurrent Major Depressive Episodes With Hypomanic Episodes); Cyclothymic Disorder; as well as depressive and bipolar disorders that are not otherwise specified, are unspecified, and are due to general medical problems or use of a substance. The chapter also provides extensive subtypes and specifiers to help the clinician record a very detailed account of the client's experiences, episodes, and disorders. Some of the specifiers, for example, are "Postpartum Onset," indicating the mood disorder began within 4 weeks of childbirth, and "Seasonal Pattern," indicating episodes of the client's mood problems correspond to seasons of the calendar.

Readers should carefully read *DSM-IV-TR* pages 345–347 for a good summary the Mood Disorders.

Anxiety Disorders. Similar to the chapter on mood disorders, this important chapter extensively covers diagnosable syndromes characterized by panic, phobia, and posttraumatic reactions, all of which are associated with affective, cognitive, behavioral, or physiological symptoms of fear and discomfort.

Several different types of anxiety problems are covered. Inside the chapter, the criteria sets for Panic Attacks and Agoraphobia first are explained. The chapter then uses these criteria sets as building blocks to form the diagnosable disorders: Panic Disorder Without Agoraphobia, Panic Disorder With Agoraphobia, and Agoraphobia Without History of Panic Disorder.

Next, the chapter presents Specific Phobias, Social Phobia, and Obsessive-Compulsive Disorder. All of these involve some form of cognitive, affective, behavioral, and physiological symptoms of fear, discomfort, and avoidance or other problematic behaviors. Then, the chapter presents Posttraumatic Stress Disorder (PTSD) and Acute Stress Disorder, both of which are diagnosed only when specific characteristic client symptoms are present, and only in response to events that meet the *DSM* definition of trauma—all of which are explained inside the chapter. Generalized Anxiety Disorder then is presented. Rounding out this class of disorders are anxiety disorders due to a general medical condition or substance use, and those anxiety disorders not specified elsewhere in the chapter.

Readers should carefully read *DSM-IV-TR* pages 429–430 for a good summary the Anxiety Disorders.

SKILL AND LEARNING EXERCISE 4.6

Becoming Familiar With Mood Disorders and Anxiety Disorders

The Mood Disorders and Anxiety Disorders are well-represented in our popular culture caseload. We recommend that you closely read these two chapters in their entirety, and then turn to our case illustrations. Remember that you are gaining an initial familiarity at this point, not detailed expertise.

To increase your understanding of diagnostic decision-making with *Mood Disorders,* take time now to closely read or reread the intake summary, diagnostic impressions, and diagnostic discussion found in the following case illustrations: Edward Cullen (Chapter 8), Cleveland Brown (Chapter 9), Lieutenant Commander Data (Chapter 10), Annie Wilkes (Chapter 12), Miss Celie (Chapter 12), and Peter Parker (Chapter 12).

To increase your understanding of diagnostic decision-making with *Anxiety Disorders,* take time now to closely read or reread the intake summary, diagnostic impressions, and diagnostic discussion found in the following case illustrations: Jamal Malik (Chapter 8), Belle (Chapter 9), Jack Bauer (Chapter 10), and Maria (Chapter 11).

It will be helpful to have your copy of the *DSM-IV-TR* available as you study the diagnostic aspects of these case illustrations.

Seven Classes of Disorders With Shared Phenomenological Features

Following the four red flags and the mood and anxiety disorders, the *DSM-IV-TR* presents a series of classes of disorders that are organized by similarity of symptoms, also referred to as shared phenomenology of features (Neukrug & Schwitzer, 2006). The idea is that we first consider whether one or more of the four critical classes found in the red flag best account for the client's presentation; then move on to next consider whether, instead, a mood disorder or anxiety disorder might be the best description; and when these are ruled out or do not fully cover the client's situation, we progress through the various classes that appear next. They include the following classes or chapters:

Somatoform Disorders, which share as a common feature the presence of physical symptoms suggesting a medical condition (a summary is found on *DSM-IV-TR* page 485; two examples are Pain Disorder, featuring physical pain associated with psychological factors, and Hypochondriasis, featuring clinically significant preoccupation with having a disease based on faulty perceptions of one's body).

Factitious Disorders, which are characterized by physical or psychological symptoms that the client intentionally produces (in self or someone under the client's care) or feigns with the specific goal of assuming the "sick patient" role (which is different from malingering and is summarized on *DSM-IV-TR* page 513).

Dissociative Disorders, which feature gradual or sudden, temporary or chronic, disruptions in previously well-functioning consciousness, memory, identity, or perception (the term *dissociation* is defined on *DSM-IV-TR* page 822, and the disorders are summarized on page 519).

Sexual and Gender Identity Disorders, all of which share characteristic disturbances in the area of sexuality (including Sexual Dysfunctions, or disturbances in sexual desire and response causing clinically significant distress or interpersonal difficulties; Paraphilias, whereby the client experiences clinically significant distress or interpersonal difficulties associated with recurrent, intense sexual urges, fantasies, or behaviors involving unusual objects, activities, or situations; Gender Identity Disorders, characterized by strong, persistent, clinically distressing cross-gender identification; and sexual disorders not otherwise specified; see *DSM-IV-TR* page 535 for a summary).

Eating Disorders, all three of which share characteristic disturbances in thoughts, feelings, behaviors, or physiology associated with eating behavior, body perceptions, and weight management (including distress and impairment meeting the criteria for Anorexia Nervosa, Bulimia Nervosa, and Eating Disorders Not Otherwise Specified; see *DSM-IV-TR* page 583 for a summary).

Sleep Disorders, all of which share characteristic disturbances in the area of sleep (including Dyssomnias, which are abnormalities in the amount, quality, timing, or restfulness of sleep, where Insomnia and Hypersomnia are examples; and Parasomnias, which are abnormal behavioral or physiological sleep experiences, where Sleep Terror Disorder and Sleepwalking Disorder are examples; see *DSM-IV-TR* pages 597–598 for a summary).

Impulse-Control Disorders Not Elsewhere Classified, which includes disorders of impulse control not classified as part of any of the disorders in the other *DSM-IV-TR* categories (they include Intermittent Explosive Disorder, Kleptomania, Pyromania, Pathological Gambling, Trichotillomania, which is impulsive and compulsive hair-pulling, and Impulse-Control Disorders Not Otherwise Specified (see *DSM-IV-TR* page 663 for a summary).

SKILL AND LEARNING EXERCISE 4.7

Becoming Familiar With Several Diagnostic Classes of Disorders

Many of these classes of diagnoses are represented in our popular culture caseload. We recommend that you closely read the various chapters in their entirety, and then turn to our case illustrations. Remember that you are gaining an initial familiarity at this point, not detailed expertise.

To increase your understanding of diagnostic decision-making with *Somatoform Disorders,* take time now to closely read or reread the intake summary, diagnostic impressions, and diagnostic discussion found in the case illustration of Elphaba (Chapter 8).

To increase your understanding of diagnostic decision-making with *Sexual and Gender Identity Disorders,* take time now to closely read or reread the intake summary, diagnostic impressions, and diagnostic discussion found in the case illustrations of Cleveland Brown (Chapter 9).

To increase your understanding of diagnostic decision-making with *Eating Disorders,* take time now to closely read or reread the intake summary, diagnostic impressions, and diagnostic discussion found in the case illustration of Claire (Chapter 8).

To increase your understanding of diagnostic decision-making with *Sleep Disorders,* take time now to closely read or reread the intake summary, diagnostic impressions, and diagnostic discussion found in the case illustration of Mario (Chapter 1).

It will be helpful to have your copy of the *DSM-IV-TR* available as you study the diagnostic aspects of these case illustrations.

Adjustment Disorders

After the diagnostic considerations found in the four red flags, frequent categories of mood and anxiety disorders, and other groups of disorders that follow, the *DSM-IV-TR* next presents the Adjustment Disorders. By definition, a diagnosable Adjustment Disorder is a "psychological response to an identifiable stressor or stressors that results in clinically significant emotional or behavioral symptoms" (APA, 2000a, p. 679). A diagnosis of Adjustment Disorder requires that the client's symptoms emerged within 3 months of the onset of the stressor. Further, the person must experience distress related to the life stressor that is beyond normally expected, typical for cultural context, and developmentally appropriate— that is, the person's distress must be clinically significant. Alternatively, reactions we consider to be "normal or expectable" can qualify for the Adjustment Disorder diagnosis when they cause clinically significant impairment in the person's ability to fulfill life roles or cause substantial dysfunction in other areas. Adjustment Disorders may occur With Depressed Mood, With Anxiety, With Mixed Anxiety and Depressed Mood, With Disturbance of Conduct, With Mixed Disturbance of Emotions and Conduct, or Unspecified—indicating which type of psychological symptoms is most prominent.

In addition, the Adjustment Disorder diagnosis is used only when the client's stressor-related concerns do not meet any of the criteria for any of the other Axis I diagnoses, and when the person's stress is not simply an exacerbation of an already-existing Axis I or Axis II problem. This is an important exclusionary criterion because it indicates to us that whenever our client's thoughts, feelings, behaviors, and physiological symptoms are sufficient for one of the red flags, frequently diagnosed classes, or another disorder, we use that diagnosis rather than Adjustment Disorder. In *DSM* language, this is an *exclusionary criterion* and the diagnosis of Adjustment Disorder is a *residual category* (Frances et al., 1995; Munson, 2001). Still, it is a very commonly needed category in many counseling settings and one we all should become experts at using (see *DSM-IV-TR* pages 679–680 for a summary).

CLINICAL SPOTLIGHT 4.2: Suicidal Behavior, Mood Disorders, and Adjustment Disorders

One of the authors (Schwitzer) was on call when he responded late at night to the local hospital to interview a man in his early 20s who was brought by ambulance to the emergency room following a suicide attempt. The man had stabbed himself multiple times in his abdomen at a deserted roadside location, and a driver passing by noticed him and called emergency services in time to save his life.

The young man's distress and suicidal behavior were in direct response to a life stressor: He had been stealing small amounts of money from his employer's cash drawer for several months, adding up to a reasonable sum. The employer had eventually noticed the loss and apprehended the young man; now, his parents and family were about to learn of his small crime, he was losing his job, he was in danger of be dismissed from school, and he faced criminal charges. Facing these pressures, the young man had been depressed for more than 2 weeks, lost all interest in academics and social life, had nearly stopped eating and sleeping, felt worthless and guilty, and ultimately attempted to take his life.

In this case, the client's symptoms clearly were in reaction to a life stressor (although of his own making) and certainly beyond what is normally expectable in such situations; however, because his symptoms met the criteria for a Major Depressive Episode, the appropriate diagnosis was Major Depressive Disorder, Single Episode, rather than Adjustment Disorder (see *DSM-IV-TR* pages 356, 375, and 683 to compare the criteria). Client cases such as these remind us of the intended purpose of moving from red flags, next to frequent mood and anxiety disorders, then to various other Axis I categories, and finally, Adjustment Disorders: It assists us to be sure we adequately describe the person's distress or impairment in order to plan the right type and level of needed treatment. It helps us avoid missing the mark for later treatment planning.

SKILL AND LEARNING EXERCISE 4.8

Becoming Familiar With Adjustment Disorders

The Adjustment Disorders are well-represented in our popular culture caseload. We recommend that you closely read the *DSM* chapter in its entirety, and then turn to our case illustrations. Remember that you are gaining an initial familiarity at this point, not detailed expertise.

  To increase your understanding of diagnostic decision-making with *Adjustment Disorders,* take time now to closely read or reread the intake summary, diagnostic impressions, and diagnostic discussion found in the following case illustrations: George Lopez (Chapter 10), Fred the Baker (Chapter 11), and the Geico Caveman (Chapter 11).

  It will be helpful to have your copy of the *DSM-IV-TR* available as you study the diagnostic aspects of these case illustrations.

Other Conditions That May Be a Focus of Clinical Attention

Axis I is the location in the multiaxial diagnostic system not only for all of the diagnosable psychological disorders (except mental retardation and personality disorders), but also for other client issues, themes, and concerns that will be one of the focuses of counseling. For convenience, the *DSM-IV-TR* text has an additional section in it that presents a wide variety of such issues and themes. Using the text's language, this section and these counseling themes are referred to as *Other Conditions That May Be a Focus of Clinical Attention.* Many counseling professionals think of this category, colloquially, as "other important counseling issues." These also are referred to colloquially as "V-Codes," which has to do with the numerical coding system of the *DSM-IV-TR* and *ICD-10* being a V-Code means the issue is not a diagnosable mental disorder. You are likely to hear this term used in case staffings and supervision.

It is important to remember that although these issues appear right in the *DSM* for our convenience, and although they are recorded on Axis I alongside the diagnosable disorders, these are not diagnosable psychological disorders. Instead, they are important areas to be addressed in counseling conforming to any of the three following situations:

- The problem is the focus of counseling or treatment, but the person is not experiencing any diagnosable mental disorder (e.g., a client seeking consultation about starting a new career, where Occupational Problem or Phase of Life Problem is listed).
- The individual is experiencing a diagnosable psychological disorder, but it is unrelated to or separate from the counseling topic (e.g., a client dealing with a lifelong ADHD who comes in for grief counseling, where Bereavement is listed).
- The client's psychological disorder is related to the counseling issue, but the topic will be an important enough focus of our work to warrant listing separately (e.g., a client who seeks counseling for Obsessive-Compulsive Disorder and also will be addressing the important topic of how her anxiety disorder is leading to marital relationship problems, where both the diagnosable disorder, Obsessive-Compulsive Disorder, and the additional counseling focus, Relational Problem, both are listed).

Counselors in various school, college and university, faith-based, community, private practice, and other outpatient and outclient settings are very likely to use these designations on Axis I along with the diagnosable disorders. Therefore, we recommend that you read the entire section, found on *DSM-IV-TR* pages 731–742, to see what is included.

SKILL AND LEARNING EXERCISE 4.9

Becoming Familiar With Other Conditions That May Be a Focus of Clinical Attention

These "other counseling issues" or "V-Codes" are well-represented in our popular culture caseload. We recommend that you closely read the *DSM* chapter in its entirety, and then turn to our case illustrations. Remember that you are gaining an initial familiarity at this point, not detailed expertise.

To increase your understanding of diagnostic decision-making with this section, take time now to closely read or reread the intake summary, diagnostic impressions, and diagnostic discussion found in the following case illustrations: Juno (Chapter 8), Cleveland Brown (Chapter 9), Waylon Smithers (Chapter 9), Jack Bauer (Chapter 10), George Lopez (Chapter 10), Lieutenant Commander Data (Chapter 10), Maria (Chapter 11), and the Geico Caveman (Chapter 11).

It will be helpful to have your copy of the *DSM-IV-TR* available as you study the diagnostic aspects of these case illustrations.

In sum, from front cover to back cover, the *DSM's* organization is intended to help guide us through the diagnostic decision-making process. The interchapter sequence is summarized in Figure 4.3

INTRACHAPTER ORGANIZATION: WHAT'S INSIDE EACH AXIS I CHAPTER?

We said above that it is important to learn about two aspects of the *DSM* in order to navigate it successfully when making Axis I diagnoses. Now that we have discussed the interchapter organization, we turn to intrachapter organization. In other words, we turn to what is inside each Axis I chapter. This is important because once the counselor has tentatively narrowed his or her diagnostic impressions to the most likely class of disorders (or a few likely classes), the next task is to compare and contrast the various diagnoses found within the class. This requires our familiarity with what is inside each chapter. As a help to clinicians, all of the various *DSM* chapters are organized almost identically. Although there are some differences—for example, the substance-related, mood, and anxiety disorder chapters use a building-block approach, so readers must be careful to distinguish what is a building block and what is a diagnosable disorder

in these chapters—for the most part, once we understand what is inside one of the chapters, we can confidently make our way through all of them.

As a brief summary, you can expect to find the following elements provided for each of the diagnoses in each Axis I chapter: Diagnostic Features; Subtypes and Specifiers; Recording Procedures; Associated Features and Disorders; and Differential Diagnosis. In addition, whenever the information is available from clinical findings or research data, you can also expect to often find the following types of information: Specific Culture, Age, and Gender Features; Prevalence; Course; and Familial Pattern. Finally, the exact Diagnostic Criteria are given again inside a set-aside box.

Diagnostic Features. The *DSM* discussion of each diagnosable disorder in each class, or chapter, of disorders begins with a detailed narrative presenting the disorder's essential features, the criteria to be considered, and other information about client presentations and the clinical picture pertaining to the diagnosis. This diagnostic narrative fully explains inclusionary criteria (exactly what features must be seen in the client's presentation, which feature are essential to the diagnosis, and how many of the various criteria must be met), exclusionary criteria (what conditions would rule out the diagnosis), minimum

Figure 4.3 *DSM-IV-TR* Helpful Axis I Interchapter Organization

Disorders Usually First Diagnosed in Infancy, Childhood, or Adolescence

This class appears at the beginning of the text and the beginning of the life span—there are 10 different categories of these disorders:

Includes Mental Retardation, Learning Disorders, Motor Skills Disorders, Communication Disorders, Pervasive Developmental Disorders, Feeding and Eating Disorders of Infancy and Early Childhood, Tic Disorders, Elimination Disorders, and Other Disorders of Infancy, Childhood, or Adolescence—which usually are seen at the beginning of the life span and, correspondingly, appear at the beginning of the *DSM.* (Note that Mental Retardation is recorded on Axis II.)

Four Red Flags (Neukrug & Schwitzer, 2006)

These four red flags appear first in text after Disorders of Infancy, Childhood, or Adolescence and are to be considered or ruled out early in diagnostic decision-making:

Delirium, Dementia, Amnesia, and Other Cognitive Disorders	Clinical disturbances in consciousness and cognition
Mental Disorders due to a General Medical Condition Not Elsewhere Classified	Psychological symptoms due to medical conditions
Substance-Related Disorders	Psychological symptoms due to substance use
Schizophrenia and Other Psychotic Disorders	Clinical disturbances predominated by psychotic symptoms such as hallucinations, delusions, or disorganized behavior

Two Frequent Outpatient Diagnostic Classes (Seligman, 2004)

These two classes appear immediately following the Four Red Flags and often are considered or ruled out next:

Mood Disorders	Includes all of the commonly diagnosed depressive and bipolar disorders
Anxiety Disorders	Includes all of the commonly diagnosed panic, anxiety, and posttraumatic disorders

Seven Classes Organized by Shared Similarity of Features

These seven classes follow the Red Flags and Frequently Diagnosed Classes in the text, and often, in diagnostic decision-making:

Somatoform Disorder	All pertain to symptoms suggesting a medical condition
Factitious Disorders	All pertain to symptoms produced to assume the sick role
Dissociative Disorders	All pertain to disruptions in consciousness, memory, identity, perception

Sexual and Gender Identity Disorders	All pertain to disruptions in sexual desire, response, behavior, or identity
Eating Disorders	All pertain to disturbances in eating-related behavior
Sleep Disorders	All pertain to disturbances in the behavior and physiology of sleep
Impulse-Control Disorders Not Elsewhere Specified	All pertain to problems involving impulse control not part of another diagnosis
Adjustment Disorders *These are the last Axis I diagnosable disorders to appear:*	
Adjustment Disorders	Clinically significant psychological responses to identifiable stressors
Other Conditions That May Be a Focus of Clinical Attention *These are important presenting concerns that do not indicate the presence of a diagnosable disorder. They appear near the end of the text after all of the diagnosable disorders have been presented:*	

Includes problems with medical conditions and medications, relationship problems, problems of neglect or abuse, and other counseling issues such as Antisocial Behavior, Borderline Intellectual Functioning, Age-Related Cognitive Decline, Bereavement, Academic Problem, Occupational Problem, Identity Problem, Religious or Spiritual Problem, Acculturation Problem, and Phase of Life Problems

duration the client must have experienced symptoms or minimum frequency of the symptoms needed for the diagnosis, symptom severity, and other features of the criteria. As examples, a diagnosis of Major Depressive Disorder requires the presence of five or more symptoms from a list, but among these five, either depressed mood or loss of interest and pleasure must be seen; a diagnosis of Generalized Anxiety Disorder requires a minimum duration of 6 months of symptoms; and a diagnosis of Schizophrenia excludes psychotic symptoms that are due to substance use.

Subtypes and Specifiers. Subtypes and specifiers are used to increase the descriptive power of our diagnoses. *Severity specifiers* are provided whenever the full criteria for a diagnosis are met, to describe the degree to which the client's concerns are causing distress or interfering with

his or her functioning. Generally, a severity specifier of "Mild" indicates the person's symptoms are not in excess of those needed to make a diagnosis; "Moderate" is a midrange indicator; and "Severe" specifies that the person's symptoms are in excess of those needed to make the diagnosis, that some of the symptoms are especially severe, or when the symptoms are especially debilitating. *Course specifiers* are used to describe the course, duration, or pattern over time of the client's concerns. Generally speaking, the course specifier "In Partial Remission" indicates the person previously was experiencing a full set of diagnostic criteria, but currently only some symptoms remain. Similarly, "In Full Remission" is added to indicate that at this time no signs of previously diagnosed disorder remain. For example, when our client has recently experienced a manic episode meeting the criteria for Bipolar I Disorder, but currently is successfully taking medication and experiencing no difficulties, it might be clinically useful to use this specifier to indicate that although the person is currently experiencing no symptoms, his or her previous symptoms are important to note.

Specifiers also are provided inside the narratives for *individual diagnoses.* For example, there are several course specifiers to help describe the situation of a client who was previously diagnosed with Substance Dependence, but who currently is not experiencing the full criteria for this diagnosis. The counselor can add: "Early" or "Sustained" Remission, indicating whether the person has been free of Substance Dependence for less than or longer than 12 months; "Partial" or "Full" Remission, indicating whether or not the person has had some symptoms or not during recovery; Remission "On Agonist Therapy" or "In a Controlled Environment," indicating whether the person has been in recovery with the treatment of an agonist medication like Antabuse, or while being in inpatient treatment or incarcerated, respectively. Counselors can find all of this information within the narrative.

Similarly, *Subtypes* are provided for many *individual diagnoses.* For example, subtypes of Adjustment Disorder are used to indicate whether the disorder is occurring "With Depressed Mood," "With Anxiety," and so on. Likewise, subtypes for the eating disorder diagnosis, Anorexia, include "Restricting Type" (indicating that weight loss is due mainly to not eating) and "Binge-Eating/Purging Type" (indicating that weight loss is due mainly to vomiting, laxative use, or similar means).

Severity, course, and subtype specifiers give the counselor greater ability to describe diagnostically the exact key features an individual is experiencing.

Recording Procedures. Usually two types of recording procedures are given for each diagnosis: one explaining how to record subtypes and specifiers, and one explaining how to record the *DSM-IV-TR/ICD-10* numerical code that goes along with each diagnosis. First, instructions

are given for writing out the subtypes and specifiers. For example, with Major Depressive Disorder, we find that the diagnosis is completed by adding the subtype and then the specifier, as follows:

- Axis I: Major Depressive Disorder, Single Episode, Moderate.

Next, instructions are given for writing out the numerical code, which is a shorthand for the Axis I and Axis II diagnoses. The codes themselves are given with the name of each diagnosis throughout the *DSM-IV-TR* and can be easily found in the text. In the example of Major Depression, adding the numerical codes would result in the following Axis I diagnosis:

- Axis I: 296.22 Major Depressive Disorder, Single Episode, Moderate.

Associated Features. Once the main diagnostic features have been explained and the instructions provided for recording the diagnosis, next the *DSM* provides information about associated features. These are clinical features that are not really criteria for a particular psychological disorder, but are known to frequently occur in association with the disorder. For example, this section tells us that for a severe eating disorder such as Anorexia, additional features might occur, including depressed mood, social withdrawal, or irritability. Knowing this information can help us more confidently and accurately evaluate and describe the client's presentation and needs. Although this information is valuable, associated features are not actually part of the diagnostic criteria for the disorder with which they are associated.

Other Information When It Is Known. Whenever it is available, the *DSM-IV-TR* provides special subheadings and narrative information explaining factors such as *Specific Culture Features, Specific Gender Features, Familial Patterns, Course,* or *Prevalence.* This information can be critical to making reliable, accurate diagnoses. For example, the *DSM-IV-TR* tells us that when considering the diagnosis of Psychotic Disorder, one Specific Culture Feature is that some religious ceremonies among certain cultures involve hearing voices, and these experiences should not be considered when making the diagnosis. Similarly, the *DSM-IV-TR* tells us in its narrative for Schizophrenia that this disorder may be over-diagnosed when working with some ethnic groups. Such information appears for many but not all disorders.

Differential Diagnoses. This subheaded section provides guidance that is critical to our diagnostic decision-making. Counseling professionals should carefully review differential diagnosis information during every diagnostic decision-making situation. Differential diagnoses are competing or alternative disorders the clinician should consider before settling on a final diagnosis. Differential diagnoses appear for every Axis I disorder and help us avoid overlooking various psychological disorders our client might be presenting. For example, when diagnosing Posttraumatic Stress Disorder, we are encouraged in the text to alternatively consider Adjustment Disorder, various other anxiety disorders, and sometimes, Malingering. Often, we are again reminded of differential diagnoses in the set-off criteria box for the diagnosis.

Diagnostic Criteria. Once we have moved through all of the narrative material described above, we reach the set-off box presenting a straightforward listing of all of the exact criteria for the diagnosis under consideration. Although certainly it is tempting to rush right to the criteria list, our view is that it is critical to explore all of the important diagnostic information found in the narrative that precedes the criteria list, in order to better understand the disorder's features, associated features, subtypes and specifiers, differential diagnoses, recording procedures—and whatever other cultural, age, gender, prevalence, course, or familial pattern information is available.

Figure 4.4 *DSM-IV-TR* Helpful Intrachapter Organization

What's Inside Each Chapter?

Diagnostic Features

Subtypes and Specifiers

Recording Procedures

Associated Features

Specific Culture, Age, Gender, Prevalence, Course, and/or Familial

Pattern Information

Differential Diagnoses

Diagnostic Criteria

A CLOSER LOOK AT AXIS II: MENTAL RETARDATION AND PERSONALITY DISORDERS

Axis II is used to record two types of diagnosable psychological disorders found in the *DSM-IV-TR:* Mental Retardation and the Personality Disorders. On Axis II, counseling professionals answer the questions:

"Does the client evidence any long-term pattern of maladaptive [personality] traits that cause significant impairment or distress?," "Does the client have [signs and symptoms that] meet criteria for any of the [personality disorders specified in the *DSM-IV-TR*]?," and "Is there evidence of mental retardation [or borderline intellectual functioning]?" (La Bruzza & Mendez-Villarrubia, 1994, p. 86)

Simply stated, the purpose of having a separate axis for these conditions is to encourage clinicians to evaluate for them. Recording these separately from the Axis I diagnoses "ensures that consideration will be given to the possible presence of Personality Disorders and Mental Retardation that might be otherwise overlooked" (APA, 2000a, p. 28) because often our attention mostly is directed to the client's immediate, more pressing, and more attention-grabbing presenting concerns characterizing an Axis I disorder rather than the Axis II concerns, which are longer-standing, sometimes underlying, and sometimes more subtle in their appearance.

Axis II also is the location in the multiaxial diagnosis for recording two types of conditions that are not diagnosable psychological disorders: Borderline Intellectual Functioning, and personality disorder features.

Mental Retardation

Mental Retardation is the very first diagnosable psychological disorder presented in the *DSM-IV-TR* and is found in the class of Disorders Usually First Diagnosed in Infancy, Childhood, or Adolescence. As with all of the other Axis I disorders, the narrative for Mental Retardation gives diagnostic features; associated features and disorders; specific culture, age, and gender features; prevalence, course, and familial patterns; and differential diagnoses. Essential features of Mental Retardation are significantly below-average intellectual functioning, along with impairment in areas of daily functioning. Evaluation for Mental Retardation requires administration of psychological test of intellectual functioning; that is, the diagnosis is based partly on IQ scores (in the case of infants who are too young for testing, clinical judgment is used), and assessment of the client's psychosocial functioning (typically reported by someone close to him or her).

The specific criteria for Mental Retardation are as follows (APA, 2000a): (a) significantly subaverage intellectual functioning, demonstrated by an IQ score of about 70 or lower on a professionally administered intelligence test; (b) deficits or impairments in everyday adaptive functioning in at least two areas, such as self-care, home living, social skills, academic skills, work, leisure, health, or safety; and (c) onset before age 18 years. Note that beyond low IQ scores, deficits in functioning are required for the diagnosis. The diagnosis "Mental Retardation" is recorded on Axis II, along with a specifier indicating whether the degree of intellectual difficulty is Mild, Moderate, Severe, Profound, or Unspecified—depending on the IQ score obtained when measuring the person's intellectual function. Mental Retardation is more fully explain on *DSM-IV-TR* pages 41–49.

Like the Learning Disorders and other disorders of childhood, child therapists, family clinicians, school counselors, and others who work extensively with individuals under age 18 years often rely heavily on the diagnosis of Mental Retardation. Of particular note, school counselors, school psychologists, and their clinical colleagues with child and adolescent caseloads often find Mental Retardation to be especially important to their diagnostic work.

SKILL AND LEARNING EXERCISE 4.10

Becoming Familiar With Mental Retardation

The diagnosis of Mental Retardation is represented in our popular culture caseload. We recommend that you closely read the *DSM* section in its entirety, and then turn to our case illustration. Remember that you are gaining an initial familiarity at this point, not detailed expertise.

To increase your understanding of diagnostic decision-making with this section, take time now to closely read or reread the intake summary, diagnostic impressions, and diagnostic discussion found in our unique take on the case of Eleanor Rigby (Chapter 11). It will be helpful to have your copy of the *DSM-IV-TR* available as you study the diagnostic aspects of this case illustration.

Personality Disorders

Personality consists of "habitual and predictable patterns of human behavior, thinking, and feeling" that are believed to result from a combination of physiological influences and psychosocial developmental influences; generally speaking, it is expected that personality undergoes a more flexible formation phase earlier in our lives, and then as we reach adolescence, early adulthood, and adulthood, our unique predictable personality pattern firms up (American Counseling Association, 2009, p. 398). When an individual's personality patterns lead to clinically significant difficulties, a Personality Disorder may be diagnosed. More specifically, a Personality Disorder comprises:

> an enduring pattern of inner experience and behavior that deviates markedly from the expectations of the individual's culture, is pervasive and inflexible, has an onset in adolescence or early adulthood, is stable over time, and leads to distress or impairment. (APA, 2000a, p. 685)

Note that as with other diagnosable mental disorders, the *DSM-IV-TR* diagnostic symptom includes only those personality difficulties that are outside what is normally expectable given the person's life context, appropriate for the person's developmental context, or acceptable given the person's cultural context. Further, diagnosable difficulties must cause clinically significant impairments in the person's intrapersonal or interpersonal life. In addition, by definition, these patterns must be long-term ones that emerge in adolescence and early adulthood and persevere through the life span, not just during times of stress or crisis.

Each diagnosis requires disruptions in cognition (ways of perceiving, thinking about, and interpreting self, others, or events), affect (range, intensity, and appropriateness of emotions), interpersonal relationship behavior, and control of impulses. Each diagnosis is made only when the pattern is not better accounted for by another diagnosable mental disorder, and when the pattern is not due to the physiological effects of substance use or a medical problem. The *DSM-IV-TR* contains 11 different diagnosable personality disorders. They

all appear together in one chapter, near the end of the diagnostic text, after all of the Axis I disorders have been presented. You can find them summarized on *DSM-IV-TR* pages 685–690.

For our convenience—to help us work our way through this class of diagnoses—the personality disorders are divided up in the *DSM-IV-TR* into three categories based on descriptive similarities among the personality disorder diagnoses. The *DSM* text calls these categories *Clusters*. In addition, there is one category for patterns that do not fall into any of the ones described. The diagnosable personality disorders are as follows:

Cluster A: Odd and Eccentric Patterns. Three specific personality disorders are in this category: Paranoid, Schizoid, and Schizotypal. The characteristic they share is that clients presenting these disorders often appear odd or eccentric.

Paranoid Personality Disorder is characterized by a long-term, maladaptive, inflexible pattern of distrust and suspiciousness. Clients presenting this disorder interpret others' motives to be malevolent.

Schizoid Personality Disorder is characterized by a long-term, maladaptive, inflexible pattern of detachment from social relationships, along with significantly restricted range of emotional expression.

Schizotypal Personality Disorder is characterized by a long-term, maladaptive, inflexible pattern of severe discomfort in close personal relationships, along with acute restriction in emotional expression.

Cluster B: Dramatic, Emotional, Erratic Patterns. The four personality disorders in this category are Antisocial, Borderline, Histrionic, and Narcissistic. The characteristic they share is that individuals experiencing these disorders often appear dramatic, emotional, or erratic in their behaviors, reactions, and relationships.

Antisocial Personality Disorder is characterized by a long-term, maladaptive, inflexible pattern of clinically significant and diagnosable disregard for, and violation, of the rights of others.

Borderline Personality Disorder is characterized by a long-term, maladaptive, inflexible pattern of unstable interpersonal relationships, unstable self-image, unstable emotional reactions, and problematic impulsiveness.

Histrionic Personality Disorder is characterized by a long-term, maladaptive, inflexible pattern of excessive emotional reaction and affective expression, and excessive attention-seeking across situations.

Narcissistic Personality Disorder is characterized by a long-term, maladaptive, inflexible pattern of grandiose self-image, need for admiration from others, and poor empathy for the situation or experiences of others.

Cluster C: Anxious and Fearful Patterns. The three personality disorders in this category are Avoidant, Dependent, and Obsessive-Compulsive. The characteristic they share is that persons dealing with these disorders often appear anxious, inhibited, or fearful.

Avoidant Personality Disorder is characterized by a long-term, maladaptive, inflexible pattern of social inhibition, feelings of being inadequate, and severe hypersensitivity to negative evaluations and reactions from others.

Dependent Personality Disorder is characterized by a long-term, maladaptive, inflexible pattern of overly submissive and problematically clinging behavior that is related to an excessive need to be taken care of in life by others.

Obsessive-Compulsive Personality Disorder is characterized by a long-term, maladaptive, inflexible pattern of being excessively preoccupied with orderliness, perfectionism, and control.

Personality Disorder Not Otherwise Specified. Along with the 10 specific disorders outlined above, the *DSM-IV-TR* provides one additional Axis II personality disorder diagnosis: Personality Disorder Not Otherwise Specified (NOS). This diagnosis is used when the client presents a disorder pertaining to personality functioning that does not meet the criteria of any other personality disorder. The person might have symptoms of several different personality disorders with do not fully meet any one criteria list, but together cause clinically significant distress and/or impairment. The person sometimes may exhibit a diagnosable personality pattern that is not captured by the ones described.

SKILL AND LEARNING EXERCISE 4.11

Becoming Familiar With Personality Disorders

The Personality Disorders are represented in our popular culture caseload. We recommend that you closely read the *DSM* chapter in its entirety, and then turn to our case illustrations. Remember that you are gaining an initial familiarity at this point, not detailed expertise.

To increase your understanding of diagnostic decision-making with this section, take time now to closely read or reread the intake summary, diagnostic impressions, and diagnostic discussion found in our unique take on two cases: Miss Piggy (Chapter 1) and Annie Wilkes (Chapter 12). It will be helpful to have your copy of the *DSM-IV-TR* available as you study the diagnostic aspects of these case illustrations.

Nondiagnosable Conditions on Axis II

Also recorded on Axis II are two types of nondiagnosable conditions that are associated with diagnosable Mental Retardation and Personality Disorders. They both are enduring life patterns that sometimes are clinically valuable to identify in our diagnostic impressions, but neither is a coded, diagnosable mental disorder.

Borderline Intellectual Functioning. Borderline Intellectual Functioning is found in the section of *DSM-IV-TR,* Other Conditions That May Be a Focus of Clinical Attention, and is defined by measured intellectual functioning reflected in an IQ score falling between 71–84, which is below average but above the threshold for a diagnosis of Mental Retardation. When one focus of the counseling relationship is to assist the client with the effects of borderline intellectual functioning, or when it may be clinically important to current or future counselors, this information is recorded on Axis II.

Personality Disorder Features. Axis II also may be used to record personality features that are prominent and maladaptive for the person but do not meet the full criteria of a personality disorder diagnosis. When one focus of the counseling relationship is to assist the person with the effects of maladaptive personality features, or when it might be clinically useful to the person's current or future counselors, these features are recorded on Axis II.

SKILL AND LEARNING EXERCISE 4.12

Becoming Familiar With Personality Features Recorded on Axis II

The diagnostic practice of recording personality disorder features on Axis II is well-represented in our popular culture caseload. We recommend that you closely read the *DSM* chapter in its entirety, and then turn to our case illustrations. Remember that you are gaining an initial familiarity at this point, not detailed expertise.

To increase your understanding of diagnostic decision-making with this section, take time now to closely read or reread the intake summary, diagnostic impressions, and diagnostic discussion found in the following case illustrations: Elphaba (Chapter 8), Tinkerbell (Chapter 9), The Beast's Belle (Chapter 9), Jack McFarland (Chapter 10), and Annie Wilkes (Chapter 12). It will be helpful to have your copy of the *DSM-IV-TR* available as you study the diagnostic aspects of these case illustrations.

A CLOSER LOOK AT AXIS III: GENERAL MEDICAL CONDITIONS

Once we have prepared Axes I and II, we turn to the remaining three axes. Among these, Axis III provides us an opportunity to list medical problems, physical complaints, and medication needs that are relevant to our client's counseling and psychological concerns. The medical situations we note on Axis III may be directly etiological to (i.e., contributing to or causing) the person's psychological concerns, or there may be another important relationship between the client's physical health problems and mental health concerns. Some examples include hypothyroidism causing a depressive disorder (illustrated in our text by the case of Eleanor Rigby), the stressful effects of having asthma on a client's adjustment, the threatening presence of hypertension (high blood pressure) in a client's medical history, or the presence of HIV infection when relevant to counseling concerns. In addition to information about physical and medical problems, Axis III also is where we can record any prescribed medications the client is taking when those medications are clinically relevant or may have psychological or psychiatric side effects. It is on Axis III that the clinician answers the questions:

"Are there any physical signs and symptoms present?," "Does the client have a documented history of any [relevant] injuries or medical disorders?," and "Could a general medical condition be causing the clinical problem noted on Axis I?" (LaBruzza & Mendez-Villarrubia, 1994, pp. 86–87)

Mental health professionals working in hospital, medical, inpatient, psychiatric, or other clinically oriented settings may be required to provide formal general medical condition

Figure 4.5   *DSM-IV-TR* Axis II Records

Mental Retardation

This diagnosable mental disorder appears in the Disorders Usually First Diagnosed in Infancy, Childhood, or Adolescence

Mild Mental Retardation	IQ level 50–55 to approximately 70 with deficits in adaptive functioning
Moderate Mental Retardation	IQ level 35–40 to 50–55 with deficits in adaptive functioning
Severe Mental Retardation	IQ level 20–25 to 35–40 with deficits in adaptive functioning
Profound Mental Retardation	IQ level below 20 or 25 with deficits in adaptive functioning

Personality Disorders

These diagnosable psychological disorders are enduring patterns traced back at least to adolescence or early adulthood

Cluster A: Odd or Eccentric	Paranoid, Schizoid, Schizotypal Personality Disorders
Cluster B: Dramatic or Erratic	Antisocial, Borderline, Histrionic, Narcissistic Personality Disorders
Cluster C: Anxious or Fearful	Avoidant, Dependent, Obsessive-Compulsive Personality Disorders

Personality Disorder Not Otherwise Specified (NOS)

Nondiagnosable Conditions on Axis II

Borderline Intellectual Functioning	IQ level between 70–84 with deficits in adaptive functioning found in Other Conditions That May Be a Focus of Clinical Attention
Personality Disorder Features	Maladaptive personality features or defenses not meeting diagnosis threshold

diagnoses on Axis III. Formal medical diagnoses are accompanied by the appropriate *ICD-10-CM* code and are formally presented. For example, formal Axis III records for a client currently experiencing a problem with an HIV infection, and another client dealing with asthma might read as follows (Neukrug & Schwitzer, 2006, pp. 181–182):

Axis III: 042 HIV infection, causing specified acute infections

and

Axis III: 493.20 Asthma, chronic obstruction

A helpful list of many of the most common general medical conditions and their *ICD* codes are provided in Appendix G of the *DSM-IV-TR*.

Conversely, it is likely that most counseling professionals working in typical outclient and outpatient settings can record acceptable information on Axis III using less formal notations, provided they are written professionally and accurately. For example, many of us in typical counseling settings would note our clients with HIV infection and asthma as follows:

Axis III: HIV-positive, causing infections

and

Axis III: Asthma

SKILL AND LEARNING EXERCISE 4.13

Becoming Familiar With Axis III General Medical Conditions

Several of the clients in our popular culture caseload present medical conditions relevant to their counseling concerns. We recommend that you closely read the *DSM* instructional section found on pages 29–30, and then turn to a few of our case illustrations. Remember that you are gaining an initial familiarity at this point, not detailed expertise.

To increase your understanding of diagnostic recordings on Axis III, take time now to closely read or reread the intake summaries, diagnostic impressions, and diagnostic discussions for Gretel (Chapter 7), Naruto (Chapter 7), Elphaba (Chapter 8), Cleveland Brown (Chapter 9), and Eleanor Rigby (Chapter 11)—and then answer the following questions:

Why was it clinically important to note Gretel's Juvenile Diabetes on Axis III? Why was it clinically relevant to record Naruto's sprained ankle on Axis III? Why was it clinically important to list Elphaba's *Emeraldia Pigmentosa (sic)* on Axis III? Why might it have been clinically relevant to list Cleveland Brown's borderline hypertension on Axis III? Why was it essential to record Eleanor Rigby's hypothyroid condition on Axis III?

What types of medical conditions do you think your own future clients are most likely to present?

A CLOSER LOOK AT AXIS IV: PSYCHOSOCIAL AND ENVIRONMENTAL PROBLEMS

Next in the multiaxial system, Axis IV provides us opportunity to list psychosocial problems and problems and conditions pertaining to the social environment that might have an impact on our client's counseling concerns, especially as they affect the Axis I diagnoses we have identified. Often these problems have an effect on how we conceptualize and plan for treatment, and the prognosis for positive counseling outcomes. It is on Axis IV that the counselor answers the questions:

"What psychosocial or environmental problem is the client facing?," "What stressors are currently taxing the client's ability to cope?," "How is the client meeting such basic needs as survival, food, shelter, clothing, safety, education, employment, friendship, affection, social interaction, and self-esteem?," and "What is the client's social support system and how well is it functioning?" (LaBruzza & Mendez-Villarrubia, 1994, p. 87)

Answering these questions, some of the stressors commonly recorded on Axis IV are losses; positive and negative life events, transitions, and changes; emotionally significant events; and anniversaries of emotionally significant events (LaBruzza & Mendez-Villarrubia, 1994). Some of the frequently recorded psychosocial and environmental difficulties are living in poverty, experiencing parental neglect or abuse, dealing with divorce, being incarcerated, or surviving traumas (Seligman, 2004). The *DSM-IV-TR* identifies several categories of common Axis IV problems. These are outlined in the *DSM* on pages 31–32 and include:

- Problems with primary support group
- Problems related to the social environment
- Educational problems
- Occupational problems
- Housing problems
- Economic problems
- Problems with access to health care services
- Problems related to crime or the legal system
- Other sorts of psychosocial and environmental problems

As a technical matter, counseling professionals most often record items on Axis IV by either listing a category and then the specific problem or by just listing the problem itself in a careful, professional manner. The following are examples of Axis IV records using both a category and a specific problem (Neukrug & Schwitzer, 2004, p. 183):

Axis IV: Problems with primary support group—disruption of family by divorce

and

Axis IV: Housing problems—unsafe neighborhood

Alternatively, the following illustrates the same records citing only the problem itself without a category:

Axis IV: Disruption of family by parents' divorce

and

Axis IV: Unsafe neighborhood

Axis IV, like Axis III, adds additional important information, when relevant, to our description of the client's experiences and life situation.

SKILL AND LEARNING EXERCISE 4.14

Becoming Familiar With Axis IV Psychosocial and Environmental Problems

Many clients in our popular culture caseload present psychosocial and environmental problems relevant to their counseling concerns. We recommend that you closely read the *DSM* instructional section found on pages 31–32, and then turn to our 30 case illustrations. Remember that you are gaining an initial familiarity at this point, not detailed expertise.

To increase your understanding of diagnostic recordings on Axis IV, take time now to briefly read or quickly reread the intake summaries and diagnostic impressions for as many cases as you can—and then answer the following questions:

What are some of most common or most important psychosocial problems found among our 30 client illustrations? What are some of the most common or most important environmental problems found among our 30 clients? Are they problems with the clients' primary support group? Educational or occupational problems? Housing, economic, or health care access problems? Crime and incarceration problems? Others?

What types of psychosocial and environmental problems do you think your own future clients are most likely to present?

A CLOSER LOOK AT AXIS V: GLOBAL ASSESSMENT OF FUNCTIONING

The fifth axis in the multiaxial system requires us to use our clinical judgment to estimate overall client functioning using a psychometric scale: the Global Assessment of Functioning, or GAF. The GAF scale is taken directly from the *DSM-IV-TR;* it is found on page 34, and instructions

for its use are printed on pages 32–33. On Axis V, counseling professionals are expected to answer the following questions:

"How well is the client currently functioning in the psychological, social, and occupational [or academic] aspects of his or her life?," "How severe are the [person's] current symptoms?" and "What score would the [client's functioning] receive on the GAF scale?" (LaBruzza & Mendez-Villarubia, 1994, p. 87)

GAF Scores

As we have mentioned previously, the GAF ranges from a high of 100 to a low of 1. Higher scores reflect better functioning and less distress, whereas the lowest scores characterize clients with severe symptoms, prominent distress, and very poor functioning. Scores in the very high range of 80 and above suggest excellent functioning and the absence of distress, whereas scores in the 70–80 range suggest the presence of minimal, transient symptoms or impairments that probably are expectable reactions to normal life stressors. Scores in the ranges from 50–70 indicate mild to moderate symptoms, with mild to moderate distressful mood and mild to moderate difficulties filling expected occupational, academic, family, or other roles. Scores in the lower ranges of 30–50 indicate progressively more serious difficulties with mood and anxiety, more serious impairment, and more need for immediate responses. At the lowest ranges, below 30, symptoms, distress, and impairment are severe, and often the client's life may be in danger.

Interestingly, the GAF score is intended to be a one-score estimate of overall functioning, as well as both *distress* (i.e., depressive mood, anxiety and panic, and other affective reactions) and *impairment* (i.e., level of success or interference with the performance of important life roles at home and school, in the family and intimate relationships, and elsewhere). To assist you in making an accurate estimate with the GAF, for each range of scores, a description of distress level is provided ("mild symptoms," "moderate symptoms," "some danger," "persistent danger," etc.); a description of impairment level is provided ("some difficulty with social functioning," "major impairment in several areas, such as work or school," "inability to function in almost all areas," etc.); examples of the corresponding distress level are provided ("difficulty concentrating after a family argument," "occasional panic attacks," "suicidal attempts," etc.); and examples of impaired behaviors corresponding to the scores are provided ("few friends, conflicts with peers," "unable to work," etc.).

As you might imagine, Axis V is useful only when there is there is good interrater agreement about what GAF scores match a particular client's clinical presentation. This means that to be successful using Axis V, you must develop expert proficiency at estimating client GAF scores in a similar way to most other peers and colleagues. This will take practice and an accumulation of experience with a wide range of client situations. Practice and consultation with the GAF will be one important topic for you during counseling supervision and case staffing meetings as you begin to develop your diagnostic skills.

SKILL AND LEARNING EXERCISE 4.15

Becoming Familiar With Axis V Global Assessment of Functioning

GAF scores are provided on Axis V on the diagnostic impressions for every client in our text's popular culture caseload. We recommend that you closely read the *DSM* instructional section found on pages 32–34, and then turn to our 30 case illustrations. Remember that you are gaining an initial familiarity at this point, not detailed expertise.

To increase your understanding of the GAF on Axis V, take time now to briefly read or quickly reread the intake summaries, diagnostic impressions, and diagnostic discussions for as many cases as you can—and then complete the following:

Find one or more case examples with GAF scores estimated in the high ranges, above 70. How do the scores for these well-functioning clients fit together with their presenting concerns, reasons for counseling, life situations, and current and past history? What does the diagnostic discussion for the case tell you about the counselor's decision-making on Axis V? Do you agree with the GAF estimated for this client, and why or why not?

(Continued)

(Continued)

Find several different case examples with GAF scores estimated in the middle ranges, from 50–70. Compare and contrast the different scores and the different client situations. What commonalities, themes, or differences do you notice that help distinguish the GAF scores? How do the scores for these clients, with symptoms varying from mild to moderate to serious, compare with one another according to their presenting concerns, reasons for counseling, life situations, and current and past history? What do the diagnostic discussions for each case tell you about the counselor's decision-making on Axis V? Do you agree with the GAF estimated for these clients, and why or why not?

Find one or more case examples with a GAF score estimated in the low and very low ranges, below 50. How do the scores for these clients with serious, impaired, or dangerous functioning fit together with their presenting concerns, reasons for counseling, life situations, and current and past history? What does the diagnostic discussion for each case tell you about the counselor's decision-making on Axis V? Do you agree with the GAF estimated for this client, and why or why not?

What range of GAF scores do you think your own future clients are likely to present most frequently?

PULLING IT ALL TOGETHER: DERIVING A MULTIAXIAL DIAGNOSIS

Read through a few of the "Discussion of Diagnostic Impressions" sections for any of the 30 popular culture cases in Part III of our text. In each discussion, you will find brief, start-to-finish examples of how the counseling professional pulls together all of his or her diagnostic skills to derive a multiaxial diagnosis. Certainly, the first step in the learning process is to become familiar with the basics: what the *DSM* system is and is not; what it does and does not do; what is covered and what is not covered; and how each of the five axes operates. For students, trainees, and beginning counseling professionals, this is the starting point! However, the next step is to begin pulling it all together and practicing diagnostic decision-making.

Determining Axis I and Axis II Diagnoses

By far, most mental health diagnostic action takes place on Axis I and II. This is where most of our concentration, attention, focus, knowledge, and skill are needed. As we have discussed, the *DSM's* limited scope, and the *DSM's* inter-chapter organization, should assist us.

Ruling Out. Most of the diagnoses found in the *DSM-IV-TR* have "rule-out-oriented" diagnostic criteria, which the system calls "exclusionary criteria" (Munson, 2001, p. 79). As we discussed earlier, usually our initial job is to rule out—or decide against—the presence of Delirium, Dementia, Amnestic, or Other Cognitive Disorders with biological etiologies; the existence of Schizophrenia or Other Psychotic Disorders; or the presence of either substance use or a medical condition that is causing the client's symptoms of a psychological disorder. We carefully "rule out" normally expectable reactions, cultural influences, and age-appropriate developmental behaviors. We also identify, and rule out from the mental disorder diagnosis, other conditions that might be causing psychological problems—such as relational problems, identity and phase of life problems, academic and occupational concerns, and neglect or physical or sexual abuse of children or others under the guardianship of another person (Munson, 2001).

Differential Diagnoses. We then move from ruling out various conditions to considering differential diagnoses. Differential diagnosis refers to differentiating one diagnosis from other disorders that have some similar presenting characteristic (APA, 2000a; Munson, 2001).

Earlier in this chapter, we recommended: first considering whether a mood disorder or anxiety disorder might be present, by attempting to match the client's data with the various depressive disorders and bipolar disorders and different anxiety disorders (panic and agoraphobia, phobias, posttraumatic stress and acute stress, obsessive-compulsive, generalized anxiety, etc.); next considering whether the client's presentation shares similarities with any of the various classes of disorders organized by area of the psychological disturbance (somatoform, dissociative, sexual and gender identity, eating, sleep, or impulse-control); and then, if none of these is a good match, or does not sufficiently capture all of the person's concerns, consider Adjustment Disorders.

Once we have identified the likely classes of disorders, we then look inside the relevant *DSM-IV-TR* chapter and use our ruling-out process and differentiation to make a closer decision about which specific disorder (if any) within the diagnostic class best matches the client's exact symptoms. For example, after we have determined our client is experiencing prominent anxiety symptoms, next we might try to match his or her recent life experiences with the diagnostic definition of a traumatic event and match his or her symptoms with the avoidance and re-experiencing symptoms of posttrauma reactions—and then differentiate further by determining that the event occurring within the past month and that the client's symptoms are mostly dissociative. On this basis, we have used a decision-making process based on *ruling out* and *differentiation* to reach a diagnosis of Acute Stress Disorder (at this point, you might want to review *DSM-IV-TR* pages 463–472 for a better picture of this Anxiety Disorder illustration).

Differential diagnosis also occurs *between* the classes of disorders. In our Acute Stress Disorder example, two additional important considerations were whether the life experience to which the person reacted met the criteria for a traumatic event, or whether it was instead a nontrauma stressful event—and whether the person's anxiety reactions were moderate or more severe. This matters to us as diagnosticians because if the event was nontraumatic but stressful, and if the

person's anxiety reactions were moderate and did not meet the criteria for posttrauma behavior, then, based on our ruling-out and differentiating process, we probably would conclude that the client was dealing with an Adjustment Disorder rather than Acute Stress Disorder. Here, it was important to understand differential diagnosis between classes of disorders (Anxiety Disorders vs. Adjustment Disorders) and within a class of disorders (PTSD vs. Acute Stress Disorder) (at this point, you might want to review *DSM-IV-TR* pages 679–683 for a better picture of this Adjustment Disorder vs. Acute Stress Disorder illustration).

The *DSM-IV-TR* provides rule-out, or exclusionary, criteria inside each diagnosis criteria set when relevant, and the text provides differential diagnosis information in every diagnosis narrative. In addition, on pages 746–757, *DSM-IV-TR* provides you with six decision trees to help you think through your ruling-out and differentiation decisions. We believe you may find the decision trees for Substance-Induced Disorders, Mood Disorders, and Anxiety Disorders to be especially helpful as you get started with mental health diagnosis. As we mentioned, we provide discussions of this sort of differential diagnosis for all 30 of our case illustrations.

More Than One Diagnosis. As you will see in many of our popular culture examples, often a client is experiencing more than one diagnosable Axis I psychological disorder, more than one Axis II disorder, both an Axis I and Axis II disorder, more than one nondiagnosable condition or focus of counseling on Axis I and/or Axis II, or a combination of multiple entries. When a person presents more than one Axis I disorder, all of these diagnoses should be recorded, with the principal or most pressing diagnosis, or main reason for the visit, listed first. When the person presents both an Axis I and an Axis II disorder, it is assumed that the Axis I condition is the primary reason for the visit, so if the Axis II diagnosis is the reason for the visit we are expected to write "Principal Diagnosis" or "Reason for Visit" following the Axis II diagnosis. For example:

Axis I: Alcohol Abuse

Axis II: Borderline Personality Disorder (Principal Diagnosis)

On each axis, diagnosable disorders are listed first, followed by nondiagnosable other conditions. For example:

Axis I: Alcohol Abuse

Occupational Problem

Partner Relational Problem

Indicating Uncertainty. Naturally, we cannot always be certain of our diagnostic impressions. When we believe a diagnosis will be needed to describe the client's needs, but we are currently uncertain about the diagnosis, we have several options. These are outlined on the *DSM-IV*-TR pages 4–5 and 743. We believe you will find three of these options most commonly used. The first option is to record our best estimated diagnosis, followed by the indicator "Provisional Diagnosis." This communicates that we have a diagnosis in mind, but believe we need further data to make a conclusion decision. For example:

Axis I: 298.9 Brief Psychotic Disorder With Marked Stressors (Provisional Diagnosis)

The second common option is to defer recording a diagnosis until a later time, such as:

Axis I: 799.9 Diagnosis or Condition Deferred on Axis I

The third common strategy is to use the category "Not Otherwise Specified." This indicates we have enough client information to narrow down the class of the disorder we believe the person is experiencing, but insufficient data to make a specific diagnosis because the client's presentation does not meet the criteria for any of the exact diagnoses within the class of diagnoses. For example:

Axis II: 301.9 Personality Disorder Not Otherwise Specified (NOS)

No Diagnosis. Finally on Axis I and Axis II, when no diagnosis at all, and no nondiagnosable other conditions at all, are to be recorded, we indicate No Diagnosis, as in the following examples:

Axis I: 309.0 Adjustment Disorder With Depressed Mood

Axis II: V71.09 No Diagnosis on Axis II

and

Axis I: V71.09 No Diagnosis or Condition on Axis I

Axis II: 318 Moderate Mental Retardation

Determining Axis III and Axis IV Diagnoses

The General Medical Conditions we record on Axis III and the Psychosocial and Environmental Problems we list on Axis IV should round out the information communicated on Axes I and II. The Axis III entries we decide to include should be coexisting medical conditions or physical problems that either are associated with the psychological disorders and conditions we recorded on Axes I and II, or if they are independent of the Axis I and Axis II diagnoses, are related to its course and treatment (Munson, 2001). The Axis IV entries we decide to include should be those psychosocial and environmental problems that have an influence on the "diagnosis, treatment, and prognosis" of the mental disorders and conditions we recorded on Axis I and Axis II (Munson, 2001, p. 73). You can review the Diagnostic Impressions and Discussion of Diagnostic Impressions for any of our case illustrations to see how the information on these axes is intended to be related to—and augment or amplify—what we know about our client based on our Axis I and Axis II information.

Determining Axis V

The GAF score we record on Axis V provides a rough estimate of a person's current overall level of functioning, and therefore the GAF we indicate should be a good fit with the diagnoses and conditions we recorded on Axes I and II. In other words, all else being equal, a modest concern on Axis I, such as a Religious or Spiritual Concern, usually is a fit with a higher GAF score in the upper ranges of some mild symptoms, transient and expectable reactions, or good functioning—whereas a more severe mental disorder on Axis I, such as Schizophrenia, usually is a fit with a lower GAF score in the moderately low and low ranges of serious symptoms, serious impairment, or danger. There should be a natural relationship between the diagnoses on the main axes and our estimate of overall functioning on Axis V.

In addition, the rating assigned to our client's functioning should be based on our estimate at the time of the evaluation, and indicated by listing the time frame in parentheses after recording the score. For example:

Axis V: GAF = 60 (at intake)

and

Axis V: GAF = 45 (at admission)

Alternatively, multiple ratings at different times can be listed when appropriate to provide further descriptive information about the client's experience. For example:

Axis V: GAF = 68 (at intake)
        GAF = 80 (at termination)
and
Axis V: GAF = 55 (at intake)
        GAF = 75 (highest in past year)

You can review the Diagnostic Impressions and Discussion of Diagnostic Impressions for any of our case illustrations to see how the GAF scores on Axis V should relate to what we know about our client based on our Axis I and Axis II information, and at specific points in time.

SKILL AND LEARNING EXERCISE 4.16

Seeing How Multiaxial Diagnoses Are Pulled Together

Refer to the cases of Juno and Claire (Chapter 8, Troubled Youth in Film and Stage), George Lopez (Chapter 10, Adults in Television Sitcoms and Drama), Fred the Baker (Chapter 11, Characters in Music, Musicals, and Advertising), Chief Bromden and Annie Wilkes (Chapter 12, Characters in Literature and Comics), located later in this text. Read the intake summary, diagnostic impressions, and discussion of the diagnosis. You may also want to have your copy of the *DSM-IV-TR* available. Working alone or with a partner, consider the following:

As we have portrayed them, as a group, these six clients present very different types of diagnosable psychological disorders and/or other focuses of counseling, varying levels of emotional need, and a range of difficulties with everyday functioning. How does the counseling reflect the client's presenting concerns and needs on Axis I and Axis II? What was ruled out by the clinician? What differential diagnoses were considered?

What information was recorded on Axis III and Axis IV? In what ways were the medical conditions, if any, related to the Axis I and Axis II diagnoses? How were the problems found on Axis IV for these clients associated with Axis I and Axis II? How do the different GAF scores found on Axis V fit with each client's Axis I and Axis II information?

Finally, what do you notice as you compare and contrast how each of these clients' multiaxial diagnosis was pulled together? Do you agree with the counselors' diagnostic decision-making?

CHAPTER SUMMARY AND WRAP-UP

This chapter started the process of learning to make a psychological disorder diagnosis. We began by putting diagnosis in context and explaining its importance in today's world of professional counseling—and introducing the *DSM-IV-TR* diagnostic classification system. We said the *DSM* provides a single, comprehensive system of diagnosis used by virtually all of today's counseling and mental health practitioners. We defined *mental disorder* and used it interchangeably with the term *psychological disorder*. We described what is and is not considered a diagnosable disorder; for instance, we said that only client situations that cause clinically significant distress or impairment may be diagnosable. Further, we said normally expectable, culturally determined, and developmentally appropriate behaviors usually are not diagnosed. We also explained the limited purpose of a diagnosis, which is to describe and communicate about the client's situation. We mentioned that a diagnosis, in and of itself, does not indicate etiology, theoretical conceptualization, professional viewpoint, or treatment. These factors were summarized in Figure 4.1. We also presented some of the major counselor reservations about making diagnoses, and described how the *DSM* system attempts to address these. Important considerations included potential for bias, potential for stigmatization or labeling, under-responsiveness to social change, overresponsiveness to payment pressure, and advanced clinical criticisms.

We then used the remainder of the chapter to learn about the *DSM-IV-TR* multiaxial diagnostic system. We presented five axes, which are five different sets of information that comprise a full diagnosis: Axis I. Clinical Disorders and Other Conditions That May Be a Focus of Clinical Attention; Axis II. Personality Disorders and Mental Retardation; Axis III. General Medical Conditions; Axis IV. Psychosocial and Environmental Problems; and Axis V. Global Assessment of Functioning (GAF). We said that Axis I answers questions about whether the client shows signs and symptoms of diagnoses and conditions contained in the *DSM*, Axis II answers questions about whether the client presents evidence of the long-term conditions of mental retardation or a

personality disorder, Axis III answers questions about the presence of physical signs and symptoms, Axis IV answers questions about what psychosocial and environmental problems and other stressors the client is facing, and Axis V answers questions about how well the client currently is functioning in the psychological and social and occupational or academic aspects of his or her life.

We explained how to use Axis I, including the *DSM-IV-TR's* interchapter and intrachapter organization, to evaluate for 15 classes of diagnosable disorders comprising more than 300 separate disorders, as well as other conditions that can be a focus of counseling. We described the diagnostic features, subtypes and specifiers, recording procedures, associated features, specific demographic information, differential diagnoses, and diagnostic criteria provided. This was summarized in Figures 4.2 and 4.3. We explained Axis II, including what the criteria are for a diagnosis of Mental Retardation and 11 different personality disorders, and summarized Axis II in Figure 4.3. We explained what to list on Axis III and what to include on Axis IV, and how to record this information on the two axes. We explained that Axis V requires us to estimate the client's functioning using the GAF scale, which is found in the *DSM-IV-TR,* and how to use the scale.

We then pulled together all of this information to show how to make a completed diagnosis. We discussed decision-making on Axis I and Axis II, including ruling-out conditions and considering differential diagnoses. We explained how to indicate more than one diagnosis, uncertainty among diagnoses, and no diagnosis on these axes. We discussed how to make determinations and what to record on Axis III and Axis IV so that this information corresponds with and enhances our Axis I and Axis II impressions. Last, we discussed how to make GAF estimations on Axis V, and how to record them, so that they also correspond with our Axis I and Axis II impressions.

Throughout the chapter, we referred the reader to specific sections and pages of the *DSM-IV-TR.* We relied extensively on our text's case illustrations: We offered many examples and learning activities that used the intake summaries, diagnostic impressions, and discussions of diagnostic impressions found in Part III of this text.

5

CASE CONCEPTUALIZATION

Making Sense of the Client's Concerns

The transition from natural helper to counseling professional takes us logically from diagnosis, which is a tool for describing client concerns, to case conceptualization, which is a tool for understanding—making sense of—client needs. Providing competent, effective counseling in today's world of mental health practice depends on our ability to select and apply a useful, valid clinical framework that helps us assess and theoretically explain the client's experiences (Hinkle, 1994; Seligman, 1996). Using case conceptualization, we take what we have learned about the different theories, models, and approaches to counseling and psychotherapy, and apply them to the needs of the specific client with whom we are working at the moment. In this way, case conceptualization skills give clinicians a rationale for the decisions they make about providing treatment (Seligman, 2004). In fact, this clinical thinking tool is so important that Meier and Davis (2005) included learning how to conceptualize client needs on the same list of important topics for new counselors as other elements of counseling like learning crisis intervention skills.

Further, as we discussed in Chapter 3, most of today's counseling professionals must become proficient with briefer psychotherapy models, integrative and eclectic counseling methods, and evidence-based practices (Budman & Gurman, 1983; Mahalick, 1990; Neukrug, 2001; Wampold, 2001). These approaches require efficient case conceptualization early on in the counseling process, usually at the earliest and moderately early stages of the counseling relationship (see Figure 3.2 for a summary). In turn, in most professional settings, assessing client concerns, developing a case conceptualization to explain these concerns, deciding on the outcomes and goals of counseling, and selecting an intervention plan usually are accomplished in just the first few sessions (Burlingame & Fuhriman, 1987; Neukrug, 2002). This can increase the pressure for good case conceptualization skills.

(Continued)

(Continued)

Certainly, all clinicians at least informally "develop ideas about what is troubling their clients and what they could be doing to help them" (Meier, 2003; Meier & Davis, 2005, p. 62; Teyber, 2000). Probably you already have made these types of informed guesses about the individuals you have assisted. However, new counselors often express confusion, ambiguity, or a lack of confidence in their case conceptualization skills when they are asked to manage the formal process of carefully, thoughtfully, and methodically applying the various professional counseling theories, models, and approaches to each new specific client situation they encounter (Glidewell & Livert, 1992; Hays et al., 2010).

To address this, in Chapter 5, we start the case-conceptualization learning process. We cover all of the information you will need to start learning to conceptualize "the complexities of working with clients" (Meier & Davis, 2005, p. 62). In the chapter, first we introduce case conceptualization in the context of today's professional practice. We define case conceptualization and explain its basic elements. Next, we use the majority of the chapter to present the Inverted Pyramid Method (IPM) of case conceptualization (Neukrug & Schwitzer, 2006; Schwitzer, 1996, 1997). This method was specially designed to give students, trainees, licensees and residents, and other new counselors a specific, four-step plan that can be used to make sense of client presentations and form a start-to-finish theoretical case conceptualization. We explain the details of each of the steps in the process, including:

- Step 1 Problem Identification
- Step 2 Thematic Groupings
- Step 3 Theoretical Inferences
- Step 4 Narrowed Inferences

Once we have explained the details of the model and each of its four steps, we pull it all together. We demonstrate how to make a fully prepared, theoretically based case conceptualization using the inverted pyramid—and explain the differences among conceptualizations that are based on a single theory, a psychotherapeutic integration of more than one theory, an eclectic mix of approaches, or a solution-focused approach. We then summarize what we have covered. We provide learning activities and professional and clinical snapshots in the chapter, and we refer to our 30 clinical cases in order to illustrate our main points about making sense of client needs via case conceptualization.

At the end of the chapter, you should be able to:

- Define case conceptualization, discuss the use of case conceptualization in today's professional counseling settings, and explain its relationship to diagnosis and treatment planning
- Identify and explain the basic elements of case conceptualization
- Discuss and explain the use of the IPM of case conceptualization
- Identify, explain, and demonstrate the use of each of the inverted pyramid approach's four steps, including:
  o Methods of assessment and problem identification at Step 1
  o Methods of forming thematic groupings at Step 2
  o Methods of forming theoretical inferences at Step 3
  o Methods of forming deeper inferences at Step 4
- Demonstrate the ability to fully prepare start-to-finish case conceptualizations based on (a) a single theory, (b) a psychotherapeutic integration of more than one theory, (c) an eclectic mix of approaches, or (d) a solution-focused approach.

CASE CONCEPTUALIZATION AND PROFESSIONAL COUNSELING

Case conceptualization is a clinical thought process that is a bridge between theory and practice. Using case conceptualization, we select from among the various theories and models we have learned about in our education and training and ongoing professional development, and then apply the theory or model we have selected to a specific client's situation. To do this, we closely observe and learn about our client, think about what we have observed and learned about his or her situation, and then represent our impressions and ideas about the client with a theoretical model (Meier & Davis, 2005). We form impressions and ideas from the point of view of a conceptual model that can help us understand the factors that may have led to the client's needs (which we will call etiological factors) as well as factors that may be maintaining the client's concerns (which we will refer to as sustaining factors).

This is an important task because, ultimately, we will use this analysis to decide how to best address, reduce, manage, or resolve the client's concerns by developing a treatment plan for tackling these concerns—either directly, or by working to mitigate the etiological factors that led to the present situation or working to mitigate the sustaining factors that are keeping the problems going, or some combination of these strategies. In other words, the way in which the clinician conceptualizes the client's case will lead to important decisions about the goals to be accomplished in counseling and about the treatment plan for accomplishing these goals (Neukrug & Schwitzer, 2006).

Specifically, case conceptualization is a clinical thinking tool that requires three basic elements (Neukrug & Schwitzer, 2006):

1. Observing, assessing, evaluating, and collecting information about the client's presenting situation.

2. Using these observations, assessments, and evaluations to distinguish patterns and themes that can be found in the client's concerns and life situation.

3. Selecting a professional counseling theory, clinical model, or conceptual approach—and then using this approach to interpret, explain, understand, make sense of, or form clinical judgments about the etiological factors (underlying or root causes) and sustaining factors (features maintaining the problem) contributing to the client's concerns.

As we noted, this process then leads to decisions about the counseling or psychotherapeutic treatment plan, including what positive changes or outcomes we and the client will work toward, and where to target our clinical work with the client to reach these changes and outcomes.

SKILL AND LEARNING EXERCISE 5.1

Three Elements of Case Conceptualization

Refer to the case of Juno, appearing in Chapter 8, Troubled Youth in Film and on Stage, located later in this text. Read the intake summary and case conceptualization. (You will see that the case conceptualization uses the IPM. Don't worry! It is not necessary for you to be familiar with the inverted pyramid to complete this exercise. The goal of this learning activity to become familiar with the three basic elements of case conceptualization described above). Working alone or with a partner, consider the following:

We introduced three basic elements required for case conceptualization. The first basic element is collecting information about the client's presenting situation. On the basis of the intake summary and case conceptualization discussion, what information did the counselor collect about (a) Juno's presenting situation, (b) Juno's background, history, past and recent experiences, life events, or other etiological factors leading to her present-day concerns, and (c) the current factors that are contributing to Juno's needs.

(Continued)

(Continued)

We said the second basic element of case conceptualization is using the information the coun-selor has collected to form themes and patterns that can be found in the client's functioning. Review again the intake summary and the "Thematic Groupings" section of the case conceptualization. You will see that, based on all of the various pieces of information collected about Juno's situation, the counselor formed three patterns or themes. What are these three themes? What symptoms or pieces of information about Juno contribute to, or go along with, each of the three groupings (in other words, how did the counselor "divide up" the presenting information to form the three theme groups)?

We then said the third basic element is applying a theoretical orientation or conceptual approach to understand, interpret, or make sense of the client information collected and the themes derived from the client data. What theoretical approach did Juno's counselor select for her conceptualiza-tion? What was her rationale for using this approach? What interpretations did the counselor reach about Juno based on the theory she applied?

Four-Step Approach

Those who are new to professional counsel-ing often feel highly challenged by the pressure to develop case conceptualizations that bridge what they learned about theory, on one hand, and their actual work with a specific client, on the other hand. Experienced practitioners are able to apply consistent, general frameworks to the job of conceptualizing the various client problems and situations they encounter. They have established for themselves a familiar way of col-lecting client information, organizing the infor-mation into meaningful patterns and groupings, and then interpreting the patterns and groupings using theory. This gives experienced practitioners a reliable way to perform case conceptualization. By comparison, new counselors (and other pro-fessionals who are not yet experienced with conceptually driven practices) tend to engage in repetitive, case-specific conceptual work that requires either starting from scratch with each new client situation or using "implicit mental models" that may not always be helpful (Meier & Davis, 2005, p. 62; Schwitzer, 1996).

Therefore, in the remainder of this chapter we introduce the IPM of case conceptualization (Neukrug & Schwitzer, 2006; Schwitzer, 1996, 1997). This is a four-step method specifically designed to give you a rational, trustworthy approach you can use for forming client concep-tualizations. We also demonstrate the method with all 30 of our case illustrations.

INVERTED PYRAMID METHOD

The IPM of case conceptualization provides you with a consistent, reliable, step-by-step process to follow when forming conceptual views of clients. The pyramid framework gives you a plan to use when you are trying to identify and under-stand client concerns. In addition, the inverted pyramid gives you a vehicle for discussing your counseling cases with clinical supervisors, in case staffing meetings and clinical team presen-tations, or in other learning environments such as with instructors or in class.

The pyramid framework is based on several psychological principles: It emphasizes having a broad, horizontal, view of the client's presenta-tion, as well as a deep, vertical, view of the etio-logical factors, roots, and underlying reasons for the client's broadly identified needs. In this way, the framework helps us illustrate the connections between presenting symptoms and concerns; additionally existing client symptoms, situations, and features; and underlying dynamics and needs.

The inverted pyramid is presented in Figure 5.1. As you can see, the framework uses four clear steps to form a total conceptualization (Neukrug & Schwitzer, 2006; Schwitzer, 1996, 1997):

1. "Casting a wide net" to broadly identify client presenting concerns, needs, and dynamics

2. Organizing all of the information about client presenting concerns, needs, and dynamics into a small number of logical groupings or functional themes

3. Tying these logical theme groups to deeper or underlying or causal interpretations or inferences based on a theory

4. Narrowing these interpretations or inferences still further to identify and explain the client's deepest dimensions or most critical areas of dysfunction

Following these four steps, the framework allows us to widely identify client concerns and narrow them down to their deeper causes as we see them (i.e., the framework lets us organize our thinking both horizontally and vertically).

This process of narrowing down client concerns to their roots is pictured diagrammatically as a funnel, or inverted pyramid. Using the approach, when we are finished with our conceptualization and have charted it on an inverted pyramid diagram, we have a graphic representation of all of the important elements influencing our client's behavior. Having this type of visual model can be extremely useful for understanding the complexities of working with a specific client (Eells, 1997; Meier, 1999, 2003).

Step 1: Problem Identification

In the first step of the pyramid approach, counselors use a wide latitude to identify the client's presenting concerns; associated concerns; and relevant aspects of the person's adjustment, functioning, and environment. Rather than adhering to theoretical assumptions, which will come later in the conceptual process, at this early information-gathering step, a wide net is cast for

Figure 5.1   Inverted Pyramid Method of Case Conceptualization

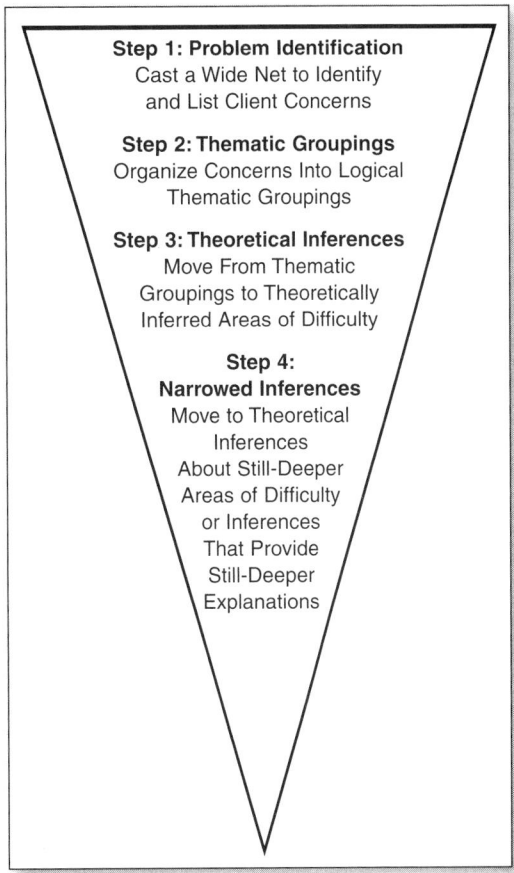

Source: Neukrug & Schwitzer, 2006; Schwitzer, 1996, 1997.

the information needed to describe the client's presenting situation as fully as possible (Dumont, 1993). Therefore, at this step, an emphasis is placed on inclusion of any potentially useful descriptive information. This material often includes data about the reason for referral; collateral reasons for counseling; family and developmental history; in-session observations and notes related to behaviors, thoughts, and affect during the interview; medical and psychiatric clinical inquiries; and/or psychological assessment. A listing then is recorded in the topmost section of the pyramid diagram (see Figure 5.1).

Step 2: Thematic Groupings

The second step of the pyramid method involves organizing client concerns and needs into intuitively logical groupings or thematic constellations. The goal of this configural step is to group together client problems, issues, and dynamics that all seem to serve similar functions or all seem to operate in the same way in the person's life. In other words, at Step 2, client information, problems, and behaviors are sorted together according to their effect on the individual's everyday life, the purposes they serve, or the ways they operate in the person's intrapersonal or interpersonal experience. As you will see in Figure 5.1, the funneling shape of the diagram emphasizes the notion that we are narrowing multiple, seemingly isolated bits and pieces of information we have collected at Step 1 into fewer, but more meaningful, configurations at Step 2. A small number of thematic groups are recorded in the upper middle section of the diagram.

Step 3: Theoretical Inferences

In contrast to Steps 1 and 2, where the practitioner uses basic professional reasoning, logical clinical thinking, and his or her general counseling knowledge base to identify and begin organizing client concerns, at Steps 3 and 4 we turn to the job of applying theory to make inferences or interpretations. At Step 3, an attempt is made to attach the thematic groups developed in the previous steps to inferred areas of difficulty according to the counselor's selected theoretical or conceptual approach. The small collection of previously identified symptom-groups or theme-groups composed in Step 2 now is refined further to reflect theoretical inferences. Moving from the widely collected

information at Step 1, to the narrower collection of groupings at Step 2, at Step 3, an attempt is made to identify an even smaller number (usually just one or two) of underlying dynamics, causal roots, or explanatory mechanisms that the selected theory indicates are the etiological and sustaining factors contributing to the client's concerns. Correspondingly, the narrowing funnel of the pyramid diagram emphasizes the organization of client-problem constellations into a still smaller number of theoretical themes that are more powerfully unifying, central, explanatory, causal, or underlying in nature (see again Figure 5.1). This small handful of theoretical inferences is recorded in the lower middle section of the diagram.

Step 4: Narrowed Inferences

Finally, at Step 4, additional theoretical work is done when needed. Staying with the same theoretical approach begun at Step 3, when it is helpful to the counselor's further understanding of the client's presentation, at Step 4, even deeper theoretical inferences about even-more-underlying areas of difficulty, or even-more-fundamentally problematic client dynamics, are identified when they exist. For example, the unifying, causal, or interpretive themes from Step 3 may be distilled further into existential, fundamental, or underlying questions, when present, of life and death (suicidal ideation or behavior, meaningfulness of life), deep-rooted shame or rage, extreme loss of identity, core faulty cognitive schemas or behavioral patterns, and the like. This step should help counselors see connections between the client's deep core faulty psychological processes, on one hand, and the more easily observable client presentations identified at Step 1, on the other hand (Mahoney, 1991). Step 4 helps identify and highlight significantly debilitating client dimensions when they exist. As shown in the figure, these are recorded in the bottommost section of the pyramid diagram.

SKILL AND LEARNING EXERCISE 5.2

Overview of the Inverted Pyramid Method of Case Conceptualization

Refer once again to the case of Juno, appearing in Chapter 8, Troubled Youth in Film and on Stage, located later in this text. This case also was the subject of Skill and Learning Exercise 5.1. Reread the intake summary and case conceptualization, and review the inverted pyramid summary diagram. Again, working alone or with a partner, reconsider some of the same questions raised in Skill and Learning Exercise 5.1, this time paying closer attention to the counselor's use of the IPM and diagram. Respond to the following:

At Step 1 of the inverted pyramid approach, what information did the counselor collect and record on the diagram? What information was collected about Juno's reason for referral? Associated needs or collateral concerns? Based on the intake summary, how exhaustive is the information recorded in the topmost portion of the diagram?

At Step 2, the counselor formed three logical theme groups. On what basis were these groups developed? What did the counselor think were the common denominators? Which data identified in Step 1 contributed to each of the three groupings (how was the information collected at Step 1 "divided up" into the three Step 2 groupings)?

At Steps 3 and 4, what theoretical approach was used? How or why did the counselor select this theory for her work with Juno? At Step 3, what theoretical inference was made? At Step 4, what deeper inference was made? How does the information in Step 3 explain or interpret the work done at Steps 1 and 2? Then, how does the additional information in Step 4 further the counselor's explanation or interpretation?

Finally, how did use of the inverted pyramid assist Juno's counselor with her case conceptualization work?

A CLOSER LOOK AT STEP 1: PROBLEM IDENTIFICATION

We have used the phrase *casting a wide net* several times now to capture the counselor's mission or assignment at Step 1 of the conceptualization process. To us, this phrase is a reminder that usually we will go beyond just the reason for referral to fully identify and describe our client's counseling needs and dynamics. In most professional counseling settings, Step 1 may be completed as the result of a semistructured counseling intake interview, psychological assessment, and mental status exam. These are summarized in Figure 5.2.

Semistructured Counseling Intake Interview

Counseling professionals in typical work settings usually conduct a beginning session with new clients that takes the form of an intake interview, screening, or evaluation session. In some clinical settings this is referred to as the "diagnostic interview" (LaBruzza & Mendez-Villarrubia, 1994, p. 103). Sometimes this stage of counseling requires multiple sessions or meetings. The primary goal of this beginning stage in the counseling relationship is to identify, describe, and gain an understanding of the client's concerns (Schwitzer, 1996, 1997). At the

Figure 5.2 Components of Inverted Pyramid Step 1: Problem Identification

Semi-Structured Counseling Interview

Presenting Problem

Behavior

Thoughts

Affect

Physiology

Additional Areas of Concern

Life Role Adjustment

Social Adjustment

Personal-Emotional Adjustment

Institutional Adjustment

In-Session Data

Thoughts

Affect

Behavior

Family and Developmental History

Parent and Family Relationships

Parent and Family History

School and Work History

Social Experiences History

Clinical Inquiries

Medical and Health Problems

Medications

Hospitalizations

Substance Use

Self-Harm and Harm to Others

Developmental Factors

Early Childhood

Middle Childhood

Early Adolescence

Adolescence/Late Adolescence

Young Adulthood

Adulthood/Middle Adulthood

Later and Older Adulthood

Cultural and Social Influences

Race

Ethnicity

Socioeconomic Class

Gender

Sexual Orientation

Religion/Spirituality

Psychological Assessment

Problem Checklists

General Personality Inventories

Specific Clinical Problems

Intelligence or Learning

Mental Status Exam

General Appearance

Attitude and Interpersonal Style

Behavior and Psychomotor Activity

Use of Speech and Language

Emotional Expression

Cognitive Function

Thought and Perception

Thought Processes

Problematic Preoccupations

Suicidality/Homocidality

Impulse Control Problems

Insight

Judgment

Reliability

same time, we use our rapport and trust-building skills at this early stage in order to begin establishing a successful therapeutic relationship with the client and instilling motivation for the counseling work ahead (Neukrug & Schwitzer, 2006). Ideally, along with gathering basic descriptive information, we are able to begin uncovering client patterns, revealing underlying dynamics, and encouraging and challenging clients toward change (Kleinke, 1994). In turn, this means that we must conduct the information-gathering process in a way that is palatable to our clients.

Intake interview content and format vary according to the needs and requirements of the specific setting, context, and professional discipline in which the assessment meeting takes place. However, generally speaking, a prototypical semistructured counseling intake interview focuses on gathering the following types of information (Neukrug & Schwitzer, 2006; Schwitzer, 1996, 1997): presenting problem, additional areas of concern, family and developmental history, in-session data, clinical inquiries, developmental factors, and cultural and societal influences. More information comes from psychological assessment and mental status exams.

Presenting Problem. The counselor usually begins the interview by inquiring about the client's reasons for seeking counseling. This includes gaining as much detailed information as the client can report about: behaviors (e.g., problematic interpersonal and relationship behaviors at home, work, or in other roles; difficulties with eating, substance use, sexuality, impulses, etc; academic or career problems, etc.); thoughts (negative self-statements, faulty beliefs, ruminations, troublesome fantasies; important questions about identity, spirituality etc.); affect (low or overly elated mood, anxiety, irritation or anger or rage, shame or guilt, etc.); and physiology (symptoms pertaining to energy level and fatigue, sleep, appetite, sexual drive, anxiety reactions, etc.).

Additional Areas of Concern. Moving beyond the stated reason for counseling, the counselor inquires about and explores additional areas of difficulty, if any, that might exist in the person's current or previous life situation. Here again, thoughts, feelings, behaviors, and physiological features are explored. To provide some structure to this line of inquiry, these additional areas can be organized as follows (adapted from Baker & Siryk, 1984): adjustment to school, work, or other major life roles or areas of functioning (job or career success, meeting school or college demands, etc.); social adjustment (family roles and relationships, intimate and romantic relationships, friendships and social relationships, work and leisure group interactions, etc.); personal-emotional adjustment (behavior, cognition, affect, and physiology in mental or physical health areas beyond the presenting problem); and institutional adjustment (satisfaction with current institutions to which the person belongs, such as work, school or college).

Family and Developmental History. Along with immediate concerns, the counselor inquires about past experiences and family systems influences, usually including: parental and family relationships and history, previous school and work experiences, previous peer and social experiences, and past intrapersonal experiences. As a rule of thumb, the clinician makes these inquiries a regular part of his or her interview routine; however, those aspects of family and developmental history that are most relevant and salient to the client's specific needs are emphasized.

In-Session Data. Observations about client presentation during the meeting sometimes provide additional clinically salient information. This information can include observations and notes about the client's expressed thoughts (thinking that is rational or irrational, optimism vs. pessimism, self-statements and self-interpretations, views of counseling, presence of delusional or psychotic thinking, etc.), expressed or demonstrated affect (facial expressions and bodily presentation, overt expressions such as teariness or loud anger, etc.), and behaviors (engaged or disengaged relationship behaviors, personal style, overtly bizarre behavior, etc.) during the meeting. Importantly, when collecting in-session data, counselors must be careful to assess client functioning in terms of psychological presentation, rather than to make moral, ethical, punitive, or other judgmental evaluations; the purpose of in-session observation is to collect material that will be helpful in conceptualizing, planning, and implementing treatment—not to make value judgments (Meier & Davis, 2005).

Clinical Inquiries. Effective intake interviews include careful, detailed routine clinical inquiries about medical and mental health factors including all of the following: medical and health problems, medical and psychiatric medications, past medical hospitalizations, past psychiatric hospitalizations, use of substances (including alcohol, other recreational and street drugs, misuse of prescription medication, and other substances), as well as self-harming, suicidal, or homicidal thoughts, feelings, impulses, and actions (we prefer to separate these out from other presenting and associated problems so that counselors are careful to assess for these, specifically, during their inquiries).

Developmental Factors. Counseling and therapy in their various forms take place with individuals across the life span, from early childhood through late adulthood. Correspondingly, developmental factors are among the various features we often must take into account during the information gathering and problem identification phases of case conceptualization.

When working with early childhood clients through about age 5 years, as well as middle childhood clients ages 6 through 11, counselors generally must assess the influences of the dramatic physical, cognitive, self-, social, and emotional developmental advances that are characteristic of these two life span phases. With these clients, counselors must be alert to typical early childhood problems centering on cooperation with others and situational issues in preschool settings and in the family, and typical middle childhood problems centering on difficulties at school and difficulties with family (such as abuse, marital discord, or divorce) and social environment (such as poverty). Likewise, when working with early adolescent clients ages 10 through 14 years, counselors generally must evaluate the influences of the rapid physical

developmental changes, and dynamic cognitive, self-, social, and emotional developmental advances that characterize this life span phase. With these clients, counselors must be alert to problems centering on management of emotions, relationship formation and discord, social behavior, and identity (cf. Vernon, 2009).

Likewise, when meeting with adolescent, late adolescent, and young adult clients, counselors generally should evaluate the influences of cognitive development, moving from dualistic to more complex thinking; identity formation, including self-definition, and self in the context of culture, sexuality, and relationships with others; intimacy, relationship formation, and management and expression of emotion; and establishing autonomy and developing competencies for the adult world. With these clients, counselors must be aware of problems centering on academic/workplace/career adjustment, social adjustment, and personal-emotional adjustment to the demands of the late adolescent, young adult, and adult worlds. With adult and middle-adult clients, further characteristic advances in the areas of cognitive development, identity formation, intimacy and relationships, and thriving in the adult world development—and adjustment problems in these areas—should be one context counselors evaluate (cf. Evans, Forney, & Guido-DiBrito, 1998). Then, when working with later and older adults, we consider again the influences of characteristic changes associated with physical, cognitive, identity, social, and emotional development and transitions at these later life span phases (cf. Schlossberg, 1995).

Although developmental factors may be more salient at certain points in the life span, attending to developmental data is potentially important with much of our clinical caseload.

Cultural and Societal Influences. As our Chapter 4 discussion of diagnosis indicated, cultural and societal influences on a person's cognitions, behaviors, affect, and physiological reactions are another important consideration when identifying and describing a client's concerns, needs, or clinical situation. Emerging from the experiences the individual has based on the characteristics associated with his or her ethnicity, race, gender, geographic origin, nationality, faith, or other factors, culture may have an impact on the person's "attitudes, habits, norms, beliefs, customs, rituals, styles, and [other aspects of adjustment and functioning that define a cultural group's adaptation to its social environment]" (McAuliffe & Associates, 2008, p. 8). These adaptations include external responses to the world around us as well as internalized dimensions of culture. McAuliffe & Associates (2008) identified six sources of cultural influence that counseling professionals might especially emphasize in their understanding of the client: race, ethnicity, class/socioeconomic status, gender, sexual orientation, and religion or spirituality.

Psychological Assessment

Under the category of psychological assessment, we include the use of written measures, formal evaluations, tests, and other instruments. These often comprise problem checklists (these usually are unique to the agency, center, or office in which the interview takes place and give the clients a method of conveying information about their concerns), general personality inventories (such as the MMPI or the California Personality Inventory), measures of specific clinical problems (such as the Beck Depression Inventory-II [BDI-II] or Eating Disorders Inventory [EDI]), and measures of intelligence or learning. Some assessment methods are not strictly written measures: for example, clinical behavioral observations, especially of children, may be included. Similarly, intelligence testing (such as using the WAIS-IV or WISC-IV) include written and other types of data collection.

Mental Status Exam

Finally among our areas of client inquiry, one important goal of Step 1: Problem Identification in typical counseling settings is to evaluate the individual's mental status. The mental status exam is an organized assessment of the client's cognitive and emotional functioning in order to systematically examine whether the person's thinking process, feeling state, and behavior may indicate that he or she is experiencing a diagnosable mental disorder (LaBruzza & Mendez-Villarrubia, 1994).

The typical mental status exam attends to all of the following (LaBruzza & Mendez-Villarrubia, 1994; Rosenberg & Kosslyn, 2011): general appearance (dress and grooming, physical characteristics relevant to the evaluation, posture and gait); attitude and interpersonal style, observable behavior and psychomotor activity, and use of speech and language (including rate or speech, normality of its volume and presentation, or any noticeable abnormalities); emotional expression (affect, presence of neurovegetative depression symptoms); cognitive functioning (conscious awareness, orientation to current situation, attention and concentration, memory for recent and distant past or report of memory problems, ability to abstract and generalize, general information level and estimate of intelligence); thought and perception (presence of disordered perceptions such as distortions, delusions, ideas of reference, or magical thinking); thought processes (including flow of ideas and quality of associations); problematic preoccupations (such as obsessions and compulsions, somatic complaints, or phobias); thoughts, feelings, and behaviors pertaining to suicidality, homocidality, or impulse control problems; and difficulties with insight, judgment, or reliability.

As you can see, the features examined in the mental status exam overlap with the other portions of the prototypical semistructured counseling intake interview. Sometimes counselors make a distinction between conducting the general interview with the goal of casting a wide net and collecting a broad range of information useful in making sense of the client's overall needs, on one hand, and specifically conducting the mental status exam with the goal of assessing client emotional and cognitive functioning for signs of mental disturbance or prominent mental disorders, on the other hand. However, when performed effectively, checking mental status according to the features we have listed above should be just one "integrated, seamless part of the whole interview" (LaBruzza & Mendez-Villarrubia, 1994, p. 104).

SKILL AND LEARNING EXERCISE 5.3

Becoming Familiar With Step 1: Problem Identification

All of the types of information gathered during semistructured counseling interviews, including use of psychological assessment and conducting mental status exams, are represented in our popular culture caseload. We invite you to read through any of the 30 cases for clear illustrations of Step 1 of the IPM. We also suggest the following:

For interesting examples of presenting problem behavior, thoughts, affect, and physiology, take time now to closely read or reread the intake summary, case conceptualization discussion, and inverted pyramid diagram found in the case illustrations of Miss Piggy (Chapter 7), Billie Jean (Chapter 11), or any other case you find compelling.

For good examples of additional areas of concern, take time now to closely read or reread the intake summary, case conceptualization discussion, and inverted pyramid diagram found in the case illustrations of Claire (Chapter 8) and Cleveland Brown (Chapter 9), emphasizing the presence of associated issues beyond the presenting concern.

For useful examples of in-session data, take time now to closely read or reread the intake summary, case conceptualization discussion, and inverted pyramid diagram found in the case illustrations of Mario (Chapter 7), Tinkerbell (Chapter 9), and Maria (Chapter 11), noting the client's thoughts, affect, and behaviors during the interview.

For poignant examples of family and developmental history, take time now to closely read or reread the intake summary, case conceptualization discussion, and inverted pyramid diagram found in the case illustrations of Naruto (Chapter 7), Belle (Chapter 9), and Miss Celie (Chapter 12), all emphasizing experiences of family and history.

For clear examples of clinical inquiries, take time now to closely read or reread the intake summary, case conceptualization discussion, and inverted pyramid diagram found in the case illustrations of Mario (Chapter 7), Eleanor Rigby (Chapter 11), and Chief Bromden and Peter Parker (Chapter 12)—emphasizing substance use, medical history, and hospitalization history.

For representative examples of developmental factors as different life span phases, take time now to closely read or reread the intake summary, case conceptualization discussion, and inverted pyramid diagram found in the case illustrations of Gretel and Naruto (Chapter 7) and Christopher Robin (Chapter 12) emphasizing childhood (Chapter 7); Claire and Elphaba (Chapter 8) and Peter Parker (12) emphasizing adolescence, late adolescence, and young adulthood; George Lopez and Jack McFarland (Chapter 10) emphasizing adulthood; and Sophia (Chapter 10) and Fred the Baker (Chapter 11) emphasizing later and older adulthood.

For clear examples of cultural and social influences, take time now to closely read or reread the intake summary, case conceptualization discussion, and inverted pyramid diagram found in the case illustrations of Jamal (Chapter 8) emphasizing socioeconomic factors, Smithers (Chapter 9) emphasizing sexual orientation, George Lopez (Chapter 10) and Maria (Chapter 11) emphasizing race and ethnicity, and the Geico Caveman (Chapter 11) emphasizing nationality.

For relevant examples using psychological assessment, take time now to closely read or reread the intake summary, case conceptualization discussion, and inverted pyramid diagram found in the case illustrations of Edward Cullen (Chapter 8), using a specific measure of depression, and Eleanor Rigby, using intelligence testing (Chapter 11).

For vivid examples emphasizing the need to conduct a mental status exam, take time now to closely read or reread the intake summary, case conceptualization discussion, and inverted pyramid diagram found in the case illustrations of Tinkerbell (Chapter 9), Annie Wilkes, and Chief Bromden (Chapter 12), all of whom presented prominent symptoms of major mental disorder.

A CLOSER LOOK AT STEP 2: THEMATIC GROUPINGS

We said earlier that Step 1 of the IPM is best captured by the phrase "casting a wide net." Correspondingly, the phrase that we find best captures the therapist's task at Step 2: Thematic Groupings is searching for common denominators. This second step involves organizing the client concerns and other information collected at Step 1 into intuitively logical groupings (or constellations) according to their commonalities and shared themes. In other words, this is a configural step, meaning we begin configuring client information in clinically useful ways. The specific goal of this configural step is to sort together, or group together, various client problems, behaviors, and other dynamics that seem to have similar effects on the person's everyday life, appear to fill similar adaptive functions for the individual, or operate similarly in the client's intrapersonal or interpersonal experience. As you can see in Figure 5.1, the narrowing of the inverted pyramid diagram as it funnels downward emphasizes that we are beginning to conceptually narrow multiple, wide-ranging, seemingly isolated bits and pieces of information (Step 1) into fewer, but more meaningful and clinically useful configurations.

At this early step in the conceptualization process, we do not yet apply theory to our understanding of the client's needs. We try to avoid having our beginning picture of the client's presentation artificially influenced by our theoretical assumptions (Dumont, 1993). Instead, at Step 2, the idea is to use professional intuitive and logical clinical judgment to begin organizing the client's issues in a way that makes the most sense. This is an important step in the conceptualization process because it helps us begin making judgments about what the important foci of counseling are and what the most critical targets for change might be.

Our popular culture case of Edward Cullen (found in Chapter 8, Troubled Youth in Film and on Stage) provides an illustration of this theory-neutral use of intuitive-logical clinical judgment to sort client data into meaningful Step 2 groupings. In this illustration, more than 20 pieces of information obtained from a clinical intake interview, psychological assessment using the Beck Depression Inventory-II (BDI-II), and mental status exam were narrowed into two clinically meaningful themes according to their effects on Edward's everyday life and the way they operate in his intrapersonal and interpersonal experience. First, the theme "Recurrent Severe Depression" was formed from wide-ranging Step 1 information such as his death and soul murder themes; sad, lost, and lonely mood; history of losses; and BDI scores. Second, the theme "Personality Dependence" was formed from data including "smothering" his girlfriend with love, needing his girlfriend as a "lifeline," and so on.

Similarly, in our popular culture case of Christopher Robin (as we have reinvented him in Chapter 12, Characters in Literature and Comics), again more than 20 bits of information collected through the clinical interview, school reports, and clinical observation were funneled into two key themes, distinguishing the problems and symptoms of "Withdrawal, Lack of Engagement, Lack of Verbal Communication" from the problem and symptoms of "All-Encompassing Preoccupation With Lives of Stuffed Animals."

In both of these examples, the counselor used clinical judgment at Step 2 to form the groupings. Later on, a theoretical approach will be applied to the interpretation or explanation of these groupings—Edward Cullen's therapist will use a combination of Cognitive Behavior Therapy and interpersonal psychotherapy, and Christopher Robin's counselor will use the expressive creative arts therapy model—but at Step 2 they rely on theory-neutral intuitive-logical clinical decision-making.

We have found four different ways counseling professionals often go about the task of forming this type of clinically valuable intuitive-logical groupings (Neukrug & Schwitzer, 2006). These include a Descriptive-Diagnostic Approach, Clinical Targets Approach, Areas of Function and Dysfunction Approach, and Intrapsychic Areas Approach. Some counseling professionals rely more exclusively on one particular approach while others use a mix of these. These approaches are summarized in Figure 5.3.

Figure 5.3 Approaches to Inverted Pyramid Step 2: Thematic Groupings

Approach	Thematic Groupings
Descriptive-Diagnostic Approach	Formed to show larger clinical problems characterized by criteria of diagnosable disorder
Clinical Targets Approach	Formed according to four aspects of experience: thoughts, feelings, behavior, and physiology
Areas of Function & Dysfunction Approach	Formed according to areas of function or dysfunction in life situations, roles, or skills
Intrapsychic Areas Approach	Formed on the basis of intrapsychic or intrapersonal themes and functioning

Descriptive-Diagnostic Approach

Using this approach to Step 2 theme formation, counselors organize the bits of client information found in Step 1—data about the client's adjustment, development, distress or dysfunction, life questions, and other counseling foci— according to the way they all related to the same diagnosable syndrome. Clinicians rely on *DSM-IV-TR* categories when using this approach. That is, counselors using the descriptive-diagnostic approach to intuitive-logical clinical thinking at Step 2 take advantage of the existing taxonomy of *DSM-IV-TR* diagnoses by sorting together different client information to show larger clinical problems characterized by the criteria and features of a diagnosable psychological disorder.

Clinical Targets Approach

Using this approach to Step 2 grouping, clinicians sort the various client data collected in Step 1 on the basis of four aspects of client experience: thoughts, feelings, behavior, and physiology. Counselors using the clinical targets approach organize together: (a) cognitions (including troubling thoughts and questions, problematic mental preoccupations, irrational thinking, faulty beliefs, schema, etc.); (b) affect (include experience of and expression of feelings, management of emotions, problematic mood, etc.); (c) behavior

(adaptive and maladaptive behavioral patterns and responses, activity in various life roles, interpersonal and relationship behaviors, etc.); and (d) physiological elements of experience (psychological and health effects of medical problems, physiological effects of substances, bodily expressions of psychological reactions such as stress or depressive symptoms, etc.).

Areas of Function and Dysfunction Approach

Using this approach to Step 2 theme formation, counselors format the client information found in Step 1 into groupings according to the their effects on the client's everyday life. Therapists using this approach find common denominators suggesting counseling concerns that can be categorized together as life situations, life themes, life roles, or life skills. Problems at work, in the client's marriage, or dealing with an illness are examples of life situations that might be formed on the basis of various client situational data. Problems across relationships with others, difficulty with decision-making in many different settings, or anger control problems are examples of life themes. Parenting concerns, career stress, learning to manage the demands of the young adult world, and academic difficulties illustrate groupings on the basis of life roles or life skills. Using this approach, the bottom line is that various, seemingly disparate symptoms or aspects of the client's presentation or situation fall together to illuminate an area of function or dysfunction.

Intrapsychic Areas Approach

Using this approach, psychotherapists construct the client information found in Step 1 into groupings according to intrapersonal life themes. That is, in contrast with the Areas of Function and Dysfunction Approach, through which we try to find common denominators according to areas of external functioning, roles, and behaviors, using the

Intrapsychic Areas Approach, counselors form symptom groups on the basis of intrapsychic or intrapersonal functioning. Applying this approach, the various pieces of information we have collected about the person's functioning or distress, adjustment, development, and other aspects of his or her presenting situation are arranged according to the ways in which they are important to the individual's internal efforts to keep up his or her self-esteem, fortify his or her sense of self, keep his or her personality intact, and handle psychoemotional threats to his or her psychological well-being. This approach emphasizes the ways in which external life affects the client's personal experience of self in the world, identity, and functioning (May, 1988).

SKILL AND LEARNING EXERCISE 5.4

Becoming Familiar With Step 2: Thematic Grouping

All four approaches to Thematic Grouping are represented in our popular culture caseload. We invite you to once again read through any of the 30 cases for interesting samples of clinical thinking at Step 2 of the IPM. To find specific illustrations using each of the four approaches, we recommend the following:

For samples of the Descriptive Diagnostic Approach, sorting client information to show large clinical problems characterized by a diagnosable disorder, take time now to read or reread the intake summary, case conceptualization discussion, and inverted pyramid diagram for these case illustrations: Naruto (Chapter 7); Edward Cullen (Chapter 8); Jessie the Cowgirl, Smithers (Chapter 9); Jack Bauer, Lieutenant Commander Data (Chapter 10); Eleanor Rigby (Chapter 11); Chief Bromden (Chapter 12).

For samples of the Clinical Targets Approach, dividing client presentations according to thoughts, feelings, behavior, and physiology, take time now to read or reread the intake summary, case conceptualization discussion, and inverted pyramid diagram for these case illustrations: Jamal (Chapter 8); Tinkerbell, the Beast's Belle (Chapter 9); Sophia (Chapter 10); Fred the Baker, Billie Jean (Chapter 11).

For samples of the Areas of Function and Dysfunction Approach, forming groups according to life situations, take time now to read or reread the intake summary, case conceptualization discussion, and inverted pyramid diagram for these case illustrations: Miss Piggy, Gretel, Snoopy (Chapter 7); Juno, Claire, Elphaba (Chapter 8); Cleveland Brown (Chapter 9); Maria (Chapter 11); Annie Wilkes, Christopher Robin (Chapter 12).

For samples of the Intrapsychic Areas Approach, forming grouping according to intrapersonal life themes, take time now to read or reread the intake summary, case conceptualization discussion, and inverted pyramid diagram for these case illustrations: Jack McFarland (Chapter 10); Miss Celie, Peter Parker (Chapter 12).

A CLOSER LOOK AT STEP 3:
THEORETICAL INFERENCES
ABOUT CLIENT CONCERNS

Up to this point in our conceptualization work, we have applied a pragmatic approach to client information-gathering at Step 1 and then an approach at Step 2 relying on rational clinical judgment to find common denominators according to the shared roles, functions, or effects the different aspects of client information seem to have on the person's everyday intrapersonal or interpersonal adjustment. Although the process is based on commonly understood psychological principles emphasizing the need to view the client's presentation both horizontally and vertically, so far our clinical thinking has been more-or-less theory-neutral. Now, at Steps 3 and 4, we are ready to apply counseling theories or models to infer, interpret, or explain the emergence of the issues we have identified in Steps 1 and 2. The phrase, applying counseling theory, best captures Step 3.

At this step, an attempt is made to tentatively attach the thematic groupings or constellations formed in the previous step to inferred areas of difficulty—such as faults or areas of need in the person's underlying thinking, behavioral response patterns, emotional reactivity, or physiological responsiveness—according to a selected theoretical perspective or counseling viewpoint. It is at Step 3 that the counselor now suggests theoretical explanations by applying the general interpretive principles that go along with one of many counseling models—for example, client-centered counseling, cognitive-behavioral therapy, psychodynamic psychotherapy, Adlerian counseling, feminist psychology, and various others—to a specific client situation. In this way, the previously identified symptom constellations are refined further to reflect inferences about the deeper aspects or causal roots of a client's difficulties or situation. Usually this means that at Step 3, even fewer themes are needed to explain the client's presenting situation.

As we said earlier, this refinement in the counselor's conceptual thinking is reflected by the placement of Step 3 farther down on the pyramid diagram. The narrowing of the funnel diagram emphasizes that at this point, a very small number of constructs—derived from theory—now are needed to explain the causal roots and sustaining factors contributing to the client's needs.

Our popular culture case of character George Lopez (found in Chapter 10, Adults in Television Sitcoms and Drama) provides an illustration of the application of an explanatory counseling theory at Step 3 to infer deeper causes of the symptom groupings formed in Step 2. In this illustration, the counselor applied Reality Therapy to an understanding of George Lopez's presenting situation. More than 20 pieces of client information were identified at Step 1, reflecting George's difficulties at work, in his family, in his marital relationship, and in cultural adjustment. These were organized using the Clinical Targets Approach into Step 2 symptom groupings.

Then, at Step 3, the general principles of the selected theory, Reality Therapy, were applied to George's specific client presentation. Reality Therapy (Choice Therapy) asserts that individuals have internal control over their choices about their reactions to life experiences, and that healthy functioning comes from approaching life situations by relying on this internal control. In contrast, according to the theory, counseling problems arise when individuals react to life events based on a belief in external control, and therefore fail to learn how to make good choices that correctly respond to their situation and needs. Applying these Reality Therapy constructs at Step 3, George's groups of distressing, disruptive, and dysfunctional symptoms (found in Step 2) were explained (or interpreted) to be derived from George "choosing paining behaviors" (and more specifically, using the language of the theory, "choosing anxietying behaviors, depressing behaviors, angering behaviors, headaching and fatiguing behaviors, and avoiding and escaping behaviors").

This explanation will become the focus as the counselor later moves from case conceptualization to treatment planning; specifically, because George's counselor believes that, on the basis of Realty Therapy, George's many current difficulties all stem from his belief in external control and the fact that he is "choosing paining behaviors," a plan for counseling will be formed that uses Reality Therapy to confront and positively change his locus of control to an internal one, and improve his choice of reactions—and, in this way, resolve the various presenting problems seen at Steps 1 and 2.

Our popular culture case of the Geico Caveman (found in Chapter 11, Characters Found in Music, Musicals, and Advertising) provides a similar illustration. In this case, more than 15 bits of client information describing Caveman's difficulties with cultural transitions and social adjustment (Step 1) are distilled into a single Step 2 theme pertaining to a pattern of anxiety, avoidance, and worry about failing, not fitting in, and not being good or desirable enough. Then, at Step 3, the general principles of the selected theory—this time, Adlerian Therapy—were applied to Caveman's specific client situation. Adlerian Therapy assumes that psychological health derives from innate drives for achievement and connection with others, and our ability to overcome normal feelings of doubt or inadequacy. In

contrast, according to the theory, counseling problems arise from unmanageable feelings of inferiority. Applying these Adlerian Therapy principles at Step 3, Caveman's constellation of anxiety, avoidance, and worry symptoms (found in Step 2) were explained (or interpreted) to derive from his "feelings of inferiority" and "low social inference" (using two constructs from the theory).

Here again, this interpretation will become the center of attention when the counselor moves from case conceptualization to treatment planning; specifically, because Caveman's therapist believes that, on the basis of Adlerian Therapy, Caveman's current difficulties stem from his feelings of inferiority and low social inference, a counseling plan will be developed that uses Adlerian Therapy to address and positively resolve these—leading to improvement in the problems presented in Steps 1 and 2.

SNAPSHOT: PROFESSIONAL PERSPECTIVE 5.1

"You Can't Buy Milk in a Hardware Store"

At Step 3 of the inverted pyramid, we begin applying the general principles of a theoretical orientation to a specific client situation. For the approach to be successful, the counseling professional must engage the client in the process. The client must find the clinician's theoretical explanation useful and valid. However, sometimes clients express ambivalence or resistance to the interpretive model we are using. For instance, one of the authors (Schwitzer) has found that clients can be hesitant to adopt the psychodynamic model he sometimes uses, through which he attempts to understand the ways in which clients' parental relationships and other developmental experiences in their families-of-origin have negatively influenced their present-day functioning in the adult world. The clients are hesitant because they do not want to "blame" their parents for their current situations—since they feel that their parents, although perhaps emotionally faulty in their ability to parent, "still did the best they could" and "at least provided me with a roof over my head and all the basics." In response, Dr. Schwitzer uses a metaphor to help clients see that the psychodynamic theoretical explanation about their families can be valid and useful in counseling, without the need to be judgmental or blaming. This is the metaphor:

According to the theory, infants, children, and adolescents have certain needs from parents, including basic food and protection, and the like, as well as emotional responses like empathy, mirroring, idealizing, and twinship—shared positive relational experiences. These are innate needs and the child is not at fault for having these practical and emotional requirements of their parents. Some parents are not well-equipped to meet these emotional requirements, due to their own family backgrounds, mental health or health needs, or environmental resource limitations (working two jobs, being deployed on military duty, etc.). Being an effective parent does require meeting the child's needs, but these parents are unable to do so given their own life circumstances.

(Continued)

(Continued)

This is similar to trying to buy milk in a hardware store. The store owner has plenty of hardware in stock, but no milk. A customer is not to blame for needing milk, but cannot purchase it from the hardware store owner. The hardware store owner provides what he or she can—the hammer and nails, and so on—and no one blames him or her for not carrying a milk supply. We can think of the customer as the child, the milk as the child's natural emotional needs from parents (or another caregiver), the hardware store owner as the parent, and the store owner's stockroom as the basic practicalities the parent is able to provide in spite of his or her emotional limitations. Just like the hardware situation, the child needed both the "milk" and the "hardware"—and although the parent successfully provided the "hardware," he or she simply did not have the "milk" in his or her stockroom. As a result, the child grew up missing an important element due to the parent's limits, leading to his or her current, adult counseling needs.

As you can see, this metaphor gives us a way to conceptualize and explain the clients' situations using the theory, without judgmentally blaming either the clients for their developmental parental requirements, or the parents, for falling short. By engaging the clients in the case conceptualization, this metaphor sets the stage for the therapeutic process that will follow, which will focus on resolving these developmental effects.

A CLOSER LOOK AT STEP 4: NARROWED INFERENCES ABOUT DEEPER CLIENT DIFFICULTIES

Step 3 moved us from pragmatic and logical clinical judgment to application of theory. Finally, at Step 4, applying the same theoretical orientation used at Step 3, the counselor forms still-deeper, more encompassing, or more incisive, causal or interpretive themes. The issues found in Step 1, sorted by common denominators in Step 2, then interpreted theoretically in Step 3, finally are distilled in Step 4 into rock-bottom fundamental inferences or underlying dynamics. These usually are even more central core interpretations of deeper difficulties in functioning, or even more central core descriptions of deeper counseling questions and life dilemmas (when these factors are not relevant, Step 4 is not needed). Correspondingly, Step 4 information is recorded in the bottommost section of the inverted pyramid diagram, and the funneling shape narrows to its endpoint. We use the phrase, applying theory to make deepest inferences, to summarize Step 4.

Figure 5.4 Characteristics of the Four Steps of the Inverted Pyramid

Steps	Characteristics
Step 1 Problem Identification Step 2 Thematic Groupings	Pragmatic approach emphasizing rational, theory-neutral clinical judgment is used to collect client information and find common denominators
Step 3 Theoretical Inferences Step 4 Deeper Theoretical Inferences	The same theoretical orientation is applied at both steps to infer, interpret, or explain the client information collected and organized at Steps 1 and 2

Core Interpretations
of Deeper Functioning

Sometimes additional interpretive explanation beyond the level provided in Step 3 is required by the theoretical orientation used. Correspondingly, Step 4 is completed whenever further interpretation or explanation is needed to fully understand the psychological world of the client and, in turn, plan for effective, responsive treatment.

For instance, using a psychodynamic theoretical approach, we might indicate in Step 3 that the problems presented by a late adolescent client with whom we are working are best understood to be the result of "autonomy conflicts" (using the language of the theory); however, we may want to go farther by continuing to apply the same theory and explaining at Step 4 that her Step 3 conflicts about separating from family and becoming a fully functioning young adult ("autonomy conflicts" according to the theory) center on, at rock bottom, the core fear that one of her parents cannot psychologically handle the daughter's successful achievement of emotional independence (a reasonable interpretation using contemporary psychodynamic theory). In this case, at Step 4, we might add the deeper interpretation, "Fear of parent's psychological disintegration" (this comes from the theory) to further and fully explain what is at the root of her Step 1 and Step 2 presenting problems.

Now having added Step 4, the combined explanation of Steps 3 and 4 will become the focus as the counselor later moves from case conceptualization to treatment planning. Specifically, interpreting the Step 1 and 2 concerns as stemming from "autonomy conflict" (Step 3), and the autonomy conflict as rooted in "parental disintegration fears" (Step 4), provides a start-to-finish picture of the client's experience that will be used as the basis for planning the direction of a psychodynamic treatment plan.

A similar illustration can be found in our text's popular culture caseload. In the case of Elphaba (Chapter 8, Troubled Youth in Film and on Stage), the therapist applied a cognitive-behavioral theoretical approach at Step 3 of her conceptualization to explain that Elphaba's various presenting concerns (listed in Step 1 and organized in Step 2) were derived from "cognitive distortions," including "magnification," "overgeneralization," and "absolutist thinking" and "problematic behavioral responses" (these are all constructs that come from the theory)—and then went on to infer at Step 4 that underlying these cognitive distortions and problematic behavioral responses was an even deeper "faulty belief." This was Elphaba's deep belief that "People must always treat me unfairly because of my pigmentation and I am helpless to change this" (see the full case in Chapter 8 for a complete discussion of this example). The additional dynamic provided at Step 4—Elphaba's deepest faulty belief, which was underlying the distortions and behaviors identified at Step 3—completed the conceptual client picture. Here again, the combined explanation of Steps 3 and 4 will become the focus when the counselor moves to cognitive-behavioral treatment planning.

Core Descriptions
of Deeper Questions

Step 4 also is used whenever further explanation is needed to theoretically capture the client's bottommost existential dilemmas and counseling questions related to deep-rooted shame or rage fueling the client's emotional presentations, extreme loss of identity, fragile personality structures, and similarly inferred deep concerns; or bottommost existential dilemmas pertaining to life and death (meaning of life, continuing to live, painfulness of life, suicidal and homicidal thoughts and feelings). For example, in our pop culture case of Lieutenant Commander Data (Chapter 10, Adults in Television Sitcoms and Drama), Step 4 is used to indicate Data is dealing with rock-bottom issues pertaining to an existential belief that his fears and anxieties about himself and the universe around him are intolerable and that he has no power to solve these fears and anxieties— and a related faulty belief that "If I can't be human I don't deserve to, or want to, exist." This type of bottommost interpretation allowed the counselor to finish the conceptual theoretical work started in Step 3 (review the entire case for a fuller discussion of Lieutenant Commander Data). Here again, the additional dynamics provided in Step 4 are needed to complete the client picture—and again the combined explanation of Steps 3 and 4 will become the focus when the counselor moves to planning treatment.

Benefits of Step 4 for New Counselors

Taken together, adding Step 4 should help you learn to recognize the connections between a client's deeper questions of self, sense of isolation, and issues of despair (Mahoney, 1991), on one hand, and the more easily recognizable, less potentially overwhelming aspects of client functioning, on the other hand. In addition, adding Step 4 gives you a reliable case conceptualization framework to use even with the most threatening or disruptive client difficulties. Further, as you can see, Steps 3 and 4 work together to help you provide a theoretical explanation of Steps 1 and 2. As we mentioned, Step 4 appears in the bottommost section of the diagram, correspondingly visually with the process of drilling down to the problems in the client's most fundamental dimensions (when they are present). When the pyramid is complete, you should be able to see how client experiences identified in the topmost portions of the pyramid are related to, or rooted in, the client's deepest dynamics.

SKILL AND LEARNING EXERCISE 5.5

Becoming Familiar With Step 3: Theoretical Inferences and Step 4: Deeper Theoretical Inferences

The use of theory to complete Step 3: Theoretical Inferences About Client Concerns, and Step 4: Narrowed Inferences About Deeper Client Difficulties, is illustrated throughout our text's popular culture caseload. In this chapter's section, "Taking a Closer Look at Step 3," we presented two such examples: The cases of George Lopez (Chapter 10, Adults in Television Sitcoms and Drama) and the Geico Caveman (Chapter 11, Characters Found in Music, Musicals, and Advertising). George Lopez's case applied Reality Therapy while the Geico Caveman's case used Adlerian Therapy as the theoretical orientation.

Take time now to closely read or reread each of these illustrations—including the intake summary, case conceptualization discussion, and inverted pyramid diagram—paying special attention to how each of these conceptualizations move from Step 3 to Step 4 of the inverted pyramid. Pay special attention to how the same theory, Reality Therapy and Adlerian Therapy, respectively, is used at both Steps 3 and 4.

Review the entire conceptualization to see how each of these cases moves from identifying client information and organizing the data according to common denominators at Steps 1 and 2, to applying theoretical inferences at Step 3 and then Step 4, in order to form a complete clinical picture of each client's psychological presentation. If you are unfamiliar with one of the theories, you might also take time now to explore the basic principles of Realty or Adlerian Therapy in order to better understand the counseling conceptualizations that are presented.

PULLING IT ALL TOGETHER: SELECTING A THEORETICAL APPROACH

We now have explored the entire case conceptualization process using the instructive IPM. At this point, you have a reliable framework for moving through the steps of collecting and meaningfully organizing client information, and then making sense of this material by applying a theoretical approach—all in preparation for the treatment planning and implementation that will follow. This is the initial step in the process of learning to form your own case conceptualizations. As you will see among the popular culture cases in Part III of the text, counseling professionals use a variety of approaches when conceptualizing (and then planning and implementing treatment for) their clients' needs. For instance, among the cases in Part III are examples of solution-focused and eclectic models as well as applications of many different single theories and combinations of theories. To pull it all together, it is necessary to discuss how therapeutic models and counseling theories are selected when working with clients.

Evidence-Based Treatment and Clinical Expertise

Generally speaking, today's counseling professionals rely on a combination of their own clinical expertise and their knowledge of evidence pertaining to treatment to make good decisions about which counseling approach might be an effective fit with a client's needs.

Evidence-based treatment refers to counseling methods that are supported by extant clinical studies and other relevant research. Some evidence-based research is used to show "absolute efficacy" (Wampold, 2001, p. 58). When we read in a professional journal or learn at a professional meeting that a treatment method shows absolute efficacy, it indicates that for the situation investigated (a particular type of presenting problem, a specific client need, a particular situation, etc.), there is solid research showing that being in counseling or psychotherapy produces better improvement in the person that no counseling or psychotherapy at all. In fact, in an extensive review of this type of research, Wampold (2001) found that, overall, counseling is "remarkably beneficial," showing an improvement rate of about 80% among clients in general (p. 119).

Other evidence-based counseling research explores "relative efficacy" (Wampold, 2001, p. 72). This type of report explains the comparative benefits of one approach versus another—for example, Dialectical Behavior Therapy versus motivational interviewing—for addressing client needs. In fact, there is a growing literature—including clinical trial-type studies and other types of research—examining the relative efficacy of different psychotherapeutic approaches for different client presentations. It is a professional requirement that we remain up to date with these findings in order to keep track of what the latest evidence tells us about the types of client changes and improvements that have been documented using various counseling interventions, and, alternatively, what approaches have been found to be counterproductive or counterindicated (Hanna & Puhakka, 1991; Hanna & Ritchie, 1995; Henry, 1998). As examples, among our case illustrations, both Miss Piggy's and Mario's counselors (Chapter 7) selected Dialectical Behavioral Therapy to address the problematic personality dynamics each of these clients presented, because outcome research has shown this approach to be one treatment method that is indicated when assisting clients with Borderline Personality Disorder (such as Miss Piggy was experiencing) and other personality difficulties (as with Mario).

Naturally, experienced counseling professionals rely on their own clinical expertise to sift through the available evidence and combine these findings with their own counseling knowledge base and the accumulated benefits of their own clinical experiences in order to make decisions about which conceptual models they will use. As counselors gain experience, they should engage in their own formal or informal process of (a) measuring the counseling outcomes they achieve, (b) identifying trends in their counseling processes and outcomes, and (c) using this data as feedback for modifying their models in order to employ increasingly more effective interventions (Hartmann, 1984; Meier & Davis, 2005; Paul, 1988). When doing so, it is expected that the therapist will make treatment decisions that are efficacious for his or her clients and are defensible on ethical, legal, and professional grounds. Among our popular culture cases are two useful examples (both found in Chapter 8):

First, Juno's counselor selected Person-Centered Therapy on the basis of her own clinical expertise, which indicated to the counselor that person-centered counseling is useful with clients such as Juno, who have the capabilities for self-understanding and self-direction, and when the desired outcomes for such clients include self-directed constructive changes and self-directed adjustment. Second, Claire's counselor selected a contemporary psychodynamic model because a combination of the literature and her own clinical practice suggested the approach was especially useful with late adolescent and young adult clinical situations such as Claire presented.

Solution-Focused, Eclectic, Purist Theoretical, and Integrative Approaches

Altogether, mental health professionals must learn to actively rely on the current evidence-based research and other professional literature (Heppner, Kivlighan, & Wampold, 1999), and judiciously draw therapeutic knowledge from their own clinical experience and expertise (Corsini, 2008). When this is done, counselors employ any of the following approaches to case conceptualization:

- Solution-focused counseling
- Eclectic mix
- Single (pure) theoretical approach
- Psychotherapeutic integration of theoretical approaches

When forming a solution-focused case conceptualization, the counselor applies a carefully chosen combination of solution-focused, solution-creating, or problem-solving tactics to his or her immediate understanding of the client's situation and then engages quickly in identifying and reaching operationalized treatment goals (Berg, 1994; de Shazer & Dolan, 2007; Gingerich & Eisengart, 2000). The focus of attention is on what the client immediately presents, wants, and needs—and which concerns will be directly

explored and addressed (Bertolini & O'Hanlon, 2002). Using the inverted pyramid, all of this information is available from Steps 1 and 2 of the conceptualization process. Therefore, when using the brief solution-focused (or problem-solving) approach, only the first two steps of the IPM are used: Problem Identification and Thematic Grouping. Further, therapists using the brief solution-focused approach are required to have a rational framework and to make carefully thought-out professional clinical decisions, rather than pulling techniques and approaches at random (Lazarus, Beutler, & Norcross, 1992; Norcross & Beutler, 2008). Correspondingly, their conceptual thinking at Steps 1 and 2 is used to guide their clinical work. Our popular culture cases of Jamal (Chapter 8), Billie Jean (Chapter 11), and Eleanor Rigby (Chapter 11) illustrate use of the inverted pyramid with solution-focused counseling.

When using an eclectic mix to form a case conceptualization, the therapist uses a varied mixture of counseling approaches and techniques (Corey, 2009). This strategy can be referred to as technical eclecticism (Datillo & Norcross, 2006; Norcross & Beutler, 2008). When applying technical eclecticism, the clinician attempts to select the most useful combination of different counseling techniques, borrowed from various theoretical orientations, without necessarily making connections between the conceptual foundations of the different orientations or necessarily subscribing to the various theories' underlying assumptions (Corey, 2009; Dattilo & Norcross, 2006; Norcross & Beutler, 2008). In other words, rather than relying on a theoretical framework, the technical eclectic approach requires the counselor to pull together his or her own "collection of techniques" based on professional judgment (Corey, 2009, p. 449; de Shazer, 1988, 1991). Therefore, when applying a technical eclectic mix, once again only the first two steps of the pyramid are used. In the case of eclectic mix, clinicians are required to use their clinical thinking at Steps 1 and 2—identifying and meaningfully organizing client information—in order to critically and systematically combine several different counseling methods. (Note that whereas solution-focused approaches operate from a specific solution-focused framework, technical eclecticism requires the professional to make rational decisions on the basis of his or her own clinical judgment; although they differ in this important way, both approaches require only Steps 1 and 2 of the pyramid.) Our popular culture case of Snoopy (as we have reinvented him in Chapter 7) demonstrates use of the inverted pyramid with an eclectic mix.

When using a purist approach, the counseling professional relies on a single therapeutic model to make sense of—to understand and explain—the client's presentation according to the model's theoretical assumptions (Neukrug & Schwitzer, 2006). The professional selects the theoretical approach on the basis of evidence-based treatment selection, his or her clinical expertise, or a combination of these. Because the primary characteristic of theory-driven case conceptualization is identifying or inferring underlying causes, etiological factors, and sustaining factors contributing to the client's situation, the bottom portions of the inverted pyramid are critical. Therefore all four steps are completed. Among our popular culture cases, we present illustrations of the IPM as it is used with cognitive behavior therapy, dialectical behavior therapy, person-centered counseling, contemporary psychodynamic psychotherapy, Adlerian Therapy, and Reality Therapy—as well as the multicomponent psychosocial intervention model, theraplay model, and expressive creative arts play therapy (see Table 1.2 to find these illustrations).

Finally among our approaches to case conceptualization, counselors very often integrate more than one theoretical approach in order to form a conceptualization (and, later, a treatment plan) that meets a specific client's needs as efficiently and effectively as possible (Dattilo & Norcross, 2006; Norcross & Beutler, 2008). This is referred to as psychotherapeutic integration (Corey, 2009). Psychotherapeutic integration is commonly used in today's professional counseling settings because it is seen as a method for flexibly tailoring clinical efforts to

"the unique needs and contexts of the individual client" (Norcross & Beutler, 2008, p. 485). Once again relying very closely on evidence-based treatment selection and clinical expertise, counselors apply psychotherapeutic integration when no single, individual model is comprehensive enough, by itself, to address the entire "range of client types," "specific problems," and "complexities" seen among their caseload (Corey, 2009, p. 450). (Note that in comparison with solution-focused counseling and technical eclecticism, we distinguish psychotherapeutic integration as a model that intentionally values and adopts the underlying theoretical assumptions of more than one counseling orientation.) As with a single, purist theoretical approach, the key characteristic of an integrative approach is combining the important assumptions of more than one theoretical orientation to identify or infer underlying causes, etiological factors, and sustaining factors contributing to the client's situation. In turn, the bottom portions of the inverted pyramid are critical, and therefore all four steps are completed. As follows, using the integration approach, constructs from all of the models used are recorded in Steps 3 and 4 of the pyramid diagram. In Part III, we illustrate a wide variety of psychotherapeutic integrations using the inverted pyramid. We show cognitive, behavioral, or cognitive behavior therapies integrated with client-centered, interpersonal, existential, brief psychodynamic, or Reality Therapy. We also show such psychotherapeutic integrations as client-centered play therapy and cognitive behavioral play therapy; behavioral and cognitive stimulation therapies; and Cognitive Behavior Therapy and cognitive remediation. We recommend that you locate these examples using Table 1.2 and review some of the discussions and diagrams.

In sum, using the IPM of case conceptualization, when solution-focused counseling or an eclectic mix is employed, Steps 1 and 2 of the IPM are needed and Steps 3 and 4 are not needed. When a single (pure) theoretical approach or a psychotherapeutic integration is employed, all four steps are fully completed.

Figure 5.5   Applying Theoretical Approaches to Case Conceptualization

Theoretical Approach	Feature	IPM Steps
Solution-focused counseling	Problem-solving tactics applied to immediate client situation Uses solution-focused conceptual framework	Steps 1 and 2 are used
Eclectic mix	Borrows from various approaches without making connections among the theoretical assumptions	Steps 1 and 2 are used
Purist theoretical approach	Relies on a single theoretical perspective to explain client presentation according to model's underlying assumptions	Steps 1, 2, 3, and 4 are used
Psychotherapeutic integration	Relies on a combination of more than one theoretical perspective to explain client presentation according to models' combined underlying assumptions	Steps 1, 2, 3, and 4 are used

SKILL AND LEARNING EXERCISE 5.6

Considering Approaches to Case Conceptualization

Counseling professionals in today's settings rely on all of the approaches to case conceptualization we have described: solution-focused, eclectic mix, purist single theory, and psychotherapeutic integration of more than one theory. Luckily, the IPM and accompanying diagram provide a reliable framework regardless which approach you use—and regardless of the specific theory or theories you select.

First, if you have not already done so, refer to Table 1.2 found in Chapter 1 of the text. Identify several cases that you find interesting. Select at least one example using a brief solution-focused approach, one or more illustrations applying a single theory, one or more applying an integration of more than one theory, and also include the case of Snoopy using an eclectic mix. What rationales are given for the choice of approach? What rationales are given for the selection of theoretical orientation? Did the counselors use evidence-based decision-making? Clinical expertise? A combination? Also notice the ways in which the pyramid diagram is completed for each approach.

Second, we suggest that you discuss these topics in a professional setting—such as in class, during counseling supervision or at a case staffing meeting, or in an interview with a practicing clinician. Discuss the differences, merits, and drawbacks of the solution-focused, eclectic, purist, and integrative approaches. Also discuss the differences, merits, and drawbacks of several of the theoretical models we present among our cases. Next, find out how others keep up with current evidence-based findings. Also find out how others track their own counseling outcomes and use the feedback to inform and improve their work.

CHAPTER SUMMARY AND WRAP-UP

This chapter moved our clinical thinking from diagnosis to case conceptualization. We started by explaining that case conceptualization is a bridge between theory and practice that allows us to understand etiological factors and sustaining factors contributing to a client's presenting situation. We outlined three elements of case conceptualization: observing, finding patterns in, and then applying an explanatory theory to, the client's concerns.

We then used the remainder of the chapter to learn about the IPM of case conceptualization. We explained that the IPM is a four-step conceptual framework specifically designed to assist new counselors with their clinical thinking about specific client scenarios. The method was summarized in Figure 5.1. We next explored each of the four steps in detail.

We characterized the purpose of Step 1: Problem Identification as "casting a wide net" to identify client needs and dynamics. We reviewed the use of the semistructured counseling intake interview (including presenting problem, additional areas of concern, family and developmental history, in-session data, clinical inquiries, developmental factors, and cultural and social influences), psychological assessment, and the mental status exam, to collect the information needed in Step 1 of the pyramid.

We described the purpose of Step 2: Thematic Grouping as "searching for common denominators" among the various client data in order to form meaningful groupings. We said this was a configural step that allowed us to see the ways in which different client problems, behaviors, and other dynamics fit together according to their impact on the client's experience. We described four pragmatic, logical-intuitive approaches to forming themes in Step 2 on the basis of rational clinical judgment: the Descriptive-Diagnostic, Clinical Targets, Areas of Function and Dysfunction, and Intrapsychic Areas approaches.

We then turned to the application of theory at Steps 3 and 4. We explained that Step 3: Theoretical Inferences About Client Concerns could be summarized by the phrase "applying counseling theory." We described the way Step 3 is used to explain the thematic groupings formed

at Step 2—including faults or areas of need pertaining to underlying thinking, behavioral response patterns, emotional reactivity, or physiological responsiveness—according to a selected theoretical orientation or counseling perspective.

This led us to Step 4: Narrowed Inferences About Deeper Client Difficulties. We said that at Step 4, we apply the same theory used at Step 3 in order to form still-deeper causal or interpretive themes. We described these as rock-bottom theoretical inferences that are either core interpretations of deeper functioning, core descriptions of deeper questions, or both. We noted that Step 4 is applied when it is relevant to our understanding of the client and mentioned the benefits of this step for those who are new to the job of forming case conceptualizations.

We highlighted the graphic value of the inverted pyramid diagram itself, which uses a funneling shape to indicate our conceptual progression from the wide net cast at Step 1 to the very narrow, deep theoretical conclusions of Step 4.

Finally, we pulled it all together. Here we reviewed the use of evidence-based decision-making and the use of clinical expertise to guide our selection of a theoretical approach or counseling perspective for use in our work with a client. We presented four common approaches to selecting a conceptual and treatment approach for use with a client: solution-focused counseling, eclectic mix (or technical eclecticism), purist application of a single theory, and psychotherapeutic integration of more than one theory. We emphasized that the IPM was equally valuable with all four approaches—and explained that the solution-focused approach and eclectic mix require only Steps 1 and 2 of the pyramid, while Steps 3 and 4 involve the entire inverted pyramid.

The diagrams, figures, professional snapshots, and exercises found in the chapter all worked together to assist readers to learn about case conceptualization with the IPM. We continued to rely extensively on our text's case illustrations: Throughout the chapter's content and though the learning activities, we offered many popular culture case examples of client information-gathering at Step 1, different approaches to thematic groupings at Step 2, and the application of various theoretical approaches at Step 3 and Step 4 of inverted pyramid.

6

TREATMENT PLANNING

Designing a Plan for Change

INTRODUCING CHAPTER 6: READER HIGHLIGHTS AND LEARNING GOALS

Using clinical thinking skills to manage the change process ultimately leads counseling and mental health professionals to treatment planning. On the basis of our description and understanding of the client's presentation, as seen in the diagnosis and case conceptualization, the treatment plan provides an intentional, carefully considered road map for the counseling experience. When forming the treatment plan, counseling professionals establish what changes ideally are expected, what interventions and counseling methods will be employed to facilitate these changes, and what sorts of measures will be used to gauge the degree of success at reaching the goals for change. Like the diagnosis and case conceptualization processes that set the stage for treatment planning, treatment planning is a required professional competency (Ackley, 1997; Reich & Kolbasovsky, 2006; Seligman, 2004).

In our discussions of diagnosis and case conceptualization, we noted that today's counseling professionals must become adept at briefer treatment models and integrative or eclectic counseling methods that emphasize evidence-based practices along with judicious use of one's own clinical expertise (Budman & Gurman, 1983; Corsini, 2008; Hanna & Puhakka, 1991; Hanna & Ritchie, 1995; Mahalick, 1990; Neukrug, 2001; Wampold, 2001). As we summarized in Figure 3.1, to accomplish all of this, counselors must form highly developed clinical thinking skills—and as we indicated in Figure 3.2, usually they must successfully complete their preparatory clinical thinking after just the first few client sessions. On the basis of this early clinical work, the treatment plan then provides the structure and direction for the counseling process that will follow (Seligman, 2004).

Successful treatment planning is expected to benefit the client and clinician—as well as other stakeholders, including the mental health professional community and the third-party payers with whom it does business (Jongsma & Peterson, 2006; Reich & Kolbasovsky, 2006). However, for treatment planning to be effective, each plan must be "tailored to the individual client's problems and needs" (Jongsma & Peterson, 2006, p. 6). In other words, "The individual's strengths and weaknesses, unique stressors, social network, family circumstances, and symptom patterns [all] must be considered in developing a treatment strategy" (Jongsma & Peterson, 2006, p. 6). For students and professionals who are new to treatment planning, this clinical thinking process sometimes can feel like an overly burdensome task (Reich & Kolbasovsky, 2006).

(Continued)

(Continued)

To assist with this, in Chapter 6, we start the treatment-planning learning process. In the chapter, first we discuss treatment planning in the context of today's professional practice. We define treatment planning and explain its basic elements. Next, we take a more detailed look at each element of a successful treatment plan. We explain all of the following:

- Behaviorally Defining the Presenting Problems
- Selecting Achievable Goals
- Determining Treatment Modes
- Demonstrating Changes and Outcomes

Once we have explored each of these elements in detail, we pull it all together. We explain and demonstrate how the diagnosis, case conceptualization, and treatment plan fit together; how to move from the case conceptualization to the treatment plan; and how to complete this work for solution-focused, eclectic, purist, and integrative theory-driven approaches to counseling and psychotherapy. We then summarize what we covered. We provide learning activities and professional and clinical snapshots throughout the chapter, and we refer to our 30 clinical cases in order to illustrate our main points about planning counseling.

By the end of the chapter, you should be able to:

- Define treatment planning, discuss the use of treatment planning in today's professional counseling practice, and explain its relationship to diagnosis and case conceptualization
- Identify, explain, and demonstrate each of the basic elements of treatment planning, including:
  o Approaches to defining presenting problems
  o Approaches to selecting goals for treatment
  o Approaches to deciding on therapeutic interventions
  o Approaches to documenting outcomes
- Demonstrate the ability to fully prepare start-to-finish treatment plans based on (a) a single theory, (b) a psychotherapeutic integration of more than one theory, (c) an eclectic mix of theories, or (d) a solution-focused approach.

TREATMENT PLANNING IN PROFESSIONAL COUNSELING PRACTICE

Counseling and psychotherapy clients experience a wide range of counseling interests, presenting concerns, and levels of need. Correspondingly, the goals of professional counseling and psychotherapy also have a wide range. This wide range includes outcomes aimed at *necessity, improvement, and potentiality* (Herron, Javier, Primavera, & Schultz, 1994). At the level of *necessity*, treatment is designed to reduce or eliminate symptoms that prevent the client from filling basic life roles and taking care of basic life responsibilities and functions. For example,

when counseling is aimed at *necessity* outcomes, goals might include helping the client to meet minimum expectations at his or her workplace, keep his or her family intact, or manage basic self-care (Ackley, 1997; Herron et al., 1994). As illustrations, our clients, Mario (Chapter 7), Sophia (Chapter 10), and Annie Wilkes (Chapter 11), presented *necessity-level* needs.

Next, at the *improvement* level, psychotherapy moves past restoring minimum levels of necessary functioning to facilitating greater psychological adjustment. The aim is to improve the underlying dynamics or situations that led to the person's needs. For example, for a client who is so depressed as to be suicidal, *necessity-level* outcomes addressing safety come first—but later, *improvement-level* counseling might address such goals as resolving the reasons for the depression, reducing the likelihood of future mood problems, and enhancing intrapersonal and interpersonal life adjustment (Ackley, 1997; Herron et al., 1994). Counseling at the *improvement level,* for instance, might focus on personality factors, relationship themes, or other areas where the person's life can be enhanced. As illustrations, our clients Cleveland Brown and Belle (both in Chapter 9) presented *improvement-level* reasons for therapy.

Then, at the level of *potentiality,* counseling goes beyond necessity and improvement, with the goal of helping the person fully reach his or her psychological and social potential. At this level, the aim is to help individuals overcome the roadblocks they are encountering or navigate the crossroads they have reached in their progress toward living and working as completely as possible (Ackley, 1997; Herron et al., 1994). At the *potentiality level,* for example, counseling might be used to reflect on important life patterns, resolve existential questions, add new dimensions to one's relationships, and increase life satisfaction. As illustrations, our clients Juno (Chapter 8)

and Smithers (Chapter 9) presented *potentiality-level* counseling interests and needs.

Fortunately, there is evidence that regardless of the levels of need and counseling interests our clients present, psychotherapy can produce successful outcomes—as long as the structure, direction, and approach to therapy that is used are a good match with the level and type of outcomes that are intended (Chambless et al., 1998; Nathan & Gorman, 2002; Seligman, 1996; Steenbarger, 1994). This is where treatment planning comes in. Designing a carefully prepared treatment plan—that is, a written plan that uses our assessment data, diagnostic impressions, and case conceptualization to establish goals and decide on the sorts of outcomes that should be expected; outlines a therapeutic approach to be employed that is well-grounded in evidence-based practice and informed by judicious use of our own clinical expertise; and states operationally how we will measure the gains accomplished—provides assurance that counseling services with a high likelihood of success will be provided (Seligman, 2006). In this way, treatment planning is a vital aspect of mental health care delivery for the wide range of client needs we are likely to encounter in our professional settings (Ackley, 2007; Reich & Kolbasovsky, 2006; Seligman, 2004).

CLINICAL SPOTLIGHT 6.1: The Case of Sneaky Pee Pee

Assessing the client's needs, determining the therapeutic approach, and establishing measurable outcomes define treatment planning. As an example, one of the authors (Rubin) recalls his treatment approach with a 6-year girl who was referred with the presenting problem of refusing to go to the bathroom while at school. During the assessment stage, the author met twice with the parents and child and gathered additional information from her teachers. He learned that the client eagerly went to school, was doing well academically and socially, was physically healthy, and up till now was on-target with all of her developmental milestones (including toilet training). Her refusal to use the school bathroom appeared to be her main concern. The girl frequently fought back the need to urinate so strongly that she either wet herself during the last period of the school day, on the car ride home, or in the house on the way to the bathroom. Her problem represented a necessity-level counseling need that was interfering with her ability to meet basic everyday functions at school.

The author determined that the client was a resourceful, emotionally expressive, creative, and intelligent child who very much wanted to solve her school bathroom problem. The author and client collaborated to name the problem "sneaky pee pee" based on the way it snuck up on her (the name "sneaky pee pee" was taken from a case by narrative therapist, Michael White (1989), called "sneaky poo"). Measurable treatment goals were set: The ultimate goal was successfully using the school bathroom.

(Continued)

(Continued)

Specific intermediate goals were set in stages: The first goal was to successfully use the bathroom in the principal's office; the next goal was to use the bathroom off the hallway; and the final goal was using the bathroom attached to her classroom. Outcome measures for change in this clinical case were the child's, parents' and teachers' reports of successful use of the bathroom at school and the absence of any toilet accidents.

Regarding treatment, counseling was provided at the school in order to minimize disruption in the girl's life. To decide on the method of intervention, the author designed a plan tailored to the individual client based on his assessment of her dynamics—and based on his extensive clinical expertise and knowledge of evidence-supported practices with these types of child client problems. Specifically, he used a therapeutic integration of Narrative Therapy and Cognitive Behavior Play Therapy. This approach was a good fit with the client because she loved storytelling—and because, interestingly, she enjoyed playing a video game in which she was reinforced for increased skill development with a series of successively colored karate belts as she defeated increasingly challenging ninja penguins.

During treatment, the counselor and client used crayons, Play-Doh, and various other arts-and-crafts materials to create scenarios both at home and at school in which she would confront "sneaky pee pee." Further, during the weekly meetings at the school, these hands-on storytelling exercises were combined with cognitive strategies to "battle her nemesis," including cognitive reframing, in vivo desensitization, and reinforcement. The reinforcements were certificates awarding her ninja karate belts for making progress toward her goal.

After a period of 3 months (seven visits), she was able to use the bathrooms anywhere in the school and had earned her the ninja black belt for defeating "sneaky pee pee"!

THE WRITTEN TREATMENT PLAN

Treatment planning is action oriented. It moves from understanding the client's concerns to deciding what to do about them. In other words, treatment planning provides a road map for reaching desired therapeutic outcomes and is the tool by which counselors put their assessment and diagnostic impressions, and case conceptualization and theoretical approach, to work (Neukrug & Schwitzer, 2006). A fully prepared treatment plan helps the clinician and client develop shared, agreed upon, realistic expectations for the counseling process; sets the specific goals and procedures to be used to track progress and determine whether the expected outcomes are being reached or, alternatively, whether changes to the counseling approach are needed; and provides the therapist with a way to demonstrate his or her effectiveness (Seligman, 2004). Secondarily, the written plan also gives the counseling professional one tool for demonstrating accountability that substantiates his or her work

(or that of his or her agency or practice setting) when communicating with stakeholders such as funders and third-party payers, or when responding to malpractice lawsuits or other legal or ethical challenges (Jongsma & Peterson, 2006; Reich & Kolbasovsky, 2006; Seligman, 2004).

The elements of a standard treatment plan are summarized in Figure 6.1. As you can see, we have included four basic components that are commonly required in today's professional counseling workplaces (Behavioral Health Network, 2005; Jongsma & Peterson, 2006; Neukrug & Schwitzer, 2006; Reich & Kolbasovsky, 2006). Exact formats and treatment plan templates vary. However, we believe that mastering the following four elements will provide the skills you need regardless of the specific format or template you might be required to use in your own specific counseling setting:

1. Behaviorally defining the counseling concerns to be addressed

2. Selecting achievable outcome goals for the counseling experience

Figure 6.1   Four Elements of a Standard Treatment Plan

Behavioral Definition of Problems	Selected from diagnostic impressions and case conceptualization
Goals for Change	Translates the selected problems into operational goals
Therapeutic Interventions	Uses the same theoretical approach found in the case conceptualization
Outcome Measures of Change	Appropriate for the selected problems, stated goals, and therapeutic approach

3. Determining the treatment approach and therapeutic interventions to be used

4. Establishing how change will be measured

Generally speaking, these elements can be presented as a written narrative or in a written table. We illustrate both approaches in each of our 30 clinical cases found in Part III of the text.

Behavioral Definitions

The first task in designing the treatment plan is to select and behaviorally define the client presentations to be addressed through treatment. Generally speaking, the most effective treatment plans can manage only a handful of identified concerns. Although the client may present a variety of problems, dynamics, counseling interests or questions, areas of growth, and other needs during the intake, assessment, or evaluation, our initial job is to select from among these concerns those that will be addressed in counseling. Here, we use our earlier clinical thinking to select our treatment targets: The problems we select come directly from those we already have described in our diagnostic impressions and delineated in our inverted pyramid case conceptualization. At the point of treatment planning, we simply move one step farther, deciding which of the various client presentations will be handled through counseling. As we form our list of concerns to be addressed, we draw directly from our diagnosis and case conceptualization—writing out the client problems operationally in a

way that captures the specific ways in which the person experiences them in his or her everyday life (Jongsma & Peterson, 2006).

Goals for Change

This step works hand in hand with selecting and behaviorally defining the problems to be addressed. Along with selecting and behaviorally defining the targets of our counseling work, treatment planning requires us to select specific, measurable outcome goals. Here, we translate the issues we have selected to work on into clear, operational statements of what we expect to be accomplished at the end of treatment. That is, whereas the first task is to select a handful of target problems from among all of the various client needs we described via our diagnostic impressions and delineated via our case conceptualization, the immediate next task is to clearly and specifically state what we and the client expect to see that will indicate that change has been accomplished. In other words, at this step, we formulate specific goals that indicate what differences in the client's thoughts, feelings, behaviors, or physiology (internal physical sensations and states) we hope to accomplish pertaining to the problems to be addressed (Jongsma & Peterson, 2006; Neukrug & Schwitzer, 2006).

Therapeutic Interventions

Once we have selected the problems to be addressed and operationally defined the goals to be accomplished, the next task is to determine therapeutic interventions. We must make critical decisions about who the service provider will be (including, for example, what setting or agencies are most appropriate, what type of professional is best prepared for the client's needs, etc.), in what treatment formats the client will participate (such as individual, group, couples or family counseling, etc.), what counseling approaches and which specific therapeutic interventions are best suited to the client's needs, and such issues as the frequency and duration of counseling we expect to be required. Here again, we rely on the case conceptualization work we already have completed: We apply the same single theoretical approach, psychotherapeutic integration of approaches, eclectic mix of approaches, or solution focus we used during case conceptualization—at this point moving from using the theory (or theories) to interpret or understand our client's presentation to using the interventions and techniques called for by the theory (or theories) to bring about change (Neukrug & Schwitzer, 2006; Seligman, 2004).

Outcome Measures of Change

To complete our treatment plan, we determine what measures will be used to demonstrate our and the client's accomplishments. This essential task allows us to track our own evolving expertise by documenting over time the results of our clinical work (Hartmann, 1984; Meier & Davis, 2005; Paul, 1988), gives clients and their counselors a method of tracking the progress of their work together (Seligman, 2004), and provides us with a means of substantiating the success and value of our clinical work when we are required to communicate with third-party payers like health maintenance organizations (HMOs) and insurance companies, other stakeholders such as our minor clients' parents, or referral sources like the court system or school personnel (Jongsma & Peterson, 2006; Reich & Kolbasovsky, 2006; Seligman, 2006). Outcome measures can include milestones or short-term gains as well as long-term expectations; pre-post, intermediate, and post measures; client reports and the reports of important others such as teachers or parents; counselor observations; psychological testing results or the results of other clinical assessments; behavioral accomplishments; and other measures. The important bottom line is to select measures that are appropriate for the selected problems, stated goals, and therapeutic approach employed.

SKILL AND LEARNING EXERCISE 6.1

Four Elements of Treatment Planning

Refer to the case of Claire, appearing in Chapter 8, Troubled Youth in Film and on Stage, located later in this text. Briefly read or reread the intake summary, diagnostic impressions, and case conceptualization, and then turn to the treatment plan. Read the narrative and table formats of the treatment plan in detail. Working alone or with a partner, consider the following:

We introduced four basic elements comprising a standard treatment plan. The first element is selecting and behaviorally defining the problems to be addressed. On the basis of the diagnostic impressions and case conceptualization, what problem or problems were selected as targets for change in the treatment plan? From where in the case conceptualization did the counselor identify this problem or these problems? Generally speaking, a treatment plan works best when only a few problems are identified. How reasonable do you find the number and nature of problems (including the main problem and subproblems) defined in the treatment plan for Claire?

We said the second basic element is translating the problems selected into operational goals for change. What goals were set according to the treatment plan? For a treatment plan to be successful, the operationalized goals should be achievable. How reasonable do you find the goals that are provided for Claire's counseling process?

We next said the third basic treatment planning element is establishing the therapeutic approach and counseling interventions. We said the approach should be the same one used in the case conceptualization. What theoretical approach did Claire's counselor select? Does it match that of the case conceptualization? How effective you believe this approach is likely to be in helping Claire reach the goals for change?

We then said the fourth element of the basic treatment plan is determining how change outcomes will be measured. What outcome measures were chosen by Claire's counselor? Do they appear appropriate for the selected target problem(s), operationalized goals, and therapeutic approach?

If you were to be Claire's counselor, how would your treatment plan—the problems to be addressed, the goals for change, the therapeutic approach to be used, the outcome measures—compare with those found in our case illustration?

A Closer Look at Behavioral Definitions and Goals for Change

As you will see by reviewing any of our 30 clinical case illustrations, the first aspects of clinical thinking that are needed when we reach the point of designing a treatment plan are selecting the problems to be addressed, stating these problems clearly and behaviorally, and then defining the specific, measurable outcome goals we expect to be achieved as we and the client work to resolve the problems selected. In fact, one of the most common criticisms of inadequate treatment plans is a lack of carefully selected problems that are translated into measurable goals (Goldman, McCulloch, & Cuffel, 2003). The details of behavioral problem definitions and measurable goals for change are summarized in Figure 6.2.

Selecting and Behaviorally Defining the Targets of Counseling

Because clients often present a variety of concerns during the early assessment stages of counseling, our first need in designing an effective plan for treatment is to sort out which problems are most salient and therefore will become the targets of treatment. To do this, the counselor organizes and prioritizes the concerns for which the client has sought assistance and sorts these into problems that are to be addressed (Jongsma & Peterson, 2006; Neukrug & Schwitzer, 2006; Seligman, 2004). Several factors are considered when narrowing in on the targets of counseling. These include characteristics of the presenting concerns, characteristics of the client, and characteristics of real-world influences. Fortunately, we can use the clinical thinking we already have applied during case conceptualization to bring these factors together as we select and define the problems targeted for treatment.

Characteristics of the Presenting Concerns. As we have discussed, individuals seek assistance for a wide range of counseling interests, presenting concerns, and levels of need—which fall along a continuum of necessity, improvement, and potentiality (Herron et al., 1994). In this chapter, we refer to all of these client interests as "target problems" (even though, strictly speaking, some of these client interests are experienced as opportunities for growth, development, and life enhancement rather than difficulty-causing problems). When deciding on the problems to be addressed via the treatment plan and counseling process that will follow,

Figure 6.2   Summarizing Behavioral Definitions and Measurable Goals

Selecting and Behaviorally Defining the Targets of Counseling	From Case Conceptualization to Treatment Plan

Characteristics of the Presenting Concerns
 	
    Urgency, Dysfunction, Impairment, and Risk
 	
    Necessity, Improvement, or Potentiality
 	
Characteristics of the Client
 	
    Self-Referred, Other-Referred, or Mandated; High, Moderate, Minimal, or No Motivation
 	
Characteristics of the Real-World Influences
 	
    Appropriate for the professional setting's mission
 	
    Achievable within the setting's services limits
 	
    Realistic given the client's accessibility
	Characteristics of the presenting concerns, client, and real-world constraints already should have been carefully evaluated during assessment, diagnosis, and case conceptualization
	
	Therefore, problem selection can be pulled directly from the Thematic Groupings found in Step 2 of the inverted pyramid
	
	Relist the Thematic Groupings directly on Treatment Plan
	
	This approach ties together all of the clinical thinking tools
	
	Selecting Measurable Goals
	
	Goes hand in hand with selection the target problems
	
	Translates each target problem into one or more operational goal
	
	Clear, measurable, objective or behavioral goals are written

clinicians first must consider *urgency, dysfunction, impairment, and risk.* Seligman (2004) referred to this as the "urgency and magnitude" of the client's various needs (p. 159). Naturally, those aspects of client need that are causing the greatest impairment and disruption in the person's ability to fulfill everyday roles and requirements, are causing the greatest psychological and emotional distress, or are causing the greatest risk for impairment or distress—including risk of harm to self or others as well as risk of severe negative consequences such as health problems, relationship problems, occupational and academic problems, or legal problems—are of the highest priority. On this basis, some client presentations receive priority and require more immediate attention in the treatment plan and during the therapeutic intervention that follows. Some areas typically receiving priority are suicidality and other forms of self-harm (e.g., anorexia or dangerous self-mutilation); harm or neglect of others; the diagnostic "red flags" we discussed in Chapter 4 (including substance-related disorders); and any other client needs causing substantial clinically significant distress or impairment. In other words, necessities usually are addressed first, then targets of improvement, and then potentiality.

For example, in our case of Mario (found in Chapter 7, Children's Characters and Video Game Characters), Mario's clinician identified two important presenting concerns: debilitating substance dependence and abuse with low motivation for change, and, secondarily, prominent sleep disturbance due to substance use. Both of these problems were described in the clinician's diagnostic impressions, and both appeared in the inverted pyramid case conceptualization. When the clinician turned next to treatment planning, he prioritized Mario's debilitating substance dependence and abuse to be most urgent and of the greatest clinical magnitude. This was the problem causing the greatest impairment and risk of negative consequences—and therefore was selected to be the treatment plan's target and focus.

Characteristics of the Client. Further, although the professional is expected to take on the role of expert authority during treatment planning, the counselor must actively collaborate with the client when selecting and defining the focus of counseling. Specifically, the client's motivation for change—and his or her motivation for addressing the concerns selected—is a critical variable in forming an effective treatment plan (Neukrug & Schwitzer, 2006; Seligman, 2004). Clients may be self-referred; referred or encouraged into counseling by significant others such as family members, intimate partners, workplace associates, or other people; referred or urged to counseling by those in institutional roles, such as teachers and school or university personnel, employers, or military superiors; or mandated by courts, case managers, probation or parole officers, and the like. Client investment may range from being highly motivated to reduce a current crisis, to highly engaged in addressing broader or deeper concerns, to modestly or minimally interested with little sense of urgency, to motivation that is so low he or she cannot successfully engage in the counseling relationship. When selecting and defining the

problems to be addressed, clinicians also must weigh these factors because the client's motivation to participate in counseling and engage in the therapeutic process depends largely on whether he or she believes the treatment plan will address his or her most pressing needs and counseling interests (Drum & Lawler, 1988; Schwitzer, 2005; Seligman, 2004).

Continuing with our case example of Mario (Chapter 7), Mario's arrival at the treatment center illustrates a situation in which our client was strongly urged into counseling by those around him in important institutional roles (his business manager and employers) rather than seeking assistance on the basis of self-referral. Mario also illustrates a client urged into treatment who is experiencing low motivation for change and little sense of urgency—which is likely to be an initial obstacle to his ability to engage in the counseling relationship. The counselor includes this important factor in the treatment plan's behavioral description of the problem by describing Mario's "minimized perception of substance abuse problem with heightened resistance to change."

Characteristics of Real-World Influences. The real-world practicalities of contemporary mental health care delivery must also be considered when selecting and defining the targets of treatment. The problems selected for counseling attention and the subsequent goals must be achievable, reasonable, and realistic, given the constraints presented by real-world influences. Generally speaking, the problems selected and goals set should be appropriate for the agency, counseling center, clinical practice, or other professional setting in which the counseling will take place. First, the goals must be achievable within the defined mission of the professional setting. For example, school counselors typically should not set goals that require intensive psychotherapeutic interventions for which their setting is not equipped. Further, the goals set must be achievable within the constraint of session limits set by the agency, counseling center, clinical practice, or setting in which the counseling will occur (or by the third-party payers supporting the agency). Other real-world limitations result from the client's access to counseling—such as realistic difficulties attending and following through with counseling due to the competing demands of his or her work, school, child-care schedule, shift work, or deployment—or the client's access to both transportation and medical insurance or other financial considerations delimiting ability to pay for services. Overall, although the counselor must work to support and advocate for the client, he or she and the client must understand the real-world constraints that will influence their work together when deciding on the problems to be addressed and goals to be achieved.

In our client, Mario's (Chapter 7) situation, the treatment plan acknowledges that Mario's presenting needs will be best addressed through inpatient treatment that includes a medical examination; individual and group counseling; and other services consistent with the mission and service offerings found in residential treatment rather than in outpatient or outclient counseling.

From Case Conceptualization to Treatment Plan. Fortunately, when the clinical thinking process we have outlined in this text is followed in detail, all of the earlier work we already have completed conducting the assessment, describing the client's presentations using diagnostic impressions, and then organizing these needs using the first two steps of the Inverted Pyramid Method of case conceptualization, fully prepares us for problem selection and definition! We should already have carefully assessed the client's presenting concerns, thoroughly evaluated the client's own characteristics, and reasonably considered the real-world influences on his or her situation and our potential work together. If we have completed all of the previous conceptual work in detail, we will not need to reinvent the wheel when we reach treatment planning. As a result, our approach to problem selection when we reach treatment planning is

a straightforward one: We pull the targets for counseling right from the thematic groupings we already have listed in our case conceptualization! Specifically, our recommended approach is to use the groups or constellations of symptoms recorded in Step 2 of the Inverted Pyramid Method of case conceptualization as our selected problems in the treatment plan. This allows us to fully capitalize on—and tightly integrate—all of our clinical thinking tools.

Once again, when he began writing the treatment plan, Mario's (Chapter 7) clinician pulled the primary problem targeted by treatment directly from the inverted pyramid case conceptualization: "debilitating substance dependence and abuse with low motivation for change." On the treatment plan, the counselor did round out the behavioral description with additional details, all of which he found directly in the assessment, diagnostic impressions, and case conceptualization he already had completed. Start to finish, the counselor's clinical thinking tools all worked together in an integrated fashion.

Selecting Measurable Goals

As we have said, this step goes hand in hand with selecting the problems to be addressed. Once we know what areas of the client's presentation will be our focus, we then list out a set of specific goals to be resolved or accomplished. These goals are written "so that it is clear . . . when the client has achieved the established objectives" (Jongsma & Peterson, 2006, p. 2). In other words, the goals we derive should be observable or measurable indicators of the outcomes we expect as a result of the therapeutic intervention process. The treatment-plan goals should state how counseling will positively change, reduce, or eliminate the ways in which the targeted problem is revealing itself in the client's life. In other words, the listed goals are objectively constructed (Jongsma & Peterson, 2006). One or more specific, operational (or behavioral) goals is required for each problem that is identified for inclusion in the treatment plan. As you may discover, this nuanced skill—thinking and then writing in terms of clear, specific, behaviorally explained problems and goals—usually requires practice and supervised experience to fully master.

Returning to the illustration, our client Mario's counselor translated the behaviorally defined problem into eight specific, objectively written outcome goals: accepting the fact of dependence, withdrawing from cocaine and alcohol, maintaining abstinence, understanding motivational obstacles, making a commitment to sobriety, acquiring coping skills, gaining an understanding of triggers to prevent relapse, and returning to a life absent of substances.

SKILL AND LEARNING EXERCISE 6.2

Becoming Familiar With Behavioral Definitions and Goals for Change

The treatment plans presented in the 30 clinical case illustrations found in Part III of the text each include Behavioral Definitions of Problems and accompanying Goals for Change. Working alone or with a partner, complete the following:

First, thinking about characteristics of the presenting problems, there are treatment plans with behaviorally defined problems ranging from necessity, to improvement, to potentiality—and varying from high to moderate to low urgency, dysfunction, impairment, and risk. Thinking about client characteristics, there are treatment plans for clients who were self-referred, other-referred, urged into counseling by others, and mandated to counseling—and treatment plans for clients with very high to very low sense of urgency and motivation for change. Thinking about characteristics of real-world constraints, there are treatment plans using brief as well as longer term counseling approaches, inpatient as well as outclient treatment, and other services that are matched with the missions of the professional settings used. Select one case from each of the six chapters in Part III—and for each case, determine the characteristics of the behaviorally defined problems, client, and real-world factors influencing the treatment planning.

Second, for each of the six cases you selected, examine how the counselor moved directly from the case conceptualization to the treatment plan's behavioral definition of the problem.

Third, for each of the six cases you selected, examine how the counselor translated the behaviorally defined problems into measurable goals for change.

Fourth, if these six clients were on your counseling caseload, how would your selection and behavioral description of the problems to be addressed, and your presentation of measurable goals for change, compare with those found in our case illustration?

A CLOSER LOOK AT THERAPEUTIC INTERVENTION

Determining the therapeutic interventions the counselor and client will employ during the counseling process is the core component of the treatment plan and is the destination to which all of our clinical thinking has been leading. This component specifies what experiences and activities will be engaged in during the "working stage" of counseling in order to reach the goals that have been set, thereby resolving or managing the problems identified—on the basis of what we have learned through our diagnostic description and conceptual understanding of the client's needs (Neukrug & Schwitzer, 2006; Schwitzer, Boyce, Cody, Holman, & Stein, 2006; Schwitzer, MacDonald, & Dickinson, 2008). Determination of the therapeutic interventions involves two sets of decisions: those pertaining to the structure of service delivery, and those about the exact psychotherapeutic or other treatment approaches to be used (Neukrug & Schwitzer, 2006; Seligman, 2004).

Decisions About the Structure of Service Delivery

Prior to deciding exactly what counseling or psychotherapeutic approaches we and the client will engage in during counseling, we must decide exactly what the delivery of services will look like. We must make decisions such as who the service provider will be, including what setting, what type of professional, and what types of auxiliary noncounseling referrals might be indicated; and what service formats are indicated (Neukrug & Schwitzer, 2006; Seligman, 2004). Figure 6.3 summarizes the decisions to be made about service delivery structure.

Selecting the Setting. Determining the structure of service delivery that will characterize the therapeutic intervention begins with decisions about which professional setting is best equipped to address the client's needs. As you probably are aware, the most common generalist outpatient or outclient settings include community counseling agencies, private practices, marriage and family practices, school counseling offices and college and university mental health centers, and the like. More specialized agencies focus on services meeting the needs of specific client populations—such as the needs of women, children, clients with low socioeconomic status, and others—or on treatments directed at specific mental health problems—such as suicide crisis centers, practices treating mood or anxiety disorders, treatment facilities for eating disorders, sleep disorder clinics, and the like. Other client presentations—for example, severe child or adolescent behavioral concerns, substance dependence, red flag problems like Schizophrenia and other impairing problems like Bipolar Disorder—sometimes are best addressed in emergency settings, residential and day treatment settings, or through brief or extended inpatient hospitalization. Among our text's case illustrations, for example, you will see services provided in independent private practices (such as Claire, Chapter 8; Cleveland Brown, Chapter 9; and Jack McFarland, Chapter 10), employee assistance programs (including Smithers, Chapter 9; and Fred the Baker, Chapter 11), day treatment (Chief Bromden, Chapter 12), and various other settings. Treatment planning starts with deciding on the most effective, efficient, and practical setting for the individual client's presentation, needs, goals, and circumstances.

Selecting the Type of Mental Health Professional. Determining the structure of service delivery often also includes decisions about which mental health professional might be best suited to work with the client based on his or

Figure 6.3   Summarizing Decisions About Structure of Service Delivery

Selecting the Service Provider

What Setting?

Outpatient Mental Health Centers and Community Agencies

Independent Private Practices

Marriage and Family Counseling Centers

School Counseling and College Counseling Centers

Employee Assistance Programs

Specialized Centers for Specific Populations

Specialized Practices for Specific Mental Health Problems

Residential and Day Treatment Settings

Substance Abuse Treatment Settings

Inpatient Hospitalization

Emergency Settings

Additional Resources

What Type of Mental Health Professional?

Generalist Professional Counselors and Psychotherapists

Family Systems Oriented Therapists and Clinical Social Workers

Doctoral-Level Licensed Psychologists

Psychiatrists

Human Services Case Workers and Chronic Care Managers

Additional Trained Professionals

What Types of Auxiliary Noncounseling Referrals?

Referrals to specialists in problems associated with health, employment, poverty, finances and debt, custody, questions of faith and spirituality, legal needs, or military deployment and reunion—such as medical practices, career consultants, social services, financial counseling, legal services, child-protective services, fleet and family support, clergy, or others

Selecting the Service Formats

Individual Counseling or Psychotherapy

Group Counseling or Psychotherapy

Structured Workshops or Specialized Groups

Couples, Marital, or Family Counseling

Child Counseling or Play Therapy

Academic or Career Counseling

Psychological Assessment and Testing

Psychiatric Evaluation and Medication

Crisis Intervention

Additional Specialized Formats

Multimodal Services

her presentation, needs, and goals. Naturally, selecting the setting and selecting the type of professional usually go hand in hand. Professional training, specializations, competencies, certifications, and licensure vary in the United States by state and community. As a shorthand summary: Some client concerns are well-matched with the skills of generalist professional counselors or psychotherapists; some clients may be best served by family-oriented and couples-oriented marriage and family therapists and family systems–oriented clinical social workers; and some may benefit from the doctoral-level education of licensed psychologists. Further, specialized services such as psychological assessment and testing require the work of a licensed professional with this expertise, who often is a clinical or school psychologist, or a professional counselor trained in these competencies—and diagnosis and evaluation for medication requires the practices of a psychiatrist (although in some cases this is performed by physicians outside the specialty of psychiatry). Case workers also often provide critical support services for clients, especially those with longer standing or chronic needs. Among our case illustrations, for example Naruto (Chapter 7) and Tinkerbell (Chapter 9) used psychiatric services while Elphaba (Chapter 8) and Billie Jean (Chapter 11) used the help of a case manager.

Selecting Auxiliary Noncounseling Services. Although we can rely on counseling to address a wide array of client needs, outside referrals to noncounseling or non–mental health professionals sometimes is an especially effective and efficient way to support, assist, or advocate for a client. For example, in school or college and university settings, referrals often are made for career counseling, academic assistance, or other student success supports. In community settings, referrals to medical centers, legal assistance, financial counseling, social services

and child protective services, mediation, and other environmental supports can provide important auxiliaries concurrent with counseling. Other, more specialized referrals also sometimes are considered: for instance, questions about religious doctrine sometimes go beyond the limits of counseling and require the assistance of a religious professional, and military family needs arising from deployment and reunion might be best addressed by a referral to fleet and family supports. Among the text's case illustrations, our client, Jack McFarland (Chapter 10), for example, might benefit from a referral for career consultation, whereas Jamal (Chapter 8) probably requires the intervention of social services along with counseling.

Selecting the Service Formats. Although typically our first thoughts usually are to equate psychological services with individual counseling, part of the job of determining the structure of treatment involves deciding from among a variety of therapeutic formats in order to identify the mode of counseling that will be "most efficacious for positive client outcomes" (Neukrug & Schwitzer, 2006, p. 235). Usually the decision about service format is made alongside our decisions about what the setting will be and who the service provider will be. Among the common general outpatient service formats are individual counseling and psychotherapy, group counseling and psychotherapy, child counseling and play therapy, and marital and family counseling. Further, more specialized individual counseling, group psychotherapy, psychoeducational programs and workshops, support groups, and other services are available for specific issues—for example, among our text's caseload, Juno (Chapter 8) might benefit from a support group for pregnant teens, Jamal (Chapter 8) may benefit from relaxation training, and both Snoopy (as we have presented him) and Naruto (both in Chapter 7) probably will require family counseling and in-school teacher consultation in addition to child counseling or play therapy.

For individuals who will be served in residential, day treatment, or inpatient hospital in order to address substance dependence, *red flag* disorders, or other seriously distressing or impairing concerns, the service formats are likely to be multimodal—combining, for instance, milieu therapy in the inpatient environment, individual psychotherapy, family counseling, psychoeducation, and postdischarge supports. For example, the needs of our clients Mario (Chapter 7), Tinkerbell (Chapter 9), and Annie Wilkes and Chief Bromden (both in Chapter 12) might be most effectively addressed with this type of multimodal service formats combination.

Decisions About the Interventions: From Case Conceptualization to Treatment Plan, Once Again

Selecting the structure of service delivery sets the stage for our and the client's actual counseling work together. Following our selection of problems and statement of measurable goals, we record the specific interventions we intend to employ directly in the written treatment plan (Jongsma & Peterson, 2006; Neukrug & Schwitzer, 2006; Reich & Kolbasovsky, 2006). It is here that we list "the actions of the clinician designed to help the client complete [his or her] objectives" (Jongsma & Peterson, 2006, p. 2). Here again, as with selecting the problems and stating the measurable goals (discussed earlier in this chapter), when the clinical thinking process outlined in this text is followed in detail, all of the earlier work we have completed leads directly to the listing of interventions on the treatment plan. We pull our therapeutic approach and specific interventions directly from the pure theory, psychotherapeutic integration of more than one theory, eclectic mix of theories and approaches, or solution-focus we have already used to form our

case conceptualization—where we already have carefully selected our therapeutic approach on the basis of evidence-based treatment recommendations and our own clinical expertise. Here again, we are able to fully capitalize on—and tightly integrate—all of our clinical thinking tools.

To do this, when completing this part of the treatment plan, we list out the interventions, actions, or behaviors indicated by our selected therapeutic approach. For example, looking at applications of a single, purist theory, because George Lopez's (Chapter 10) counselor used Reality Therapy in the case conceptualization, you will find that the interventions selected during treatment planning all come from the Reality Therapy approach; and because Jessie's (Chapter 9) therapist used Theraplay in the case conceptualization, you will see that the interventions recorded on the treatment plan each are derived from the Theraplay model. Looking at examples of psychotherapeutic integrations, because Miss Celie's (Chapter 12) counselor relied on an integration of Feminist Therapy and Schema-Focused Cognitive Therapy, you will notice that the interventions found in the treatment plan all come from either Feminist Therapy or Schema-Focused Cognitive Therapy; and since Peter Parker's (Chapter 12) therapist applied a psychotherapeutic integration of Reality Therapy and Cognitive Behavior Therapy during case conceptualization, each of the interventions found on the treatment plan were derived from Reality Therapy or Cognitive Behavioral methods. Similarly, since Snoopy's (Chapter 7) counselor used an eclectic mix of DIR/Floortime Model, Behavior Therapy, and Expressive Creative Arts Play Therapy, an eclectic mixture of techniques from these three approaches forms the therapeutic interventions in Snoopy's treatment plan; and since Billie Jean's (Chapter 11) therapist used a brief solution-focused approach during case conceptualization, the treatment plan also presents brief solution-focused interventions.

CLINICAL SPOTLIGHT 6.2: The Girl Who Was Into Everything

Developing a treatment plan is an important task that requires the counseling professional to use his or her best skills and judgment in order to form a proposed plan for therapy. However, it is important to remember that even the most effectively designed treatment plan can be successfully implemented through counseling only when the client agrees with the plan, collaborates with the counselor, and engages in the therapeutic process. The experience of one of the authors (Rubin) provides a good illustration.

As a licensed psychologist, along with providing counseling and psychotherapy, Dr. Rubin also performs psychological testing. He finds this to be an advantage when he is fortunate enough to continue to work with a client after an evaluation has been completed, because he has the benefit of access to a great deal of biopsychosocial information regarding the client as well as the client's family, which he can incorporate into his case conceptualization and—ultimately—the treatment plan. Such was the situation when he was asked to perform a psychoeducational evaluation in order to assess the intellectual, academic, information processing, and personality functioning of an 11-year-old girl who was in the seventh grade of a small private school. The girl was referred for the evaluation because she was having particular difficulty paying attention in class, remaining on task, following through with assignments both in class and at home, and containing her high energy level. Although her parents appeared to be very loving and caring, they were struggling to effectively provide discipline for their daughter and to provide a calm, organized, and consistent household for her and themselves.

Over the course of the evaluation, the author was able to determine that this client was highly intelligent, creative, energetic, and importantly, on her grade level academically. However, she struggled to hold information in her memory and was easily distracted, impulsive, and a poor planner. Her behaviors met the *DSM-IV-TR* diagnostic criteria for Attention-Deficit/Hyperactivity Disorder (ADHD), Combined Type. On the basis of the diagnosis and case conceptualization resulting from the evaluation, a treatment plan was developed.

The treatment plan took into account not only the assessment findings, but also information gained from consultation with the girl's parents and teachers. First, the treatment plan presented a behavioral definition of the problem based on the *DSM-IV-TR* criteria for ADHD, Combined Type. Next, the author prioritized measurable outcome goals. These included improved attention span and planning skills, enhanced concentration and memory functioning, and reduced impulsivity. It was critical to include goals of helping the parents to better organize their household and schedule and to assist them to improve their overall parental effectiveness.

On the basis of evidence-based best practices and the author's extensive clinical expertise, he determined that the therapeutic approach to be employed in counseling would be Multicomponent Psychosocial Intervention, which is designed to target multiple areas of a client's (and, in this case, the family's) biopsychosocial functioning. Following this theoretical approach, the therapeutic interventions designated in the treatment plan were as follows: parent effectiveness training and family counseling; Cognitive Behavior Therapy; as well as academic remediation targeting memory, and planning and organization skill training.

Outcome measures of change identified in the treatment plan would be as follows: parent and teacher report of improved functioning in class and at home; positive pre-post changes in scores on the Conners-3 Inventory and the Behavior Rating Inventory of Executive Functioning (BRIEF); and clinician observation of increased parental effectiveness and of better organization within the home.

All in all, the treatment plan was closely derived from the assessment, diagnostic impressions, and conceptualization. The problems to be targeted were carefully selected and behaviorally defined, and the goals for change were for critical ones that were measurably presented. The intervention approach was competently chosen, and the interventions were well-rounded and comprehensive. The outcome measures were thorough. The author worked diligently to inform, engage, and motivate the parents. Unfortunately, the couple decided not to pursue counseling. For reasons that remain unclear to the author, they declined the treatment plan and the family did not return to therapy—an occurrence that is not uncommon in professional counseling work.

A Closer Look at Outcome Measures of Change

With the problems to be targeted selected and behaviorally defined, measurable outcome goals delineated, and therapeutic interventions determined, the final step needed to complete the treatment plan is establishing the outcome measures of change to be used to demonstrate the degree to which counseling has successfully met the intended outcome goals. These measures of change provide information that is useful to us as we evaluate the effectiveness of our work; feedback that is valuable to the client as he or she considers his or her progress, and data that are critical to third-party payers and other stakeholders (including the client's parents or family). It is also useful in providing needed information to referral sources and mandating entities (such as courts or schools and others) who require evidence that the resources invested in the counseling process were worthwhile.

Change can be assessed by a combination of subjective and objective measures. Further, some treatment plans include measures of change at designated milestone points along the way during the counseling process, in the form of short-term or intermediate outcomes, as well as measures of end goals, while other treatment plans include only measures of end goals. Naturally, the dynamics of the client, the nature of the presenting concerns, the features of the intended outcome goals, and the structural factors and therapeutic interventions defining the counseling process each can have an influence on exactly what outcome measures of change are most appropriate (Jongsma & Peterson, 2006; Neukrug & Schwitzer, 2006; Seligman, 2004). The exact needs of the intended audience—whether primarily the clinician and client themselves, third-party payers, referral agents, or additional stakeholders—also can influence the selection of outcome measures (Goldman et al., 2003; Reich & Kolbasovsky, 2006). Taken together, some of the most commonly employed methods are: client record and self-report, report by observers, in-session counselor observation, clinician rating and clinical estimate, and pre-post comparisons or post scores alone onpsychometric instruments and psychological tests (Jongsma & Peterson, 2006; Neukrug & Schwitzer, 2006; Seligman, 2004).

Commonly Used Measures of Change

A combination of outcome measures usually is used in successful treatment. This combination relies on client report, reports of observers, counselor observations, clinician ratings, and/or psychological measures.

Figure 6.4 Summarizing Outcome Measures of Change

Measurements of Change Can Occur	Commonly Used Measures Include
At midpoints and milestones measuring short-term gains	Client record and self-report of behavioral change
At termination as measures of end-goal attainment	Reports of observers (parents, teachers, case managers, others)
At both midpoints and endpoints	Counselor in-session observations of behavior change
	Counselor's clinical ratings (using the GAF or another measure)
	Change scores or post scores on psychological instruments

Client Report. Naturally, evaluating the effectiveness of our therapeutic intervention in meeting the goals for treatment begins with the client. Correspondingly, client self-report typically is used as one measure of change. Client self-report can take any of these forms:

- Systematic client verbal report of status, changes, and noticeable outcomes during the counseling interview
- Self-reflective notes or scheduled diary reports kept in between meetings and shared at sessions
- More structured logs and checklists kept in between meetings and shared at sessions
- Other forms of client sharing

You might indicate as outcome measures that clients will report positive outcomes related to necessity-level improvements (experiencing reductions in, or elimination of, symptoms that previously prevented the client from filling basic life roles and taking care of basic life functions), improvement-level gains (bolstering, adding defenses or compensations against, or resolving the underlying dynamics or situations that, at intake, had led to or sustained the person's presenting needs), or potentiality-level change advances (clarifying and improving important life patterns, resolving existential questions, adding new dimensions to one's relationships, or increasing life satisfaction). Depending on the treatment goals, clients may be asked to report about changes in thoughts, affect or mood, behaviors (including interpersonal behaviors), and/or physiological signs. Similarly, they might report on outcomes as experienced in family and home, intimate and social relationships, work and academic settings, and/or other domains as they relate to the behaviorally defined goals.

Observer Reports. In some client and treatment circumstances, observers who fill critical roles and relationships in the person's life might also be utilized as observers and reporters of change. When this approach is included among our outcome measures, observers may be asked to: provide systematic verbal reports about the client's status, changes, and noticeable outcomes

during the counseling interview or by another means of communicating with the counselor; by providing the clinician with observational descriptive notes or scheduled diary reports; or using more structured logs and checklists. Some examples of observers who might be tapped included:

- Parents, guardians, or caretakers
- Teachers, instructors, or school or institutional administrators
- Professionals such as case managers, counseling and psychotherapy group leaders, residential treatment or inpatient staff members, and consulting psychiatrists
- Professionals outside the allied counseling and health fields, such as probation and parole officers, and the like

Counseling professionals must be cautious when using such observers to ensure they are reliable observers and are invested advocates for the person's improvement. Further, all reliance on—and communication with—observers must conform with all relevant ethical codes, professional best practices and guidelines, and legal statutes.

Counselor Observations. We expect the counseling relationship to provide one sample or snapshot of the client's experiences, presentations, adjustment, and functioning. As follows, we typically use the counseling professional's observations and records during interviews and sessions as a measure of change. Counselors observe changes in the client's:

- Cognitive functioning, thought process, thought content, and expressions of thought
- Underlying affective states, current mood, and expression of feelings
- Expressive behaviors, interpersonal relationship behaviors, and other client activity
- Physiological signs associated with thought, mood, or behavior

According to the goals for change, client dynamics, and nature of the counseling process, clinicians might regularly record observations about client outcomes after each session, at other specified intervals, or at termination. These observations should be direct, specific assessments closely tied to the behavioral goals for change—rather than the more general, global notes we often keep as a routine record of the counseling process.

Clinician Ratings. As an alternative to, or supplement to, narrative records of our session-by-session observations, counselors also may rely on systematic ratings of client outcomes. These can take the form of:

- Recording using more structured logs and checklists
- Use of reliable or valid behavioral measures
- Reliance on a widely used measure such as the *DSM-IV-TR's* Global Assessment of Functioning (GAF)

Here again, these records should be direct, specific assessments closely tied to the behavioral goals for change—rather than the more general, global notes we often keep as a routine record of the counseling process. Psychotherapists might regularly record observations about client outcomes after each session, at other specified intervals, or at termination. When these measures are used, the expected amount of improvement in scores, the type of changes to be seen in the results, or changes in the profile to be produced should be stated ahead of time—the increment or quality of change that is hoped for should be written down when the measurable outcomes of change are listed in the treatment plan.

Psychological Measures. Clients, observers, and clinicians each can complete observational logs and checklists. Psychotherapists also may complete structured, formalized clinical ratings such as the GAF. Further data used to document changes in thoughts, feelings, behaviors, and physiological presentations can be obtained by including expected changes in scores from reliable and valid standardized psychological tests and clinical assessment tools. As with clinician rating systems, when reliable and valid psychological measures are used, the expected amount of improvement in scores, the type of changes to

be seen in the results, or changes in the profile to be produced should be indicated ahead of time among the measurable outcomes of change that are written into the treatment plan. Psychological measures fall into several categories:

- General measures of psychological or personality functioning (e.g., the MMPI-2, California Psychological Inventory, or Millon inventories)
- Measures of specific problem areas (e.g., the Beck Depression Inventory-2 measuring depression, Eating Disorders Inventory measuring eating-related concerns, or MAST measuring substance use-related needs) or specific foci of counseling (e.g., the Strong Campbell Interest Inventory examining career development)
- Measures of intellectual and academic ability and functioning (e.g., the WAIS-IV, WISC-IV, other intelligence tests producing an IQ score; and standardized individually administered measures of ability in specified academic domains, such as math, reading, or written expression. The Wechsler Individual Assessment Test [WIAT-3] or academic portion of the Woodcock Johnson Psychoeducational Battery [WJ-3] would meet this particular assessment need).

It should be noted that not only must the psychological measures selected be appropriate for the client experiences to be assessed, but that they also must be appropriately sensitive to change for the time frame in which they are to be used. Further, the goals set must reflect the measures' sensitivity to change, and the change associated with the client capabilities or characteristic to be measured. For example, IQ scores normally are expected to remain relatively stable after early childhood developmental stages, and therefore usually are not good outcome measures of change in most outpatient or outclient settings. These goals can include expected pre-post comparisons or post-treatment-only measurements.

Finally, in addition, structured observational evaluations associated with play therapy or creative expressive arts may be used to produced outcomes of change associated with child counseling clients; these might be grouped with clinical observations, clinician ratings, or psychological measures, depending on the form, content, and statistical characteristics of the measure which employed.

Timelines for Measuring Change

Outcomes can be measured at midpoints and as milestones throughout the counseling process to show short-term gains, at termination to document end-goal attainment, or at both midpoints and endpoints. When they are used, midpoint and milestone measures can be made: (a) following each counseling session, (b) according to the calendar (weekly, monthly, every 6 months, etc.), (c) according to another relevant calendar (e.g., using the academic calendar, at the beginning, middle, and end of a semester; using an occupational calendar, at the start of a new job, again at the end of the new employee probation period, and again after one year of employment; or using a probation or parole calendar, at the time of release to the custody of the probation or parole officer, and again at the time of each scheduled probation or parole meeting), or according to another relevant schedule. Regardless of which

midpoint schedule, if any, is used, the frequency and timeline for measures of outcomes should be stated in the treatment plan at the time it is written. We believe that whenever feasible, setting milestone goals that are assessed by midpoint measures provides valuable ongoing clinical information that is useful to the counselor and client and, often, other interested constituencies.

This chapter's Clinical Spotlight 6.2 presented a useful illustration: in the real-life case example, the therapist's treatment plan used a combination of parent and teacher report of improved functioning in class and at home (observations of others), positive pre-post changes in scores on the Conners-3 Inventory and the Behavior Rating Inventory of Executive Functioning (BRIEF) (psychological measures), and clinician observation of increased parental effectiveness and of better organization within the home (counselor observations) measured at two points in time (following intake and prior to termination) to measure change outcomes. Throughout the case illustrations found in Part III of the text, you will find many different combinations of outcome measures relying on assessment at a variety of time points.

Becoming Familiar With Outcome Measures of Change

The treatment plans presented in the 30 clinical case illustrations found in Part III of the text each include Outcome Measures of Change. Working alone or with a partner, complete the following:

First, review again the 30 cases and identify at least one illustration that employed as an outcome measure of change: client reports, observer reports, counselor in-session observations, clinician ratings, and psychological measures. Among these, include some cases utilizing milestones or short-term gains along with ultimate gains to be observed at termination.

Second, for each of the cases you selected, examine how the counselor moved directly from the treatment plan's behavioral definition of the problem and measurable goals for change to the outcome measures of change. On what basis were milestone or short-term outcome measures selected? On what basis were the endpoint measures selected?

Third, if the various clients you identified were on your counseling caseload, how would your choice of measurable outcomes of change compare with those found in our case illustrations?

PULLING IT ALL TOGETHER: THE TREATMENT PLAN NARRATIVE OR TABLE

Pulling the treatment plan together really means that we have reached the point of pulling together *all* of our clinical thinking, beginning with our assessment work and diagnostic impressions, moving to identifying and organizing the client's presentations via the first steps of case conceptualization, on to using a single or combined set of theories to explain the contributing causal and sustaining factors via the latter steps of case conceptualization—and now reaching the point of behaviorally setting out the goals for counseling; specifically stating the counseling intervention approaches to be used during the counseling relationship; and listing the ways in which you, the client, and other interested parties will measure the counseling process's success. Pulling together the treatment plan indicates you have employed the full range of clinical thinking tools and applied your full range of clinical thinking competences in order to set the stage for the important work in which you and the client will engage.

Many different formats, templates, and paper or electronic forms are used in today's world of professional mental health care delivery. The exact format to be followed often depends on the type of professional setting (outpatient treatment, school counseling, college mental health, etc.), the specific agency or center (the community agency in your location, the school building, the practice, or the campus at which you work), client population (the need level, types of concerns, reimbursement factors), and specifications of interested constituencies (third-party payers like HMOs and insurance groups, referring schools or courts, etc.). It is important to learn about the format to be used before writing up your treatment thoughts into the formalized written plan. Once you are ready to turn to the writing, then it is important for the plan to be "clearly identifiable" in your written records (Reich & Kolbasovsky, 2006, p. 79).

We offer two generic approaches to treatment plan preparation: The first generic approach is to use a narrative model in which the treatment plan itself is clearly titled, each of the four elements (Behavioral Definition of Problems, Goals for Change, Therapeutic Interventions, and Outcome Measures of Change) are clearly subheaded, and contents in each of these four sections is presented in list form. Our 30 case illustrations each include this type of narrative listing highlighted with a shaded background. The second basic strategy is to construct a treatment plan table. To do this, we clearly title the treatment plan, provide the behavioral definition of problems, and then present a three-column table containing: Goals for Change, Therapeutic Interventions, and Outcome Measures of Change. Each of the text's cases also presents a table-style treatment plan.

CHAPTER SUMMARY AND WRAP-UP

This chapter concluded our introduction of the clinical thinking tools that are required competencies in today's professional counseling and psychotherapy world. We characterized treatment planning as the culmination of a clinical thinking process that moves from diagnosis to case conceptualization to intervention. We began the chapter by discussing the role of treatment planning in today's clinical practices, and said that it helps ensure that counseling services with a high likelihood of success will be provided to clients with widely ranging levels of need. We introduced four elements essential to a basic written treatment plan: behaviorally defining the counseling concerns to be addressed, selecting achievable outcome goals for the counseling experience, determining the treatment approach and therapeutic interventions to be used, and establishing how change will be measured. These were summarized in Figure 6.1.

We next examined each element in detail. We explained that Selecting and Behaviorally Defining the Targets of Counseling required us to consider factors including characteristics of the presenting concerns, the client, and real-life influences. We then described how to go from the selected problems to Selecting Measurable Goals, and explained that these two steps work hand in hand. The discussion also focused on how to use the clinical thinking already completed during case conceptualization—forming logical groupings of client presentations and needs at Step 2 of the inverted pyramid—to readily select the problems and behaviorally define the goals of change.

We then examined the Therapeutic Intervention element of treatment planning. We explained that first to be considered usually are Decisions About the Structure of Service Delivery. Here the clinician determines the setting for counseling, the type of mental health professional, auxiliary noncounseling services required, and various service formats to be engaged. As we explained, building on this foundation, we then make decisions about the actual interventions. We said that when completing this part of the treatment plan, counselors list out the interventions, actions, or behaviors indicated by the single therapeutic approach, integration of two or more approaches, eclectic mix of approaches, or solution-focus found in our case conceptualization. In this way, both the problem and the therapeutic interventions for the treatment plan are drawn from the case conceptualization.

We completed the treatment plan by examining Measurable Outcomes of Change. We explained the timeline for measures—which can include measurements of short-term gains at midpoints and milestones, measures of endpoint successes, or both. We also explained the sorts of measures usually used in combination to complete this part of the plan. We said these can include the use of client observations, observations of others, counselor in-session observations, clinician estimates and ratings, and psychological measures. Details for each of these approaches were provided in the chapter.

To finish the chapter, we pulled all of this material together by suggesting two generic formats for constructing the actual written treatment plan: a narrative format, which is illustrated in each of the text's Part III case examples and can be found in gray shading for easy access; and a three-column table format, also illustrated in each of the text's 30 cases.

The chapter's figures, professional snapshots, and learning exercises all worked together to help readers build their treatment planning skills. The chapter made extensive use of the text's case illustrations, both in the chapter material itself, and in the learning activities. This chapter wrapped up our intensive presentation of the clinical thinking skills needed in the transition to professional counseling and psychotherapy: diagnosis, case conceptualization, and treatment planning.

PART III

DIAGNOSIS, CASE CONCEPTUALIZATION, AND TREATMENT PLANNING

Thirty Case Illustrations

7

Children's Characters and Video Game Characters

The Cases of Miss Piggy, Mario, Gretel, Naruto, and Snoopy

Preview: Popular Culture Themes

In this first chapter of five cases, you will meet a group of characters who have gained popularity through a range of mediums such as television, film, literature, comic books, and video games. Although as you will see in their "clinical cases" that they experience widely varying and deeply challenging life circumstances and clinical presentations, each of them is either a child, or childlike, and have thus been brought together in order to highlight clinical themes that are unique to this age group.

Each one of these young characters compels us to examine our preconceived and commonly accepted beliefs about children as they are depicted through the various media of popular culture, and the way in which the various mediums influence our relationships with children. For example, Rose (1995) noted that television's "narratives have become playgrounds for children's depictions of their needs and struggles" (p. 60), and, as such, provide metaphors for them to live by and through which we can understand and communicate with them therapeutically. Since television and film are so ubiquitous in our society, they also exert a very

powerful influence on our perceptions, and in particular, by furnishing consumers (adults and children) with "explicit identity models not of who to be but of how to be" (Ott, 2003, p. 58). Not as positive perhaps, is the way that television's different depictions of boys and girls have reinforced the boundary between masculinity and femininity (Marinucci, 2005). With regard to the depiction of mental illness in children in the media, it has been argued that over the last two decades, particularly since the demise of the *Cosby Show,* that fairy-tale families and idyllic children have lost their appeal to increasingly sophisticated audiences who demand more reality-based, and often edgier, flawed and even fragile characters, particularly children and teens (Johnson, 2006). The downside of this trend is that as in most other forms of popular media, television and film depictions of the mentally ill are laced with stereotypes of violence (Diefenbach, 1997) and often sensationalize psychopathology (Wedding, 2005). Finally, with the advent of social networking and electronic media, the Internet and video games are replete with disturbing and disturbed images of children and teens (Singer & Singer, 2007).

With regard to the specific characters in this section, Miss Piggy, whom we call Clarissa "Miss Piggy" Porciness, was one of the original Muppets, whose love for Kermit the Frog was surpassed only by her self-admiration. She graduated from the provincial constraints of the world of The Muppets to star in major motion pictures, children's literature, and the Ice Capades. In our presentation, Miss Piggy struggles with Borderline Personality Disorder. Mario, whom we call "Mario Alito," is the iconic mainstay of the Nintendo video game empire whose bold and daring digital escapades have made him a hero. Although he is best known for his many video game incarnations, Mario has also leapt to lunch boxes, clothing and even vitamins. In our presentation, Mario struggles with a severe substance-abuse problem. Gretel, whom we rename "Gretel Gerstenhagen," is the sister of Hansel in the beloved fairy-tale story of two impish children who light out into the frightening adult world. The story of *Hansel and Gretel* has traveled across oceans and generations and been retold in numerous cartoons and movies. In our presentation, Gretel struggles with Oppositional Defiant Disorder. Naruto Uzumaki had his start in Japanese manga and anime, and soon crossed the continents as the multimedia star of television cartoons, film, and video games. In our presentation, Naruto struggles with both Attention-Deficit/Hyperactivity Disorder (ADHD) and Conduct Disorder. And finally, there is Snoopy, central character, along with his perennial pal Charlie Brown, in Charles Schulz's famous *Peanuts* comic strip. Like some of the other characters in this section, the tenacious pup has starred in full-length motion pictures, in numerous children's books, and has appeared on consumer products too numerous to mention. In our presentation, Snoopy struggles with Autistic Disorder.

Although a strange assortment, the characters in this section share many of the same behavioral, emotional, and social challenges common to young people in contemporary society. Often feeling misunderstood by adults, they seek the camaraderie of peers. In the process, they experience powerful and long-lasting feelings of rejection, and even abandonment, which leads them to question the safety and security of the adult world. They struggle to regulate themselves in the face of stress, both inner and outer, and in doing so, often make life-changing decisions—sometimes for the better, and other times not. The thin line that separates reality and fantasy for children often presents a challenge for these particular characters, who must gain confidence in themselves in order to cope with very real challenges. Miss Piggy, Mario, Gretel, Naruto, and Snoopy will offer you lessons for learning about our youngest clients.

APPROACHES TO LEARNING

As you learn about this group of characters, pay attention to:

- The manner in which the popular culture representations of children and adults with mental health problems reflects the balance between their vulnerability and resilience.
- How children and adults with mental health problems are depicted in the media, particularly in the movies, and based upon your clinical knowledge, whether those depictions appear realistic.
- How media depictions reflect society's perception of mental health problems in children and adults.
- Whether or not the mental health problems of children and adults depicted in popular culture are consistent or inconsistent with your understanding of the various *Diagnostic and Statistical Manual of Mental Disorders, Fourth Edition, Text Revision (DSM IV-TR)* categories found in this chapter.

CASE 7.1 *THE MUPPET SHOW'S* MISS PIGGY

INTRODUCING THE CHARACTER

Miss Piggy is the porcine star of the long-running children's television entertainment and educational program *The Muppet Show.* Starting her illustrious career as a bit character on *The Muppet Show,* Miss Piggy, by virtue of her charisma, many musical and dramatic talents, and, of course, what became known as her powerful "karate chop," gained instant celebrity among children and adults around the globe. So popular was the porcine beauty that she often appeared outside *The Muppet Show* on television as well as in variety shows and movies with real-life stars, including the likes of Sylvester Stallone, Dolly Parton, and Herb Alpert of the Tijuana Brass. More recently, Miss Piggy and her perennial love interest, Kermit the Frog, appeared on *American Idol.* Her comedic, satiric, and dramatic talents have made her a recognizable and unforgettable mainstay of popular culture. Building on our impressions of Miss Piggy's character portrayal, the following basic case summary and diagnostic impressions describe concerns we imagine she has been experiencing at least since early adulthood, characterized by instability in interpersonal relationships, self-perceptions, and affect; and impulsivity.

Meet the Client

You can assess the client in action by viewing clips of Miss Piggy's video material at the following websites:

- http://www.youtube.com/watch?v=hCN KggRYW2I Miss Piggy on *The View*
- http://www.youtube.com/watch?v= BeuekMbXClw Miss Piggy and Kermit
- http://www.youtube.com/watch?v=b7HY YKEbfLk Miss Piggy singing "I Will Survive"
- http://www.spike.com/video/miss-piggy-pizza-hut/2691925 Miss Piggy dishes it for Pizza Hut
- http://www.youtube.com/watch?v=XhbF5 u9yMkU Miss Piggy meets Joan Rivers

You can also watch the following movie:

- Frawley, J. (Director). (1979). *The Muppet movie.* [Motion Picture]. Argentina: Henson Associates.

BASIC CASE SUMMARY

Identifying Information. Clarissa "Miss Piggy" Porciness is a 32-year-old Porcine American woman who resides in an urban center in Chicago. Miss Piggy currently is employed as the artistic director of Le Muppetrie Center for Artistic Studies in downtown Chicago. Currently she lives alone, following a divorce 3 years ago that ended her second marriage. She was dressed appropriately for the interview in a style that typically would be described as highly socially stylish and would be perceived as somewhat dramatic and seductive.

Presenting Concern. Clarissa Porciness set up an initial intake appointment at the Downtown Counseling Center at the urging of her assistant, Kermit Frogere, who reported that he was concerned about her changes in mood at work and in her interpersonal relationships, and her recent expressions of suicidal thoughts following the sudden ending of a romantic relationship. At times during the interview, Clarissa appeared to be experiencing low mood, was tearful, and expressed self-doubting thoughts, primarily when describing the rejection she felt at the ending of a recent romance, and during two divorces. At other times during the interview, she appeared upbeat, confident, and solicited the therapist's agreement that she was physically attractive and could likely attract "a new man any time I am ready."

Background, Family, and Relevant History. Clarissa Porciness was born the only child in a moderate income household in New Orleans, Louisiana. Clarissa's parents, Maurice and Claire Porciness, worked as street performers and on tourist stages in the city's French Quarter, and according to Clarissa's memory, they were "thrilled at having a daughter whom they hoped could carry on the family tradition," as she apparently demonstrated exceptional musical and singing talent at the age of 4. As a toddler and onward throughout childhood, Clarissa accompanied her parents to street festivals and clubs and was billed as the "Little French Marionette."

She attended magnet schools for the performing arts in the New Orleans school system. She reports that beginning in her later high school years, she began engaging in secretive romantic, and later, sexual relationships with same-age male peers at a neighboring school; secretive, brief relationships with same-age female peers at her own school; and, increasingly, short romantic relationships with college-aged men and, occasionally, women, she encountered while working in tourist venues.

She was married briefly at age 19 while attending a local college for the performing arts. She described the marriage as conflictual. She married again at age 26, which she described as both "exciting" and conflictual. This marriage also ended in divorce. Clarissa reported that she and each partner were "still attracted to each other" but also each having sexual affairs with others, and that she eventually realized that she "felt unloved by my ex-husband, or anyone else." She has been successfully employed in her occupational field throughout adulthood.

Problem and Counseling History. Clarissa Porciness reports that she is ambivalent about the need for counseling, but reports that she is open to beginning counseling "if it will help me learn to choose and keep the right man, or maybe woman, and feel more in control." She also agrees with her assistant, Kermit, that her mood ranges substantially from elation and extremely high self-confidence when "work and relationships are going great" on one hand, to depression accompanied by self-demeaning thoughts and dramatic suicidal fantasies, usually in response to changes in romantic relationships, on the other hand. She also reports having some concerns about her use of alcohol in order "to feel better" and her difficulties managing angry outbursts when her creative work is underappreciated and her angry and rejected feelings when "my best friends and new boyfriends desert me."

Along with alcohol use, she reports "sometimes being a little worried" about impulsive shopping, especially for expensive high-fashion clothing and household items like new furniture and kitchen appliances, when she "isn't feeling so good about myself." She reports that "sometimes I am so angry and under so much pressure I feel like I'm dreaming, like I'm just watching myself go through the motions." She denies any current such thoughts or feelings. Overall, her problem history indicates a sometimes exhausting pattern of unreliable self-worth, relationship-seeking, and defending herself against extreme highs and lows in mood and adjustment via alcohol abuse, irresponsible shopping and spending, and reckless sexual relationships.

Goals for Counseling and Course of Therapy to Date. Miss Porciness is ambivalent about continued counseling and reported that she probably would rather see a medical doctor who could perhaps "give me something to calm my nerves" rather than a "head shrink who just wants to creep into my brain and dissect me like some sort of high school biology pig project." However, she voiced enjoying "having someone to listen to me" and agreed to return for at least several more meetings.

Diagnostic Impressions

Axis I.   V71.09 No Diagnosis or Condition on Axis I

Axis II.   301.83 Borderline Personality Disorder

Axis III.   None

Axis IV.   Problems with primary support group—History of two divorces

Problems related to the social environment—Romantic relationship disruptions

Axis V.   GAF = 50 (at intake)

GAF = 65 (highest level past year)

DISCUSSION OF DIAGNOSTIC IMPRESSIONS

Miss Piggy made an appointment at the Downtown Counseling Center because, at the moment, she was experiencing depressed mood, suicidal thoughts, and feelings of rejection following the ending of a romantic relationship. In the interview, along with and in spite of her depressive mood symptoms, she emphasized her own attractiveness and ability to "attract a man." She also reported long-standing problems with dramatic fantasies about herself, use of alcohol to mitigate feelings of abandonment, instability (changes in affect lasting moments, hours, or days) and reactivity (angry outbursts, brief depressed episodes) of mood, impulsivity (in expensive shopping), highs and lows in self-worth, and on occasion, dissociative symptoms ("watching myself go through the motions").

The purpose of a *DSM-IV-TR* diagnosis is to describe a client's symptoms in order to communicate with other mental health professionals about the clinical picture the client is experiencing. A multiaxial diagnosis presents all the various diagnosable disorders and other conditions that might be a focus of clinical attention on Axis I except for the Personality Disorders and Mental Retardation, which are reported on Axis II. In other words, Axis II answers the questions: "Does the client evidence any long-term pattern of maladaptive character traits that cause significant impairment or distress?" and "Does the client [present symptoms and experiences that] meet the criteria for any of the [diagnosable] personality disorders?" as well as whether mental retardation is present (LaBruzza & Mendez-Villarrubia, 1994, p. 86). Before moving on to a discussion of differential diagnosis for Miss Piggy, it is important for counselors to be aware that diagnostic labels and the expectations they create may communicate gender bias. This may be particularly so in the case of certain personality disorders that reinforce traditional stereotyped perception of men and women (Antisocial Personality Disorder for men and Dependent Personality Disorder for women), and anxiety and eating disorders, which are disproportionately assigned to women (Eriksen & Kress, 2008).

As we have portrayed her presenting concerns, we imagined Miss Piggy to have been experiencing an enduring, stable pattern of inner experience and behavior, present at least since early adulthood, characterized by problematic impulsive behaviors, together with instability in interpersonal relationships, self-perceptions, and affect, which are causing clinically significant distress as well as impairment in her work and personal relationships. Her long-term functioning is characterized by problematic patterns present across her young adult and adult life span, which is the central feature of a personality disorder. Specifically, Miss Piggy's symptoms center around unstable relationships, reactive mood, unstable sense-of-self moving from idealizing to devaluing and impulsiveness, alcohol abuse, and problematic sexuality. These suggest a diagnosis of Borderline Personality Disorder.

Differential diagnoses might include one of the Axis I Mood Disorders; Substance-Related Disorders; as well as Delirium, Dementia, and Amnestic and Other Cognitive Disorders. However, her mood symptoms do not meet the full criteria for a diagnosable depressive disorder (such as Major Depressive Disorder or Dysthymia); there is not enough information to warrant an additional diagnosis of Alcohol Abuse beyond the criteria already provided for Borderline Personality Disorder; and her occasional dissociative symptoms are transient and in reaction to relationship stresses, which also are a part of the Borderline Personality Disorder diagnosis.

To round out the diagnosis, Miss Piggy's relationship stressors are emphasized on Axis IV, and on Axis V her functioning is represented by Global Assessment of Functioning (GAF) scores ranging from the presence of only mild symptoms in the recent past, to the current, more serious symptoms that led to her appointment. The information on these axes is consistent with a diagnosis of Borderline Personality Disorder.

CASE CONCEPTUALIZATION

When Miss Piggy came into the Downtown Counseling Center for her first meeting, her counselor collected as much information as possible about the problems that led to her appointment. The counselor first used this information to develop diagnostic impressions. Miss Piggy's concerns were described by Borderline Personality Disorder. Next, the counselor developed a case conceptualization. Whereas the purpose of diagnostic impressions is to *describe* the client's concerns, the goal of case conceptualization is to better *understand* and clinically *explain* the person's experiences (Neukrug & Schwitzer, 2006). It helps the counselor understand the etiology leading to Miss Piggy's Borderline Personality Disorder and the factors maintaining the concern. In turn, case conceptualization sets the stage for treatment planning. Treatment planning then provides a "road map" that plots out how the counselor and client expect to move from presenting concerns to positive outcomes (Seligman, 1993, p. 157)—helping Miss Piggy better manage her emotions, relationships, impulses, and self-perceptions.

When forming a case conceptualization, the clinician applies a purist counseling theory, an integration of two or more theories, an eclectic mix of theories, or a solution-focused combination of tactics, to his or her understanding of the client. In this case, Miss Piggy's counselor based her conceptualization on a purist theory that is an extension of Cognitive Behavior Therapy, Dialectical Behavior Therapy. The counselor selected this approach based on her knowledge of current outcome research with clients experiencing Borderline Personality Disorder and other personality problems (Critchfield & Smith-Benjamin, 2006; Feigenbaum, 2007; Livesley, 2007; Looper & Kirmayer, 2002). According to the research, Dialectical Behavior Therapy is one treatment approach indicated when assisting clients with borderline personality symptoms (Feigenbaum, 2007). The approach also is consistent with this counselor's professional therapeutic viewpoint and the services offered at the Downtown Counseling Center.

The counselor used the Inverted Pyramid Method of case conceptualization because this method is especially designed to help clinicians more easily form their conceptual pictures of their clients' needs (Neukrug & Schwitzer, 2006; Schwitzer, 1996, 1997). The method has four steps: Problem Identification, Thematic Groupings, Theoretical Inferences, and Narrowed Inferences. The counselor's clinical thinking can be seen in Figure 7.1.

Step 1: Problem Identification. The first step is Problem Identification. Aspects of the presenting problem (thoughts, feelings, behaviors, physiological features), additional areas of concern besides the presenting concern, family and developmental history, in-session observations, clinical inquiries (medical problems, medications, past counseling, substance use, suicidality), and psychological assessments (problem checklists, personality inventories, mental status exam, specific clinical measures) all may contribute information at Step 1. The counselor "casts a wide net" in order to build Step 1 as exhaustively as possible (Neukrug & Schwitzer, 2006, p. 202). As can be seen in Figure 7.1, the counselor included an extensive list of Miss Piggy's mood symptoms (mood volatility, elation vs. depression, angry reactions, etc.), romantic relationship dynamics (divorce, rejection, excessive sexual features, etc.), use of fantasies and impulses to self-regulate (including shopping and alcohol), occasional dissociation, and aspects of her developmental history (objectifying parents, etc.) at Step 1. She attempted to go beyond just listing the main reason for referral and to be as complete as she could.

Step 2: Thematic Groupings. The second step is Thematic Groupings. The clinician organizes all of the exhaustive client information found in Step 1 into just a few intuitive-logical clinical groups, categories, or themes, on the basis of sensible common denominators (Neukrug & Schwitzer, 2006). Four different ways of forming the Step 2 theme groups can be used: Descriptive-Diagnosis Approach, Clinical Targets Approach, Areas of Dysfunction Approach, and Intrapsychic Approach. As can be seen in the figure, Miss Piggy's counselor selected the Areas of Dysfunction Approach. This approach sorts together all of the Step 1 information into "areas of dysfunction according to important life situations, life themes, or life roles and skills" (Neukrug & Schwitzer, 2006, p. 205).

The counselor grouped together (a) Miss Piggy's unstable mood, mood changes, and mood reactivity into the theme "Emotional instability with highs and lows in mood and self-evaluation"; (b) her romantic relationship issues into the theme "Romantic relationship instability with overvaluing and devaluing"; (c) her fantasies, expensive shopping, alcohol use, and dissociation into the theme "Impulsive and reckless behaviors and self-mitigating behaviors"; and (d) her problematic family emotional dynamics into the theme "History of objectification by parents." Her conceptual work at Step 2 gave the counselor a way to begin understanding and explaining Miss Piggy's many concerns as a narrower list of a few clear, meaningful areas of negative functioning.

So far, at Steps 1 and 2, the counselor has used her clinical assessment skills and her clinical judgment to begin meaningfully understanding Miss Piggy's needs. Now, at Steps 3 and 4, she applies the theoretical approach she has selected. She begins making theoretical inferences to interpret and explain the processes or roots underlying Miss Piggy's concerns as they are seen in Steps 1 and 2.

Step 3: Theoretical Inferences. At Step 3, concepts from the counselor's selected theory, Dialectical Behavior Therapy, are applied to explain the experiences causing, and the mechanisms maintaining Miss Piggy's intrapersonal and interpersonal difficulties. The counselor tentatively matches the theme groups in Step 2 with this theoretical approach. In other words, the symptom constellations in Step 2, which were distilled from the symptoms in Step 1, now are combined using theory to show what are believed to be the underlying causes or psychological etiology of Miss Piggy's current needs (Neukrug & Schwitzer, 2006; Schwitzer, 2006, 2007).

According to Dialectical Behavior Therapy (Linehan, 1993a; Morgan, 2005), a blend of behavioral and psychodynamic factors lead to clients' difficulties. These factors primarily center on the environment in which a child develops. Specifically, the theory suggests that when a child has a strong need for validation of his or her highly sensitive emotional core, but the

child's parental or family environment does not provide adequate validation (i.e., the child grows up in an "invalidating and/or abusive environment"), then he or she may develop specific problems with the expression of emotions, engaging in experiences as they are, and engaging in relationships from a rational perspective (Linehan, 1993a, 1993b).

As can be seen in Figure 7.1, when the counselor applied these Dialectical Behavior Therapy concepts, she explained at Step 3 that the various issues noted in Step 1 (unstable mood, etc.), which can be understood to be themes of (a) emotional instability, (b) romantic relationship instability, (c) impulsive and self-mitigating behaviors, and (d) parental objectification (Step 2), are understood to be a group of five problems with Regulation of Emotions and Behaviors drawn from the theory: (a) emotional inhibition, (b) emotional over expressiveness, (c) separation of self from events, (d) seeing reality with distortions, and (e) not accepting experiences without hanging on or getting rid of them. These are detailed more fully on Figure 7.1.

Step 4: Narrowed Inferences. At Step 4, the clinician's selected theory continues to be used to address still-deeper issues when they exist (Schwitzer, 2006, 2007). At this step, "still-deeper, more encompassing, or more central, causal themes" are formed (Neukrug & Schwitzer, 2006, p. 207). Continuing to apply Dialectical Behavior Therapy concepts at Step 4, Miss Piggy's counselor presented a single, deepest, most-fundamental etiological inference that she believed to be most explanatory and causal regarding Miss Piggy's reasons for referral: experience of an invalidating environment in which her parents did not meet psychosocial development needs by validating her emotional core. When all four steps are completed, the client information in Step 1 leads to logical-intuitive groupings on the basis of common denominators in Step 2; the groupings then are explained using theory at Step 3; and then, finally, at Step 4, further deeper explanations are made. From start to finish, the thoughts, feelings, behaviors, and physiological features in the topmost portions are connected on down the pyramid into deepest dynamics.

The completed pyramid now is used to plan treatment, through which the counselor and Miss Piggy will address her deficits in regulation of emotions and behaviors stemming, more deeply, from her experience of an invalidating environment.

TREATMENT PLANNING

At this point, Miss Piggy's clinician at the Downtown Counseling Center has collected all available information about the problems that have been of concern to her and Mr. Frogere. Based upon this information, the counselor developed a five-axis *DSM-IV-TR* diagnosis and then, using the "inverted pyramid" (Neukrug & Schwitzer, 2006; Schwitzer, 1996, 1997), formulated a working clinical *explanation* of Miss Piggy's difficulties and their etiology that we called the *case conceptualization.* This, in turn, guides us to the next critical step in our clinical work, called the *treatment plan,* the primary purpose of which is to map out a logical and goal-oriented strategy for making positive changes in the client's life. In essence, the treatment plan is a road map *"*for reducing or eliminating disruptive symptoms that are impeding the client's ability to reach positive mental health outcomes" (Neukrug & Schwitzer, 2006, p. 225). As such, it is the cornerstone of our work with not only Miss Piggy, but with all clients who present with disturbing and disruptive symptoms and/or personality patterns (Jongsma & Peterson, 2006; Jongsma, Peterson, & McInnis, 2003a, 2003b; Seligman, 1993, 1998, 2004).

A comprehensive treatment plan must integrate all of the information from the biopsychosocial interview, diagnosis, and case conceptualization into a coherent plan of action. This *plan* comprises four main components, which include: (1) a behavioral definition of the problem(s), (2) the selection of achievable goals, (3) the determination of treatment modes, and (4) the documentation of how change will be measured. The *behavioral definition of the problem(s)* consolidates the

results of the case conceptualization into a concise hierarchical list of problems and concerns that will be the focus of treatment. The *selection of achievable goals* refers to assessing and prioritizing the client's concerns into a *hierarchy of urgency* that also takes into account the client's motivation for change, level of dysfunction and real-world influences on his or her problems. The *determination of treatment modes* refers to selection of the specific interventions, which are matched to the uniqueness of the client and to the client's goals and clearly tied to a particular theoretical orientation (Neukrug & Schwitzer, 2006). Finally, the clinician must establish how change will be measured based upon a number of factors, including client records and self-report of change, in-session observations by the clinician, clinician ratings, results of standardized evaluations such as the Beck Depression Inventory (Beck, Steer, & Brown, 1996), pre-post treatment comparisons, and reports by other treating professionals.

The four-step method discussed above can be seen in Figure 6.1 (p. 109) and is outlined below for the case of Miss Piggy, followed by her specific treatment plan.

Step 1: Behavioral Definition of Problems. The first step in treatment planning is to carefully review the case conceptualization, paying particular attention to the results of Step 2 (Thematic Groupings), Step 3 (Theoretical Inferences), and Step 4 (Narrowed Inferences). The identified clinical themes reflect the core areas of concern and distress for the client, while the theoretical and narrowed inferences offer clinical speculation as to their origins. In the case of Miss Piggy, there are two primary areas of concern. The first, "deficits in regulation of emotions and behaviors," refers to her unstable mood, quick shifting from idealizing to devaluing herself and others, occasional impulsive and reckless behavior, suicidal ideation, and the use of alcohol. The second, "romantic relationship instability," refers to her quick shifting from idealizing to devaluing others, and overvaluing sexuality and

Figure 7.1 Miss Piggy's Inverted Pyramid Case Conceptualization Summary: Dialectical Behavior Therapy

1. IDENTIFY AND LIST CLIENT CONCERNS

Unstable mood, angry outbursts
Occasional dissociation
Mood changes at work ("watching myself
  go through the motions")
Mood changes in personal relationships
Periods of elation and grandiosity
Periods of depression and self-demeaning
Moves from idealizing to devaluing self and
  others
Occasional suicidal ideation
History of being objectified by parents
History of being showcased child actress
"Little French Marionette" as toddler

Adult history of 2 divorces
Adult history of romantic rejections
Overvaluing of sexuality
Overvaluing own sexual attractiveness
Adolescent sexuality with older partners
Ambiguous sexual relationships with female
  partners
Dramatic, grandiose fantasies about self
Use of alcohol to mitigate abandoned feelings
Use of expensive shopping to mitigate
  devalued feelings

2. ORGANIZE CONCERNS INTO LOGICAL THEMATIC GROUPINGS

1. Emotional instability with highs and lows in mood and self-evaluation
2. Romantic relationship instability with overvaluing and devaluing
3. Impulsive and reckless behaviors and self-mitigating behaviors
4. History of objectification by parents

3. THEORETICAL INFERENCES: ATTACH THEMATIC GROUPINGS TO INFERRED AREAS OF DIFFICULTY

Deficits in Regulation of Emotions and Behaviors

1. Emotional inhibition in attempt
   to be accepted
2. Emotional overexpressiveness in attempt
   to have feelings understood
3. Separates self from ongoing events
   and interactions
4. Does not see reality without
   distortions
5. Does not accept experiences
   without attempting to hang on
   to or get rid of them

4. NARROWED INFERENCES: SUICIDALITY AND DEEPER DIFFICULTIES

Deeper Etiological Inference
Invalidating Environment:
Parental environment
did not validate
sensitive emotional
core

promiscuous and seductive behaviors. These symptoms and personality patterns are consistent with the diagnosis of Borderline Personality Disorder (APA, 2000a; Linehan, Heard, & Armstrong, 1993; Paris, 2000).

Step 2: Identify and Articulate Goals for Change. The second step is the selection of achievable goals, which is based upon a number of factors, including the most pressing or urgent behavioral, emotional, and interpersonal concerns and symptoms as identified by the client and clinician, the willingness and ability of the client to work on those particular goals, and the realistic (real-world) achievability of those goals (Neukrug & Schwitzer, 2006). At this stage of treatment planning, it is important to recognize that not all of the client's problems can be addressed at once, so we focus initially on those that cause the greatest distress and impairment. New goals can be created as old ones are achieved. In the case of Miss Piggy, the goals are divided into two prominent clusters. Her "deficits in regulation of emotions and behaviors" requires that we enhance her ability to accurately label and express feelings, achieve balance between idealizing and devaluing herself, understand and eliminate dangerous and impulsive behavior, and reduce the frequency of her suicidal ideation and behavior. Her romantic relationship instability requires that we assist her to identify relationship triggers that lead to overvaluing and devaluing of others, to recognize and control her use of sex to manipulate others, to become comfortable with her own sexuality, and to decrease dependence on others to meet own needs while building confidence and assertiveness.

Step 3: Describe Therapeutic Interventions. This is perhaps the most critical step in the treatment planning process because the clinician must now integrate information from a number of sources, including the case conceptualization, the delineation of the client's problems and goals, and the treatment literature, paying particular attention to

empirically supported treatment (EST) and *evidence-based practice* (EBP). In essence, the clinician must align his or her treatment approach with scientific evidence from the fields of counseling and psychotherapy. Wampold (2001) identifies two types of evidence-based counseling research: studies that demonstrate "absolute efficacy," that is, the fact that counseling and psychotherapy work, and those that demonstrate "relative efficacy," that is, the fact that certain theoretical/technical approaches work best for certain clients with particular problems (Psychoanalysis, Gestalt Therapy, Cognitive Behavior Therapy, Brief Solution-Focused Therapy, Cognitive Therapy, Dialectical Behavior Therapy, Person-Centered Therapy, Expressive/Creative Therapies, Interpersonal Therapy, and Feminist Therapy) and when delivered through specific treatment modalities (individual, group, and family counseling). In the case of Miss Piggy, we have decided to use Dialectical Behavior Therapy because of its demonstrated effectiveness with clients experiencing Borderline Personality Disorder (Binks et al., 2009; Feigenbaum, 2007; Linehan, 1993a, 1993b; Linehan et al., 1993). This therapeutic approach relies on a combination of methods (cognitive behavior modification, mindfulness training, transference work and dialectics) that target the common factors of personality disorder treatment (therapeutic structure, relationships) (Livesley, 2007) and the deficits that are specific to borderline conditions. Specific techniques for Miss Piggy will include strengthening of the client-therapist relationship, development of self-esteem enhancement techniques, exploring family-of-origin relationships, and group counseling to enhance relationship skills.

Step 4: Provide Outcome Measures of Change. This last step in treatment planning requires that we specify how change will be measured and indicate the extent to which progress has been made toward realizing these goals (Neukrug & Schwitzer, 2006). The counselor has considerable flexibility in this phase and may choose from a number of objective domains (psychological tests and measures of self-esteem, depression, psychosis, interpersonal relationship, anxiety, etc.), quasi-objective measures (the *DSM-IV-TR's* Axis V GAF scale; pre-post clinician, client, and psychiatric ratings), and subjective ratings (client self-report, clinician's in-session observations). In Miss Piggy's case, we have included a number of these, including decreased client-reported frequency of impulsive and suicidal acts, clinician observation of stabilized mood, gradual increase in her GAF, and decrease of drinking in response to stress.

The completed treatment plan is now developed through which the counselor and Miss Piggy will begin their shared work to modify and hopefully decrease her prominent symptomatolgy, build coping skills, improve the quality of her relationships, and move in the direction of overall positive change. Miss Piggy's treatment plan follows and is summarized in Table 7.1.

TREATMENT PLAN

Client: Clarissa "Miss Piggy" Porciness

Service Provider: Downtown Counseling Center—Female Individual Counselor

BEHAVIORAL DEFINITION OF PROBLEMS:

1. Deficits in regulation of emotions and behaviors—Unstable mood; rapid changes from sadness to elation, shifts quickly from idealizing to devaluing self, occasional impulsive and reckless behavior, suicidal ideation, use of alcohol and shopping to mitigate devalued feelings

2. Romantic relationship instability—Shifts quickly from idealizing to devaluing others, over-valuing of sexuality, promiscuous and seductive behavior

GOALS FOR CHANGE:

1. Deficits in regulation of emotions and behaviors

   - Enhance ability to accurately label and express feelings
   - Achieve balance between idealizing and devaluing self
   - Understand and eliminate dangerous and impulsive behavior
   - Reduce frequency of suicidal ideation and behavior

2. Romantic relationship instability

   - Identify relationship triggers that lead to overvaluing and devaluing of other
   - Recognize and control the use of sex to manipulate others
   - Become comfortable with own sexuality
   - Decrease dependence on others to meet own needs; build confidence, and assertiveness

(Continued)

(Continued)

THERAPEUTIC INTERVENTIONS:

An intermediate- to long-term course of individual counseling (6 months to a year) using key elements of Dialectical Behavior Therapy (DBT), supplemented by group intervention to address alcohol abuse and relationship issues

1. Deficits in regulation of emotions and behaviors

   - Encourage discussion of emotions, both positive and negative
   - Develop cognitive and behavioral strategies for enhancing self-esteem
   - Identify experiences that lead to positive self-regard and cognitions that interfere with it
   - Recognize relationship between internal states and the need to shop and drink
   - Identify emotional and behavioral triggers for impulsive behavior
   - Recognize the rewards and negative consequences for impulsive behavior
   - Develop a strategy for seeking help when feeling suicidal
   - Refer for evaluation to determine the need for medication
   - Refer to psychoeducational group for alcohol abuse

2. Romantic relationship instability

   - Discuss importance of working collaboratively with therapist around needs for dependency and boundaries
   - Explore family of origin relationship, particularly the devaluing and objectification by parents
   - Identify triggers for feelings of abandonment and their relationship to suicidal feelings and impulsive behaviors
   - Assign client to group counseling to build relationship effectiveness skills, including assertiveness and the expression of needs
   - Develop cognitive and behavioral skills to identify and correct distorted perceptions in relationship to valuation of self and others

OUTCOME MEASURES OF CHANGE:

The development of enhanced ability to regulate mood, self-esteem, and relationship stability will be measured by:

- Client's regular attendance in counseling and positive assessment of her ability to clearly communicate her thoughts and feelings
- Gradual stabilization of clinician's rating of client's GAF to the mild range (>70)
- Increased scores on standardized self-esteem inventory as well as client's self-report and clinician's recording of positive self-statements
- Decreased client-reported frequency of impulsive acts and suicidal thoughts
- Gradual decrease of stress-related and emotionally motivated drinking
- Client report of reduced interpersonal conflicts and improved communication and problem-solving within romantic relationships
- Clinician observation of client's stabilized mood along with pre-post measures of improvement on Beck Depression Inventory-II

Table 7.1   Miss Piggy's Treatment Plan Summary: Dialectical Behavior Therapy

Goals for Change	Therapeutic Interventions	Outcome Measures of Change
Deficits in regulation of emotions and behaviors	Deficits in regulation of emotions and behaviors	The development of enhanced ability to regulate mood, self-esteem, and relationship stability will be measured by:
Enhance ability to accurately label and express feelings	Encourage discussion of emotions, both positive and negative	Client's regular attendance in counseling and positive assessment of her ability to clearly communicate her thoughts and feelings
Achieve balance between idealizing and devaluing self	Develop cognitive and behavioral strategies for enhancing self-esteem	
Understand and eliminate dangerous and impulsive behavior	Identify experiences that lead to positive self-regard and cognitions that interfere with it	Gradual stabilization of clinician's rating of client's GAF to the mild range (>70)
Reduce frequency of suicidal ideation and behavior	Recognize relationship between internal states and the need to shop and drink	Increased scores on standardized self-esteem inventory as well as client's self-report and clinician's recording of positive self-statements
Romantic relationship instability	Identify emotional and behavioral triggers for impulsive behavior	
Identify relationship triggers that lead to overvaluing and devaluing of others	Recognize the rewards and negative consequences for impulsive behavior	
Recognize and control the use of sex to manipulate others	Develop a strategy for seeking help when feeling suicidal	Decreased client-reported frequency of impulsive acts and suicidal thoughts
Become comfortable with own sexuality	Refer for evaluation to determine the need for medication	Gradual decrease of stress-related and emotionally motivated drinking
Decrease dependence on others to meet own needs, build confidence and assertiveness	Refer to psychoeducational group for alcohol abuse	
Romantic relationship instability	Romantic relationship instability	Client report of reduced interpersonal conflicts and improved communication and problem-solving within romantic relationships
Identify relationship triggers that lead to overvaluing and devaluing of other	Discuss importance of working collaboratively with therapist around needs for dependency and boundaries	
Recognize and control the use of sex to manipulate others	Explore family of origin relationships, particularly the devaluing and objectification by parents	Clinician observation of client's stabilized mood along with pre-post measures of improvement on the Beck Depression Inventory-II
Become comfortable with own sexuality	Identify triggers for feelings of abandonment and their relationship to suicidal feelings and impulsive behaviors	
Decrease dependence on others to meet own needs, build confidence, and assertiveness	Assign client to group counseling to build relationship effectiveness skills, including assertiveness and the expression of needs	
	Develop cognitive and behavioral skills to identify and correct distorted perceptions in relationship to valuation of self and others	

CASE 7.2 NINTENDO'S MARIO

INTRODUCING THE CHARACTER

Mario is the iconic star of Nintendo's globally known video game series of the same name. The character—a diminutive, Italian, mustachioed plumber complete with overalls—was created by Japanese manga artist Shigeru Miyamoto, was first introduced in 1981 as "Jump Man" in the early video game Donkey Kong, and by now has starred in more than 100 Nintendo games.

The many incarnations of the original video game featuring Mario were loosely based upon the Disney cartoon, Popeye. Mario, who has incredible jumping ability, continually battles against his nemesis, Bowser, to rescue Princess Peach from a variety of dangerous situations. Mario has appeared in many video games; has crossed over into television shows, comic books, and movies; has been imprinted on lunch boxes, T-shirts, magazines, and shampoo bottles; and has even been incarnated as a plush toy. Considered by many to be as recognizable as Mickey Mouse, Mario is Nintendo's mascot and has earned seven world records in the 2008 gamers' edition of *Guinness World Book of Records*. These records include: best-selling video games series of all time, first movie based on an existing video game, and the most prolific video game character. Expanding on what is known about the Mario character, the following basic case summary and diagnostic impressions fill in more of our own imagined details about Mario and describe areas of dysfunction we believe he has been confronting since adolescence and throughout adulthood, stemming from his problematic use of cocaine and alcohol, along with some self-aggrandizing personality features.

> ### Meet the Client
>
> You can assess the client in action by viewing clips of Mario's video material at the following websites:
>
> - http://www.youtube.com/watch?v=82TS WzOsPYc Mario hard at work
> - http://www.youtube.com/watch?v=iO 10_IbDUBU Mario, the intergalactic star

BASIC CASE SUMMARY

Identifying Information. Mario Alito, born Nunzio Alito, is a 44-year-old European American of Italian family heritage who resides in both South Beach, Florida, and Beverly Hills, California. Mario currently is employed as a photographic and action model, working primarily as the image of Mario of the Nintendo games, and as "Mario the Romancer," whose visage has been featured on the cover of more than 200 teen romance novels. In this occupational role, he is known as the "Fabio of video games." His appearance was appropriate for the interview.

Presenting Concern. Mario arrived at this private Beverly Hills Drug Rehabilitation Center at the urging of his agent, following what was described as a "2-week cocaine binge" that resulted in the threat of losing his video game contract and primary source of income. His agent first referred him as contestant on the television reality show, *Celebrity Rehab,* but he was rejected for the show because his condition was assessed as being too fragile. At the center, his intake was performed by a multidisciplinary team comprising a psychiatrist, a psychologist, a milieu specialist, and the substance-abuse coordinator. Up to this most recent incident, Mario insisted he had used cocaine "only recreationally," but had decided to "let it all go" soon after discovering that his contracts with both Nintendo and Teen Heart Publishing might not be renewed.

Background, Family Information, and Relevant History. Mario Alito was born in Miami, Florida. His family of origin included his father, mother, and two siblings; both of his older sisters were in middle school at the time of his birth. Mario described his parents as devout Catholics who had hopes that he would become a priest. He attended private Catholic schools in Miami where, according to the client, his "charm, stunning good looks, and athletic prowess" garnered him popularity among male and female peers as well as his teachers. He described academic difficulties during his elementary and middle school years that may have been associated with an undetected learning disability, and reported compensating by developing facility at cheating as well as manipulating more vulnerable students to do his work for him. Apparently his parents knew nothing of these negative activities and believed instead that their son was living up to all of their expectations for him.

During high school, Mario excelled at gymnastics and won the State high-jump championship during each of his 4 years, which earned him the attention of the media. In addition, by the time he was a sophomore, Mario was working occasionally in modeling for local fashion magazines and on television commercials. Mario reports he was popular and highly socially active with male peers and socially and sexually active with high school girlfriends. At the same time, it appears he began sometimes alienating friends and teachers by dwelling on his accomplishments, talents, and what he saw as an unlimited future of success and wealth. During his junior year in high school, Mario began drinking alcohol on weekends at football games, parties, and other social events, usually becoming at least mildly intoxicated and usually driving himself and dates or friends home. He reports being introduced to cocaine in the summer before his senior year, and he said in retrospect "I loved the rush . . . the parties got better, girls really noticed me, and I was one of the coolest kids." He reports that his use increased to weekly, usually on weekends. When he was arrested at age 17 for a minor cocaine possession, his parents denied that their son was involved in drugs, quickly bailed him out of jail, and took him to the mandatory 6-week drug-abuse counseling program, where he essentially manipulated the therapist into believing that he had used cocaine on only several occasions.

During a gymnastics competition in his senior year, Mario was approached by a talent agent who was well connected with the video game industry. In fact, an advertising representative from the Nintendo Corporation noticed Mario and believed that his image would be perfect for the prototype of an Italian video game character that was in development and was based on the cartoon character Popeye. Within 2 years, Mario's athletic prowess was transformed into what would become the most famous video game character of all time, Mario. As a sideline, he capitalized on his physical attractiveness and unique looks by modeling for teen romance novel covers. By that time, Mario was in his late 30s, wealthy, famous, and world renown. He apparently engaged in a lifestyle described by his agent as "week-long cocaine binges, jet setting, and womanizing." After recently being arrested for public indecency and intoxication, his contracts with both Nintendo and Teen Heart Publishing were in jeopardy of being canceled. Over this time period, Mario has had diminishing contact with his parents and adult sisters; friends, colleagues, and professional contacts other than his agent appear to have distanced themselves from him.

Problem and Counseling History. With the exception of his brief psychoeducational intervention during high school, Mario has neither received nor sought counseling services for his substance use. He made it quite clear from the outset that "I don't really think I have a problem. . . . If you were losing your livelihood, what would you do?" Mario sat impatiently throughout the intake interview, seemingly more interested in entertaining the interviewers and providing a resume than he was in disclosing relevant personal information about himself. He spoke frequently and intensely about his fame and popularity and the "enormous pressure that comes with being an icon."

Information gathered suggests that Mario's alcohol use has increased since his early high school years. His weekend use appears to have increased during his teen years and early 20s to half-week use, often from Wednesdays through Sunday or Monday. However, it appears that this use has remained about the same or diminished some in recent years as he has increasingly used powder cocaine. His present alcohol use seems most present when he is unable to locate cocaine, his drug of choice (e.g., when he is traveling by airplane between his two home cities). It is notable that he has missed several video game filmings and photo obligations due to hangover symptoms, in spite of warnings from his employers and agent. However, outside of minor hangovers, he does not report losing interest or giving up other social or life activities and does not seem to have increased his use beyond long weekends or "in between" cocaine episodes.

Information gathered also suggests that Mario's cocaine use has increased since his early high school years. His weekend use appears to have increased during his teen years and early 20s to half-week use, and at times, week-long use, especially in between work obligations. He reports that "although I certainly don't have a problem," he has several times attempted to curb use at the request of a romantic partner or his agent, but generally found himself unable to "just cut down." In fact, he appears to be spending more of his income, and a greater amount of his time, locating and using increasing amounts of cocaine (in comparison with his steady alcohol use rates). He says the increase is so that "I can still feel that great rush." Further, he seems to use this substance at unplanned times to ward off extreme tiredness, nightly trouble sleeping, and feeling agitated and irritated when he stops use. Of note, he finds that sleep becomes difficult when he is using cocaine and then does not return to normal, and he said he rarely sleeps through the night; the client attributes his sleep deficits and fatigue to jet lag.

Goals for Counseling and Course of Therapy to Date. When asked if he would like to once again admit himself into the clinic's substance-abuse rehab program for treatment beyond the intake screening, Mario adamantly denied having "a problem with drugs." He did agree to short-term counseling "as long as I can get back on my feet, clean up my image, and get back out there on stage where I belong."

Diagnostic Impressions

Axis I.   304.3 Cocaine Dependence with Physiological Dependence

292.89 Cocaine-Induced Sleep Disorder, Insomnia Type, With Onset During Intoxication

305.00 Alcohol Abuse

Axis II. V71.09 No Diagnosis on Axis II

Axis III. None

Axis IV. Occupational Problems—Threat of job loss

Problems with Primary Support Group—Unstable relationships

Axis V. GAF = 52 (at admission)

GAF = 65 (highest level past year)

DISCUSSION OF DIAGNOSTIC IMPRESSIONS

Mario's arrival at the Beverly Hills Drug Rehabilitation Center was prompted by a cocaine binge that resulted in the threat of job loss.

Although during his evaluation Mario denied "having a problem," his history indicates that his cocaine use has steadily increased since it began during his high school years. He describes feeling agitated and irritable when he stops use, which are signs of withdrawal. According to his history, his pattern of use includes periods during which he was unsuccessful at cutting down his use despite his efforts to do so; his spending excessive time, effort, and money to obtain cocaine; and continued use despite his knowledge that it is interfering with his intimate relationships and work obligations. In addition, his history of recurrent alcohol use has resulted in missed work obligations, and drinking to the point of having hangovers, despite his knowledge of these ill effects. Finally, Mario disclosed in the interview that he has prominent disturbances in sleep that developed during his cocaine use and withdrawal.

The Substance-Related Disorders of the *DSM-IV-TR* comprise all of the Substance Use Disorders (Dependence and Abuse) and Substance Induced Disorders (Intoxication, Withdrawal, and substance-induced disruptions in mood, sleep, and sexual function) related to the use of 11 classes of drugs (including alcohol), medications, and toxins. Diagnosable *DSM-IV-TR* Substance-Related Disorders do not address nonproblematic experimentation and the social or recreational use of alcohol or other drugs; rather, diagnosable disorders pertain only to abuse and dependence and other clinically significant patterns of substance-related behavior resulting in negative life consequences (Inaba & Cohen, 2000). These disorders are listed on Axis I.

Expanding on his video game persona by filling in our own imagined details, we described Mario as presenting problematic use of cocaine and alcohol, including negative effects on his sleep. His cocaine use comprises a maladaptive pattern in which he experiences unsuccessful efforts to cut down, commitment of substantial time to use and recovery, and persistence even in light of negative consequences in his interpersonal and work life. This kind of substance use pattern indicates a diagnosis of Cocaine Dependence. The diagnosis is subtyped With Physiological Dependence because Mario experiences characteristic withdrawal symptoms when he occasionally reduces or ceases his heavy, prolonged use. His alcohol use comprises a maladaptive pattern in which he continues

drinking despite his knowledge of negative consequences at work and in other areas of his life. Finally, his sleep disruption seems sufficiently problematic as to interfere with his daily functioning and therefore warrants a diagnosis. His sleep problems developed during cocaine intoxication and are not better accounted for by another cause, indicating a diagnosis of Cocaine-Induced Sleep Disorder. Mario's problem is trouble maintaining sleep rather than excessively sleeping and began during cocaine use rather than withdrawal; therefore, the diagnosis is subtyped Insomnia Type and the specifier With Onset During Intoxication is used.

Differential diagnoses might include Alcohol Dependence rather than Alcohol Abuse; and, regarding sleep, Circadian Rhythm Sleep Disorder, Jet Lag Type. However, unlike Mario's cocaine use, his alcohol use pattern meets the criteria for the less advanced diagnosis, abuse, rather than the more advanced diagnosis, dependence. Likewise, although the client attributes his sleep difficulties to a mismatch between his sleep-wake schedule due to jet travel, there is no evidence to support this, and his insomnia is better accounted for by his substance use.

To complete the diagnosis, Mario's work and relationship stressors are emphasized on Axis IV, and on Axis V his functioning is represented by GAF scores ranging from mild symptoms in the recent past to the current, moderately serious symptoms that led to his arrival at the center. This information is consistent with the substance-related diagnostic pattern on Axis I.

CASE CONCEPTUALIZATION

When Mario came into the private Beverly Hills Drug Rehabilitation Center, he participated in an initial screening and assessment process conducted by a multidisciplinary evaluation team. During the process, as much information as possible was collected about the symptoms and situations leading to Mario's referral. Included among the intake materials were a thorough psychosocial, medical, and substance use history;

client report; team observations; and other reports. Based on the evaluation, his counselor and the team developed diagnostic impressions, describing his presenting concerns by Cocaine Dependence, the insomnia type of Cocaine-Induced Sleep Disorder, and Alcohol Abuse. A case conceptualization next was developed. Whereas the purpose of diagnostic impressions is to *describe* the client's concerns, the goal of case conceptualization is to better *understand* and clinically *explain* the person's experiences (Neukrug & Schwitzer, 2006). It helps the counselor understand the etiology leading to Mario's substance use and related problems, and the factors maintaining these concerns. In turn, case conceptualization sets the stage for treatment planning. Treatment planning then provides a road map that plots out how the counselor and client expect to move from presenting concerns to positive outcomes (Seligman, 1993, p. 157)—helping Mario reduce or eliminate his problematic substance use and improve his sleep.

When forming a case conceptualization, the clinician applies a purist counseling theory, an integration of two or more theories, an eclectic mix of theories, or a solution-focused combination of tactics to his or her understanding of the client. In this case, Mario's counselor and the intake team based the conceptualization on psychotherapeutic integration of two theories (Corey, 2009). Psychotherapists very commonly integrate more than one theoretical approach in order to form a conceptualization and treatment plan that will be as efficient and effective as possible for meeting the client's needs (Dattilo & Norcross, 2006; Norcross & Beutler, 2008). In other words, counselors using the psychotherapeutic integration method attempt to flexibly tailor their clinical efforts to "the unique needs and contexts of the individual client" (Norcross & Beutler, 2008, p. 485). Like other counselors using integration, Mario's clinician chose this method because he had not found one individual theory that was comprehensive enough, by itself, to address all of the "complexities," "range of client types," and "specific problems" seen among his everyday caseload (Corey, 2009, p. 450).

Specifically, Mario's counselor selected an integration of (a) the Multicomponent Psychosocial Intervention Theory and (b) Motivational Interviewing. He selected this approach based on the client's presentation of long-standing substance dependence with physiological consequences such as sleep disruption, and long-standing alcohol abuse patterns. Multicomponent Psychosocial Intervention often is indicated when a combination of symptoms will be targeted via residential and community-based treatment, group therapy and self-help groups, as well as family therapy (Crits-Christoph et al., 1999; Higgins et al., 1993; Higgins & Silverman, 1999; Humpreys & Moos, 2007; Moos & Timko, 2008; Saatcioglu, Erim, & Cakmak, 2006; Stanton & Shadish, 1997), whereas an integrated approach emphasizing Motivational Interviewing is indicated for addressing the personal dynamics related to changing substance using behaviors and choices (Baer & Peterson, 2002; Miller & Rollnick, 2002). Mario's counselor is comfortable theoretically integrating these approaches, and it is the model commonly employed at the Beverly Hills center he selected for Mario.

The counselor used the Inverted Pyramid Method of case conceptualization because this method is especially designed to help clinicians more easily form their conceptual pictures of their clients' needs (Neukrug & Schwitzer, 2006; Schwitzer, 1996, 1997). The method has four steps: Problem Identification; Thematic Groupings; Theoretical Inferences; and Narrowed Inferences. The counselor's clinical thinking can be seen in Figure 7.2.

Step 1: Problem Identification. The first step is Problem Identification. Aspects of the presenting problem (thoughts, feelings, behaviors, physiological features), additional areas of concern besides the presenting concern, family and developmental history, in-session observations, clinical inquiries (medical problems, medications, past counseling, substance use, suicidality), and psychological assessments (problem checklists, personality inventories, mental status exam, specific clinical measures) all may contribute information at Step 1. The counselor "casts a wide net" in order to build Step 1 as exhaustively as possible (Neukrug & Schwitzer, 2006, p. 202). As can be seen in Figure 7.2, the counselor and the evaluation team identified: Mario's cocaine use symptoms, factors, and consequences; Mario's alcohol use symptoms, factors, and consequences; immediate social concerns (threat of job loss, etc.); information about his history of use; his sleep symptoms; as well as strengths, accomplishments, and areas of successful adjustment. The problem description in Step 1 attempted to go beyond just the current events leading to Mario's referral in order to be fully descriptive.

Step 2: Thematic Groupings. The second step is Thematic Groupings. The clinician organizes all of the exhaustive client information found in Step 1 into just a few intuitive-logical clinical groups, categories, or themes, on the basis of sensible common denominators (Neukrug & Schwitzer, 2006). Four different ways of forming the Step 2 theme groups can be used: Descriptive-Diagnosis Approach, Clinical Targets Approach, Areas of Dysfunction Approach, and Intrapsychic Approach. As can be seen in the figure, Mario's counselor selected the Areas of Dysfunction Approach. This approach sorts together all of the Step 1 information into "areas of dysfunction according to important life situations, life themes, or life roles and skills" (Neukrug & Schwitzer, 2006, p. 205).

The counselor grouped together (a) all of Mario's substance use behaviors, consequences, and motivational factors associated with both cocaine and alcohol into the theme: Debilitating substance dependence and abuse with low motivation for change; and (b) Mario's single concern pertaining to sleep into the stand-alone theme: Prominent sleep disturbance due to substance use. His conceptual work at Step 2 gave the counselor a way to begin understanding and explaining the client's many concerns as a narrower list of just two, clear, meaningful areas of negative functioning. As a substance-abuse counseling specialist, he based his groupings on the literature suggesting

that (a) clients and patients experiencing abuse or dependence of more than one substance see better outcomes when their concerns are conceptualized and treated together, as a polysubstance abuse problem, rather than as individual problems, and (b) clients with substance-use problems and an additional mental health concern respond better when the additional mental health problem also is addressed (Project MATCH Research Group, 1997).

So far, at Steps 1 and 2, the counselor has used his clinical assessment skills and clinical judgment to begin meaningfully understanding Mario Alito's needs. Now, at Steps 3 and 4, he applies the theoretical approach he has selected. He begins making theoretical inferences to interpret and explain the processes or roots underlying Mario Alito's concerns as they are seen in Steps 1 and 2.

Step 3: Theoretical Inferences. At Step 3, concepts from the counselor's theoretical integration of two approaches—Multicomponent Psychosocial Intervention and Motivational Interviewing—are applied to explain the experiences surrounding, and the mechanisms maintaining, Mario's problematic substance use and its consequences. The counselor tentatively matches the theme groups in Step 2 with this theoretical approach. In other words, the symptom constellations in Step 2, which were distilled from the symptoms in Step 1, now are combined using theory to show what are believed to be the underlying causes or psychological etiology of Mario Alito's current needs (Neukrug & Schwitzer, 2006; Schwitzer, 2006, 2007).

First, Multicomponent Psychosocial Intervention Therapy was applied primarily to Mario's abuse and dependence behaviors. According to the model, there are interpersonal and community antecedents, and social consequences, of substance use; consequently, these social factors are necessary to understand a person's substance use behaviors and then target treatment (National Institute on Drug Abuse, 2008). Along these lines, the counselor inferred that there are multiple social, interpersonal, and community antecedents and consequences of Mario's substance use.

Second, Motivational Interviewing was applied primarily to Mario's intrapersonal experience of his use, especially as it related to his motivation for change. According to the model, individuals exist and may move through a series of predictable stages of change, including Precontemplation, Contemplation, Preparation, Action, and Maintenance (Prochaska, Norcross, & DiClemente, 1994). Conceptually, understanding where a client exists in the process of contemplating and enacting change provides a guide to treatment planning using the nondirective social influence methods of Motivational Interviewing (Markland, Ryan, Tobin, & Rollnick, 2005; Miller & Rollnick, 2002). Along these lines, the counselor inferred that: Mario is in a stage of very low readiness for change.

Step 4: Narrowed Inferences. At Step 4, the clinician's selected theory continues to be used to address still-deeper issues when they exist (Schwitzer, 2006, 2007). At this step, "still-deeper, more encompassing, or more central, causal themes" are formed (Neukrug & Schwitzer, 2006, p. 207). Mario's counselor continued to use psychotherapeutic integration of two approaches.

First, continuing to apply Multicomponent Psychosocial Intervention concepts at Step 4, Mario's counselor presented a pair of narrowed theoretical inferences, which he believed to be most explanatory and causal regarding Mario's problematic substance use: (a) Mario responds to multiple social factors that are antecedents to his substance use and is experiencing multiple interpersonal and community consequences as a result of his use; and, correspondingly, (b) Mario must change his substance-use behavior in multiple social, interpersonal, and community contexts in order to control his cocaine and alcohol us and to avoid the social consequences of his use. Second, continuing to apply Motivational Interviewing, the counselor presented another, complementary, narrowed theoretical inference: Mario is in the Precontemplation stage with temporary motivation for change due to current

interpersonal pressures (Prochaska et al., 1994). When all four steps are completed, the client information in Step 1 leads to logical-intuitive groupings on the basis of common denominators in Step 2, the groupings then are explained using theory at Step 3, and then, finally, at Step 4, further deeper explanations are made. From start to finish, the thoughts, feelings, behaviors, and physiological features in the topmost portions are connected on down the pyramid into deepest dynamics.

TREATMENT PLANNING

At this point, Mario's clinician at the Beverly Hills Drug Rehabilitation Center has collected all available information about the problems that have been of concern to him and the treatment team that performed Mario's assessment. Based upon this information, the counselor developed a five-axis *DSM-IV-TR* diagnosis and then, using the "inverted pyramid" (Neukrug & Schwitzer, 2006; Schwitzer, 1996, 1997), formulated a working clinical *explanation* of Mario's difficulties and their etiology that we called the *case conceptualization.* This, in turn, guides us to the next critical step in our clinical work, called the *treatment plan,* the primary purpose of which is to map out a logical and goal-oriented strategy for making positive changes in the client's life. In essence, the treatment plan is a road map "for reducing or eliminating disruptive symptoms that are impeding the client's ability to reach positive mental health outcomes" (Neukrug & Schwitzer, 2006, p. 225). As such, it is the cornerstone of our work with not only Mario, but with all clients who present with disturbing and disruptive symptoms and/or personality patterns (Jongsma et al., 2003a, 2003b; Jongsma & Peterson, 2006; Seligman, 1993, 1998, 2004).

A comprehensive treatment plan must integrate all of the information from the biopsychosocial interview, diagnosis, and case conceptualization into a coherent plan of action. This *plan* comprises four main components, which include

Figure 7.2   Mario's Inverted Pyramid Case Conceptualization Summary: Psychotherapeutic Integration of Multicomponent Psychosocial Intervention and Motivational Interviewing

1.   IDENTIFY AND LIST CLIENT CONCERNS

Recent cocaine binge prompting referral
Declined by *Celebrity Rehab* due to severity
Recent threat of job loss due to cocaine use
Cocaine use interferes with intimate relationships
Cocaine use interferes with friendships
Alcohol abuse behavior
Fails to meet work obligations due to
   alcohol use
Drinks alcohol to point of hangovers
Continues drinking despite
   consequences and finances

Steadily increasing cocaine use since high school
Affective withdrawal signs: Agitated, irritable
   when stops using cocaine
Periods of being unable to cut down or stop
   use despite efforts
Expends increasing time, money, effort to obtain cocaine
Hesitant, resistant to change
Minimizes perception of substance-related problems
Significant sleep disturbance attributable to cocaine
Popular, athletic, sexually attractive, success at career
Successful history despite substance use

2.   ORGANIZE CONCERNS INTO LOGICAL THEMATIC GROUPINGS

   1.   Debilitating substance dependence and abuse with low
         motivation for change
   2.   Prominent sleep disturbance due to substance use

**3.   THEORETICAL INFERENCES: ATTACH THEMATIC
       GROUPINGS TO INFERRED AREAS OF DIFFICULTY**
       Psychotherapeutic Integration

Multicomponent Psychosocial Intervention
Theoretical Inference:
There are multiple social, interpersonal, and
community antecedents and consequences
of Mario's substance abuse

Motivational Interviewing
Theoretical Inference:
Mario is in a stage of very
ready for change

**4.   NARROWED INFERENCES: SUICIDALITY
       AND DEEPER DIFFICULTIES**
       Psychotherapeutic Integration

Multicomponent Psychosocial
Intervention
Narrowed Theoretical Inferences:
1.   Mario responds to multiple social
      factors that are antecedents to his
      substance use, and is experiencing
      multiple interpersonal and community
      consequences as a result of his use
2.   Mario must change his substance
      use behavior in multiple social,
      interpersonal, and community contexts
      in order control his cocaine and alcohol
      use and to avoid the social consequences
      of his use

Motivational Interviewing
Narrowed Theoretical Inferences:
Mario is in the Precontemplation
stage with temporary motivation
for change due to current
interpersonal pressures

(1) a behavioral definition of the problem(s), (2) the selection of achievable goals, (3) the determination of treatment modes, and (4) the documentation of how change will be measured. The *behavioral definition of the problem(s)* consolidates the results of the case conceptualization into a concise hierarchical list of problems and concerns that will be the focus of treatment. The *selection of achievable goals* refers to assessing and prioritizing the client's concerns into a *hierarchy of urgency* that also takes into account the client's motivation for change, level of dysfunction, and real-world influences on his or her problems. The *determination of treatment modes* refers to selection of the specific interventions, which are matched to the uniqueness of the client and to his or her goals and clearly tied to a particular theoretical orientation (Neukrug & Schwitzer, 2006). Finally, the clinician must establish how change will be measured, based upon a number of factors including client records and self-report of change, in-session observations by the clinician, clinician ratings, results of standardized evaluations such as the Beck Depression Inventory-II (Beck & Steer, 1990) or a family functioning questionnaire, pre-post treatment comparisons, and reports by other treating professionals.

The four-step method discussed above can be seen in Figure 6.1 (p. 109) and is outlined below for the case of Mario Alito, followed by his specific treatment plan.

Step 1: Behavioral Definition of Problems. The first step in treatment planning is to carefully review the case conceptualization, paying particular attention to the results of Step 2 (Thematic Groupings), Step 3 (Theoretical Inferences), and Step 4 (Narrowed Inferences). The identified clinical themes reflect the core areas of concern and distress for the client, while the theoretical and narrowed inferences offer clinical speculation as to their origins. In the case of Mario, there is one primary and overarching area of concern. "Debilitating substance dependence and abuse with low motivation for change and sleep disturbance" refers to his steadily increasing cocaine and alcohol use since high

school; continued drinking and cocaine use despite consequences; failure to meet work, family and relationship obligations when hung-over from alcohol or coming down from a cocaine binge; expending increasing amounts of time and money to obtain cocaine; minimized perception of substance-abuse problem with heightened resistance to change despite efforts; and significant sleep disturbance directly attributable to cocaine use and affective withdrawal signs, including agitation and irritability upon cocaine cessation. These symptoms and stresses are consistent with the diagnosis of Cocaine Dependence With Physiological Dependence; Cocaine-Induced Sleep Disorder, Insomnia Type, With Onset During Intoxication; Alcohol Abuse (APA, 2000a; Gordek & Folsom, 2006; Grant et al., 2006; Inaba & Cohen, 2000; Jaffe, Rawson, & Ling, 2005; NIDA, 2008; Substance Abuse and Mental Health Services Organization, 2006).

Step 2: Identify and Articulate Goals for Change. The second step is the selection of achievable goals, which is based upon a number of factors, including the most pressing or urgent behavioral, emotional, and interpersonal concerns and symptoms as identified by the client and clinician, the willingness and ability of the client to work on those particular goals, and the realistic (real-world) achievability of those goals (Neukrug & Schwitzer, 2006). At this stage of treatment planning, it is important to recognize that not all of the client's problems can be addressed at once, so we focus initially on those that cause the greatest distress and impairment. New goals can be created as old ones are achieved.

In the case of Mario, the goals flow directly from his primary problem, "debilitating substance dependence and abuse with low motivation for change and sleep disturbance." This complex, long-standing, and multidimensional problem requires that we design an intervention that is equally multidimensional so as to address all of the components of his substance-abuse problem. Based upon the assumption that Mario's long-standing abuse of drugs and alcohol originated and evolved within a social context, it follows that there have been, and continue to be, a number of intrapersonal, interpersonal, and community factors that shape, reinforce, and maintain his behavior. Some of these may include his faulty cognitions around substance abuse, the maladaptive behavioral pattern that has developed through which he acquires and uses cocaine and alcohol, the adverse physical and physiological effects on him of these substances (including sleep problems), drug/alcohol-based and drug/alcohol-centered casual and intimate relationships, the reciprocal impact of career and celebrity status on his substance use, the perception of himself as a high-power and "untouchable" celebrity, and the impact of his numerous altercations, arrests, and failed rehabilitative efforts on both his self-image and the image of him in the public eye. This complex array of etiological and maintaining factors requires that we help Mario to accept the fact of his chemical dependence and the destructive effect it has had in all areas of his life, to help him withdraw from cocaine and alcohol and stabilize him physically and emotionally, to establish and maintain total abstinence while increasing his knowledge of the addictive process and lifestyle, to acquire the necessary intrapersonal and interpersonal coping skills to maintain long-term sobriety, to develop an understanding of his personal pattern of relapse by identifying internal, interpersonal, and community triggers for relapse, and to achieve a high quality of life, absent substance abuse. Additionally, given that Mario's substance abuse is both long-standing and pervasive, it is important, if we are to help him achieve the above goals, to assess his motivation for change. We know that he is in a stage of "very low readiness for change," so we will need to clarify obstacles to motivation and then help him to strengthen his resolve and commitment to attain and maintain sobriety.

Step 3: Describe Therapeutic Interventions. This is perhaps the most critical step in the treatment planning process because the clinician must now integrate information from a number of sources, including the case conceptualization, the delineation of the client's problems and goals, and the treatment literature, paying particular attention to *empirically supported treatment* (EST) and *evidence-based practice* (EBP). In essence, the clinician must align his or her treatment approach with scientific evidence from the fields of counseling and psychotherapy. Wampold (2001) identifies two types of evidence-based counseling research: studies that demonstrate "absolute efficacy," that is, the fact that counseling and psychotherapy work, and those that demonstrate "relative efficacy," that is, the fact that certain theoretical/technical approaches work best for certain clients with particular problems (Psychoanalysis, Gestalt Therapy, Cognitive Behavior Therapy, Brief Solution-Focused Therapy, Cognitive Therapy, Dialectical Behavior Therapy, Person-Centered Therapy, Expressive/Creative Therapies, Interpersonal Therapy, and Feminist Therapy); and when delivered through specific treatment modalities (individual, group, and family counseling).

In the case of Mario, we have decided to use a two-pronged "integrated" approach comprised of Multicomponent Psychosocial Intervention and Motivational Interviewing. Multicomponent Psychosocial Intervention relies on a combination of techniques, modalities, and therapeutic venues to address the complex array of physiological, psychological (cognitive, behavioral and emotional), interpersonal, and community factors that are related to, reinforce, and maintain substance abuse. These include Cognitive Behavior Therapy, family therapy, and psychoeducation delivered in a combination of outpatient and residential individual and group format (Anton, O'Malley, & Ciraulo, 2006; Crits-Christoph et al., 1999; NIDA, 2008). Techniques that we will sequentially use with Mario as he moves from residential to outpatient counseling include referral for a medical examination of substance-related damage and monitoring during period of acute withdrawal; individual and group substance abuse psychoeducation; regular attendance in Narcotics Anonymous (NA); family counseling to identify the role members play in maintaining his substance abuse; identify physiological, emotional, and interpersonal triggers for substance use; identify and refute irrational thoughts related to his self-image as well as to substance abuse and celebrity; develop nonsubstance-related self-regulation/coping skills, including deep breathing, muscle relaxation, assertiveness, self-affirmation, and mindfulness. Upon discharge, Mario will continue to receive group counseling at the center supplemented with individual and family counseling in the community. Techniques, in addition to those selected from his inpatient stay, will include assignment of a sponsor for abstinence support, development of a list of ways that sobriety could positively impact his life, plan social and recreational activities that are not associated with substance use, bibliotherapy for substance-abuse recovery, establishment of a mechanism for random drug screening, development of hierarchy of routines and activities to avoid relapse triggers, maintaining regular contact with sponsor and NA attendance upon discharge, assisting him in identifying and avoiding situations and people associated with substance use and psychiatric referral for possible psychopharmacotherapy (anxiety/depression).

We will also use Motivational Interviewing (MI), which asserts that the very notion of the "unmotivated client," Mario in this case, is largely a myth. According to MI (Markland et al., 2005; Miller & Rollnick, 2002), "The client is viewed as an individual who waxes and wanes in his or her motivation, and one who can become motivated under the right circumstances" (Neukrug, 2011, p. 472). MI's basic tenets are in line with "self determination theory [SDT]" (Markland et al., 2005), which advocates competence, autonomy, and relatedness, and suggests that motivation is multidimensional, dynamic and fluid, modifiable and a key to change, and is in turn effected by the clinician's style and capacity to elicit and enhance motivational states. The clinician's role is to identify the "stage" or readiness for change that the client is in (precontemplation, contemplation, preparation, action, and maintenance) and to then selectively use both directive (cognitive behavioral) and nondirective (open-ended questions, affirmations, reflective listening and summarizing [OARS], empathy and affirmation) skills to help the client move forward in his or her commitment to change. This technique, albeit relatively new,

has been found to be effective in the treatment of a number of behavioral problems, including substance abuse and other "addictive" disorders (Arkowitz & Miller, 2008; Carrol et al., 2006). It is particularly suited for Mario, whose motivation has historically been erratic and undermined by a myriad of psychosocial and cognitive factors and who is beginning to understand the destructive effects of substance abuse on all facets of his life. The specific techniques that will be used with him are designed to enhance his competence, autonomy, and relatedness and include open-ended questions around his drug use, perceptions of himself and goals, genuine and congruent affirmations highlighting his strengths, reflective and empathetic listening to his concerns and motivational obstacles, "rolling with his resistance" rather than directly confronting and challenging it, highlighting and summarizing the discrepancies in his narrative that maintain his substance use and undermine his motivation, and exploring options.

Step 4: Provide Outcome Measures of Change. This last step in treatment planning requires that we specify how change will be measured and indicate the extent to which progress has been made toward realizing these goals (Neukrug & Schwitzer, 2006). The counselor has considerable flexibility in this phase and may choose from a number of objective domains (psychological tests and measures of self-esteem, depression, psychosis, interpersonal relationship, anxiety, etc.), quasi-objective measures (the *DSM-IV-TR-TR's* Axis V GAF scale; pre-post clinician, client and psychiatric ratings), and subjective ratings (client self-report, clinician's in-session observations). In Mario's case, we have implemented a number of these, including client self-reported alcohol and cocaine abstinence, a pre-post improved measure on the Alcohol Use Inventory (Horn, Wanberg, & Foster, 1990), a 3-month post measure of GAF functioning in the mild-moderate range (60–70), and a 6–12 month measure of functioning in the mild range (>70), 6–12 month substance-free urine tests, client self-report, and clinician observed improvement in motivation to remain abstinent.

The completed treatment plan is now developed through which the counselor and Mario will work through his substance-abuse problem. The treatment plan appears below and is summarized in Table 7.2.

TREATMENT PLAN

Client: Mario Alito

Service Provider: Beverly Hills Drug Rehabilitation Center

BEHAVIORAL DEFINITION OF PROBLEMS:

1. Debilitating substance dependence and abuse—Steadily increasing cocaine and alcohol use since high school, continued drinking and cocaine use despite consequences, failure to meet work, family, and relationship obligations when hungover from alcohol or coming down from a cocaine binge, expending increasing amounts of time and money to obtain cocaine, minimized perception of substance-abuse problem with heightened resistance to change despite efforts, significant sleep disturbance directly attributable to cocaine use, and affective withdrawal signs, including agitation and irritability upon cocaine cessation.

GOALS FOR CHANGE:

1. Debilitating substance dependence and abuse

- Accept the fact of chemical dependence and its destructive effect
- Withdraw from cocaine and alcohol and stabilize physically, behaviorally, and emotionally
- Establish and maintain total abstinence while increasing knowledge of the addictive process and lifestyle
- Clarify obstacles to change motivation
- Strengthen his motivation, resolve, and commitment to attain and maintain sobriety
- Acquire the necessary intrapersonal and interpersonal coping skills to maintain long-term sobriety
- Develop an understanding of personal pattern of relapse by identifying internal, interpersonal, and community triggers for relapse
- Achieve a high quality of life absent the use of substances

THERAPEUTIC INTERVENTIONS:

A moderate-term course of individual Multicomponent Psychosocial Intervention and Motivational Interviewing (6–9 months)

1. Debilitating substance dependence and abuse

Inpatient/Residential

- Referral for a medical examination of substance-related damage and monitoring during period of acute withdrawal
- Individual and group substance-abuse psychoeducation

(Continued)

(Continued)

- Regular attendance in Narcotics Anonymous (NA)
- Family counseling to identify the role members play in maintaining substance abuse
- Identify physiological, emotional, and interpersonal triggers for substance use
- Identify and refute irrational thoughts related to self-image as well as to substance abuse and celebrity
- Develop non-substance-related self-regulation/coping skills, including deep breathing, muscle relaxation, assertiveness, self-affirmation, and mindfulness

Outpatient

- Assignment of a sponsor for abstinence support
- Development of a list of ways that sobriety could positively impact life
- Plan social and recreational activities not associated with substance use
- Bibliotherapy for substance-abuse recovery
- Establishment of a mechanism for random drug screening
- Development of hierarchy of routines and activities to avoid relapse triggers
- Maintain regular contact with sponsor
- NA attendance
- Assist in identifying and avoiding situations and people associated with substance use
- Psychiatric referral for possible psychopharmacotherapy (anxiety/depression).

Motivational Interviewing Techniques

- Open-ended questions around drug use, self-perceptions, and goals
- Genuine and congruent affirmations highlighting strengths
- Reflective and empathetic listening to concerns and motivational obstacles
- "Rolling with resistance" rather than directly confronting and challenging it
- Highlighting and summarizing discrepancies in narrative that maintain substance use and undermine motivation
- Exploration of options

OUTCOME MEASURES OF CHANGE:

The immediate cessation of substance use and establishment and maintenance of total abstinence and long-term adaptive functioning as measured by:

- Client self-reported alcohol and cocaine abstinence
- Pre-post improved measure on the Alcohol Use Inventory
- 3-month post measures of GAF functioning in the mild-moderate range (60–70)
- 6–12 month measure of functioning in the mild range (>70)
- 12 month arrest-free police record
- 6–12 month substance-free urine tests
- Client self-report and clinician observation of improved quality of life and positive attitude and motivation to remain substance-free

Table 7.2   Mario's Treatment Plan Summary: Psychotherapeutic Integration of Multicomponent Psychosocial Intervention and Motivational Interviewing

Goals for Change	Therapeutic Interventions	Outcome Measures of Change
Debilitating substance dependence and abuse	Debilitating substance dependence and abuse	The immediate cessation of substance use and establishment and maintenance of total abstinence and long-term adaptive functioning as measured by:
Accept the fact of chemical dependence and its destructive effects	*Inpatient/Residential* Referral for a medical examination of substance-related damage and monitoring during period of acute withdrawal	Client self-reported alcohol and cocaine abstinence
Withdraw from cocaine and alcohol and stabilize physically, behaviorally, and emotionally	Individual and group substance-abuse psychoeducation	Pre-post improved measure on the Alcohol Use Inventory
Establish and maintain total abstinence while increasing knowledge of the addictive process and lifestyle	Regular attendance in Narcotics Anonymous (NA) Family counseling to identify the role members play in maintaining substance abuse	3-month post measures of GAF functioning in the mild-moderate range (60–70)
Clarify obstacles to change motivation	Identify physiological, emotional, and interpersonal triggers for substance use	6–12 month measure of functioning in the mild range (>70)
Strengthen his motivation, resolve, and commitment to attain and maintain sobriety	Identify and refute irrational thoughts related to self-image as well as to substance abuse and celebrity	12-month arrest-free police record
Acquire the necessary intrapersonal and interpersonal coping skills to maintain long-term sobriety	Develop nonsubstance-related self-regulation/coping skills, including deep breathing, muscle relaxation, assertiveness, self-affirmation, and mindfulness	6–12 month substance-free urine tests
Develop an understanding of personal pattern of relapse by identifying internal, interpersonal, and community triggers for relapse	*Outpatient* Assignment of a sponsor for abstinence support	Client self-report and clinician observation of improved quality of life and positive attitude and motivation to remain substance-free
Achieve a high quality of life absent the use of substances	Development of a list of ways that sobriety could positively impact life	
	Plan social and recreational activities not associated with substance use	
	Bibliotherapy for substance-abuse recovery	
	Establishment of a mechanism for random drug screening	
	Development of hierarchy of routines and activities to avoid relapse triggers	

(Continued)

Table 7.2 (Continued)

Goals for Change	Therapeutic Interventions	Outcome Measures of Change
	Maintain regular contact with sponsor	
	NA attendance	
	Assist in identifying and avoiding situations and people associated with substance use	
	Psychiatric referral for possible psychopharmacotherapy (anxiety/ depression)	
	Motivational Interviewing Techniques	
	Open-ended questions around drug use, self-perceptions, and goals	
	Genuine and congruent affirmations highlighting strengths	
	Reflective and empathetic listening to concerns and motivational obstacles	
	"Rolling with resistance" rather than directly confronting and challenging it	
	Highlighting and summarizing discrepancies in narrative that maintain substance use and undermine motivation	
	Exploration of options	

CASE 7.3   *HANSEL AND GRETEL'S* GRETEL

INTRODUCING THE CHARACTER

Gretel is the young protagonist in the Brothers Grimm fairy tale *Hansel and Gretel,* which first appeared in print centuries ago and has since been depicted in a variety of media, including: short films, television cartoons, and an 1893 opera of the same name by 19th-century play-wright Engelbert Humperdinck. *Hansel and Gretel* is a beloved fairy tale about a woodcutter's children who suffer the loss of their mother and who must then endure an evil stepmother (despite the common occurrence of blended families in contemporary life, stepparents often are stereotyped as "evil" in traditional fairy

tales). As often happens in such old-school fairy tales, the woodcutter, about whom we know little other than that he is a hard worker, falls prey to his new wife's desires to be rid of Hansel and Gretel. She convinces him to cast them into the woods where they find a magical gingerbread house inhabited by a witch. Although the witch welcomes the children, they soon discover that she plans to eat them. Upon discovering her nefarious plan, Hansel pushes the witch into the oven. Thinking that the witch is dead, the children remain in the cottage and eat candy and sweets for days before finding their way home thanks to a marked path that they had cleverly left behind. The father, who was heartbroken over the loss of his children, eagerly welcomes them back and rids the family, once and for all, of his evil-doing wife. *Hansel and Gretel* is a timeless tale about parental loss, betrayal, and the resourcefulness and resiliency of children. Using *Hansel and Gretel* as our starting point, the following basic case summary and diagnostic impressions explore a clinically significant pattern of hostile and defiant behaviors we believe a similar 10-year-old girl named Gretel might be experiencing.

Meet the Client

You can assess the client in action by viewing clips of Gretel's video material at the following websites:

- http://www.youtube.com/watch?v=Kxk IGXVwZTM Hansel and Gretel
- http://www.youtube.com/watch?v=n7 ZMFLyZ4BU Mickey and Minnie as Hansel and Gretel

BASIC CASE SUMMARY

Identifying Information. Gretel Gerstenhagen is a 10-year-old Austrian girl who is a fourth-grade student at the Gingerbread Learning Academy. Currently she lives at home with her fraternal twin, Hansel, her father, and her stepmother, who only recently became a member of the family. In appearance, Gretel can be characterized as "a rosy-cheeked, blue-eyed girl with curly blond hair." She was dressed in a traditional Germanic child's outfit, left over from a school play in which she starred, which she reported wearing "because it annoys my stepmother." She lives in a socioeconomically lower middle-class neighborhood, her father is a skilled carpenter, and her stepmother works in the home.

Presenting Concern. Gretel was sent to the school counselor's office for an initial meeting by the assistant principal because she has several times stolen another student's lunchbox "as a joke," and refused her teacher's request to return the hidden lunchbox at lunchtime. Gretel had been sent to the principal's office on several occasions for similar behavior, which seemed to have escalated soon after her father remarried to a woman the child referred to as a "witch." Gretel also has been diagnosed with juvenile diabetes.

Background, Family Information, and Relevant History. Gretel and her fraternal twin Hansel were born in Vienna, Austria, to a fourth-generation military family headed by a father who worked as a skilled carpenter and traveled frequently, following house-building demand across the region, and a mother who was bedridden throughout her pregnancy and sick for the first 2 years of the children's lives. Reports indicate that Gretel and her brother were only allowed to visit their mother at her bedside for short periods. A day before their third birthday, their mother died, and soon after the father brought an au pair into the house. Apparently, unbeknownst to the father, the au pair was bringing men into the family home when the father was away. Gretel and her brother learned early how to manipulate this woman, whom they referred to as the "evil witch" and who reciprocated in kind with harsh punishment and withdrawal of privileges. Gretel recalled how the au pair used to bake gingerbread houses and eat them herself while the children watched and begged. One day during a rare outing to the park, one of the neighbors noticed the harsh manner in which the au pair treated the children, and reported directly to their father, who immediately fired her.

Following this experience, he decided to spend more time with the children in order to make up for his many absences. By that time, the children were 7 years of age, and he decided that it would be beneficial to move to the United States where he took a job with a contractor firm. Although Gretel was upset at leaving the familiarity of Austria and the friends that she had made, she soon found a safe and secure haven at the Gingerbread Learning Academy, where she and Hansel were enrolled in the third grade. Soon after the relocation, Hansel and Gretel's father married for a second time to a woman who had never wanted children but who fell in love with their father.

Several months after marrying, Gretel and Hansel's father returned to his busy work life, leaving the children primarily in the care of their new stepmother, who like the au pair they had in Austria, put her needs before those of the children. She would spend long hours on the phone talking to friends, neglecting the children, leaving them to fend for themselves, do their own homework, and even make their own food. Gretel became very adept at sneaking candy from the cupboards as well as stealing it from the small grocery at the corner of their street. Gretel also developed what teachers and her father described as a "short fuse," becoming touchy in response to even very minor adult feedback about her behavior, loudly angry at perceived insults, and argumentative at home, in class, and in the Gingerbread Afterschool Program. When household chores such as cleaning the playroom were left undone, she wrongly blamed her brother; at school, she blamed classmates for incidents on the playground. Increasingly, she yelled at her stepmother at home, muttered under her breath at her classroom teacher, and made a clear point of being out of her seat during classroom quiet time. Characteristically, after a particularly unpleasant evening with the stepmother, Gretel and Hansel ran away from home, living in a small park by the home, and subsisting only on the candy and cookies that they had pirated away before their departure, which Gretel said she did "to show that witch!" It was at that point that Gretel and Hansel's father were summoned to the school and told that unless he took immediate action to control his daughter (and son), that they would be removed from the school and possibly even the home. Upon hearing this and realizing that their plan had failed, Gretel told her teacher "maybe I'll just kill myself . . . that'll teach her."

Goals for Counseling and Course of Therapy to Date. Several days after the meeting with the children, Mr. Gerstenhagen and his wife visited with the school counselor and the district school psychologist in order to develop a plan of action. It was decided that Gretel and Hansel would undergo psychological evaluations and review by a planning team, after which a decision would be made determining whether individual or family counseling or both would be implemented.

Diagnostic Impressions

Axis I.   313.81 Oppositional Defiant Disorder

Axis II.   V71.09 No Diagnosis on Axis II

Axis III. Type II Juvenile Diabetes

Axis IV. Problems with primary support group—Death of mother, remarriage of father, relational tension with stepmother

Problems related to social environment—Geographic relocation to United States

Axis V.   GAF = 64 (Current)

GAF = 70 (Highest level past school year)

Discussion of
Diagnostic Impressions

Gretel was mandated to visit the school counselor's office after repeatedly hiding another student's lunchbox as a deliberately annoying joke and refusing her teacher's demands to return the lunchbox. Likewise, she has engaged in purposefully annoying behavior at home (such as dressing in odd costumes). Her parents and teachers report that she has a "short-fused" temper, is often argumentative, easily feels resentment, and at times seems spiteful. She also blames other children (e.g., her brother) or adults (e.g., her mother) for her own misbehavior.

The Disorders Usually First Diagnosed in Infancy, Childhood, or Adolescence is a far-reaching section of the *DSM-IV-TR*. It is organized into many groupings of disorders that all share the feature of beginning early in the life cycle. One of these groupings that is especially important to the everyday practice of counseling professionals who work with children and adolescents in school and community settings is called Attention-Deficit and Disruptive Behavior Disorders. Attention-Deficit/Hyperactivity Disorder, Conduct Disorder, and Oppositional Defiant Disorder all are in this group.

Using *Hansel and Gretel* as our starting point in this case example, we presented a 10-year-old girl named Gretel who was experiencing a clinically significant pattern of hostile and defiant behaviors beyond what is normally expected among her age and cultural peer group. Her behaviors have been persistent for many months, and they have become sufficiently problematic to impair Gretel's family relationships at home, her relationships with teachers and peers at school, and her ability to perform and succeed in the classroom. Gretel's behaviors suggests a diagnosis of Oppositional Defiant Disorder, the key feature of which is a pattern of "negativistic, hostile, and defiant behavior" lasting for at least 6 months, typically in a child under 18 years old.

One differential diagnosis might be Conduct Disorder, Childhood-Onset Type. This is another diagnosis found among the group of Disruptive Behaviors diagnoses in the *DSM-IV-TR's* Disorders Usually First Diagnosed in Infancy, Childhood, or Adolescence. This diagnosis is ruled out, however, since Gretel's behaviors, although negative and defiant, do not feature the aggressiveness to people and animals, destructiveness, deceitfulness, and serious rule violations characteristic of a Conduct Disorder. Another consideration is No Diagnosis on Axis I because oppositional behavior is normally typical of certain developmental stages such as early childhood and adolescence. In turn, the Oppositional Defiant Disorder diagnosis is appropriate "only if behaviors occur more frequently and have more serious consequences than is typically observed in other individuals of comparable developmental stage and lead to significant impairment in social, academic, or occupational functioning" (APA, 2000a, p. 102). Gretel's behaviors meet this standard.

To round out the diagnosis, Gretel's diabetes is listed on Axis III because its presence may have impacted significantly upon the family system. Further, her family and social stressors are emphasized on Axis IV, and on Axis V her functioning is represented by GAF scores indicating mild symptoms causing some difficulty in social and school functioning (like occasional theft and similar conduct). The information on these axes is consistent with the Axis I diagnosis portrayed by Gretel in this scenario.

Case Conceptualization

When Gretel came into the Gingerbread Learning Academy's school counseling office, her counselor first conducted an intake meeting in order to collect as much information as he could about the symptoms and situations leading to Gretel's referral. Included in the intake materials were a developmental history, client report, counselor observations, child-oriented clinical interview, play observation, parent report inventories, and information shared by Gretel's school principal and teachers (Knell, 1993, 1994). Based on the intake, Gretel's counselor developed diagnostic impressions, describing her presenting concerns by Oppositional Defiant Disorder. A case conceptualization next was developed. Whereas the purpose of diagnostic impressions is to *describe* the client's concerns, the goal of case conceptualization is to better *understand* and clinically *explain* the person's experiences (Neukrug & Schwitzer, 2006). It helps the counselor understand the etiology leading to Gretel's Oppositional Defiant behaviors, and the factors maintaining these concerns. In turn, case conceptualization sets the stage for treatment planning. Treatment planning then provides a road map that plots out how the counselor and client expect to move from presenting concerns to positive outcomes (Seligman, 1993, p. 157)—helping Gretel manage her oppositional behaviors and defiant thoughts and attitudes, and improving her interpersonal interactions.

When forming a case conceptualization, the clinician applies a purist counseling theory, an integration of two or more theories, an eclectic mix of theories, or a solution-focused combination of techniques, to his or her understanding of the client. In this case, Gretel's counselor based his conceptualization on psychotherapeutic integration of two theories (Corey, 2009). Psychotherapists very commonly integrate more than one theoretical approach in order to form a conceptualization and treatment plan that will be as efficient and effective as possible for meeting the client's needs (Dattilo & Norcross, 2006; Norcross & Beutler, 2008). In other words, counselors using the psychotherapeutic integration method attempt to flexibly tailor their clinical efforts to "the unique needs and contexts of the individual client" (Norcross & Beutler, 2008, p. 485). Like other counselors using integration, Gretel's school counselor chose this method because he had not found one individual theory that was comprehensive enough, by itself, to address all of the "complexities," "range of client types," and "specific problems" seen among his everyday student caseload (Corey, 2009, p. 450).

Specifically, Gretel's counselor selected an integration of (a) Child-Centered Play Therapy and (b) Cognitive Behavioral Play Therapy. He selected this approach based on Gretel's presentation of problematic behaviors and his knowledge of current outcome research and recommended practice literature with clients experiencing these types of concerns (Kazdin & Weisz, 2003; Lawrence, Condon, Jacobi, & Nicholson, 2006; Mowder, Rubinson, & Yasik, 2009). According to the research, Cognitive Behavioral Play Therapy is one treatment approach indicated when assisting clients who might benefit from a combination of cognitive and behavior change, whereas an integrated approach emphasizing Child-Centered Play Therapy is indicated when the counselor expects to facilitate the child's own problem-solving capacity (Knell, 1993, 1994; Landreth, 1991). The Gingerbread Child Guidance Clinic counselor is comfortable theoretically integrating these approaches.

The counselor used the Inverted Pyramid Method of case conceptualization because this method is especially designed to help clinicians more easily form their conceptual pictures of their clients' needs (Neukrug & Schwitzer, 2006; Schwitzer, 1996, 1997). The method has four steps: Problem Identification, Thematic Groupings, Theoretical Inferences, and Narrowed Inferences. The counselor's clinical thinking can be seen in Figure 7.3.

Step 1: Problem Identification. The first step is Problem Identification. Aspects of the presenting problem (thoughts, feelings, behaviors, physiological features), additional areas of concern besides the presenting concern, family and developmental history, in-session observations, clinical inquiries (medical problems, medications, past counseling, substance use, suicidality), and psychological assessments (problem checklists, personality inventories, mental status exam, specific clinical measures) all may contribute information at Step 1. The counselor "casts a wide net" in order to build Step 1 as exhaustively as possible (Neukrug & Schwitzer, 2006, p. 202). As can be seen in Figure 7.3, the counselor thoroughly noted not just all of Gretel's current oppositional and defiant behaviors occurring at school and at home, all of Gretel's aggressive and disrespectful behaviors occurring with peers in various school and neighborhood settings, and her running away and challenge of adults—but also, as much important information as he could find regarding Gretel's earlier developmental experiences, childhood life transitions, and parental and caretaker experiences. He attempted to go beyond just listing the main behaviors that precipitated the referral and to be as complete as he could.

Step 2: Thematic Groupings. The second step is Thematic Groupings. The clinician organizes all of the exhaustive client information found in Step 1 into just a few intuitive-logical clinical groups, categories, or themes, on the basis of sensible common denominators (Neukrug & Schwitzer, 2006). Four different ways of forming the Step 2 theme groups can be used: Descriptive-Diagnosis Approach, Clinical Targets Approach, Areas of Dysfunction Approach, and Intrapsychic Approach. As can be seen in Figure 7.3, Gretel's counselor selected the Areas of Dysfunction Approach. This approach sorts together all of the Step 1 information into "areas of dysfunction according to important life situations, life themes, or life roles and skills" (Neukrug & Schwitzer, 2006, p. 205).

The counselor formed two groupings. He grouped together all of Gretel's negative parental and family experiences (loss of mother, au pair difficulties, relocation, stepmother difficulties, absent father, etc.) into the theme: History of absent, emotionally absent, neglectful, and/or punitive parents and adult caretakers since pre-age 3. Likewise, he grouped together all of the remaining Step 1 items—Gretel's many past and current hostile and problematic behaviors and attitudes—into the theme: Current oppositional and defiant attitudes and behaviors in school, home, and neighborhood.

So far, at Steps 1 and 2, the counselor has used his clinical assessment skills and his clinical judgment to begin critically describing Gretel's needs. Now, at Steps 3 and 4, he applies the theoretical approach he has selected. He begins making theoretical inferences to explain the factors leading to, and maintaining, Gretel's issues as they are seen in Steps 1 and 2.

Step 3: Theoretical Inferences. At Step 3, concepts from the counselor's theoretical integration of two approaches—Child-Centered Play Therapy and Cognitive Behavioral Play Therapy—are applied to the factors causing, and the mechanisms maintaining, Gretel's reasons for referral. The counselor tentatively matches the theme groups in Step 2 with this theoretical approach. In other words, the symptom constellations in Step 2, which were distilled from the symptoms in Step 1, now are combined using theory to show what are believed to be the underlying processes or psychological mechanisms of Gretel's current needs (Neukrug & Schwitzer, 2006; Schwitzer, 2006, 2007).

First, Child-Centered Play Therapy was applied primarily to Gretel's attitudes and use of behaviors for self-expression. According to the Child-Centered Play Therapy conceptual model, adult-child relationships characterized by warm, genuine, unconditional positive regard set the conditions for the child to develop his or her natural "innate human capacity" to "strive toward growth and maturity," become "constructively self-directing," and able to responsibly and realistically express his or her thoughts, feelings, and attitudes (Landreth & Sweeney, 1997, p. 17). Without these relationship conditions, or with contradictory conditions, the child may not develop a positive striving, constructive self-direction, and responsible and realistic self-expression; instead, she may develop in problematic or frustrating directions (Landreth, 1991; Landreth & Sweeney, 1997). Correspondingly, as can be seen in Figure 7.3, Gretel's counselor made the theoretical inference that "Gretel is engaging in hostile types of attitudes and behaviors in order to express negative, ambivalent, and anxious feelings she has toward parents, adults, and peer targets."

Second, Cognitive Behavioral Play Therapy was applied primarily to Gretel's learned behaviors.

According to the Cognitive Behavioral Play Therapy model, cognitive and behavioral learning principles apply to children so that the child's behaviors often may be understood as stemming from faulty learning or faulty beliefs; his or her thoughts, feelings, fantasies, and environment all may contribute to inaccurate learned behaviors and reactions (Knell, 1993, 1994). As also can be seen in Figure 7.3, when Gretel's counselor additionally applied these concepts, he developed a further Step 3 inference, as follows: Gretel has learned through her history of relationship experiences with parents, stepparents, and other adults that she is unsuccessful at communicating her thoughts and feelings through realistic positive, responsible expressions and actions.

Step 4: Narrowed Inferences. At Step 4, the clinician's selected theory continues to be used to address still-deeper issues when they exist (Schwitzer, 2006, 2007). At this step, "still-deeper, more encompassing, or more central, causal themes" are formed (Neukrug & Schwitzer, 2006, p. 207). Gretel's counselor continued to use psychotherapeutic integration of two approaches.

First, continuing to apply Child-Centered Play Therapy concepts at Step 4, the counselor presented a single, deepest theoretical inference that he believed to be most fundamental for Gretel from a child-centered perspective: Gretel has failed to experience the types of attending, encouraging, unconditionally positive parental and adult relationships needed to promote her responsible, positive, self-directed expression of self and management of self; instead, she has experienced the types of nonattending, discouraging, conditional, negative parental and adult relationships that promote irresponsible, negative, un-self-managed expressions of self through hostile attitudes and behaviors. Second, continuing to apply Cognitive Behavioral Play Therapy concepts, Gretel's counselor presented an additional, complementary deep theoretical inference, as follows: Gretel maintains the faulty belief that using hostile, negative behaviors is the only method she has for successfully expressing her attitudes, thoughts, and feelings. These two narrowed inferences, together, form the basis for understanding Gretel's current counseling situation as we have written her imagined clinical case illustration.

When all four steps are completed, the client information in Step 1 leads to logical-intuitive groupings on the basis of common denominators in Step 2, the groupings then are explained using theory at Step 3, and then, finally, at Step 4, further deeper explanations are made. From start to finish, the thoughts, feelings, behaviors, and physiological features in the topmost portions are connected on down the pyramid into deepest dynamics.

TREATMENT PLANNING

At this point, Gretel's clinician at the Gingerbread Child Guidance Clinic has collected all available information about the problems that have been of concern to her and the psychological team that performed her assessment. Based upon this information, the counselor developed a five-axis *DSM-IV-TR* diagnosis and then, using the "inverted pyramid" (Neukrug & Schwitzer, 2006; Schwitzer, 1996, 1997), formulated a working clinical *explanation* of Gretel's difficulties and their etiology that we called the *case conceptualization*. This, in turn, guides us to the next critical step in our clinical work, called the *treatment plan*, the primary purpose of which is to map out a logical and goal-oriented strategy for making positive changes in the client's life. In essence, the treatment plan is a road map "for reducing or eliminating disruptive symptoms that are impeding the client's ability to reach positive mental health outcomes" (Neukrug & Schwitzer, 2006, p. 225). As such, it is the cornerstone of our work with not only Gretel, but with all clients who present with disturbing and disruptive symptoms and/or personality patterns (Jongsma & Peterson, 2006; Jongsma, Peterson, & McInnis, 2003a, 2003b; Seligman, 1993, 1998, 2004).

A comprehensive treatment plan must integrate all of the information from the biopsychosocial

Figure 7.3 Gretel's Inverted Pyramid Case Conceptualization Summary: Psychotherapeutic Integration of Child-Centered Play Therapy and Cognitive Behavioral Play Therapy

1. IDENTIFY AND LIST CLIENT CONCERNS

Repeated hiding lunchbox as practical joke
Deliberately annoying classroom behavior
Deliberately annoying home behavior (costumes)
Blames other children for her misbehavior
"Short-fused" temper
Impaired classroom relationships
Argumentative
Impaired family relationships
Easy resentment
Spiteful, hostile
Mutters at teachers

Age 3 bedridden, absent mother
Death of mother at age 3
Age 3–7 punitive au pair
Au pair bringing men to house
Age 7 relocation to U.S.
Geographic and personal adjustment
Yells at stepmother
Stepmother emotionally neglectful
Stepmother neglectful of children's
    caretaking needs
Has recently run away
Absent father

2. ORGANIZE CONCERNS INTO LOGICAL THEMATIC GROUPINGS

1. History of absent, emotionally absent, neglectful,
   and/or punitive parents and adult caretakers since age 3
2. Current oppositional and defiant attitude and behaviors
   in school, home, and neighborhood

**3. THEORETICAL INFERENCES: ATTACH THEMATIC
GROUPINGS TO INFERRED AREAS OF DIFFICULTY**
Psychotherapeutic Integration

Child-Centered Play Therapy
Gretel is engaging in hostile types of
  attitudes and behaviors in order to
express negative, ambivalent, and
anxious feelings she has toward
parents, adults, and peer targets

Cognitive-Behavioral Play Therapy
Gretel has learned through her history of
relationship experiences with parents,
stepparents, and other adults that she is
unsuccessful communicating her thoughts
and feelings through realistic positive,
responsible expressions and actions

**4. NARROWED INFERENCES:
SUICIDALITY AND DEEPER
DIFFICULTIES**
Psychotherapeutic Integration

Child-Centered Play Therapy
Gretel has failed to experience the
types of attending, encouraging,
unconditionally positive parental and
adult relationships needed to
promote her responsible self and
management of self; instead she has
experienced the types of nonattending, discouraging, conditional,
negative parental and adult
relationships that promote
irresponsible, negative, un-self-
managed expressions of self through
hostile attitudes

Cognitive Behavioral Play
Gretel maintains the faulty belief that using
hostile, negative behaviors is the only
method she has for successfully expressing
her attitudes, thoughts, and feelings, and
behaviors

interview, diagnosis, and case conceptualization into a coherent plan of action. This *plan* comprises four main components, which include (1) a behavioral definition of the problem(s), (2) the selection of achievable goals, (3) the determination of treatment modes, and (4) the documentation of how change will be measured. The *behavioral definition of the problem(s)* consolidates the results of the case conceptualization into a concise hierarchical list of problems and concerns that will be the focus of treatment. The *selection of achievable goals* refers to assessing and prioritizing the client's concerns into a *hierarchy of urgency* that also takes into account the client's motivation for change, level of dysfunction, and real-world influences on his or her problems. The *determination of treatment modes* refers to selection of the specific interventions, which are matched to the uniqueness of the client and to his or her goals and clearly tied to a particular theoretical orientation (Neukrug & Schwitzer, 2006). Finally, the clinician must establish how change will be measured, based upon a number of factors, including client records and self-report of change, in-session observations by the clinician, clinician ratings, results of standardized evaluations such as the Conners 3 (Conners, 2008) or a family functioning questionnaire, pre-post treatment comparisons, and reports by other treating professionals.

The four-step method discussed above can be seen in Figure 6.1 (p. 109) and is outlined below for the case of Gretel, followed by her specific treatment plan.

Step 1: Behavioral Definition of Problems. The first step in treatment planning is to carefully review the case conceptualization, paying particular attention to the results of Step 2 (Thematic Groupings), Step 3 (Theoretical Inferences) and Step 4 (Narrowed Inferences). The identified clinical themes reflect the core areas of concern and distress for the client, while the theoretical and narrowed inferences offer clinical speculation as to their origins. In the case of Gretel, there are two primary areas of concern. The first, "history of absent, emotionally absent, neglectful and/or punitive parents and

adult caretakers since age 3," refers to the terminal illness and death of her mother when she was 3 years old, being raised by a punitive au pair between the ages of 3 and 7, the father's remarriage to an emotionally and behaviorally neglectful stepmother, and the subsequent absence of her father from the home for long periods. The second, "current oppositional and defiant attitudes and behaviors at school, home and neighborhood," refers to repeatedly hiding a lunchbox as practical joke, deliberately annoying classroom and home behavior, blaming other children for her misbehavior, a short-fused temper, argumentativeness, resentfulness, spitefulness and hostility, yelling at her stepmother, muttering at her teachers, running away from home, and impaired classroom and family relationships. These symptoms are consistent with the diagnosis of Oppositional Defiant Disorder (APA, 2000a; Matthys & Lochman, 2010; Parritz & Troy, 2011).

Step 2: Identify and Articulate Goals for Change. The second step is the selection of achievable goals, which is based upon a number of factors, including the most pressing or urgent behavioral, emotional, and interpersonal concerns and symptoms as identified by the client and clinician, the willingness and ability of the client to work on those particular goals, and the realistic (real-world) achievability of those goals (Neukrug & Schwitzer, 2006). At this stage of treatment planning, it is important to recognize that not all of the client's problems can be addressed at once, so we focus initially on those that cause the greatest distress and impairment. New goals can be created as old ones are achieved. In the case of Gretel, the goals are divided into two prominent areas. The first, "history of absent, emotionally absent, neglectful and/or punitive parents and adult caretakers since age 3," requires that we help Gretel to successfully grieve the loss of her mother, to begin reinvesting in relationships with others, and to resolve her feelings of sadness and anger that are associated with the loss. Successful achievement of this goal also requires that we help Gretel's father and stepmother understand and support Gretel through this grief process, while also strengthening their marital relationship and parent effectiveness. The second, "current oppositional and defiant attitudes and behaviors at school, home, and neighborhood," requires that we help Gretel to reduce the frequency and intensity of hostile and defiant behaviors toward adults, terminate her defiant and aggressive behavior and replace it with controlled, respectful, and obedient behavior, to resolve the conflict that underlies anger, hostility, and defiance, and to improve her relationship with peers, teachers, and parents. In order to achieve these goals, we must also help her parents and teachers to more effectively discipline her and to communicate with each other regarding her behavior at home and in school.

Step 3: Describe Therapeutic Interventions. This is perhaps the most critical step in the treatment planning process because the clinician must now integrate information from a number of sources, including the case conceptualization, the delineation of the client's problems and goals, and the treatment literature, paying particular attention to *empirically supported treatment* (EST) and *evidence-based practice* (EBP). In essence, the clinician must align his or her treatment approach with scientific evidence from the fields of counseling and psychotherapy. Wampold (2001) identifies two types of evidence-based counseling research: studies that demonstrate "absolute efficacy," that is, the fact that counseling and psychotherapy work, and those that demonstrate "relative efficacy," that is, the fact that certain theoretical/technical approaches work best for certain clients with particular problems (Psychoanalysis, Gestalt Therapy, Cognitive Behavior Therapy, Brief Solution-Focused Therapy, Cognitive Therapy, Dialectical Behavior Therapy, Person-Centered Therapy, Expressive/Creative Therapies, Interpersonal Therapy, and Feminist Therapy); and when delivered through specific treatment modalities (individual, group, and family counseling).

In the case of Gretel, we have decided to use an Integrative Approach to counseling that combines Child-Centered Play Therapy (CCPT) and Cognitive Behavior Play Therapy, supplemented with Family Play Therapy. It is important to note that "specific interventions proposed for clinical disturbances . . . have included individual psychotherapy for the child and/or caregiver, parent training with emphasis on developmental expectations and sensitive responsiveness, family therapy or caregiver/child dyadic therapy" (Zeanah & Boris, 2005, p. 365). CCPT is a humanistic and nondirective approach to child counseling that derives from the work of Carl Rogers (Rogers, 1961, 1977) and Virginia Axline (1947). It is based upon the premise that children have an inherent capacity for self-understanding, self-expression, positive relationships, and mental health, which can be nurtured and facilitated under the therapeutic conditions of attuned empathy, congruence, and unconditional positive regard. In the nonjudgmental and nonhurried playspace that provides the child access to toys, materials, and activities for the full expression of thoughts, feelings, and behaviors, he or she can work through conflicts, gain self-acceptance, and develop effective coping skills for living in the world (Landreth, 2002; Moustakas, 1959; Nordling, Cochran, & Cochran, 2010). It has been effectively applied to a wide range of child behavior and emotional problems, including the symptoms of Oppositional Defiant Disorder (Baggerly, Ray, & Bratton, 2010; VanFleet, Sywulak, Caporaso, Sniscak, & Guerney, 2010). Specific techniques that will be drawn from this approach will include using unconditional positive regard, acceptance, attuned empathy, focused tracking, and selective limit-setting with Gretel as she engages with the different materials and activities in the playroom (arts and crafts, puppets, dollhouse, drawing, storytelling, role-playing). With regard to Gretel's Conduct Disorder symptoms, techniques drawn from this approach will include using unconditional positive regard, acceptance, attuned empathy, focused tracking, and selective limit-setting in the therapeutic playroom as she engages with different materials and activities (arts and crafts, puppets, dollhouse, drawing, storytelling, role-playing).

Cognitive Behavior Play Therapy was originally devised as a means of applying the empirically proven methods of cognitive and behavior therapy to working with children, particularly in the playroom (Knell, 1993, 1994). This approach relies on a variety of cognitive techniques (reframing, challenging irrational thoughts, and cognitive restructuring) and behavioral techniques (reinforcement for and shaping of adaptive behavior, extinction of maladaptive behaviors, systematic desensitization, exposure with response prevention). However, the cognitive behavioral play therapist may also use artistic and expressive playroom materials, such as board games, puppets, dolls, drawing, storytelling, and the sandtray to achieve these ends. An example would be engaging a child through the use of puppets in a conversation about angry feelings and defiant behavior for the purpose of refuting irrational thoughts and/or shaping positive behavior. This technique has been effectively applied to a variety of childhood emotional and behavioral problems, including symptoms of Oppositional Defiant Disorder (Drewes, 2009). Specific techniques drawn from this approach will include using puppets and role-play to address Gretel's oppositional defiant behavior, shaping prosocial behavior through sandtray miniature play, and creating cartoon-strip stories around the themes of opposition and positive engagement.

Family Play Therapy is a means of engaging and problem-solving with the entire family using the methods and materials of play therapy. Reliant upon play and playful interaction, it provides a comfortable medium for children and adults, engages family members in a common pleasurable task, allows for a deeper level of communication, facilitates a broad scope of diagnostic information, and encourages family relatedness (Lowenstein, 2008, 2010). Although the empirical evidence base for Family Play Therapy is evolving, techniques drawn from this modality have been effectively applied with children and families struggling with a wide range of problems, including bereavement communication difficulties and behavioral problems (Ariel, 2005; Gil, 1984; Schaefer & Carey, 1994). With regard to the case of Gretel, the therapist will use the family play genogram, family puppet play, family drawing, family house-building, and family sculpting.

Additionally, both parents and teachers will be given psychoeducation in child bereavement and Oppositional Defiant Disorder, the means with which to communicate with each other about Gretel's behavior, and Parent Effectiveness Training [PET] (Gordon, 2000).

Step 4: Provide Outcome Measures of Change. This last step in treatment planning requires that we specify how change will be measured and indicate the extent to which progress has been made toward realizing these goals (Neukrug & Schwitzer, 2006). The counselor has considerable flexibility in this phase and may choose from a number of objective domains (psychological tests and measures of self-esteem, depression, psychosis, interpersonal relationship, anxiety, etc.), quasi-objective measures (the *DSM-IV-TR's* Axis V GAF scale; pre-post clinician, client, and psychiatric ratings), and subjective ratings (client self-report, clinician's in-session observations). In Gretel's case, we have implemented a number of these, including pre-post measures of behavior including conduct problems and impulse control on the parent and teacher version of the Conners 3 (Conners, 2008), sustained post-only measures of GAF functioning in the mild range (>70), client self-report of friendly and prosocial relationships with peers at school, teacher- and parent-reported improvement in behavior, compliance; impulse, behavior, and emotional control, and parent and teacher report of improved daily communication between home and school.

The completed treatment plan is now developed through which the counselor, Gretel, and her parents (and teachers) will begin their shared work of building an effective behavioral management system at home and at school, enhancing communication channels between parents and teachers, modifying and then reducing the impact of her Oppositional Defiant Disorder, and helping Gretel to effectively grieve her losses. Gretel's treatment plan is as follows and is summarized in Table 7.3.

TREATMENT PLAN

Client: Gretel

Service Provider: Gingerbread Child Guidance Clinic

BEHAVIORAL DEFINITION OF PROBLEMS:

1. History of absent, emotionally absent, neglectful, and/or punitive parents and adult caretakers since age 3—Terminal illness and death of mother at 3 years of age, raised by a punitive au pair between the ages of 3 and 7, father's remarriage to an emotionally and behaviorally neglectful stepmother, subsequent absence of father from the home for long periods

2. Current oppositional and defiant attitudes and behaviors at school, home, and neighborhood—Repeatedly hiding lunchbox as practical joke, deliberately annoying classroom and home behavior, blaming other children for own misbehavior, a short-fused temper, argumentativeness, resentfulness, spitefulness and hostility, yelling at stepmother, muttering at teachers, running away from home, and impaired classroom and family relationships

GOALS FOR CHANGE:

1. History of absent, emotionally absent, neglectful, and/or punitive parents and adult caretakers since age 3

   Goals for Gretel

   - Successfully grieve the loss of mother
   - Begin reinvesting in relationships with others
   - Resolve her feelings of sadness and anger that are associated with the loss

   Related Goals for Parents

   - Understand and support Gretel through grief process
   - Strengthening the marital relationship

2. Current oppositional and defiant attitudes and behaviors at school, home, and neighborhood

   Goals for Gretel

   - Reduce the frequency and intensity of hostile and defiant behaviors toward adults and peers
   - Terminate defiant and aggressive behavior and replace with controlled, respectful, and obedient behavior
   - Resolve the conflict that underlies anger, hostility, and defiance
   - Improve relationship with peers, teachers, and parents

   Goals for Parents and Teachers

   - Guide parents and teachers to more effective discipline practices
   - Communicate with each other regarding behavior at home and in school

(Continued)

(Continued)

THERAPEUTIC INTERVENTIONS:

A moderate-term course (4–6 months) of Integrated Counseling including Child-Centered, Cognitive Behavior, and Family Play Therapy, supplemented with Parent Effectiveness Training

1. History of absent, emotionally absent, neglectful, and/or punitive parents and adult caretakers since age 3

Techniques for Gretel

- Using unconditional positive regard, acceptance, attuned empathy, focused tracking, and selective limit-setting in the therapeutic playroom as client engages with different materials and activities (arts and crafts, puppets, dollhouse, drawing, storytelling, role-playing)

Techniques for Adults and Gretel

- Family play genogram
- Family puppet play
- Family drawing
- Family house-building
- Family sculpting

2. Current oppositional and defiant attitudes and behaviors at school, home, and neighborhood

Techniques for Gretel

- Using unconditional positive regard, acceptance, attuned empathy, focused tracking, and selective limit-setting in the therapeutic playroom as client engages with different materials and activities (arts and crafts, puppets, dollhouse, drawing, storytelling, role-playing)
- Using puppets and role-play to address oppositional defiant behavior
- Shaping prosocial behavior through sandtray miniature play
- Creating cartoon-strip stories around the themes of opposition and positive engagement

Techniques for Adults

- Psychoeducation in oppositional defiant behavior
- Parent effectiveness training
- Psychoeducation in child bereavement
- Daily communication report between home and school

OUTCOME MEASURES OF CHANGE:

Reduced oppositional defiant behavior, increased behavioral and emotional compliance as well as prosocial behavior, and effective grieving as measured by:

- Pre-post measures of behavior, including conduct problems and impulse control on parent and teacher version of the Conners 3
- Sustained post-only measures of GAF functioning in the mild range (>70)
- Clinician and client self-report of friendly and prosocial relationships with peers at school
- Clinician observation of effective grieving through play
- Teacher- and parent-reported improvement in compliance; impulse, behavior, and emotional control
- Parent and teacher report of improved daily communication between home and school
- Parent report of improved communication and relationship (including father's presence in home)

Table 7.3   Gretel's Treatment Plan Summary: Psychotherapeutic Integration of Child-Centered Play Therapy and Cognitive Behavioral Play Therapy

Goals for Change	Therapeutic Interventions	Outcome Measures of Change
History of absent, emotionally absent, neglectful, and/or punitive parents and adult caretakers since age 3	History of absent, emotionally absent, neglectful, and/or punitive parents and adult caretakers since age 3	Reduced oppositional defiant behavior, increased behavioral and emotional compliance as well as prosocial behavior, and effective grieving as measured by:
Goals for Gretel	*Techniques for Gretel*	
Successfully grieve the loss of mother	Using unconditional positive regard, acceptance, attuned empathy, focused tracking, and selective limit-setting in the therapeutic playroom as client engages with different materials and activities (arts and crafts, puppets, dollhouse, drawing, storytelling, role-playing)	Pre-post measures of behavior, including conduct problems and impulse control on parent and teacher version of the Conners 3
Begin reinvesting in relationships with others		
Resolve her feelings of sadness and anger that are associated with the loss		Sustained post-only measures of GAF functioning in the mild range (>70)
Related Goals for Parents	*Techniques for Adults and Gretel*	
Understand and support Gretel through grief process	Family play genogram	Clinician and client self-report of friendly and prosocial relationships with peers at school
Strengthening the marital relationship	Family puppet play	
	Family drawing	
	Family house-building	Clinician observation of effective grieving through play
	Family sculpting	
Current oppositional and defiant attitudes and behaviors at school, home, and neighborhood	Current oppositional and defiant attitudes and behaviors at school, home, and neighborhood	Teacher- and parent-reported improvement in compliance; and impulse, behavior, and emotional control
Goals for Gretel	*Techniques for Gretel*	
Reduce the frequency and intensity of hostile and defiant behaviors toward adults and peers	Using unconditional positive regard, acceptance, attuned empathy, focused tracking, and selective limit-setting in the therapeutic playroom as client engages with different materials and activities (arts and crafts, puppets, dollhouse, drawing, storytelling, role-playing)	Parent and teacher report of improved daily communication between home and school
Terminate defiant and aggressive behavior and replace with controlled, respectful, and obedient behavior		Parent report of improved communication and relationship (including father presence in home)
Resolve the conflict that underlies anger, hostility, and defiance	Using puppets and role-play to address oppositional defiant behavior	
Improve relationship with peers, teachers, and parents	Shaping prosocial behavior through sandtray miniature play	
Goals for Parents and Teacher	Creating cartoon-strip stories around the themes of opposition and positive engagement	
Guide parents and teachers to more effective discipline practices	*Techniques for Adults*	
	Psychoeducation in oppositional defiant behavior	
	Parent effectiveness training	
Communicate with each other regarding behavior at home and in school	Psychoeducation in child bereavement	
	Daily communication report between home and school	

CASE 7.4   JAPANESE ANIME'S NARUTO

INTRODUCING THE CHARACTER

Naruto Uzumaki is the main character in the Japanese manga and anime juggernaut of the same name. The manga, a Japanese print comic or cartoon popular art form, was first introduced in 1999 in Japan's *Shonen Jump Magazine* and introduced to North America in television and movie form by VIZ Media in 2005. Naruto has received numerous awards and is one of the most popular anime and manga characters in the world.

Naruto's story begins in the tiny Japanese village of Konohagakure, which is tyrannized by the dreaded "nine-tailed demon fox" who randomly and viciously kills villagers. A military leader of the village is able to subdue the demon fox and seal it inside the orphaned newborn Naruto. However, because this otherwise innocent child now contains the essence of evil, he is spurned by the village, regarded as an enemy, and ostracized. Naruto embarks on a series of pranks, ostensibly attention getting, but that only serve to further ostracize him from the village. Naruto is taken under the wing of martial arts teacher, Kakashe Hatake, who brings him into the protective circle of the village military school. There he befriends Sasuke Uchiha and Sakura Haruno, who together with Naruto form the powerful Team 7. The stories that follow chronicle the adventures of Team 7 and Naruto as he grows into a powerful, respected, and feared ninja who learns the importance of self-control, being a team player, and the true meaning of valor. The following basic case summary and diagnostic impressions describe what we portray as Naruto's childhood concerns associated with patterns of inattention and hyperactivity, and the violation of others' rights and age-appropriate norms.

Meet the Client

You can assess the client in action by viewing clips of Naruto's video material at the following websites:

- http://www.hulu.com/watch/35645/ naruto-enter-naruto-uzumaki#s-p12-n1- so-i0 Naruto's origin story
- http://www.hulu.com/watch/35628/ naruto-sasuke-and-sakura-friends-or- foes#s-p11-n1-so-i0 Naruto and friends
- http://www.hulu.com/watch/35657/ naruto-the-land-where-a-hero-once- lived#s-p10-n1-so-i0 A hero's journey
- http://www.hulu.com/watch/60872/ naruto-the-closed-door#s-p11-so-i0 The Closed Door

BASIC CASE SUMMARY

Identifying Information. Naruto Uzumaki is a 9-year-old Japanese boy who lives in London, England. He attends school and receives martial arts training at the Shonen Jump Academy on the outskirts of the city. His appearance is notable for his athletic build.

Presenting Concern. Naruto was referred to the London Clinic by the Shonen Jump Academy headmaster, Nigel Englander, who has become increasingly frustrated with the boy's hyperactive, impulsive, and destructive behaviors around the school as well as his seemingly uncontrollable preoccupation with becoming a "ninja master." Although the instructors at the school recognize that Naruto has had a very difficult life, they now fear for the safety of the other students and have observed that in spite of his martial arts training,

Naruto often seems incapable of appropriately channeling his aggressive impulses.

Background, Family Information, and Relevant History. Naruto was born in a small fishing village on the outskirts of Tokyo where, soon after his birth, he was abandoned, primarily because the strange birthmark on his neck frightened his young and deeply spiritual parents. Naruto spent the first 2 years of his life in the care of extended family who noticed from the start that "the boy was unique" and possessed what was described as a "mystical aura." By the time Naruto was 4 years old, he proved almost ungovernable, and family members began to suspect that he was somehow possessed by an evil spirit.

According to a social services report, the elders feared for the welfare of the family and therefore decided to bring Naruto to the Tokyo Orphanage where, because of his alluring physical features, he was quickly placed with a Japanese-British couple who had lost their first child in a drowning incident. Naruto's transition to this new family and living in Great Britain were apparently difficult from the start; he cried almost incessantly, was difficult to soothe, and initially made little eye contact with his newly adopted family. Over time, Naruto's adjustment and relation to his new family appear to have improved.

Naruto's parents enrolled him for school in London's Shonen Jump Academy, where he initially thrived but soon became a concern to his teachers. A second-grade psychological evaluation indicated that "in summary, Naruto is a very bright and academically gifted child who has had great difficulty adjusting to the demands of a structured classroom environment . . . his impulsivity, distractibility, and almost uncontrollable activity level pose a danger to his classmates and it is therefore recommended that he be transferred to the Special Education Program." Once

placed in that program with other children who had similar difficulties, Naruto became notably more unmanageable, aggressive, and indiscriminately violent toward his classmates.

Once Naruto began aggressing toward his adoptive parents, they attempted psychiatric intervention; however, the child was highly resistant to taking medication. The parents began quarreling late into the evening, lamenting that they had waited so long for a child, but that Naruto was coming between them. It was at that point that they had to decide whether to keep the child or return him to the state system. After weeks of deliberation and spiritual counseling, they decided that Naruto had spent too much time disconnected from family and had experienced too many upsetting transitions and that they would therefore commit to remaining his parents.

Problem and Counseling History. Naruto was first observed in several of his classes, both in the morning and afternoon, once from behind a one-way mirror and on multiple occasions by an in-class evaluator. He was observed during both seat work and free play within the classroom as well as when shadowed during two of the school day's recesses. In comparison with the other children in his class, Naruto was highly active, easily distracted, occasionally and seemingly randomly aggressive toward other children, and unaffected by his teacher's numerous attempts at maintaining his attention or holding him accountable for his behavior.

His teachers expressed concerns that although he is a bright student, he performs very poorly at math because of careless mistakes beyond those usually made by his age group. His teachers also reported that in spite of his abilities, he earned low grades in many subjects because he would fail to follow straightforward instructions, seemed unable to carefully organize his thoughts and writing, had almost daily challenges "just staying on the topic" or "listening to me when I speak to him." In addition, they rarely collected completed homework from Naruto, who reported to his teachers that "I hate this hard stuff and I don't want to do it."

After 3 days of observation, Naruto was visited by the school counselor and engaged in a number of creative activities, including drawing, sculpting, and storytelling. During these visits, his attention was more easily maintained, likely due to the changing and creative nature of the activities. However, when the evaluator attempted to hold short conversations without play or activities, he was unable to pay attention, drummed his fingers, and squirmed. Further, when the evaluator announced the imminent ending of the sessions, Naruto became irritable, verbally aggressive, and ran about the room saying, "You can't catch me, you can't catch me. I'm a Ninja." He then drew a picture of himself dressed in an orange ninja outfit killing both his teacher and the evaluator. As he left the room, Naruto shouted, "You'll never get me to stay . . . I have the power of the nine-tailed fox, and I can clone myself into fifteen copies."

His parents report similar behaviors in the home and that Naruto repeatedly lost house keys, sports equipment, and other items. They said he could not be relied on to do age-appropriate jobs at home like taking out the trash, even when they tried implementing a chart of chores and a reward system. They also reported that they suspected he was "terrorizing the neighbor children" by threatening to "beat them up with my ninja powers," bringing his martial arts weapons onto the playground, and stealing their schoolbooks. Although his peers are hesitant to identify him, it is relatively certain that he is responsible for a head wound sustained by one classmate during a "game." His parents report that neighborhood parents no longer will allow their children to play with Naruto, and outside of school, most avoid him.

Both teachers and parents observe that Naruto has difficulty staying in his seat in the classroom or, for example, at the dinner table, at home; and echo that it is "nearly impossible to get him to be still for a few minutes!" At home, his father is unable to engage Naruto is quiet tasks such as fishing or soccer drills; at school, monitors are unable to allow him to eat in the main cafeteria because he "runs around like his clock is wound too tight." In classes he enjoys, when he does pay attention, his teachers report that he is so noisy and so quick to jump into discussions, that other children are intimidated or outshouted.

Goals for Counseling and Course of Therapy to Date. The observation team met with Naruto's parents a week after the last visit and determined that he had a multitude of psychosocial needs. The team's decision was that Naruto's most immediate needs were for a therapeutic connection through which he could form a secure bond and, as characterized by the lead counselor, "Begin the long therapeutic journey." Specific short-term and long-term goals will be provided in the accompanying treatment plan.

Diagnostic Impressions

Axis I.   314.01 Attention-Deficit/Hyperactivity Disorder, Combined Type

   312.81 Conduct Disorder, Childhood-Onset Type, Moderate

Axis II.   V71.09 No Diagnosis on Axis II

Axis III.   Mild ankle sprain (athletic injury)

Axis IV.   Problems with primary support group—Removal from the home, multiple home placements, adoption

   Problems related to social environment—Geographic relocation to Great Britain

Axis V.   GAF = 51 (Current)

   GAF = 65 (Highest level past year)

DISCUSSION OF
DIAGNOSTIC IMPRESSIONS

Naruto was referred to the London Clinic by the academic headmaster in response to his hyperactive, impulsive, and destructive school behaviors. A previous psychological report similarly identified his impulsivity, distractibility, and "almost uncontrollable" activity level. When observed in class, he did, indeed, appear highly active and easily distracted. His parents reported that at home he lost important items like keys, failed to follow through on chores like taking out the trash, and almost had an inability to "sit still" at the dinner table. Further, his teachers and headmaster found his bullying, physical fights with other children, and intimidation of his classmates worrisome; and at home, his parents similarly worry that he has been "terrorizing" neighborhood children. He also has stolen and probably caused another child's head wound.

The section of the *DSM-IV-TR* titled "Disorders Usually First Diagnosed in Infancy, Childhood, or Adolescence" has a wide reach. The section is organized into a large number of groupings of disorders that all share the feature of occurring early in the life cycle. The grouping known as the Attention-Deficit and Disruptive Behavior Disorders is especially important to the everyday practice of counseling professionals who work with children and adolescents in school and community settings (Reif, 2005). Attention Deficit/Hyperactivity Disorder (ADHD), Conduct Disorder (CD), and Oppositional Defiant Disorder all are in this group.

We portrayed Naruto's childhood concerns to include a pattern of inattention and hyperactivity, and a pattern of violating others' rights and age-appropriate norms. His problematic behavior has been persistent for at least a year. Naruto's inattentive and hyperactive-impulsive behaviors have occurred both at school and at home. These behaviors are characteristic of ADHD. This diagnosis is suggested when abundant inattention symptoms are present, abundant hyperactive symptoms are present, or when both sets are present, so much so that they undermine the child's functioning. Naruto is experiencing both sets of maladaptive behaviors about equally, indicating a subtype of Combined Type.

One differential diagnosis that might be considered is No Diagnosis on Axis I because "in early childhood, it may be difficult to distinguish symptoms of Attention-Deficit/Hyperactivity Disorder from age-appropriate behaviors in active children such as 'running around or being noisy'" (APA, 2000a, p. 91). However, Naruto's behaviors clearly lead to clinically significant impairment in social and occupational functioning, occur in more than one setting (school and home) as required for the diagnosis, and are excessive for both his age and developmental level.

In Naruto's childhood concerns, we also portrayed a second pattern of violating the basic rights of others, especially those of his peers, and age-appropriate norms by engaging in bullying and intimidation, using his martial arts tools as weapons, and stealing. These behaviors are characteristic of CD. Naruto is less than 10 years old, indicating Childhood-Onset Type. He displayed sufficient symptomatology to warrant the diagnosis, and since his actions have led to another child's injury and to his peer's "terror," we also assigned the subtype of Moderate Severity.

Another diagnosis that may be considered in Naruto's case is Oppositional Defiant Disorder, which is also found among the group of Disruptive Behaviors diagnoses in the *DSM-IV-TR's* Disorders Usually First Diagnosed in Infancy, Childhood, or Adolescence. However, Naruto's behaviors are better accounted for by CD, indicating a pattern of violating rules and norms and others' rights, than by Oppositional Defiant Disorder, which more narrowly refers to only negative, defiant attitudes and behaviors. Another differential consideration is whether a second diagnosis is needed at all in addition to ADHD. Although the hyperactive and impulsive behavior of children with ADHD often is disruptive, this behavior by itself is not characterized by violating age-appropriate social norms, and so the additional diagnosis is needed to describe and communicate about this pattern in Naruto's behavior.

To complete the diagnosis, Naruto's ankle sprain is listed on Axis III, his family and social stressors are emphasized on Axis IV, and on Axis V his functioning is represented by GAF scores ranging from the presence of only mild symptoms within the past year, to the current, moderately serious symptoms affecting school and other functioning that led to his referral. The information on these axes is consistent with the Axis I diagnosis describing Naruto's patterns.

CASE CONCEPTUALIZATION

When Naruto came in to the London Clinic, he first participated in an intake and evaluation meeting. The intake counselor collected as much information as possible about the problematic situations in school and outside of school that led to Naruto's referral. The counselor first used this information to develop diagnostic impressions. Naruto's concerns were described by the combined type of ADHD, along with moderate CD. Next, the counselor developed a case conceptualization. Whereas the purpose of diagnostic impressions is to *describe* the client's concerns, the goal of case conceptualization is to better *understand* and clinically *explain* the person's experiences (Neukrug & Schwitzer, 2006). It helps the counselor understand the etiology leading to Naruto's presenting concerns and the factors maintaining these behaviors. In turn, case conceptualization sets the stage for treatment planning. Treatment planning then provides a road map that plots out how the counselor and client expect to move from presenting concerns to positive outcomes (Seligman, 1993, p. 157)—helping Naruto increase his abilities to attend appropriately and manage his behavioral activity levels, and reduce his negative actions toward peers and adults.

When forming a case conceptualization, the clinician applies a purist counseling theory, an integration of two or more theories, an eclectic mix of theories, or a solution-focused combination of tactics, to his or her understanding of the client. In this case, Naruto's counselor based her conceptualization on a purist theory applicable to the behavioral needs of child clients, the Multicomponent Psychosocial Intervention

Approach. She selected this approach based on her knowledge of current outcome research and the best practice literature pertaining to child clients dealing with ADHD and conduct and related disorders (DuPaul & Stoner, 2003; Henggeler, Schoenwald, Borduin, Rowland, & Cunningham, 1998; Kazdin, 1995; Kazdin & Weisz, 2003). The Multicomponent Psychosocial Intervention Approach also is the London Clinic's treatment mode of choice for clients with these types of concerns, and the theory is consistent with this counselor's professional therapeutic viewpoint.

The counselor used the Inverted Pyramid Method of case conceptualization because this method is especially designed to help clinicians more easily form their conceptual pictures of their clients' needs (Neukrug & Schwitzer, 2006; Schwitzer, 1996, 1997). The method has four steps: Problem Identification; Thematic Groupings; Theoretical Inferences; and Narrowed Inferences. The counselor's clinical thinking can be seen in Figure 7.4.

Step 1: Problem Identification. The first step is Problem Identification. Aspects of the presenting problem (thoughts, feelings, behaviors, physiological features), additional areas of concern besides the presenting concern, family and developmental history, in-session observations, clinical inquiries (medical problems, medications, past counseling, substance use, suicidality), and psychological assessments (problem checklists, personality inventories, mental status exam, specific clinical measures) all may contribute information at Step 1. The counselor "casts a wide net" in order to build Step 1 as exhaustively as possible (Neukrug & Schwitzer, 2006, p. 202). As can be seen in the figure, the counselor thoroughly noted not just all of Naruto's hyperactive and inattention behaviors occurring at school and at home, all of Naruto's aggressive, violent, and intruding behaviors occurring with peers in various school and neighborhood settings, and his challenge of adults—but also, as much important information as she could find regarding Naruto's earlier developmental experiences, childhood life transitions, strengths and talents, and physical medical notes. She attempted to go beyond just listing the main behaviors, causing the referral and to be as complete as she could.

Step 2: Thematic Groupings. The second step is Thematic Groupings. The clinician organizes all of the exhaustive client information found in Step 1 into just a few intuitive-logical clinical groups, categories, or themes, on the basis of sensible common denominators (Neukrug & Schwitzer, 2006). Four different ways of forming the Step 2 theme groups can be used: Descriptive-Diagnosis Approach, Clinical Targets Approach, Areas of Dysfunction Approach, and Intrapsychic Approach. As can be seen in the figure, Naruto's counselor selected the Descriptive-Diagnosis Approach. This approach sorts together all of the various Step 1 information about the client's adjustment, development, distress, or dysfunction "to show larger clinical problems as reflected through a diagnosis" (Neukrug & Schwitzer, 2006, p. 205).

The counselor formed two themes by grouping together all of Naruto's behavioral challenges comprising ADHD (attention and hyperactivity in school, home, peer, and other social settings—occurring since an early age and throughout family changes, orphanage, and adoption transitions) and all of Naruto's behavioral challenges comprising CD (aggressive, uncontrolled behavior violating peers' rights and adults' authority—occurring since an early age and throughout family changes, orphanage, and adoption transitions). The counselor's conceptual work at Step 2 gave her a way to begin thinking about Naruto's functioning and concerns more insightfully.

So far, at Steps 1 and 2, the counselor has used her clinical assessment skills and clinical judgment to begin critically understanding Naruto's needs. Now, at Steps 3 and 4, she applies the selected theoretical approach. She begins making theoretical inferences to explain the factors leading to, and maintaining, Naruto's issues as they are seen in Steps 1 and 2.

Step 3: Theoretical Inferences. At Step 3, concepts from the counselor's selected theory, the Multicomponent Psychosocial Intervention Approach, are applied to explain the experiences causing, and the mechanisms maintaining Naruto's problematic behaviors. The counselor tentatively matches the theme groups in Step 2 with this theoretical approach. In other words, the symptom constellations in Step 2, which were distilled from the symptoms in Step 1, now are combined using theory to show what are believed to be the underlying causes or psychological etiology of Naruto's current needs (Neukrug & Schwitzer, 2006; Schwitzer, 2006, 2007).

Like family systems theory, the Multicomponent Psychosocial Intervention Approach is based on the assumption that a child's disruptive attending, hyperactive, and problematic conduct behaviors occur in social contexts: in school, in the family, in the neighborhood, and with peers (Henngeler et al., 1998). In turn, according to the theory, antecedents and behavioral consequences in various psychosocial contexts are important in maintaining the child's challenging behaviors (Barkley, 2006). Changes, therefore, are needed to modify and generalize new behavior across settings (Barkley, 2006; DuPaul & Stoner, 2003), including new self-management skills (Barkley, 2006; DuPaul & Stoner, 2003), new social skills (DuPaul & Weyandt, 2006), new teacher and classroom responses in school contexts (Barkley, 2006), and new responses from parents and in the family (Barkley, 2006; Hosie & Erik, 1993). Of course, counselors using this conceptual approach also often pay attention to predisposing biological factors, and may seek psychopharmacological consultations beyond their psychosocial conceptualization (Chacko et al., 2005; Frankel, Cantwell, Myatt, & Feinberg, 1999).

As can be seen in Figure 7.4, when the counselor applied this Multicomponent Psychosocial Intervention Approach, she made three theoretical inferences at Step 3 to explain the issues identified in Step 1, leading to the themes at Step 2: (a) Given his biological predispositions and background social history, Naruto has learned to employ hyperactive, inattentive, aggressive, and violating behaviors in his school context as a primary method of adjusting, coping, responding, and/or interacting with others; (b) given his biological predispositions and background social history, Naruto has learned to employ hyperactive, inattentive, aggressive, and violating behaviors in his family system as a primary method of adjusting, coping, responding, and/or interacting with others; and (c) given his biological predispositions and background social history, Naruto has learned to employ hyperactive, inattentive, aggressive, and violating behaviors in his neighborhood, peer, and other everyday social environments as a primary method of adjusting, coping, responding, and/or interacting with others. These are presented on Figure 7.4.

Step 4: Narrowed Inferences. At Step 4, the clinician's selected theory continues to be used to address still-deeper issues when they exist (Schwitzer, 2006, 2007). At this step, "still-deeper, more encompassing, or more central, causal themes" are formed (Neukrug & Schwitzer, 2006, p. 207). Continuing to apply Multicomponent Psychosocial Intervention concepts at Step 4, Naruto's counselor presented a single, most-fundamental construct, which she believed to be most explanatory and causal regarding Naruto's reasons for referral: the deeper inference that Naruto engages in predisposed and learned hyperactive, inattentive, aggressive, and violating behaviors in multiple component psychosocial systems, and therefore changes in multiple component systems are needed to promote new learning and changed behaviors. When all four steps are completed, the client information in Step 1 leads to logical-intuitive groupings on the basis of common denominators in Step 2, the groupings then are explained using theory at Step 3, and then, finally, at Step 4, further deeper explanations are made. From start to finish, the thoughts, feelings, behaviors, and physiological features in the topmost portions are connected on down the pyramid into deepest dynamics.

The completed pyramid now is used to plan treatment to assist Naruto in multiple psychosocial systems.

TREATMENT PLANNING

At this point, Naruto's clinician at the London Clinic has collected all available information about the problems that have been of concern to her and the evaluation team that performed the assessment. Based upon this information, the counselor developed a five-axis *DSM-IV-TR* diagnosis and then, using the "inverted pyramid" (Neukrug & Schwitzer, 2006; Schwitzer, 1996, 1997), formulated a working clinical *explanation* of Naruto's difficulties and their etiology that we called the *case conceptualization.* This, in turn, guides us to the next critical step in our clinical work, called the *treatment plan,* the primary purpose of which is to map out a logical and goal-oriented strategy for making positive changes in the client's life. In essence, the treatment plan is a road map *"for reducing or eliminating disruptive symptoms that are impeding the client's ability to reach positive mental health outcomes"* (Neukrug & Schwitzer, 2006, p. 225). As such, it is the cornerstone of our work with not only Naruto, but with all clients who present with disturbing and disruptive symptoms and needs (Jongsma & Peterson, 2006; Jongsma et al., 2003a, 2003b; Seligman, 1993, 1998, 2004).

A comprehensive treatment plan must integrate all of the information from the biopsychosocial interview, diagnosis, and case conceptualization into a coherent plan of action. This *plan* comprises four main components, which include (1) a behavioral definition of the problem(s), (2) the selection of achievable goals, (3) the determination of treatment modes, and (4) the documentation of how change will be measured. The *behavioral definition of the problem(s)* consolidates the results of the case conceptualization into a concise hierarchical list of problems and concerns that will be the focus of treatment. The *selection of achievable goals* refers to assessing and prioritizing the client's concerns into a *hierarchy of urgency* that also takes into account the client's motivation for change, level of dysfunction, and real-world influences on his or her problems. The *determination of treatment modes* refers to selection of the specific interventions, which are matched to the uniqueness of the

Figure 7.4   Naruto's Inverted Pyramid Case Conceptualization Summary: Multicomponent
Psychosocial Intervention Approach

1. IDENTIFY AND LIST CLIENT CONCERNS

Born with frightening birthmark
Referred to special education to protect classmates
Rejected by parents
Aggressive with classmates, peers
Unmanageable at age 4
Assigned to Tokyo orphanage
Overly aggressive sports play
British parent adoption and relocation
Does not stay "on task"
Has harmed, "beaten up" classmates
Bright, intellectually gifted, athletically gifted

Extremely hyperactive at school
Inattentive at school
Inability to "sit in one place"
Aggressive toward parents
Hyperactive at home
Difficulty with dinner table, etc.
Fighting
Fails to complete chores
Loses keys and personal items
Ankle sprain sports injury

2. ORGANIZE CONCERNS INTO LOGICAL THEMATIC GROUPINGS

1. Attention Deficit/Hyperactivity Disorder: Inattention and
    hyperactivity in school, home, peer, and other social
    settings occurring since an early age and throughout family
    changes, orphanage, and adoption transitions
2. Conduct Disorder: Aggressive, uncontrolled behavior
    violating peers' rights and adults' authority, occurring since
    an early age and throughout family changes, orphanage,
    and adoption transitions

**3. THEORETICAL INFERENCES: ATTACH THEMATIC
     GROUPINGS TO INFERRED AREAS OF DIFFICULTY**

Psychotherapeutic Integration

Multiple Component Psychosocial Systems in
Which Difficulties Occur

1. Given his biological predispositions and background social history, Naruto has learned to employ
    hyperactive, inattentive, aggressive, and violating behaviors in his school context as a primary method
    of adjusting, coping, responding, and/or interacting with others
2. Given his biological predispositions and background social history, Naruto has learned to employ
    hyperactive, inattentive, aggressive, and violating behaviors in his family system as a primary method
    of adjusting, coping, responding, and/or interacting with others
3. Given his biological predispositions and background social history, Naruto has learned to employ
    hyperactive, inattentive, aggressive, and violating behaviors in his neighborhood, peer, and other
    everyday social environments as a primary method of adjusting, coping, responding, and/or
    interacting with others

**4. NARROWED INFERENCES: SUICIDALITY AND
     DEEPER DIFFICULTIES**

Psychotherapeutic Integration

Deeper Multicomponent Psychosocial Inference

Naruto engages in predisposed and learned hyperactive, inattentive, aggressive,
and violating behaviors in multiple component psychosocial systems and therefore
changes in multiple component systems are needed to promote new learning and
changed behaviors

client and to his or her goals and clearly tied to a particular theoretical orientation (Neukrug & Schwitzer, 2006). Finally, the clinician must establish how change will be measured, based upon a number of factors including client records and self-report of change, in-session observations by the clinician, clinician ratings, results of standardized evaluations such as the Conners 3 (Conners, 2008) or a family functioning questionnaire, pre-post treatment comparisons, and reports by other treating professionals.

The four-step method discussed above can be seen in Figure 6.1 (p. 109), and is outlined below for the case of Naruto, followed by his specific treatment plan.

Step 1: Behavioral Definition of Problems. The first step in treatment planning is to carefully review the case conceptualization, paying particular attention to the results of Step 2 (Thematic Groupings), Step 3 (Theoretical Inferences), and Step 4 (Narrowed Inferences). The identified clinical themes reflect the core areas of concern and distress for the client, while the theoretical and narrowed inferences offer clinical speculation as to their origins. In the case of Naruto, there are two primary areas of concern. The first, Attention-Deficit/Hyperactivity Disorder, refers to his extreme hyperactivity and inattention at school and at home, difficulty staying on task and completing chores and assignments, inability to sit in one place, and regular loss of his keys and other personal items. The second, Conduct Disorder, refers to his aggressiveness with classmates, peers, and parents, nonprovoked fighting, use of his "ninja powers," defiance of authority, and violation of the rights of others. These symptoms and stresses are consistent with the diagnosis of ADHD, Combined Type; CD, Childhood-Onset Type, Moderate (APA, 2000a; Barkley, 2006; Conners, 2008; Kazdin, 1995; Tippins & Reiff, 2004).

Step 2: Identify and Articulate Goals for Change. The second step is the selection of achievable goals, which is based upon a number of factors, including the most pressing or urgent behavioral, emotional, and interpersonal concerns and symptoms as identified by the client and clinician, the willingness and ability of the client to work on those particular goals, and the realistic (real-world) achievability of those goals (Neukrug & Schwitzer, 2006). At this stage of treatment planning, it is important to recognize that not all of the client's problems can be addressed at once, so we focus initially on those that cause the greatest distress and impairment. New goals can be created as old ones are achieved. In the case of Naruto, the goals are divided into two prominent areas. The first, Attention-Deficit/Hyperactivity Disorder, requires that we help Naruto to sustain attention and concentration for consistently longer periods of time, to increase the frequency of on-task behaviors, to demonstrate improvement in his impulse control, to regularly take medication to decrease impulsivity, hyperactivity, and distractibility, and to improve his self-esteem. It also requires that we help his teachers and parents better understand the symptoms of ADHD, including the role of medication, to develop and use effective behavioral management strategies in the classroom, and for his parents to effectively structure his home life using positive rewards and effective consequences. The second, Conduct Disorder, requires that we help Naruto to comply with rules and expectations in the home, school, and community, eliminate antisocial behavior, cease acts of violence and aggression, demonstrate improvement in impulse control, express anger in a controlled manner, resolve the core conflicts that contribute to aggressive feelings, thoughts, and behaviors, and to build prosocial attitudes and behaviors. It also requires that we help his teachers and parents better understand the symptoms of CD as well as to establish and maintain clear limits around aggressive behavior.

Step 3: Describe Therapeutic Interventions. This is perhaps the most critical step in the treatment planning process because the clinician must now

Chapter 7 Children's Characters and Video Game Characters • 179

integrate information from a number of sources, including the case conceptualization, the delineation of the client's problems and goals, and the treatment literature, paying particular attention to *empirically supported treatment* (EST) and *evidence-based practice* (EBP). In essence, the clinician must align his or her treatment approach with scientific evidence from the fields of counseling and psychotherapy. Wampold (2001) identifies two types of evidence-based counseling research: studies that demonstrate "absolute efficacy," that is, the fact that counseling and psychotherapy work, and those that demonstrate "relative efficacy," that is, the fact that certain theoretical/technical approaches work best for certain clients with particular problems (Psychoanalysis, Gestalt Therapy, Cognitive Behavior Therapy, Brief Solution-Focused Therapy, Cognitive Therapy, Dialectical Behavior Therapy, Person-Centered Therapy, Expressive/Creative Therapies, Interpersonal Therapy, and Feminist Therapy); and when delivered through specific treatment modalities (individual, group, and family counseling).

In the case of Naruto, we have decided to use a Multicomponent Psychosocial Intervention Approach, which addresses the biological, psychological, and social factors that contribute to and maintain the child's disruptive behavior, which in Naruto's case, centers on his ADHD and CD symptoms. This multicomponent and contextualized intervention makes use of medication to address the biologically based deficits in self-regulation, behavioral management within the home, school, and community, as well as individualized psychological strategies with the child (Arnold et al., 1997; Miranda, Presentacion, Garcia, & Siegenthaler, 2009; Wells et al., 2000). More specifically, the counselor provides psychoeducation to teachers and parents so that they are better prepared to understand the causes, symptoms, and treatment needs for children with ADHD and CD, hands-on parent-training that involves contingency management strategies, and the use of self-monitoring, shaping, modeling, social-skill building, and reinforcement for

the child both in-session and in their natural environment. Although Multicomponent Psychosocial Intervention refers to an overall approach to treatment that has been implemented on a larger large multisite scale, it relies, in essence, on the use of empirically validated and effective techniques for management of the symptoms of disruptive behavior disorders (ADHD and CD) (Barkley, 2006; Chacko et al., 2005; DuPaul & Stoner, 2003; Frankel et al., 1999; Henggeler et al., 1998; Hosie & Erik, 1993).

With regard to Naruto's ADHD symptoms, techniques drawn from this approach will include caretaker and teacher psychoeducation (including bibliotherapy) about the symptoms of ADHD and the use of medication; assisting parents and teachers in the construction of a behavioral management system using shaping, effective consequences, and reward for on-task behavior, regulated impulsivity and reduced distractibility; developing effective communication channels between parents and teachers through use of a progress chart; teaching Naruto self-control and relaxation skills, including "stop, look and listen," deep breathing, and progressive muscle work; helping him to identify internal and external triggers and stressors for off-task behavior; and shaping through positive and modeling on-task behavior using drawings, puppets, and action figures to create positive behavioral stories.

With regard to Naruto's CD symptoms, techniques drawn from this approach will include caretaker and teacher psychoeducation (including bibliotherapy) about causes, symptoms, and medication management, building effective communication channels between home and school, assisting parents and teachers in construction of an effective behavioral management system; assisting Naruto in making connections between feelings and aggressive reactions, identifying triggers for aggressive behavior, teaching him relaxation-based self-control strategies, including deep breathing and muscle control, shaping his prosocial behavior using creative methods in-session as well as in group, and reinforcing him for positive behavior, self-awareness, and social interaction.

Provide Outcome Measures of Change. This last step in treatment planning requires that we specify how change will be measured and indicate the extent to which progress has been made toward realizing these goals (Neukrug & Schwitzer, 2006). The counselor has considerable flexibility in this phase and may choose from a number of objective domains (psychological tests and measures of self-esteem, depression, psychosis, interpersonal relationship, anxiety, etc.), quasi-objective measures (the *DSM-IV-TR's* Axis V GAF scale; pre-post clinician, client and psychiatric ratings), and subjective ratings (client self-report, clinician's in-session observations). In Naruto's case, we have implemented a number of these, including pre-post measures of attention, concentration, and improved impulse control on parent and teacher version of the Conners 3 (Conners, 2008), sustained post-only measures of GAF functioning in the mild range (>70), clinician and client self-report of friendly and prosocial relationships with peers at school, teacher- and parent-reported improvement in attention, impulse, behavior, and emotional control, parent and teacher report of improved daily communication between home and school, and compliance with psychopharmacotherapy.

The completed treatment plan is now developed through which the counselor, Naruto, his parents, and teachers will begin their shared work of building an effective behavioral management system at home and at school, enhancing communication channels between parents and teachers, modifying and then reducing the impact of his ADHD, eliminating his aggressive behavior, building his prosocial behavior, and enhancing his overall self-esteem. Naruto's treatment plan appears below, and a summary can be found in Table 7.4.

TREATMENT PLAN

Client: Naruto Uzumaki

Service Provider: London Clinic

BEHAVIORAL DEFINITION OF PROBLEMS:

1. ADHD—Extreme hyperactivity and inattention at school and at home, difficulty staying on task and completing chores and assignments, inability to sit in one place, and regular loss of keys and other personal items

2. CD—Aggressiveness toward classmates, peers, and parents, nonprovoked fighting, use of his "ninja powers," defiance of authority, and violation of the rights of others

GOALS FOR CHANGE:

1. ADHD

- Sustain attention and concentration for consistently longer periods of time
- Increase the frequency of on-task behaviors
- Demonstrate improvement in his impulse control
- Improve self-esteem development
- Help teachers and parents better understand the symptoms of ADHD
- Help teachers develop and use effective behavioral management strategies

- Help parents to effectively structure home life using positive rewards and effective consequences
- Regularly take medication to decrease impulsivity, hyperactivity, and distractibility

2. CD

- Comply with rules and expectations in the home, school, and community
- Eliminate antisocial behavior
- Cease acts of violence and aggression
- Demonstrate improvement in impulse control
- Express anger in a controlled manner
- Resolve the core conflicts that contribute to aggressive feelings, thoughts, and behaviors
- Build prosocial attitudes and behaviors
- Help teachers and parents better understand the symptoms of CD
- Help teachers and parents to establish and maintain clear limits around aggressive behavior

THERAPEUTIC INTERVENTIONS:

A moderate-term course (6–9 months) of Multicomponent Psychosocial Intervention at home, school, and in the community directed at client, parents, and teachers

1. ADHD

Parent/Teacher Intervention

- Caretaker and teacher psychoeducation (including bibliotherapy) about the symptoms of ADHD and the use of medication
- Assisting parents and teachers in the construction of a behavioral management system using shaping, effective consequences, and reward for on-task behavior, regulated impulsivity, and reduced distractibility
- Building effective communication channels between parents and teachers through use of a daily progress chart
- Developing a signaling system to alert client to off-task behavior
- Encourage participation in ADHD support group

Direct Intervention With Client

- Teaching self-control and relaxation skills, including "stop, look, and listen," deep breathing, and progressive muscle work
- Strengthening executive functioning through tasks targeted at working memory, internalized speech, and self-regulation
- Identify internal and external triggers and stressors for off-task behavior
- Shaping through positive and modeling on-task behavior
- Use of a self-control checklist for on-task and focused behavior
- Using drawings, puppets, and action figures to create positive behavioral stories
- Encouraging and reinforcing medication compliance
- Reinforce attendance in after-school ADHD skills and socialization group

(Continued)

(Continued)

2. CD

Parent/Teacher Intervention

- Caretaker and teacher psychoeducation (including bibliotherapy) about the symptoms of CD and the use of medication
- Assisting parents and teachers in the construction of a behavioral management system using shaping, effective consequences, and reward for nonaggressive and helpful/compliant behavior
- Building effective communication channels between parents and teachers through use of a progress chart focused on positive behavior
- Monitor caretaker reactivity to client's aggressiveness

Direct Intervention With Client

- Assist client in making connection between feelings and aggressive reactive behaviors
- Identify triggers for aggressive perceptions, feelings, and behaviors
- Teaching self-control and relaxation skills, including "stop, look, and listen," deep breathing, and progressive muscle work
- Shaping prosocial behavior through positive reinforcement and modeling
- Using drawings, puppets, and action figures to create positive social/behavioral stories
- Reinforce client for positive, conciliatory, and helpful social behavior
- Family counseling using role-playing of positive interactions
- Encouraging and reinforcing medication compliance

OUTCOME MEASURES OF CHANGE:

Improved on-task, attentive, and prosocial attitudes and behavior both at home and in school as measured by:

- Pre-post measures of improved attention, concentration, and impulse control on the parent and teacher version of the Conners 3
- Sustained post-only measures of GAF functioning in the mild range (>70)
- Clinician-, teacher-, and parent-reported improvement in attention, impulse, behavior, and emotional control as well as social interactions
- Client-reported awareness of triggers for emotional and behavioral dyscontrol
- Client self-report of friendly and prosocial relationships with peers at school
- Parent and teacher report of improved daily communication between home and school
- Compliance with psychopharmacotherapy

Table 7.4 Naruto's Treatment Plan Summary: Multicomponent Psychosocial Intervention

Goals for Change	Therapeutic Interventions	Outcome Measures of Change
ADHD Sustain attention and concentration for consistently longer periods of time Increase the frequency of on-task behaviors Demonstrate improvement in his impulse control Improve self-esteem development Help teachers and parents better understand the symptoms of ADHD Help teachers develop and use effective behavioral management strategies Help parents to effectively structure home life using positive rewards and effective consequences Regularly take medication to decrease impulsivity, hyperactivity, and distractibility Conduct Disorder Comply with rules and expectations in the home, school, and community Eliminate antisocial behavior Cease acts of violence and aggression Demonstrate improvement in impulse control Express anger in a controlled manner Resolve the core conflicts that contribute to aggressive feelings, thoughts, and behaviors	ADHD *Parent/Teacher Intervention* Caretaker and teacher psychoeducation (including bibliotherapy) about the symptoms of ADHD and the use of medication Assisting parents and teachers in the construction of a behavioral management system using shaping, effective consequences, and reward for on-task behavior, regulated impulsivity, and reduced distractibility Building effective communication channels between parents and teachers through use of a daily progress chart Developing a signaling system to alert client to off-task behavior Encourage participation in ADHD support group *Direct Intervention With Client* Teaching self-control and relaxation skills, including "stop, look, and listen," deep breathing, and progressive muscle work Strengthening executive functioning through tasks targeted at working memory, internalized speech, and self-regulation Identify internal and external triggers and stressors for off-task behavior Shaping through positive and modeling on-task behavior Use of a self-control checklist for on-task and focused behavior Using drawings, puppets, and action figures to create positive behavioral stories Encouraging and reinforcing medication compliance Reinforce attendance in after-school ADHD skills and socialization group	Improved on-task, attentive, and prosocial attitudes and behavior both at home and in school as measured by: Pre-post measures of improved attention, concentration, and impulse control on the parent and teacher version of the Conners 3 Sustained post-only measures of GAF functioning in the mild range (>70) Clinician-, teacher-, and parent-reported improvement in attention, impulse, behavior, and emotional control as well as social interactions Client-reported awareness of triggers for emotional and behavioral dyscontrol Client self-report of friendly and prosocial relationships with peers at school Parent and teacher report of improved daily communication between home and school Compliance with psychopharmacotherapy

(Continued)

Table 7.4 (Continued)

Goals for Change	Therapeutic Interventions	Outcome Measures of Change
Build prosocial attitudes and behaviors Help teachers and parents better understand the symptoms of ADHD Help teachers and parents to establish and maintain clear limits around aggressive behavior	Conduct Disorder *Parent/Teacher Intervention* Caretaker and teacher psychoeducation (including bibliotherapy) about the symptoms of CD and the use of medication Assisting parents and teachers in the construction of a behavioral management system using shaping, effective consequences, and reward for nonaggressive and helpful/compliant behavior Building effective communication channels between parents and teachers through use of a progress chart focused on positive behavior Monitor caretaker reactivity to client's aggressiveness *Direct Intervention With Client* Assist client in making connection between feelings and aggressive reactive behaviors Identify triggers for aggressive perceptions, feelings, and behaviors Teaching self-control and relaxation skills, including "stop, look, and listen," deep breathing, and progressive muscle work Shaping prosocial behavior through positive reinforcement and modeling Using drawings, puppets, and action figures to create positive social/behavioral stories Reinforce client for positive, conciliatory, and helpful social behavior Family counseling using role-playing of positive interactions Encouraging and reinforcing medication compliance	

CASE 7.5   *PEANUTS'* SNOOPY

Introducing the Character

Snoopy is a dog who first appeared in the *Peanuts* comic strip, featuring Charlie Brown and his gang, drawn by Charles Schulz in 1950. Since his newspaper comic-strip introduction, Snoopy has appeared in television cartoons, full-length animated movies, in countless *Peanuts* and Charlie Brown books, and even as a life-size Ice Capades character. Additionally, the famous beagle has appeared on a wide range of popular culture merchandise, including lunchboxes, clothing, stationary, cereal boxes, Halloween masks, and telephones. Since his introduction as a shy and homeless dog adopted by a suburban family, Snoopy has evolved into a bold, self-confident, and imaginative character who chooses to live his life on top of—rather than inside—the proverbial dog house. Best friend and lifelong companion to the loveable yet struggling Charlie Brown, Snoopy has fashioned himself as a World War I dogfighter, a detective, a dancer, and an international lover. His good-natured and playful antics are often juxtaposed with sarcasm, arrogance, and narcissistic self-assurance that have entertained children of all ages for six decades.

In the basic case summary and diagnostic impressions that follow, we take a different look at Snoopy's behaviors, from a clinical perspective that examines features including impaired development in social interaction and restricted interests and activities. You will see that, for the purposes of this case, dogs are allowed in school!

Meet the Client

You can assess the client in action by viewing clips of Snoopy's video material at the following websites:

* http://www.youtube.com/watch?v= gKxXAwBRuVo Snoopy in a bad mood
* http://www.youtube.com/watch?v=r NremK0cBEg Snoopy vs. the Red Barron
* http://www.youtube.com/watch?v= hUQX2B67KL4 Snoopy loves dancing
* http://www.youtube.com/watch?v= pq9hBEvFNlM Snoopy kisses Lucy
* http://www.youtube.com/watch?v= iyIxW-ouwAg Snoopy and Charlie Brown

Basic Case Summary

Identifying Information. Snoopy Brown is a 12-year-old Canine American youth who resides in a middle-class suburban home in Austin, Texas, with an intact family comprising two parents, a brother, Charlie, and a sister, Sally.

Presenting Concern. Snoopy Brown has been a student at Charles Schulz Elementary School for the past 2 years, having transferred from a parochial school in a nearby city. Since being at the school, his teachers have been increasingly concerned about behavior that is highly atypical for children with whom they have worked. These behaviors include difficulty with expressive language, spinning, tapping, pacing, and other self-stimulating habits; inappropriate touching of the other students; occasional wetting of himself; and an inordinate preoccupation with fantasy. Snoopy was referred for evaluation by the school administrator, who says she has become increasingly frustrated by Snoopy's "strange behavior" and the increasing drain this has placed on her teachers to simultaneously meet both his and his classmates' needs.

Background, Family Information, and Relevant History. Snoopy was born several weeks prematurely to parents who had undergone fertility treatments in order to expand their family; however, Snoopy appeared to readily advance and begin making normally expected developmental progress through his first 3 years. At the same time, in comparison with other same-age peers, he appeared to have less interest in his parents or making eye contact with others, smiled less, and did not always come when called or attend to his parents' voices. However, his parents did not immediately identify these as concerns. As he continued to age in years 3 and beyond, his parents did begin to notice that he did not seem to seek relationships with peers as normally expected; did not engage his parents or adults with eye contact, body postures, or emotional expressions, as did Charlie and Sally. It became clearer he was more interested in repetitive and sensorimotor rather than symbolic and representational play, was more interested in playing with his toys—balls, rubber toys shaped like bones and mailmen, tugging ropes, and so on—than in engaging in play with people. He increasingly preferred to be alone in the backyard, basement, or his "house" out back.

By the time he was 6 years old, Snoopy's language skills had sufficiently developed so that he could communicate in simple phrases with his parents and Charlie and Sally. However, he was uncomfortable verbalizing with members outside of the family, and the parents decided to enroll him in a special education program within the public school system. There, he largely kept to himself, refused to do his work, and instead, sat quietly on floor fantasizing about being a World War I flying ace. By that time, Snoopy was working with both a speech therapist and an occupational therapist. Although these professionals noted a minimal increase in his social interactions, occupational therapy was unsuccessful in reducing his growing obsession with toy objects. These professionals recommended to his parents that they limit Snoopy's time playing with his balls, rubber toys, and tugging ropes, and limit the time he spent engaged in his stereotypical ritual of watching out the window for birds and watching out the front door for the mailman. However, his protests were so vociferous that his parents ultimately conceded. Snoopy spent hours in his room pretending he was Snoopy, the World War I flying ace, and seemed happiest when left alone with his fantasy life. By the time he was 9, the parents had enrolled him in the Charles Schulz Learning Academy, which specialized in services for students with developmental delays, a designation that his parents struggled with but

finally accepted. At the beginning of the school year, he was referred to the assessment team for a comprehensive developmental evaluation.

Problem and Counseling History. Mr. and Ms. Brown's primary concern was with Snoopy's almost complete lack of verbal human language, for which he compensated by movements and head-shaking and alternative sounds. Along the same lines, they and his teachers were worried about his inability to sustain an engaged conversation of more than a few moments. They also were concerned about his repetitive self-stimulating play to the exclusion of interest in socializing with others his age. Although he played and had an imagination, his internal fantasy life was unvaried and dealt almost exclusively with pretending to be a World War I air combat pilot. Although they believed Snoopy to be highly intelligent based on the extent of his play and fantasy life, they were worried that in the absence of an interest in other children, his adolescent years would be extremely stressful. Along with his rituals of looking out the window and out the front door, he engaged in repetitive behaviors, including digging purposelessly in the backyard. Past therapeutic efforts were dedicated largely to increasing the range of his reciprocal interactive capacities, but were individual rather than group based. For this reason, his parents were now interested in providing whatever services were necessary.

Goals for Counseling and Course of Therapy to Date. As of this writing, Mr. and Mrs. Brown were confident in their decision to proceed with the comprehensive evaluation and in the treatment team's ability to successful assess and develop a treatment plan for Snoopy's pattern of concerns. They saw this as an opportunity to finally understand their child and set in motion the necessary resources to provide for his developmental and psychological needs.

Diagnostic Impressions

Axis I.   299.00 Autistic Disorder

Axis II.   V71.09 No diagnosis on Axis II

Axis III.   None reported

Axis IV.   None

Axis V.   GAF = 41 (current)

GAF = 50 (highest level past year)

DISCUSSION OF DIAGNOSTIC IMPRESSIONS

Snoopy was referred by his school administrator because she and his teachers at Charles Schultz Elementary School had become worried about his behavior, which was highly atypical for children with whom they usually work. Snoopy's behaviors included: difficulty with expressive language, spinning, tapping, pacing, and other self-stimulating habits; inappropriate touching of the other students; occasional wetting of himself; and an inordinate preoccupation with fantasy.

The far-reaching section of the *DSM-IV-TR* titled "Disorders Usually First Diagnosed in Infancy, Childhood, or Adolescence" is organized into a large number of groupings of disorders that all share the feature of occurring early in the life cycle. Two of the diagnoses found in the grouping known as the Pervasive Developmental Disorders are Autistic Disorder and Asperger's Disorder. Increasingly, being able to identity, evaluate, and diagnose and provide treatment and support for students with these disorders are important clinical skills for counseling professionals who work with children, adolescents, young adults, and adults in school, college and university, and community settings (Adreon & Durocher, 2007; Van Bergeijk, Klin, & Volkmar, 2008).

We looked at Snoopy's behavior from a unique clinical perspective that examined features including impaired development in social interaction and restricted interests and activities. The primary symptoms that Snoopy is experiencing include qualitative impairment in social interaction, as seen as by his absence of interest in same-age peers, impairment in the use of normally expected nonverbal behavior like facial expressions, and lack of engaged conversations or social reciprocity; qualitative impairment in communication, as seen by his almost total lack of spoken language; and inflexible behavior patterns centering on his imaginary role as a World War I pilot, and purposeless repetitive behavior such as digging in the backyard. Onset was by age 2 or 3 years, with clear abnormal functioning in social interaction, language, and Snoopy's imaginative play. In such cases of impairment in social interaction, impairment in communication, and restricted repetitive behavior, the diagnosis is Autistic Disorder.

Regarding differential diagnoses, Asperger's Disorder might be considered. Like all of the Pervasive Developmental Disorders, both Autism and Asperger's Disorders are characterized by problems with social interactions. However, Autistic Disorder requires delay or impairment in early language development (as seen in our look at Snoopy) not found with Asperger's

Disorder. Further, when making the diagnosis of Autistic Disorder, Rett's Disorder, and Childhood Disintegrative Disorder both must be ruled out; the essential feature of these two disorders is developmental deficits (Rett's Disorder) or regression in functioning (Childhood Disintegrative Disorder) following an early period of normal development. Both can be ruled out in Snoopy's case.

To round out the diagnosis, the absence of clinically significant personality features, medical problems, or psychosocial stressors (beyond those interpersonal stresses already covered by a diagnosis of Autistic Disorder) are indicated on Axes II, III, and IV. Snoopy's serious symptoms and serious impairment in school and social functioning are represented by the GAF scores seen on Axis V, which are consistent with the diagnosis listed on Axis I.

CASE CONCEPTUALIZATION

During Snoopy's first meeting in the counseling office, his counselor conducted an intake meeting in order to collect as much information as she could about the symptoms and situations leading to Snoopy's referral. Included in the intake materials were a developmental history, client report, counselor observations, child-oriented clinical interview, play observation, parent report inventories, and information shared by his school principal and teachers (Knell, 1994). Based on the intake, Snoopy's counselor and the school's treatment team developed diagnostic impressions, describing Snoopy's presenting concerns as Autistic Disorder. A case conceptualization next was developed.

When forming a case conceptualization, the clinician applies a purist counseling theory, an integration of two or more theories, an eclectic mix of theories, or a solution-focused combination of tactics to his or her understanding of the client. In this case example, Snoopy's counselor based her conceptualization on an eclectic combination of counseling approaches and techniques (Corey, 2009). Dattilo and Norcross (2006) and Norcross and Beutler (2008) referred to this strategy as

technical eclecticism. Clinicians using technical eclecticism attempt to select the best possible combination of treatment techniques from different theoretical approaches without necessarily making connections between the conceptual foundations of the different approaches or necessarily subscribing to the theories' underlying theoretical positions (Corey, 2009; Dattilo &Norcross, 2006; Norcross & Beutler, 2008). Whereas solution-focused approaches operate from a specific solution-focused framework, and psychotherapeutic integration is based on integrating the underlying theories of more than one compatible model, the technical eclectic approach requires clinicians to put together a number of techniques that derive from their clinical experience and professional judgment (Corey, 2009; de Shazer, 1988, 1991). To be effective with this approach, clinicians must critically and systematically combine methods using a rational decision-making process based on their training and supervision, clinical experience, and professional development (Corey, 2009; Neukrug & Schwitzer, 2006). Being effective at technical eclecticism requires well-formed knowledge and skill (Lazarus, Beutler, & Norcross, 1992; Norcross & Beutler, 2008).

Although the purpose of diagnostic impressions is to *describe* the client's concerns, the goal of case conceptualization when using technical eclecticism is to better *understand* and clinically *arrange* the person's experiences in preparation for applying a selection of interventions. It helps the counselor understand the etiology leading to Snoopy's autistic behaviors, and the factors maintaining these concerns. In turn, case conceptualization sets the stage for treatment planning. Treatment planning then provides a "road map" that plots out how the counselor and client expect to move from presenting concerns to positive outcomes (Seligman, 1993, p. 157)—helping Snoopy improve his levels of intrapersonal and interpersonal functioning.

Snoopy's counselor used the Inverted Pyramid Method of case conceptualization because this method is especially designed to help clinicians more easily form their conceptual pictures of their clients' needs (Neukrug & Schwitzer, 2006; Schwitzer, 1996, 1997). Generally speaking, when the Inverted Pyramid Method is used with a purist theory-based conceptual model or a theoretical integration of psychotherapies, there are four steps: Problem Identification, Thematic Groupings, Theoretical Inferences, and Narrowed Inferences. However, when the eclectic approach is used, only the first two steps are needed: Problem Identification and Thematic Grouping. From an eclectic perspective, it is these two steps that set the stage for rationally combining a set of techniques to target the client's needs.

Snoopy's counselor was aware that the most effective treatments for the problems associated with Autistic Disorders are very intensive and address multiple needs (Amos, 2004; Rogers, 1998). In turn, she selected an eclectic mix of the DIR/Floortime Model (Developmental, Individual-Difference, Relationship-Based Model) (Greenspan & Wieder, 2006), Cognitive Behavior Therapy (Knell, 1993, 1994), and Expressive Creative Arts Play Therapy (Gladding, 1995, 2005). Snoopy's counselor's eclectic clinical thinking can be seen in Figure 7.5.

Step 1: Problem Identification. The first step is Problem Identification. Aspects of the presenting problem (thoughts, feelings, behaviors, physiological features), additional areas of concern besides the presenting concern, family and developmental history, in-session observations, clinical inquiries (medical problems, medications, past counseling, substance use, suicidality), and psychological assessments (problem checklists, personality inventories, mental status exam, specific clinical measures) all may contribute information at Step 1. The counselor "casts a wide net" in order to build Step 1 as exhaustively as possible (Neukrug & Schwitzer, 2006, p. 202). As can be seen in Figure 7.5, the counselor identified Snoopy's current and recent problematic repetitive, purposeless, and stereotypical behaviors at school and home (odd play, fantasy games, etc.), solitary social preferences (lack of engaging parents, preferring playing alone, etc.), details of early and recent developmental

history, and speech and occupational therapy history. The counselor attempted to go beyond just the presenting symptoms in order to be as descriptive as she could.

Step 2: Thematic Groupings. The second step is Thematic Groupings. The clinician organizes all of the exhaustive client information found in Step 1 into just a few intuitive-logical clinical groups, categories, or themes, on the basis of sensible common denominators (Neukrug & Schwitzer, 2006). Four different ways of forming the Step 2 theme groups can be used: Descriptive-Diagnosis Approach, Clinical Targets Approach, Areas of Dysfunction Approach, and Intrapsychic Approach. As can be seen in the figure, Snoopy's counselor selected the Areas of Dysfunction Approach. This approach sorts together all of the Step 1 information into "areas of dysfunction according to important life situations, life themes, or life roles and skills" (Neukrug & Schwitzer, p. 205). She believed this approach would best set the stage for selecting an eclectic mix of counseling techniques to target Snoopy's different needs.

Snoopy's counselor first grouped together all of his symptoms, presentations, and history related to social isolation and solitary preferences into the theme: Lack of social interests, social interactions, and verbal communications due to Autistic Disorder. The counselor then grouped together all of Snoopy's symptoms, presentations, and history related to stereotypical behaviors, stereotypical play preferences, and stereotypical fantasies into the next theme: solitary, repetitive, stereotypical, and purposeless behaviors and play due to Autistic Disorder.

With this two-step conceptualization completed, the client information in Step 1 leads to logical-intuitive groupings on the basis of common denominators in Step 2, and the counselor is ready to engage the client in planning and implementing technical eclecticism in order to address Snoopy's current counseling situation as we have written his imagined clinical case illustration.

Figure 7.5   Snoopy's Inverted Pyramid Case Conceptualization Summary: Eclectic Combination of DIR/Floortime Model, Behavior Therapy, and Expressive Creative Arts Play Therapy

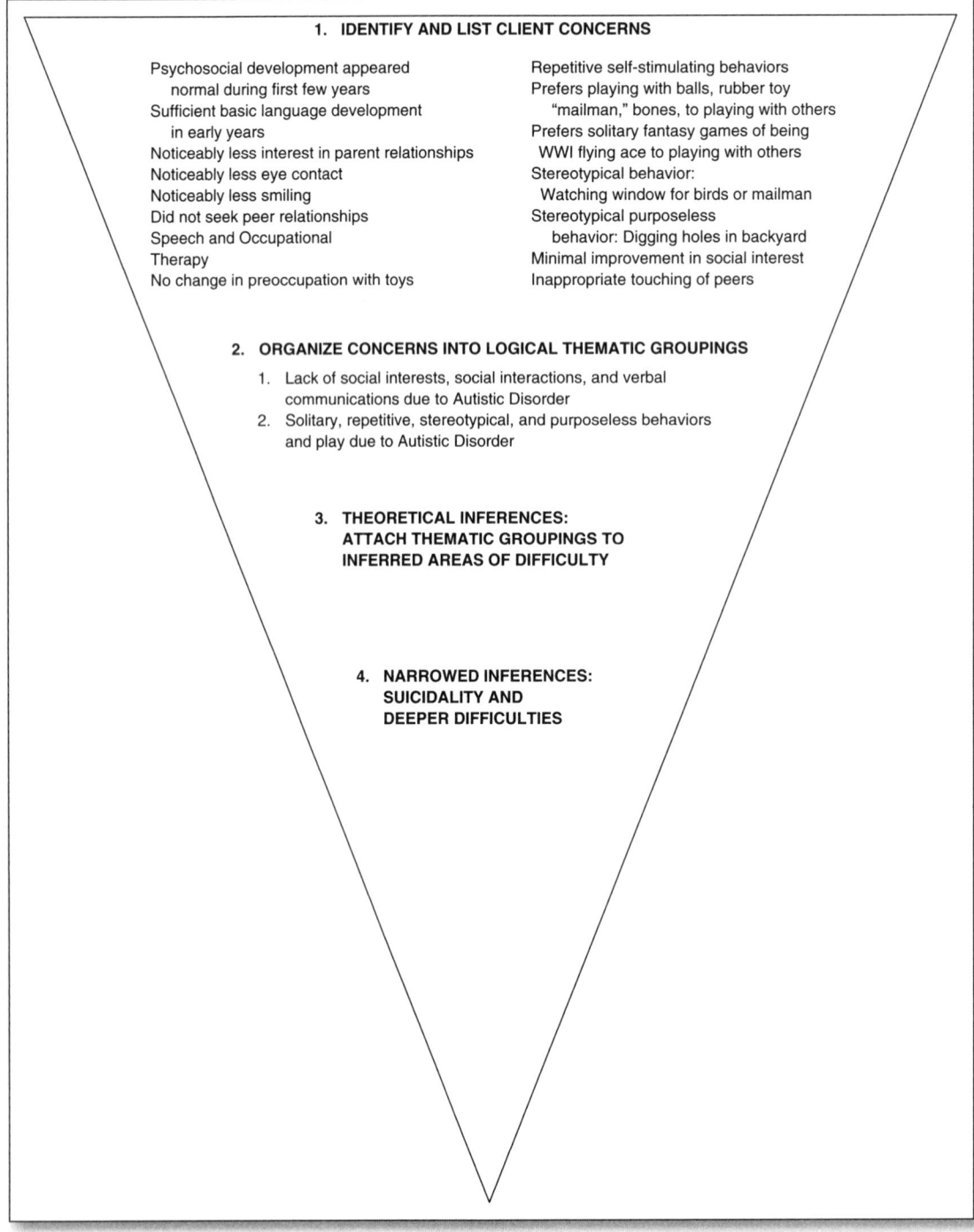

1. IDENTIFY AND LIST CLIENT CONCERNS

Psychosocial development appeared
   normal during first few years
Sufficient basic language development
   in early years
Noticeably less interest in parent relationships
Noticeably less eye contact
Noticeably less smiling
Did not seek peer relationships
Speech and Occupational
Therapy
No change in preoccupation with toys

Repetitive self-stimulating behaviors
Prefers playing with balls, rubber toy
   "mailman," bones, to playing with others
Prefers solitary fantasy games of being
   WWI flying ace to playing with others
Stereotypical behavior:
   Watching window for birds or mailman
Stereotypical purposeless
   behavior: Digging holes in backyard
Minimal improvement in social interest
Inappropriate touching of peers

2. ORGANIZE CONCERNS INTO LOGICAL THEMATIC GROUPINGS

1. Lack of social interests, social interactions, and verbal
   communications due to Autistic Disorder
2. Solitary, repetitive, stereotypical, and purposeless behaviors
   and play due to Autistic Disorder

**3. THEORETICAL INFERENCES:
   ATTACH THEMATIC GROUPINGS TO
   INFERRED AREAS OF DIFFICULTY**

**4. NARROWED INFERENCES:
   SUICIDALITY AND
   DEEPER DIFFICULTIES**

TREATMENT PLANNING

At this point, Snoopy's clinician at the Charles Schultz Elementary School has collected all available information about the problems that have been of concern to him and the treatment team that performed his assessment. Based upon this information, the counselor developed a five-axis *DSM-IV-TR* diagnosis and then, using the "inverted pyramid" (Neukrug & Schwitzer, 2006; Schwitzer, 1996, 1997), formulated a working clinical *explanation* of Snoopy's difficulties and their etiology that we called the *case conceptualization*. This, in turn, guides us to the next critical step in our clinical work, called the *treatment plan,* the primary purpose of which is to map out a logical and goal-oriented strategy for making positive changes in the client's life. In essence, the treatment plan is a road map "for reducing or eliminating disruptive symptoms that are impeding the client's ability to reach positive mental health outcomes" (Neukrug & Schwitzer, 2006, p. 225). As such, it is the cornerstone of our work with not only Snoopy, but with all clients who present with disturbing and disruptive symptoms and needs (Jongsma & Peterson, 2006; Jongsma et al., 2003a, 2003b; Seligman, 1993, 1998, 2004).

A comprehensive treatment plan must integrate all of the information from the biopsychosocial interview, diagnosis, and case conceptualization into a coherent plan of action. This *plan* comprises four main components, which include (1) a behavioral definition of the problem(s), (2) the selection of achievable goals, (3) the determination of treatment modes, and (4) the documentation of how change will be measured. The *behavioral definition of the problem(s)* consolidates the results of the case conceptualization into a concise hierarchical list of problems and concerns that will be the focus of treatment. The *selection of achievable goals* refers to assessing and prioritizing the client's concerns into a *hierarchy of urgency* that also takes into account the client's motivation for change, level of dysfunction, and real-world influences on his or her problems. The *determination of*

treatment modes refers to selection of the specific interventions, which are matched to the uniqueness of the client and to his or her goals and clearly tied to a particular theoretical orientation (Neukrug & Schwitzer, 2006). Finally, the clinician must establish how change will be measured, based upon a number of factors including client records and self-report of change, in-session observations by the clinician, clinician ratings, results of standardized evaluations such as the Conners 3 (Conners, 2008) or a family functioning questionnaire, pre-post treatment comparisons, and reports by other treating professionals.

The four-step method discussed above can be seen in Figure 6.1 (p. 109) and is outlined below for the case of Snoopy, followed by his specific treatment plan.

Step 1: Behavioral Definition of Problems. The first step in eclectic treatment planning is to carefully review the case conceptualization, paying particular attention to the results of Step 2 (Thematic Groupings). The identified clinical themes reflect the core areas of concern and distress for the client. In the case of Snoopy, there are two primary areas of concern. The first, "lack of social interests, social interactions and verbal communication," refers to his current deficiency in verbal communication despite early basic language development, noticeably less interest in parent relationships with minimal eye contact or smiling, disinterest in seeking out peer relationships, and minimal improvement in social interest or verbal communication despite speech and occupational therapy. The second, "solitary, repetitive, stereotypical and purposeless behaviors and play," refers to his repetitive self-stimulating behaviors, preference for play with balls, rubber toys, and military aviator fantasies over peer-based interactive play, ceaseless digging in the backyard, watching out the window and door for birds or the mailman, and inappropriate touching of peers. These symptoms and stresses are consistent with the diagnosis of Autistic Disorder (APA, 2000a; Hersen & Ammerman, 2000; Parritz & Troy, 2011; Sicile-Kira & Grandin, 2004).

Step 2: Identify and Articulate Goals for Change. The second step is the selection of achievable goals, which is based upon a number of factors, including the most pressing or urgent behavioral, emotional, and interpersonal concerns and symptoms as identified by the client and clinician, the willingness and ability of the client to work on those particular goals, and the realistic (real-world) achievability of those goals (Neukrug & Schwitzer, 2006). At this stage of treatment planning, it is important to recognize that not all of the client's problems can be addressed at once, so we focus initially on those that cause the greatest distress and impairment. New goals can be created as old ones are achieved. In the case of Snoopy, the goals are divided into two prominent areas. The first, "lack of social interests, social interactions and verbal communication," requires that we help Snoopy to strengthen his basic language skills and the ability to communicate simply with others, to strengthen the basic emotional bond with his parents, to engage in reciprocal and cooperative interactions with others on a regular basis, and to help his parents, teachers, and peers to develop a level of understanding and acceptance of Snoopy's capabilities and to set realistic expectations for his behavior. The second, "solitary, repetitive, stereotypical and purposeless behaviors and play," requires that we help Snoopy to reduce self-stimulatory and repetitive behaviors, to shape symbolic play behaviors, to assist him in tolerating changes in his routine or immediate environment, and to attain the highest, most realistic level of overall functioning.

Step 3: Describe Therapeutic Interventions. This is perhaps the most critical step in the treatment planning process because the clinician must now integrate information from a number of sources, including the case conceptualization, the delineation of the client's problems and goals, and the treatment literature, paying particular attention to *empirically supported treatment* (EST) and *evidence-based practice* (EBP). In essence, the clinician must align his or her treatment approach with scientific evidence from the fields of counseling and psychotherapy. Wampold (2001) identifies two types of evidence-based counseling research: studies that demonstrate "absolute efficacy," that is, the fact that counseling and psychotherapy work, and those that demonstrate "relative efficacy," that is, the fact that certain theoretical/technical approaches work best for certain clients with particular problems (Psychoanalysis, Gestalt Therapy, Cognitive Behavior Therapy, Brief Solution-Focused Therapy, Cognitive Therapy, Dialectical Behavior Therapy, Person-Centered Therapy, Expressive/Creative Therapies, Interpersonal Therapy, and Feminist Therapy); and when delivered through specific treatment modalities (individual, group, and family counseling).

In the case of Snoopy, we have decided to use an Eclectic Intervention Approach based upon the DIR/Floortime Model, elements of behavioral and expressive/creative therapies, and supplemented with family counseling, psychoeducation, and social skills training. Because of the complexity of Autism and the pervasiveness of its impact, intervention must be multifaceted and target neurological, psychological, and social factors (Rosenberg & Kosslyn, 2010). Although current treatments do not directly target neurological factors in Autism, psychotropic medication may be used to address associated behavioral and emotional features, including disruptive behaviors, aggression, agitation, inattention, and hyperactivity (des Portes, Hagerman, & Hendren, 2003; Meyers, Plauche-Johnson, & Council on Children With Disabilities, 2007). Therefore, we will refer Snoopy's parents to a pediatric psychiatrist who specializes in the treatment of pervasive developmental disorders. It will also be important to refer Snoopy for a comprehensive speech/language evaluation as well as an occupational therapy assessment in order to determine the current level of his daily living skills competencies.

In order to address Snoopy's behavioral and social skill deficits, we will use a combination of Applied Behavior Analysis (ABA) and the DIR/Floortime Model. It is important to note that "specific interventions proposed for clinical disturbances . . . have included individual psychotherapy for the child and/or caregiver, parent training with emphasis on developmental expectations and sensitive responsiveness, family therapy or caregiver/child dyadic therapy" (Zeanah & Boris, 2005, p. 365). Applied Behavior Analysis (Lovaas et al., 1987) uses procedures derived from the principles of operant conditioning (reinforcement, extinction, shaping) in order to decrease the frequency of inappropriate and maladaptive behaviors while increasing the likelihood and frequency of desired and adaptive behaviors (social, communicative, and play skills in Snoopy's case). ABA relies heavily upon parents working alongside the therapist both in the clinic/school and at home in order maximize behavioral gains and to generalize them in the client's daily life. ABA has been found to be effective in enhancing daily living, play, social, communicative, and self-care skills in children with Autistic Spectrum Disorders (Cooper, Heron, & Heward, 1987; Eikeseth, Smith, Jahr, & Eldevik, 2002; Howlin, Magiati, & Charman, 2009; Meyers et al., 2007). In Snoopy's case, the Applied Behavior analyst will work with the parents to employ frequent use of praise and positive reinforcement to increase Snoopy's verbalizations and social communication, to implement a response-shaping program to facilitate his language and social interaction skills, to use a token economy at home and in the school to build interactive play and social communication skills, to teach the parents effective contingency management to decrease Snoopy's idiosyncratic and purposeless play, and to help them to extinguish Snoopy's repetitive and purposeless play by reinforcing engagement with a broader array of play materials and activities.

The DIR/Floortime Model (Greenspan & Weider, 2006) is a highly hands-on and interactive assessment and intervention program, the objective of which is to increase opportunities for back-and-forth communication and engagement with the child that provide learning opportunities to enhance social communication skills.

Based upon the premise that clinicians must honor the unique ways that autistic children experience their world, interact, and develop, the DIR/Floortime Model relies on the use of highly trained therapists to interact with the child and parent through increasingly challenging sensory, communicative, and social activities. It has been used extensively in working with children on the autism spectrum (Greenspan & Weider, 2006). Because effective use of this model requires extensive and highly specialized training, we will refer Snoopy's parents to the Schulz Development Resources Academy, which specializes in the DIR/Floortime Model.

More recently, creative techniques, that is, those that employ art, music, dance, drama, and play, have been used to enhance sensory integration, social skills, communication, and symbolic thinking. Social Stories (Gray & Garand, 1983) is one such methodology that relies upon the use of picture stories to teach social problem-solving skills, and it has been found to be useful in working with children with Autism Spectrum Disorders (Kokina & Kern, 2010). Another play-based intervention that has been found to be both useful and effective with these children is Lego therapy (LeGoff, 2004), which uses Legos to teach social skills. Lego toys are naturally attractive and sensorily appealing, and as such can capture the attention of autistic children for long periods. The play therapist works with children individually or in groups to build Lego-based social scenarios through which clients can interact. In Snoopy's case, we will use elements of both Social Stories and Lego therapy to enhance his social and communication skills.

Finally, and working directly with Snoopy's parents, we will provide family counseling aimed at strengthening their relationship so they may work intensively with Snoopy, refer them to an autism support group, and encourage them to join the Autism Society of America to expand their knowledge and support.

Step 4: Provide Outcome Measures of Change. This last step in treatment planning requires that we specify how change will be measured and indicate the extent to which progress has been made toward realizing these goals (Neukrug & Schwitzer, 2006). The counselor has considerable flexibility in this phase and may choose from a number of objective domains (psychological tests and measures of self-esteem, depression, psychosis, interpersonal relationship, anxiety, etc.), quasi-objective measures (the *DSM-IV-TR*'s Axis V GAF scale; pre-post clinician, client and psychiatric ratings), and subjective ratings (client self-report, clinician's in-session observations). In Snoopy's case, we have implemented a number of these, including pre-post measures of adaptive functioning on the Gilliam Autism Rating Scale (Gilliam, 2006); clinician, teacher, and parent-reported improvement in verbal communication, social interaction, and creative/ expressive play, parent and teacher report of improved communication between home and school; and compliance with psychopharmacotherapy.

The completed treatment plan is now developed through which the counselor, Snoopy, his parents, and teachers will begin their shared work of improving communication channels between home and school, connecting with autism support organizations, and, most importantly, helping him to communicate and interact more effectively and play in a nonrepetitive and more creative fashion at home and at school. The treatment plan is described below and summarized in Table 7.5.

TREATMENT PLAN

Client: Snoopy

Service Provider: Charles Schulz Elementary School Counseling Department

BEHAVIORAL DEFINITION OF PROBLEMS:

1. Lack of social interests, social interactions, and verbal communication—Current deficiency in verbal communication despite early basic language development, noticeably less interest in parent relationships with minimal eye contact or smiling, disinterest in seeking out peer relationship, minimal improvement in social interest or verbal communication despite speech and occupational therapy

2. Solitary, repetitive, stereotypical, and purposeless behaviors and play—Repetitive self-stimulating behaviors, preference for play with balls, rubber toys, and military aviator fantasies over peer-based interactive play, digging in the backyard, watching out the window for birds or the mailman, and inappropriate touching of peers

GOALS FOR CHANGE:

1. Lack of social interests, social interactions, and verbal communication

   - Strengthen basic language skills and the ability to communicate simply with others
   - Strengthen the basic emotional bond with parents
   - Engage in reciprocal and cooperative interactions with others on a regular basis
   - Help parents, teachers, and peers to develop a level of understanding and acceptance of client's capabilities and to set realistic expectations for behavior

2. Solitary, repetitive, stereotypical, and purposeless behaviors and play

   - Reduce self-stimulatory and repetitive behaviors
   - Shape symbolic play behaviors
   - Assist in tolerating changes in routine and immediate environment
   - Attain the highest, most realistic level of overall functioning

THERAPEUTIC INTERVENTIONS:

An ongoing course of eclectic intervention targeting neurological, psychological, and social/interpersonal factors drawn from DIR/Floortime, behavior, and artistic/expressive therapies, supplemented with psychoeducation and group support for parents and teachers

Targeting Neurological Factors (agitation, inattention, hyperactivity, disruptiveness)

- Referral to pediatric psychiatrists for management of related behavioral and emotional symptoms
- Referral for speech/language and occupational therapy evaluation

Targeting Psychological Factors (solitary, repetitive and purposeless play)

- Use effective contingency management to decrease idiosyncratic and purposeless play
- Extinguish repetitive and purposeless play by reinforcing engagement with a broader array of play materials and activities
- Referral for DIR/Floortime training
- Lego and Social Stories

Targeting Social Interactions and Communication

- Employ frequent use of praise and positive reinforcement to increase Snoopy's verbalizations and social communication
- Use a token economy at home and in the school to build interactive play and social communication skills
- Implement a response-shaping program to facilitate his language and social interaction skills
- Referral for DIR/Floortime training
- Lego and Social Stories

Targeting Parenting

- Provide family counseling aimed at strengthening relationship
- Referral to an autism support group
- Encouragement to join the Autism Society of America to expand knowledge and support base
- Referral for DIR/Floortime training

OUTCOME MEASURES OF CHANGE:

Improved social, communicative, and adaptive behavior both at home and in school as measured by:

- Improved scores on the Gilliam Autism Rating Scale-II
- Clinician-, teacher-, and parent-reported improvement in verbal communication, social interaction, and creative/expressive play
- Parent and teacher report of improved daily communication between home and school
- Compliance with psychopharmacotherapy

Table 7.5   Snoopy's Treatment Plan Summary: Eclectic Combination of DIR/Floortime Model, Behavior Therapy, and Expressive Creative Arts Play Therapy

Goals for Change	Therapeutic Interventions	Outcome Measures of Change
Lack of social interests, social interactions, and verbal communication	Lack of social interests, social interactions, and verbal communication	Improved on-task, attentive, and prosocial attitudes and behavior both at home and in school as measured by:
Strengthen basic language skills and the ability to communicate simply with others	Solitary, repetitive, stereotypical, and purposeless behaviors and play	Clinician-, teacher-, and parent-reported improvement in verbal communication, social interaction, and creative/expressive play
Strengthen the basic emotional bond with parents	*Targeting Neurological Factors (agitation, inattention, hyperactivity, disruptiveness)*	
Engage in reciprocal and cooperative interactions with others on a regular basis	Referral to pediatric psychiatrists for management of related behavioral and emotional symptoms	Parent and teacher report of improved daily communication between home and school
Help parents, teachers, and peers to develop a level of understanding and acceptance of client's capabilities and to set realistic expectations for behavior	Referral for speech/language and occupational therapy evaluation	Compliance with psychopharmacotherapy
	Targeting Psychological Factors (solitary, repetitive, and purposeless play)	
Solitary, repetitive, stereotypical, and purposeless behaviors and play	Use effective contingency management to decrease idiosyncratic and purposeless play	
Reduce self-stimulatory and repetitive behaviors	Extinguish repetitive and purposeless play by reinforcing engagement with a broader array of play materials and activities	
Shape symbolic play behaviors	Referral for DIR/Floortime training	
Assist in tolerating changes in routine and immediate environment	Lego and Social Stories	
Attain the highest, most realistic level of overall functioning	*Targeting Social Interactions and Communication*	
	Employ frequent use of praise and positive reinforcement to increase verbalizations and social communication	
	Use a token economy at home and in the school to build interactive play and social communication skills	
	Implement a response-shaping program to facilitate his language and social interaction skills	
	Referral for DIR/Floortime training	
	Lego and Social Stories	
	Targeting Parenting	
	Provide family counseling aimed at strengthening relationship	
	Referral to an autism support group	
	Encouragement to join the Autism Society of America to expand knowledge and support base	
	Referral for DIR/Floortime training	

FOLLOW-UP: DIAGNOSIS, CASE CONCEPTUALIZATION, AND TREATMENT PLANNING THEMES—CHAPTER SUMMARY

This chapter presented a challenging clinical caseload comprising two adult clients, Miss Piggy and Mario, and three children, Gretel, Naruto, and Snoopy. The caseload had a gender balance of two female clients and three males. Among the caseload's diversity were three American clients (whom, along with Mario, who has an Italian American cultural heritage, we described as Porcine American with a French American cultural heritage and Canine American) and two children who experienced international relocations: Gretel, an Austrian girl whose father relocated to the United States and married an American, and Naruto, a Japanese boy adopted in London by British parents. Upper, upper-middle, and middle socioeconomic statuses were represented by this group of clients. One of the adults, Mario, is heterosexual, and we characterized the other adult, Miss Piggy, as having a bisexual orientation.

One of the adults, Miss Piggy, sought counseling services at an independent outpatient client practice, the Downtown Counseling Center of Chicago, and the other adult, Mario, sought inpatient treatment at a private Beverly Hills Drug Rehabilitation Center; all three children were referred for counseling in their communities by their school counselor, assistant principal, or headmaster.

Among the adult concerns presented by our clients making up this chapter's caseload, Miss Piggy sought assistant for concerns characterized diagnostically as Borderline Personality Disorder, and Mario required assistance with Cocaine Dependence, Cocaine-Induced Sleep Disorder, and Alcohol Abuse. Looking at the counseling theories represented, their counselors formed case conceptualizations and then treatment plans based on Dialectical Behavior Therapy, and a psychotherapeutic integration of Multicomponent Psychosocial Intervention and Motivational Interviewing, respectively. The younger clients were referred for a range of childhood concerns, described diagnostically as Oppositional Defiant Disorder, Attention-Deficit/Hyperactivity Disorder, Conduct Disorder, and Autistic Disorder. Looking at theoretical approaches, their counselors formed case conceptualizations and then treatment plans based on a psychotherapeutic integration of Child-Centered Play Therapy and Cognitive Behavioral Play Therapy; Multicomponent Psychosocial Intervention; and an eclectic mix of DIR/Floortime Model, Behavior Therapy, and Expressive Creative Arts Play Therapy.

In their treatment plans, these clients' counselors expressed hopes that their clients would achieve such as outcomes as being able to better regulate mood, self-esteem, and relationship stability (Miss Piggy); immediate cessation of substance use and establishment and maintenance of total abstinence and long-term adaptive functioning (Mario); reduced oppositional defiant behavior, increased behavioral and emotional compliance, prosocial behavior, and effective grieving (Gretel); and improved on-task, attentive, and prosocial attitudes and behavior at home and in school (Naruto and Snoopy).

STUDY QUESTIONS AND LEARNING ACTIVITIES

Based on your understanding of this chapter's cases, consider and respond to these Study Questions and Learning Activities:

1. This caseload is a challenging one.

   a. If you were assigned this group of clients, what would be your initial reactions to their individual characteristics and differences? Working with both adults and children? Their reasons for referral?

   b. What would you identify as your greatest strengths for assisting these five clients? Your areas of greatest need for growth?

2. In their Basic Case Summaries, this chapter's counselors focused on their clients' earlier developmental and family experiences, presenting concerns, assessment of current distress, and areas and life roles in which they were experiencing difficulties, client strengths, and

hopes for change. There was an emphasis on: Miss Piggy's family and development history; patterns, severity, and consequences of Mario's substance use; Gretel's earliest and formative negative developmental experiences as well as the effects of problematic behaviors in multiple settings inside and outside of school; Naruto's developmental experiences and early life transitions, his strengths and talents, medical notes, and distinguishing his violent and aggressive behaviors from his attention deficits and hyperactivity; and for Snoopy, information from developmental history, counselor observations, play observation, parent report, information from school, and the interview itself.

a. Keeping in mind that the initial counseling meeting, screening session, or intake interview usually requires the counselor to balance rapport and trust-building, on one hand, and assessment and information-gathering, on the other hand, what would you identify as your greatest strengths when engaging these five clients in the counseling process, and gathering the clinical information needed to conceptualize and plan for their counseling process? Your areas of greatest need for growth?

b. Looking at the five Basic Case Summaries, how does this type of clinical writing differ from your everyday thinking and conversation about people? What are your levels of comfort, skill, and experience in this type of professional writing? What steps can you take to further develop or improve these skills?

c. What suggestions would you have for one or more of the counselors in this chapter regarding missing, overlooked, or underemphasized—or overemphasized—information gathered and reported in the Basic Case Summaries? What would you like to have known more about? What methods could be used—clinical interview questions, observations, psychological measures, or other means—to find the additional information you would seek?

3. This chapter illustrated *DSM-IV-TR* diagnoses found in the following sections: Disorders Usually First Diagnosed in Infancy, Childhood, or Adolescence; Substance-Related Disorders; and Personality Disorders.

a. How familiar are you with these sections of the *DSM-IV-TR?* What is your comfort level using the *DSM-IV-TR* to explore these sets of concerns? Which of these groups of disorders are likely to be most important to you in the practicum, internship, residency, or professional practice settings in which you hope to work?

b. What are your attitudes, reactions, or thoughts concerning diagnosis of childhood disorders? Concerning the diagnosis of behavioral consequences of problematic substance use? Concerning diagnosing lifelong patterns characterized as personality disorders? How can you further explore or develop your professional attitudes about diagnosis of these types of concerns?

c. What will be your next steps in gaining greater comfort and skills at diagnosis of the attention-deficit and disruptive behavior disorders of childhood? Substance-use and substance-induced disorders? Personality disorders?

d. What are your attitudes, reactions, or thoughts concerning use of Axis IV to record psychosocial and environmental stressors (such as Miss Piggy's history of divorces) and Axis V to record general medical problems (such as Naruto's ankle sprain)? What will be your next steps in gaining greater comfort and skills with these axes?

e. Among this group of clients, Axis V Global Assessment of Functioning (GAF) scores ranged from 41 (Snoopy's serious symptoms) to 64 (Gretel's mild symptoms). What are your attitudes, reactions, or thoughts concerning use of Axis V GAF scores to estimate the client's overall level of functioning? Do you agree with the counselors' estimates found in this chapter? What will be your next steps in gaining greater comfort and skills estimating Axis V GAF scores?

4. This chapter's cases included two examples of case conceptualization and treatment planning using purist counselor theories, two examples of psychotherapeutic integration, and one use of an eclectic mix of theories.

a. What is your level of familiarity with the various adult counseling theories illustrated in this chapter: Dialectical Behavior Therapy? Multicomponent Psychosocial Intervention? Motivational Interviewing?

What is your level of familiarity with the various child-counseling theories illustrated in this chapter: Child-Centered Play Therapy, Cognitive Behavioral Play Therapy, Child-Oriented Behavior Therapy, Expressive Creative Arts Play Therapy, and DIR/Floortime Model? What do you believe are their relative strengths and weaknesses? For which individuals do they seem to be a good match? For what types of client concerns do they seem to be potentially effective? What do the evidence and discussions found in the current literature say about this?

b. Which of these theories seem to be a good fit with your own attitudes and skills? Which interest you the most?

c. To learn more, review the resources and references cited in the chapter, interview a practicing counselor who uses these theories in his or her everyday work, seek clinical supervision from a supervisor experienced with the approach, enroll in a special-topics class, or look for continuing education workshops and conference presentations covering these approaches.

d. What are your thoughts, reactions, and comfort level integrating multiple psychotherapeutic approaches to address the needs of your clients? Which theories are you most likely, or least likely, to consider integrating into your approach? How will you decide when, with whom, and in what ways, to integrate multiple approaches? To consider and learn more about integrating approaches such as Multicomponent Psychosocial Intervention and Motivational Interviewing, interview a practicing counselor who uses an integration of these theories in his or her everyday work, seek clinical supervision from a supervisor experienced with psychotherapeutic integration of these theories, or seek other professional consultations and learning opportunities.

e. What are your thoughts, reactions, and comfort level eclectically mixing multiple psychotherapeutic approaches to address the needs of your clients? What are the differences between psychotherapeutic integrating, and eclectically mixing, theories? What knowledge or skills will you need to be an effective eclectic counselor?

f. Which theories are you most likely, or least likely, to consider eclectically mixing? How will you decide when, with whom, and in what ways to integrate multiple approaches? To consider and learn more about integrating approaches such as Multicomponent Psychosocial Intervention and Motivational Interviewing, interview a practicing counselor who uses an integration of these theories in his or her everyday work, seek clinical supervision from a supervisor experienced with psychotherapeutic integration of these theories, or seek other professional consultations and learning opportunities.

5. The case conceptualizations found in this chapter began with casting a wide net for client concerns and dynamics, next forming intuitive-logical groupings to begin better understanding the clients' presentations, and then applying counseling theories to make clinical inferences about the clients' situations.

a. How does this type of professional clinical thinking differ from your everyday thinking, conversation, and analysis about people? What are your levels of comfort, skill, and experience at this type of clinical thinking? What steps can you take to further develop or improve your conceptualizing skills?

b. What are your thoughts, reactions, and critique of the ways these counselors grouped together: Miss Piggy's emotional, romantic, impulsive, and developmental issues? Mario's substance-use behaviors and sleep disturbance? Gretel's historical and current, issues? Naruto's Attention-Deficit/Hyperactivity and Conduct Disorders? Snoopy's social concerns and solitary behavior concerns due to Autistic Disorder? Do you agree with each of these thematic groupings? How might you have organized these differently, more usefully, or more effectively?

c. What are your thoughts and reactions pertaining to the ways the counselors applied the various theoretical approaches in order to explain, make inferences about, and prepare for treatment planning with these clients? What were your reactions to the counselors' presentations of Miss Piggy's deficits in regulation of emotions and behaviors and deeper inference of an invalidating environment

(Dialectical Behavior Therapy)? The social context of Mario's substance use (Multicomponent Psychosocial Intervention), and his readiness for change (Motivational Interviewing)? Gretel's hostile behaviors and lack of positive parental experiences (Child-Centered Play Therapy) and learned experiences and faulty beliefs (Cognitive Behavioral Play Therapy)? Naruto's difficulties in multiple component systems (Multicomponent Psychosocial Intervention)? Snoopy's problems with social interactions and repetitive behaviors due to Autisim (eclectic mix of DIR/Floortime, Behavior, and Expressive Creative Arts Play Therapy)? Do you agree with the ways the counselor used the various theories with these clients? How might you have applied the theories differently, more usefully, or more effectively?

6. A fully developed treatment plan was presented for each of the individuals comprising this chapter's caseload. The treatment plans provide goals for change, interventions, and outcome measures.

   a. How does this type of clinical writing, thinking, and preparation for the professional counseling process differ from your everyday approach to engaging in helpful relationships with people? What are your levels of comfort, skill, and experience with this type of professional writing, thinking, and preparation? What steps can you take to further develop or improve your treatment planning skills for the types of practicum, internship, residency, or work settings that are of most interest to you?

   b. This chapter's treatment plans first list goals for change for each "client" character, next apply the selected counseling theory to clearly state the interventions and approaches to be used, and finally identify ways to measure the expected changes. What are your thoughts, reactions, and critique of the ways this chapter's counselors prepared Miss Piggy's, Mario's, Naruto's, Gretel's, and Snoopy's treatment plans? What interests

you most about these plans? What raises questions for you?

   c. What are your thoughts and reactions pertaining to the dialectical behavioral interventions (Miss Piggy), multiple components of psychosocial inpatient and outclient treatment and motivational interviewing techniques (Mario), child-centered, cognitive behavioral, and family-oriented play therapies and use of parent effectiveness training (Gretel), multiple component psychosocial methods at school, home, and other contexts (Naruto), and mixture of child therapies (Snoopy) outlined as interventions? With which are you most familiar? Least familiar? Unfamiliar? Which will you select to learn more about through further reading, clinical supervision, or other professional development? Alternatively, which do not seem to be close fits with your own preferred approach?

   d. These clients' counselors used counselor observation, client report, change scores on psychological measures and the GAF, behavioral reports, and other means to measure outcomes. As you review the outcome measures found on Miss Piggy's, Mario's, Gretel's, Naruto's, and Snoopy's treatment plans, consider these questions: Do the measures seem realistic and accomplishable? Are they concrete and specific enough to indicate change? Are they sensitive to the needs of the client? Which of these measures will become a regular part of your own repertoire, which might you decline to use, and what additional measures might you add to your own list? What new skills and competencies might you need to develop in order to effectively report on your own clients' outcomes?

7. Now, working independently, with a partner, or in a small group, select your own "client" from among the pop culture world of Children's Characters and Video Game Characters. Develop your own narrative about the client's arrival at counseling. Then, prepare a fully completed Basic Case Summary, Diagnostic Impressions, Case Conceptualization, and Treatment Plan!

8

TROUBLED YOUTH IN FILM AND ON STAGE

The Cases of Edward Cullen, Jamal, Juno, Claire, and Elphaba

PREVIEW: POPULAR CULTURE THEMES

In this second chapter of cases, you will meet a group of characters who have become mainstays in popular culture through their initial and then enduring presence in film and on the live stage. Although they differ widely in race, gender, and even species, as well as in their initial believability (one is a witch and another a vampire), each of these indelible characters will offer you an opportunity to appreciate the contemporary adolescent experience.

The depiction of troubled youth in popular culture, particularly in film and on stage, dates to the early part of the 20th century. Dramatized representations of alienated, angst-ridden, disenfranchised, and hypersexed youth have both captured our collective imaginations and led us to reflect on the often tenuous relationship between adults and teens. Popular magazines, comic books, and advertising perpetuate the stereotype that young men are primarily sexual while young women are primarily relational and subordinate to the sexual needs of their male partners (Farvid & Braun, 2006; Holmberg, 1998; Young, 1993). This dichotomy is further reinforced by the sexualized, hypercompetitive, and idealized representation of teens and young adults in television programming (Tiggerman, 2005), through popular sport (McLeod, 2006) and music, in which the additional elements of pathos and rage are prominent (Best & Kellner, 1999; Lacourse, Claes, & Vilenueve, 2001). And finally, film has been a powerful stage upon which the identity struggles, family discord, and relationship battles of youth have been dramatically enacted (Robertie, Weidenbenner, Barrett, & Poole, 2008).

With regard to the specific characters in this section, Edward Cullen, along with his mortal Bella, comes to us through the vivid imagination of teen author Stephenie Meyers and her wildly popular four-installment *Twilight* Saga Collection. In addition to his presence on the silver screen and in novels, the morose and yearnful teen Edward's visage has appeared on every possible piece of clothing. In our presentation, Edward struggles with Major Depressive Disorder and Dependent

Personality Features. Jamal Malik, the main character in the Oscar-winning film *Slumdog Millionaire,* first came to our attention through a novel of the same name by Vikas Swarup. In both incarnations, Jamal faced unbelievable adversity, and his story has won the hearts and imaginations of a worldwide audience. In our presentation, Jamal struggles with Acute Stress Disorder. Juno MacGuff, the unlikely title character of the slice-of-life film *Juno,* is a teen who struggles with a life-changing decision to carry her baby to term. Although her character has not yet crossed over to other mediums, the actor who played her, Ellen Page, has starred in television commercials for Cisco Systems. In our presentation, Juno struggles with Parent-Child Relational Problems. Claire Standish is one of an ensemble cast of teens in the 1980's teen classic *The Breakfast Club,* which became anthemic for a generation. In our presentation, Claire struggles with Cannabis Abuse, Eating Disorder NOS, and Trichotillomania. Finally, there is Elphaba Thropp, the green-skinned witch from Gregory Maguire's revisionist novel *Wicked: The Life and Times of the Wicked Witch of the West.* It was later adapted into a Broadway musical. In our presentation, Elphaba struggles with Body Dysmorphic Disorder and Antisocial Personality Features.

The plots surrounding these particular characters vary considerably, from not-so-thinly disguised teen romances to slice-of-life stories of seemingly everyday adolescents to fantastical tales of the supernatural, which just happen to star young people. At a deeper level, however, their stories are about the core challenges of the teen years, including the need to cling to the innocence of childhood while at the same time venturing out into the confusing borderland of adolescence, and the struggle to develop and then assert identity. Theirs are the stories of surviving physically, sexually, and emotionally in relationships that are often confusing and painful, and of having to make life-altering decisions that vault them to a precarious and unfamiliar new place in their developmental trajectory. The stories of Edward, Jamal, Juno, Claire, and Elphaba will offer opportunities that will guide you in your clinical work with the most challenging population—that of adolescents and young adults.

APPROACHES TO LEARNING

As you learn about this group of characters, pay attention to:

- The ways in which the symptoms of these characters are consistent with your understanding of adolescent and young adult clients' needs.
- Whether the diagnosis of personality disorder or personality disorder features is clinically useful and developmentally appropriate.
- How the depiction of disorders in this age group has changed over time.
- The ways that popular media perpetuate gender, race, and sexual stereotypes about youth, particularly those with mental illness.

CASE 8.1   VAMPIRE ANTHOLOGY'S EDWARD CULLEN

INTRODUCING THE CHARACTER

Edward Cullen is the main character in Stephenie Meyers's four-volume vampire anthology, which includes *Twilight* (2005), *New Moon* (2006), *Eclipse* (2007), and *Breaking Dawn* (2008). Although initially written for a teen readership, the widespread popularity and cross-generational appeal of these books resulted in their cinematic adaptation. The stories chronicle the experiences of the Cullens, a band of powerful vampiric immortals who struggle among themselves, against a neighboring band of werewolves, and with greater human society for their very survival.

At the heart of the Cullen clan is Edward, who is the member most recently "turned" into a vampire by the group's leader, Carlisle, who did so in 1918 in order to save him from the fatal ravages of the Spanish influenza. Edward is depicted as a sullen and tormented perpetual teenager who in spite of artistic genius, limitless strength, and searing intellect, yearns to love and be loved. His romance with Bella, the object of his affections, conjures themes of Shakespearean romance and tragedy and leads both reader and moviegoer to ponder the existential issues of meaning, mortality, significance, love, and death. Ultimately, Edward's relationship with Bella forces upon him choices that he would rather not have to make. The following basic case summary and diagnostic impressions describe Cullen's mood problems, characterized by recurrent episodes of depression and related symptoms.

Meet the Client

You can assess the client in action by viewing clips of Edward Cullen's video material at the following websites:

- http://www.youtube.com/watch?v=bfY tIQG-xNQ Edward saves Bella and first reveals himself
- http://www.youtube.com/watch?v= 6VUUdy7Eh18 Edward turned into a vampire
- http://www.youtube.com/watch?v=Vc1 UqeHhjeo Edward and Bella first conversation

BASIC CASE SUMMARY

Identifying Information. Edward Cullen is a 17-year-old Caucasian male who is a senior at Forks High School in Washington state. He lives with his legal guardian, Carlisle, and his extended family. Edward excels in all academic subjects. Although it has been reported that he is athletically gifted and multitalented in the arts, he participates in neither team sports nor any of the school's social organizations. In appearance, he is a tall, lanky young man who would be described as physically attractive. During the interview, he displayed an engaging demeanor.

Notably to the interviewer, his piercing golden eyes seemed to suggest pathos and wisdom beyond his years. Edward scheduled an evening appointment after sundown and arrived on time.

Presenting Concern. Edward was referred by his school counselor, Anne Lestat, who became concerned that some of Edward's art projects were graphically violent, and that many of the poems and short stories he produced in his English class were infused with juxtaposed themes of love, death, and soul murder. The counselor was concerned these themes might be indicative a depressive disorder and suicidality.

Background, Family Information, and Relevant History. Edward Anthony Masen was born in 1901 to Edward and Elizabeth Masen of Chicago, Illinois. He described an uneventful and seemingly happy childhood and a very close relationship with both of his parents, who worked long hours in one of the city's many meat-packing plants. The plant was subsequently closed for health reasons and he vaguely recalled "people dying all around me, including my parents." Subsequently, he spent several years in an orphanage where, around age 17, he contracted the Spanish influenza. On the day of his death, Edward was visited by one of the hospital's benefactors, Carlisle Cullen, who "turned" him into a vampire and thus gave him immortality.

Over the next several decades and into the present, Edward has lived with the Cullen clan, a band of biologically unrelated, yet perpetually joined vampires that includes Carlisle and Esmee, their daughter Rosalie and her husband Emmett; Edward, Alice, his sister, and her brother, Jasper. Being immortal, Edward has been unable to attend any particular high school for a full 4 years lest his agelessness be suspected. As a result, the clan has frequently relocated, and Edward has been deprived of the opportunity, among others, of long-term friends or intimate relationships beyond those of his clanmates. Edward appears to have struggled with his immortality as it has isolated him from the normally expected experiences of both life and love. For this reason, he vowed never to "turn" girlfriends into immortals, that is, until he met Bella. It has only been she to whom he has revealed his immortality and with whom he has shared the depth of his longing to be an average and ordinary teenager. In spite of his many gifts, Edward describes himself as feeling sad, lonely, and "lost."

Problem and Counseling History. Edward agreed to come to counseling on the referral of his school counselor and at the urging of his current girlfriend, Bella. According to the client, his girlfriend is concerned about his recurring periods of sadness and sense of detachment from the world around him. He indicated that the girlfriend also is worried about "being smothered with his love." Along these lines, Edward was almost singular in his focus during the interview on "my eternal love for Bella" and described her worries as primary motivator for seeking counseling.

Edward agreed with his school counselor's and girlfriend's assessment that his mood often was low. Based on his written responses to an intake questionnaire and responses to the Beck Depression Inventory II, his self-report, and his presentation during the interview, it appears that, at present, Edward is experiencing a major depressive episode. He reports that he has been feeling "really, really down" for the past 3 weeks, and has little interest in daily activities, including the school projects and clan activities that ordinarily he would enjoy. Over this time, he reports having difficulty falling asleep and staying asleep in his bed, which he describes as a "coffin." His appetite is low and he made the unusual comment that he "had lost his taste for blood" lately. Cognitively, he appears to dwell on what he sees as his and his life's shortcomings. He referred to Bella as his "lifeline." Although his strangely golden eyes seemed to glow almost preternaturally when talking about her, he was otherwise lackluster, apathetic, and monosyllabic when describing his life, that at points during the interview, he wished would end. Edward lamented that he was tired of living as he saw no end to his suffering and felt trapped between life and death. He added that Bella was his only link to life, which he described as unobtainable.

Edward and his school counselor agree that he has experienced similar periods of low mood several times during his tenure at his current high school, each lasting several weeks and then mostly but not completely subsiding. He can remember a time period several years ago, prior to his first experience of low mood: "back then I sort of remember feeling great, like you're supposed to." He says at that time his mood began what he experienced as a gradual decline, lasting about 6 months, before "plummeting into self-doubt and angst, like now." He reports no memories of periods of elation or unusually heightened mood, although he said "sometimes when I feel better it is almost like a high." Notably, this current event seems unusually difficult to Edward, and he reports "seeing the dead walking around" and "hearing death trying get at me from the other side of the door." He denies having had these perceptions on a regular basis, but does report they have been present "for days now." He also reports that unlike "most times when I'm feeling morose," he is having difficulty feeling even transient moments of relief, such as during a funny movie or even when spending time with his girlfriend.

Goals for Counseling and Course of Therapy to Date. To date, two intake sessions have been conducted, one with Edward and one with him and Bella. When asked if he believed his family would be interested in attending counseling, Edward was quick to say "they really go their own way and don't believe in therapy." Although Edward did not perceive himself to be as distressed or depressed as either Bella or his school counselor did, he acquiesced to a course of counseling in order to "make Bella happy." In this context, he reiterated that he would die for her. Given his seeming preoccupation death as well as Bella's concern for his welfare, Edward was asked if he would be willing to participate in a psychiatric evaluation so that he may consider the possibilities of medical treatment or in-patient hospitalization. He was resistant to both options but again reiterated that he would do anything for Bella. He denied that his absence of self-focus, moroseness, and preoccupation with both Bella and death were a problem, but agreed to continue in counseling. Edward denied any intention to act on his suicidal ideation, was reassuring that he would not follow through with any self-harming actions, and agreed to return.

Diagnostic Impressions

Axis I.   296.34 Major Depressive Disorder, Recurrent (Without Full Interepisode Recovery), Current Episode, Severe With Mood-Congruent Psychotic Features

Axis II.   Dependent Personality Features

Axis III.   Immortality

Axis IV.   Problems related to the social environment—Conflicts with neighborhood members

Axis V.   GAF = 50 (current)

GAF = 70 (highest level past year)

DISCUSSION OF DIAGNOSTIC IMPRESSIONS

Edward Cullen was referred by the school counselor, who suspected he might be experiencing a depressive disorder because he was producing work reflecting recurrent thoughts of death. Likewise, his girlfriend, Bella, was worried about his recurring periods of sadness and detachment; and his intake materials, including Beck Depression Inventory-II (BDI-II) scores, supported the presence of depressive symptoms. In fact, Edward reported periods of very low mood and diminished interest in school and other usually enjoyable activities, along with difficulties with sleep and appetite, dwelling on his "shortcomings," and observably apathetic, slowed speech, and actions.

The *Diagnostic and Statistical Manual of Mental Disorders, Fourth Edition, Text Revision's (DSM-IV-TR)* Mood Disorders section includes all of the diagnosable disorders that feature a disturbance in mood. The mood disorders and the anxiety disorders, which share a high comorbidity in general, probably comprise the client concerns most commonly seen by counseling professionals. The Mood Disorders include Depressive Disorders (in which the client experiences "unipolar" depression), Bipolar Disorders (in which the client experiences manic, hypomanic, or mixed episodes), and mood disorders that are due to substance use or a medical condition.

In this case, we characterized Edward Cullen's mood problems to be comprised of recurrent

episodes of depression and related symptoms. In the absence of any evidence of abuse of a substance (such as alcohol) or effects of medical problem (like hypothyroidism), Edward's current low mood and low social interests, physiological symptoms (pertaining to appetite, sleep, and energy), cognitive symptoms (pertaining to self-reproach and thoughts of death) meet the criteria for a Major Depressive Episode. Mood Episodes are used as building blocks for making a mood disorder diagnosis.

Edward has experienced no history of either Manic or Hypomanic Episodes; in turn, the diagnosis is Major Depressive Disorder rather than Bipolar Disorder. He has experienced a series of depressive episodes, and in between the episodes he has some but not full relief from his symptoms. In turn, the course is specified as Recurrent (Without Full Interepisode Recovery). Finally, and with regard to his current episode: His experiences satisfy multiple criteria for a Major Depressive Episode, well beyond the minimum needed to make the diagnosis; further, he is experiencing psychotic experiences in the form of visual hallucinations in which he sees "the dead walking around." Death themes are consistent with depression, and as such are considered to be congruent with the condition. The severity specifier, Severe With Mood-Congruent Psychotic Features, is therefore the best fit.

One differential diagnosis regarding mood that might be considered is Dysthymic Disorder, since

Edward continues to have depressive symptoms even when his major episodes lift. Dysthymic Disorder describes a persistent experience of mild or moderate depression. However, this diagnosis requires at least 2 years of symptoms prior to the person's first Major Depressive Episode, which Edward does not report. Another possible differential consideration is a separate diagnosis for Edward's hallucinations. However, the psychotic symptoms occur exclusively during the course of the Depressive Disorder, rather than independent of it. For example, Spitzer et al. (1994, pp. 415–416) reported a poignant case illustration of this phenomenon in which a 15-year-old girl with Major Depressive Disorder "often [heard] the voice of a young child crying for help."

On Axis II, problematic personality features and defenses can be listed even when they do not reflect a diagnosable Personality Disorder—if these personality characteristics are important to understanding the client's functioning and are maladaptive for the person. We provided the notation, Dependent Personality Features, to describe Edward's submissive attitudes and clinging behaviors in his intimate relationship, which have some maladaptive qualities "related to an excessive need to be taken care of" (APA, 2000a, p. 685).

To complete the diagnosis, Edward's medical condition *(sic)*, "immortality," is listed on Axis III, his social stressors are emphasized on Axis IV, and on Axis V his functioning is represented by Global Assessment Functioning (GAF) scores ranging from the presence of only mild symptoms in the recent past, in between episodes, to the current, more serious symptoms that led to his referral. The information on these axes is consistent with a diagnosis of Major Depressive Disorder, Recurrent.

CASE CONCEPTUALIZATION

When Edward Cullen arrived at counseling, his intake counselor collected as much information as possible about the symptoms and situations leading to Edward's referral. Included among the intake materials were a thorough history, client report, counselor observations, and Beck Depression Inventory-II (BDI-II) findings. Based on the intake, Edward Cullen's counselor developed diagnostic impressions, describing his presenting concerns as recurrent Major Depressive Disorder, and Dependent Personality Features. A case conceptualization next was developed. Whereas the purpose of diagnostic impressions is to *describe* the client's concerns, the goal of case conceptualization is to better *understand* and clinically *explain* the person's experiences (Neukrug & Schwitzer, 2006). It helps the counselor understand the etiology leading to Edward's depressive disorder and personality features, and the factors maintaining these concerns. In turn, case conceptualization sets the stage for treatment planning. Treatment planning then provides a road map that plots out how the counselor and client expect to move from presenting concerns to positive outcomes (Seligman, 1993, p. 157)—helping Edward Cullen improve his low mood and related symptoms, and reducing the problematic aspects of psychological dependence.

When forming a case conceptualization, the clinician applies a purist counseling theory, an integration of two or more theories, an eclectic mix of theories, or a solution-focused combination of tactics to his or her understanding of the client. In this case, Edward's counselor based his conceptualization on psychotherapeutic integration of two theories (Corey, 2009). Psychotherapists very commonly integrate more than one theoretical approach in order to form a conceptualization and treatment plan that will be as efficient and effective as possible for meeting the client's needs (Dattilo & Norcross, 2006; Norcross & Beutler, 2008). In other words, counselors using the psychotherapeutic integration method attempt to flexibly tailor their clinical efforts to "the unique needs and contexts of the individual client" (Norcross & Beutler, 2008, p. 485). Like other counselors using integration, Edward's clinician chose this method because he had not found one individual theory that was comprehensive enough, by itself, to address all of the "complexities," "range of client types," and "specific problems" seen among his everyday caseload (Corey, 2009, p. 450).

Specifically, Edward Cullen's counselor selected an integration of (a) Cognitive Behavior Therapy and (b) Interpersonal Psychotherapy. He selected this approach based on Edward's presentation of intrapersonal mood concerns along with interpersonal personality features, and his knowledge of current outcome research with clients experiencing these types of concerns (Critchfield & Smith-Benjamin, 2006; Fochtmann & Gelenberg, 2005; Hollon, Thase, & Markowitz, 2007; Westen & Morrison, 2001). According to the research, Cognitive Behavior Therapy is one treatment approach indicated when assisting clients with depressive disorders (Fochtmann & Gelenberg, 2005; Hollon et al., 2002; Westen & Morrison, 2001), whereas an integrated approach emphasizing Interpersonal Psychotherapy is indicated for treatment of personality dynamics such as Edward's (Critchfield & Smith-Benjamin, 2006; Livesley, 2007). Cullen's counselor is comfortable theoretically integrating these approaches.

The counselor used the Inverted Pyramid Method of case conceptualization because this method is especially designed to help clinicians more easily form their conceptual pictures of their clients' needs (Neukrug & Schwitzer, 2006; Schwitzer, 1996, 1997). The method has four steps: Problem Identification, Thematic Groupings, Theoretical Inferences, and Narrowed Inferences. The counselor's clinical thinking can be seen in Figure 8.1.

Step 1: Problem Identification. The first step is Problem Identification. Aspects of the presenting problem (thoughts, feelings, behaviors, physiological features), additional areas of concern besides the presenting concern, family and developmental history, in-session observations, clinical inquiries (medical problems, medications, past counseling, substance use, suicidality), and psychological assessments (problem checklists, personality inventories, mental status exam, specific clinical measures) all may contribute information at Step 1. The counselor "casts a wide net" in order to build Step 1 as exhaustively as possible (Neukrug & Schwitzer,

2006, p. 202). As can be seen in Figure 8.1, the counselor identified Edward Cullen's primary concerns (major depression and related symptoms and data); additional concerns (relationship dependency features); and past concerns (history of losses and adjustments to vampire existence). He attempted to go beyond just the current events leading to Edward's referral in order to be descriptive as he could.

Step 2: Thematic Groupings. The second step is Thematic Groupings. The clinician organizes all of the exhaustive client information found in Step 1 into just a few intuitive-logical clinical groups, categories, or themes on the basis of sensible common denominators (Neukrug & Schwitzer, 2006). Four different ways of forming the Step 2 theme groups can be used: Descriptive-Diagnosis Approach, Clinical Targets Approach, Areas of Dysfunction Approach, and Intrapsychic Approach. As can be seen in the figure, Edward Cullen's counselor selected the Descriptive-Diagnosis Approach. This approach sorts together all of the various Step 1 information about the client's adjustment, development, distress, or dysfunction "to show larger clinical problems as reflected through a diagnosis" (Neukrug & Schwitzer, 2006, p. 205).

The counselor grouped together all of Edward's various affective, cognitive, behavioral, and physiological symptoms of recurrent mood disorder into the overarching descriptive-diagnostic theme, recurrent severe depression. Likewise, he grouped Edward's "smothering" behavior and other romantic relationship dynamics into a second theme, personality dependence. The counselor's conceptual work at Step 2 gave him a way to think about Edward's functioning and concerns more insightfully.

So far, at Steps 1 and 2, the counselor has used his clinical assessment skills and his clinical judgment to begin critically understanding Edward's needs. Now, at Steps 3 and 4, he applies the theoretical approach he has selected. He begins making theoretical inferences to explain the factors leading to Edward's issues as they are seen in Steps 1 and 2.

Step 3: Theoretical Inferences. At Step 3, concepts from the counselor's theoretical integration of two approaches—Cognitive Behavior Therapy and Interpersonal Psychotherapy—are applied to explain the experiences causing, and the mechanisms maintaining, Edward Cullen's problematic thoughts, feelings, and behaviors. The counselor tentatively matches the theme groups in Step 2 with this theoretical approach. In other words, the symptom constellations in Step 2, which were distilled from the symptoms in Step 1, now are combined using theory to show what are believed to be the underlying causes or psychological etiology of Edward Cullen's current needs (Neukrug & Schwitzer, 2006; Schwitzer, 2006, 2007).

First, Cognitive Behavior Therapy was applied primarily to Edward's depressive needs. According to Cognitive Behavior Therapy (Beck, 1995, 2005; Ellis, 1994, 2004; Ellis & MacLaren, 2005), irrational thinking, faulty beliefs, or other forms of cognitive errors lead individuals to engage in problematic behaviors and to experience negative moods and attitudes. As can be seen in Figure 8.1, when the counselor applied these Cognitive-Behavior Therapy concepts, he explained at Step 3 that the various issues noted in Step 1 (issues of death and soul death, depressed mood, etc.), which can be understood in Step 2 to be a theme of recurrent severe depression, are rooted in or caused by: (a) negative view of self, (b) negative interpretation of experiences, and (c) negative perceptions about the future.

Second, Interpersonal Psychotherapy was applied primarily to Edward's needs as expressed in his to romantic dependence. According to Interpersonal Psychotherapy, problematic, repetitive, rule-bound communication and transactional patterns in a person's family of origin can be the source of many long-standing young and adult intrapersonal personality dynamics and problematic interpersonal relationship behaviors

(Teyber, 1992; Wenar, 1990). According to the theory, family transactional patterns are highly emotionally charged and powerful, and occur repetitively. Correspondingly, "These repetitive patterns of family interaction, roles, and relationships are internalized and become the foundation of our sense of self and the social world" (Teyber, 1992, p. 13). More specifically, conflictual, disapproving, rejecting, or ambivalent parental and family interpersonal responses cause the cognitive and emotional strain that leads to problematic interpersonal behaviors (Wenar, 1990). As also can be seen in the figure, when the counselor applied these interpersonal psychotherapy concepts, he additionally explained at Step 3 that the various Step 1 issues (viewing girlfriend as a lifeline, etc.) that can be understood in Step 2 to be a theme of personality dependence, are rooted in or caused by (a) early loss of opportunities for parental affective learning in family of origin due to parents' deaths, and (b) repetitive, negative/mixed/ambivalent transactional patterns in his adopted vampiric family and community relationships.

Step 4: Narrowed Inferences. At Step 4, the clinician's selected theory continues to be used to address still-deeper issues when they exist (Schwitzer, 2006, 2007). At this step, "still-deeper, more encompassing, or more central, causal themes" are formed (Neukrug & Schwitzer, 2006, p. 207). Edward Cullen's counselor continued to use a psychotherapeutic integration of two approaches.

First, continuing to apply Cognitive Behavior Therapy concepts at Step 4, Edward's counselor presented a single, deepest, most-fundamental negative distortion that he believed to be most explanatory and causal regarding Edward's primary reasons for referral: the deepest irrational self-statement that "I don't believe I will ever be able to feel good about myself or enjoy my existence ever again now that I cannot be a normal, mortal teenager." Second, continuing to apply Interpersonal Psychotherapy, the counselor presented a single, most deeply rooted characterological conflict and habitual response pattern: "Due to early losses and the strain of repeated negative transactions during his development, the client must hold onto his romantic relationships 'at all costs' to avoid the anxieties and depression of self-rejection." These two narrowed inferences, together, form the basis for understanding the etiology and maintenance of Edward's difficulties.

When all four steps are completed, the client information in Step 1 leads to logical-intuitive groupings on the basis of common denominators in Step 2, the groupings then are explained using theory at Step 3, and then, finally, at Step 4, further deeper explanations are made. From start to finish, the thoughts, feelings, behaviors, and physiological features in the topmost portions are connected on down the pyramid into deepest dynamics.

TREATMENT PLANNING

At this point, Edward's clinician at the Forks Counseling Center has collected all available information about the problems that have been of concern to him and his school counselor. Based upon this information, the counselor developed a five-axis *DSM IV-TR* diagnosis and then, using the "inverted pyramid" (Neukrug & Schwitzer, 2006; Schwitzer, 1996, 1997), formulated a working clinical *explanation* of Edward's difficulties and their etiology that we called the *case conceptualization.* This, in turn, guides us to the next critical step in our clinical work, called the *treatment plan,* the primary purpose of which is to map out a logical and goal-oriented strategy for making positive changes in the client's life. In essence, the treatment plan is a road map *"for reducing or eliminating disruptive symptoms that are impeding the client's ability to reach positive mental health outcomes"* (Neukrug & Schwitzer, 2006, p. 225). As such, it is the cornerstone of our work with not only Edward, but with all clients who present with disturbing and disruptive

symptoms and/or personality patterns (Jongsma & Peterson, 2006; Jongsma, Peterson, & McInnis, 2003a, 2003b; Seligman, 1993, 1998, 2004).

A comprehensive treatment plan must integrate all of the information from the biopsychosocial interview, diagnosis, and case conceptualization into a coherent plan of action. This *plan* comprises four main components, which include (1) a behavioral definition of the problem(s), (2) the selection of achievable goals, (3) the determination of treatment modes, and (4) the documentation of how change will be measured. The *behavioral definition of the problem(s)* consolidates the results of the case conceptualization into a concise hierarchical list of problems and concerns that will be the focus of treatment. The *selection of achievable goals* refers to assessing and prioritizing the client's concerns into a *hierarchy of urgency* that also takes into account the client's motivation for change, level of dysfunction, and real-world influences on his or her problems. The *determination of treatment modes* refers to selection of the specific interventions, which are matched to the uniqueness of the client and to his or her goals and clearly tied to a particular theoretical orientation (Neukrug & Schwitzer, 2006). Finally, the clinician must establish how change will be measured, based upon a number of factors, including client records and self-report of change, in-session observations by the clinician, clinician ratings, results of standardized evaluations such as the Beck Anxiety Inventory (Beck & Steer, 1990) or a family functioning questionnaire, pre-post treatment comparisons, and reports by other treating professionals.

The four-step method discussed above can be seen in Figure 6.1 (p. 109), and is outlined below for the case of Edward Cullen, followed by his specific treatment plan.

Step 1: Behavioral Definition of Problems. The first step in treatment planning is to carefully review the case conceptualization, paying particular attention to the results of Step 2 (Thematic

Figure 8.1   Edward Cullen's Inverted Pyramid Case Conceptualization Summary: Psychotherapeutic Integration of Cognitive Behavior Therapy and Interpersonal Psychotherapy

1. IDENTIFY AND LIST CLIENT CONCERNS

Violent death themes in art projects
Death, eternal love, and soul murder themes
Writing
Feeling sad, "down"
Feeling "lost," lonely
Feelings of detachment
Loss of interest in daily activities
Apathy, lackluster presentation
BDI II Scores
Angst about self
Poor self-appraisal
Recurrent periods of depression
Hearing conversations of the dead

History of death of parents
History of death of others near him
History of death and loss entering vampire family
Adjustment and loss associated with vampiric existence
"Smothering" girlfriend with love
Motivated for change by love relationship
Views girlfriend as "lifeline"

2. ORGANIZE CONCERNS INTO LOGICAL THEMATIC GROUPINGS

1. Recurrent severe depression
2. Personality dependence

3. THEORETICAL INFERENCES: ATTACH THEMATIC GROUPINGS TO INFERRED AREAS OF DIFFICULTY

Psychotherapeutic Integration

Cognitive Behavior Therapy

1. Negative view of self
2. Negative interpretation of experiences
3. Negative perceptions about the future

Interpersonal Psychotherapy

1. Early loss of positive affective learning in family due to parents' death
2. Repetitive, negative/mixed transactional patterns in adopted vampire family relationships

4. NARROWED INFERENCES: SUICIDALITY AND DEEPER DIFFICULTIES

Psychotherapeutic Integration

Cognitive Behavior Therapy
Deepest Negative Distortion:
"I don't believe I will ever be able to feel good about myself or enjoy my existence ever again now that I cannot be a normal, mortal teenager"

Interpersonal Psychotherapy
Characterological Conflict and Habitual Response Pattern:
Due to early losses and the strain of repeated negative transactions during his development, Edward must hold onto his romantic relationship "at all costs" to avoid the anxieties and depression of self-rejection

Groupings), Step 3 (Theoretical Inferences), and Step 4 (Narrowed Inferences). The identified clinical themes reflect the core areas of concern and distress for the client, while the theoretical and narrowed inferences offer clinical speculation as to their origins. In the case of Edward, there are two primary areas of concern. The first, "recurrent severe depression," refers to his feeling sad, detached, down, lonely, and lost; his loss of interest in daily activities, lackluster appearance, self-doubt, and poor self-appraisal as well as the violent death and immortality themes in his art projects, including seeing and hearing walking dead. The second, "personality dependence," refers to smothering his girlfriend with love, viewing her as a lifeline, and his motivation for change by the love relationship. These symptoms and stresses are consistent with the diagnosis of Major Depressive Disorder, Recurrent (Without Full Interepisode Recovery), Current Episode Severe With Mood-Congruent Psychotic Features and Dependent Personality Features (Andrews, Slade, Sunderland, & Anderson, 2007; APA, 2000a; Critchfield & Smith-Benjamin, 2006; Dobson, 1989; Hollon, Thase, & Markowitz, 2002; Livesley, 2007).

Step 2: Identify and Articulate Goals for Change. The second step is the selection of achievable goals, which is based upon a number of factors, including the most pressing or urgent behavioral, emotional, and interpersonal concerns and symptoms as identified by the client and clinician, the willingness and ability of the client to work on those particular goals, and the realistic (real-world) achievability of those goals (Neukrug & Schwitzer, 2006). At this stage of treatment planning, it is important to recognize that not all of the client's problems can be addressed at once, so we focus initially on those that cause the greatest distress and impairment. New goals can be created as old ones are achieved. In the case of Edward, the goals are divided into two prominent areas. The first, "severe recurrent depression," requires that we help Edward to understand the basis for his depression, identify its triggers, replace negative with positive self-talk, use behavioral strategies to overcome depression,

learn and implement problem-solving strategies to avoid depressive outcome, learn and implement relapse prevention strategies and to develop positive, life-affirming activities and a supportive social network The second, "personality dependence," requires that we help Edward to understand the basis of his dependent style in his family of origin and earlier life circumstances, to develop confidence in himself so that he may meet his own needs and tolerate being alone, and to achieve a healthy balance between interpersonal dependence and independence.

Step 3: Describe Therapeutic Interventions. This is perhaps the most critical step in the treatment planning process because the clinician must now integrate information from a number of sources, including the case conceptualization, the delineation of the client's problems and goals, and the treatment literature, paying particular attention to *empirically supported treatment* (EST) and *evidence-based practice* (EBP). In essence, the clinician must align his or her treatment approach with scientific evidence from the fields of counseling and psychotherapy. Wampold (2001) identifies two types of evidence-based counseling research: studies that demonstrate "absolute efficacy," that is, the fact that counseling and psychotherapy work, and those that demonstrate "relative efficacy," that is, the fact that certain theoretical/technical approaches work best for certain clients with particular problems (Psychoanalysis, Gestalt Therapy, Cognitive Behavior Therapy, Brief Solution-Focused Therapy, Cognitive Therapy, Dialectical Behavior Therapy, Person-Centered Therapy, Expressive/Creative Therapies, Interpersonal Therapy, and Feminist Therapy); and when delivered through specific treatment modalities (individual, group, or family counseling).

In the case of Edward, we have decided to use a two-pronged Integrated Approach to therapy. This is comprised first of Cognitive Behavior Therapy (CBT) (Beck, 1995, 2005; Ellis, 1994, 2004; Ellis & MacLaren, 2005), which has been found to be highly effective in counseling and psychotherapy with adolescents (and adults) who experience the symptoms of Major Depressive Disorder (Fochtmann & Gelenberg, 2005; Hollon et al.,

212 • PART III THIRTY CASE ILLUSTRATIONS

2002; Westen & Morrison, 2001). CBT relies on a variety of cognitive techniques (reframing, challenging irrational thoughts, and cognitive restructuring) and behavioral techniques (reinforcement for and shaping of adaptive behavior, extinction of maladaptive behaviors, systematic desensitization, exposure with response). Interpersonal Therapy, which has also been found to be effective with clients struggling with depression centered on early relationship and loss issues (APA, 2000b; Depression Guideline Panel, 1993; Klerman & Weissman, 1993; Weissman, Markowitz, & Klerman, 2000), relies upon an eclectic mix of techniques to help clients to understand and resolve conflicting and self-limiting thoughts, feelings, and behaviors as well as interpersonal deficits in their adults life that have origins in early as well as ongoing family roles, conflicts, and losses. Specific techniques for Edward that are drawn from these approaches include expressing painful feelings of loss related to early life experiences, identifying triggers for depressive thoughts, feelings, and behaviors, engaging in a regular schedule of life-affirming activities, understanding his dependent style, refuting irrational beliefs about relationships, and building self-esteem.

Step 4: Provide Outcome Measures of Change. This last step in treatment planning requires that we specify how change will be measured and indicate the extent to which progress has been made toward realizing these goals (Neukrug & Schwitzer, 2006). The counselor has considerable flexibility in this phase, and may choose from a number of objective domains (psychological tests and measures of self-esteem, depression, psychosis, interpersonal relationship, anxiety, etc.), quasi-objective measures (the *DSM-IV-TR's* Axis V GAF scale; pre-post clinician, client and psychiatric ratings), and subjective ratings (client self-report, clinician's in-session observations). In Edward's case, we have implemented a number of these, including pre-post measure on the Beck Depression Inventory-II, post-only measures of GAF functioning in the mild range (>70), clinician-observed and client-reported use of positive self-talk, client-reported increased self-reliance and reduced dependency, resolution of grief, and compliance with psychopharmacological treatment

The completed treatment plan is now developed through which the counselor and Edward will begin their shared work of reducing his depression and dependency and building a healthy self-image and relationship style. Edward Cullen's treatment plan follows and is summarized in Table 8.1.

TREATMENT PLAN

Client: Edward Cullen

Service Provider: Forks Counseling Center

BEHAVIORAL DEFINITION OF PROBLEMS:

1. Recurrent Severe Depression—Feeling sad, detached, down, lonely, and lost; loss of interest in daily activities, lackluster appearance, self-doubt and poor self-appraisal; violent death and immortality themes in art projects, including seeing and hearing walking dead

2. Personality Dependence—Smothering girlfriend with love, views girlfriend as lifeline, motivated for change by love relationship

GOALS FOR CHANGE:

1. Recurrent severe depression

   - Grieve death of his parents and a "normal" life
   - Develop a healthy balance between dependence and independence
   - Alleviate depressed mood and return to a previous level of functioning
   - Learn and implement problem-solving strategies to avoid depressive outcome
   - Learn and implement cognitive and behavioral relapse prevention strategies
   - Develop a positive self-image, life-affirming activities, and a supportive social network
   - Effectively use psychotropic medication

2. Personality dependence

   - Understand the basis of his dependent style in his family of origin and earlier life circumstances
   - Develop confidence in himself so that he may meet his own needs and tolerate being alone
   - Achieve a healthy balance between interpersonal dependence and independence

THERAPEUTIC INTERVENTIONS:

A short-to-moderate-term course of individual cognitive-behavior counseling (3–6 months)

1. Recurrent severe depression

   - Express painful feelings related to early life experiences that reinforce and maintain depression
   - Identify triggers for depressive thoughts, feelings, and behaviors
   - Replace negative with positive self-talk
   - Use behavioral strategies to overcome depression
   - Bibliotherapy for depression
   - Psychopharmacology for depression
   - Develop and engage in regular schedule of activities

2. Personality dependence

   - Verbalize and understand relationship between early losses, roles, and life transitions and dependent personality style
   - Describe the style of interpersonal dependence through family counseling
   - Recognize and refute irrational statements contributing to dependency
   - Identify his own emotional and behavioral needs and practice strategies for fulfilling them
   - Role-playing conversations with lost loved ones
   - Identify triggers for dependence-seeking and reinforcing behaviors

OUTCOME MEASURES OF CHANGE:

The development of healthy, positive, and self-affirming attitudes toward himself with decreased dependence upon Bella, and the ability to engage with others in social situations as measured by:

- Pre-post measures on the Beck Depression Inventory-II
- Post measures of GAF functioning in the mild range (>70)
- Client self-report of increased involvement in nonmacabre and life-affirming activities such as hobbies, clubs, and social activities
- Client-reported increased self-reliance and involvement in other nonromantic relationships
- Clinician-observed and client-reported elimination of negative self-talk and negative interpretations of experiences
- Clinician-observed and client-reported use of positive self-talk
- Compliance with psychopharmacological treatment

Table 8.1   Edward Cullen's Treatment Plan Summary: Psychotherapeutic Integration of Cognitive Behavior Therapy and Interpersonal Therapy

Goals for Change	Therapeutic Interventions	Outcome Measures of Change
Recurrent severe depression	Recurrent severe depression	The development of healthy, positive and self-affirming attitudes toward himself with decreased dependence upon Bella and end the inability to engage with others in social situations as measured by:
Grieve death of his parents and a "normal" life	Express painful feelings related to early life experiences that reinforce and maintain depression	
Develop a healthy balance between dependence and independence	Identify triggers for depressive thoughts, feelings, and behaviors	Pre-post measures on the Beck Depression Inventory
Alleviate depressed mood and return to a previous level of functioning	Replace negative with positive self-talk	Post measures of GAF functioning in the mild range (>70)
	Use behavioral strategies to overcome depression	
Learn and implement problem-solving strategies to avoid depressive outcome	Bibliotherapy for depression	Client self-report of increased involvement in nonmacabre and life-affirming activities such as hobbies, clubs, social activities
	Psychopharmacology for depression	
Learn and implement cognitive and behavioral relapse prevention strategies	Develop and engage in regular schedule of activities	Client-reported increased self-reliance and involvement in "other" nonromantic relationships
	Personality dependence	
Develop a positive self-image, life-affirming activities, and a supportive social network	Verbalize and understand relationship between early losses, roles, and life transitions and dependent personality style	Clinician-observed and client-reported elimination of negative self-talk and negative interpretations of experiences
Effectively use psychotropic medication	Describe the style of interpersonal dependence through family counseling	
Personality dependence	Recognize and refute irrational statements contributing to dependency	Clinician-observed and client-reported use of positive self-talk
Understand the basis of his dependent style in his family of origin and earlier life circumstances	Identify his own emotional and behavioral needs and practice strategies for fulfilling them	Compliance with psychopharmacological treatment
Develop confidence in himself so that he may meet his own needs and tolerate being alone	Role-playing conversations with lost loved ones	
Achieve a healthy balance between interpersonal dependence and independence	Identify triggers for dependence-seeking and reinforcing behaviors	

CASE 8.2 *SLUMDOG MILLIONAIRE'S* JAMAL MALIK

INTRODUCING THE CHARACTER

Jamal Malik is the main character in the internationally acclaimed Oscar-winning film *Slumdog Millionaire* (Boyle & Tandan, 2008), which first appeared as the novel *Q & A* by Indian author Vikas Swarup (2008). The story follows the orphan street hustler, Jamal Malik, through his unlikely success as a contestant on the Indian version of the popular American game show, *Who Wants to Be a Millionaire?*

At the beginning of the film, the audience watches Jamal being tortured by local Mumbai police who are pressuring him to confess that he has been cheating on the television show *Who Wants to Be a Millionaire?* Of great interest to the police, but of even greater interest to the game show producers, is how this otherwise impoverished, uneducated, and itinerant young man knows the answers to the increasingly complex questions he is being asked before a live audience and millions of Indian TV viewers. Over the course of the narrative, it becomes clear that Jamal knows the answers to the various questions because in one way or another, and over the course of his young life, he has either directly or indirectly experienced situations that he is later able to parlay into answers to the game show questions.

Orphaned at birth, he, along with his older brother, Salim, learned to survive on the tough and gang-infested streets of the Juhu slums in Mumbai, India. There, he meets and falls in love with Latika, who in turn falls prey to the Mumbai gangs and who, over the course of her own tormented childhood and adolescence, connects deeply with Jamal. The story is an intricate tapestry, weaving together issues of politics, social class, religion, and the power of capitalism and Western greed to transform, not only a single individual, but a society. It is also a story of hope. The following basic case summary and diagnostic impressions describe what we portray as Jamal's clinically significant negative reactions to his exposure to the traumatic experience of police capture and torture.

Meet the Client

You can assess the client in action by viewing clips of Jamal Malik's video material at the following websites:

- http://www.youtube.com/watch?v=Ak70 AEHw1as Malik on *Who Wants to Be a Millionaire*
- http://www.youtube.com/watch?v=AIz bwV7on6Q Movie trailer
- http://www.youtube.com/watch?v=__ HQGvSqZ5I Growing up on the streets

BASIC CASE SUMMARY

Identifying Information. Jamal Malik is a homeless 17-year-old Indian youth who was orphaned at birth and who has been living in the Juhu neighborhood (characterized as a slum) of urban Mumbai with his brother, Salim. Jamal has labored in sweat shops, stolen food, engaged in robbery, and has prostituted himself. He has nevertheless been able to remain uninvolved with the local gangs that have claimed the loyalty of his brother. In appearance, he is a tall, slender, athletically built young man who could be described as having "chiseled features" and "piercing dark brown eyes." Regarding religious identity important to his context, although Jamal is of the Muslim faith, he reports that he does not believe in God and professes a deep conviction that "I watch out for myself" and that he will "work my way out of these miserable slums no matter what it takes."

Presenting Concern. Jamal Malik was referred to the Government Community Services Center of Mumbai by staff of the Center for Spiritual Enlightenment. Jamal's brother initially brought him to the Center once he noticed that his brother appeared to be "in a daze" almost all day long, and at night either could not sleep, or called out during repeated nightmares. His brother also said he could not be induced to walk anywhere near the local police station or jail building, and that he turned corners to avoid walking down the same streets as police on patrol. His brother estimated that Jamal had been "like this" since his experience appearing on *Who Wants to Be a Millionaire?* which ended about 15 days ago. When interviewed, Jamal said he "really couldn't remember too much about all of that," although it was exciting. He seemed overly sensitive to noises and distractions during the interview, and said he "wasn't quite feeling like himself."

Background, Family, and Relevant History. The onset of Jamal's presenting concerns appears to be recent, extending back about 2 weeks. Background and relevant history prior to onset include his developmental experiences growing up parentless is severe poverty, briefly in government facilities and then since about age 7 to the present, homeless on the streets with his brother and peers. Jamal was originally seen at the Center for Spiritual Enlightenment, where the staff described his symptoms as *jiryan* or *dhat*, which are culturally-specific folk diagnoses (APA, 2000a); however, a spiritual advisor at the center who had obtained a master's degree in counseling in Dublin recommended referring him to the Government Community Services Center for what appeared to be symptoms of what Western mental health professionals would describe as Posttraumatic Stress Disorder or Acute Stress Disorder.

Although stressful, appearing on the recent game show does not meet the criteria for a traumatic event.

However, it appears that Jamal has experienced captivity and torture by the local police, during which he was threatened with death and actually physically and mentally tortured. Along with the presenting symptoms of sleep difficulties, what appears to be hypervigilance (he seems to startle easily), and a lack of emotional response about his recent major life events (his brother described him as "in a daze"), Jamal said that at times during the day he feels as though the city around him "just isn't really real . . . it's just moving along around me" or as though he is now a detached observer of his behavior as he watches "the world bump along." His various symptoms and experiences appear consistent with negative reactions to a traumatic event.

Goals for Counseling and Course of Therapy to Date. Based on Jamal's brother's description, referral data provided by the Center, and Jamal's intake, it appears that he is experiencing clinically significant reactions to recent events to which he reacted with intense fear and other distressful responses. To date he has participated in two meetings at Center for Enlightenment and one intake here at the Government Services Center. Jamal agreed to our recommendation that he remain a client at this Center primarily due to the encouragement of his brother. The immediate plan includes: (a) follow-up assessment to make a final determination of diagnosis and treatment plan, (b) ongoing treatment at this Center, and (b) referral to the social services wing of the Government Community Services Center for assistance with housing and basic needs.

Diagnostic Impressions

Axis I.   308.3 Acute Stress Disorder

Axis II.   V71.09 No Diagnosis on Axis II

Axis III.   None

Axis IV.   Problems related to the social environment—Recent incarceration and violent interrogation by police

Economic problems—Extreme poverty, difficulty collecting game show winnings

Housing problems—Homelessness, unsafe neighborhood

Axis V.   GAF = 51 (current)

GAF = 85 (highest level past 2 months)

DISCUSSION OF
DIAGNOSTIC IMPRESSIONS

Jamal Malik was referred to the Government Community Services Center because his brother and the referring counselor were concerned about him "being in a daze," not sleeping or at other times having nightmares, staying away from the local police building and jail and avoiding police on patrol, and seeming overly vigilant about the goings-on around him. In the interview, Jamal reported that, in fact, he could not remember much about his *Millionaire* adventure beyond its excitement. He also said he that along with being in a daze, at times the city around him seems unreal. As the case discussed, he recently survived police capture and torture during an interrogation.

The predominant feature shared by all of the diagnosable conditions found in the Anxiety Disorders section of the *DSM-IV-TR* is the presence of increased arousal, excessive worry, or other signs of anxiety that cause distress or impairment, including, at times, panic. Among these are Acute Stress Disorder and Posttraumatic Stress Disorder, both of which, by definition, occur only in the aftermath of, or as a result of, a traumatic life event that is either directly experienced or witnessed.

This case described what we portrayed as Jamal's clinically significant negative reactions to his exposure to the traumatic experience of police capture and torture. Jamal experienced an event characterized by threat to his physical integrity (he was held against his will), was subjected to painful torture and physical injury, and the threat of serious physical damage or possibly death; he reacted with intense helplessness and fear. These characteristics meet the *DSM-IV-TR* definition of a traumatic event. Following the event, Jamal has been experiencing dissociative symptoms, including reduced awareness of his surroundings (he feels "in a daze"), derealization (his external worlds seem unreal and mechanical), and some amnesia (failure to fully recall the event). He has been re-experiencing the event during nightmares. He has also been avoiding places (i.e., the police station and jail) and people (i.e., police patrols)

reminiscent of the event. He has signs of anxiety, including sleep disruption. According to the case timeline, it has been 15 days since the traumatic event. These factors indicate a diagnosis of Acute Stress Disorder. Differential diagnoses might include Posttraumatic Stress Disorder (PTSD) or Adjustment Disorder. However, PTSD requires more than 1 month of symptoms, whereas Acute Stress Disorder fits when symptoms occur within 1 month of a severe stressor and have not lasted beyond 4 weeks. Acute Stress Disorder describes the concerns of individuals "who have immediate and intense stress reactions to traumatic events and need immediate clinical attention rather than waiting more than a month [for the symptoms of PTSD]" (Munson, 2001, p. 185). Should Jamal's symptoms persist, the diagnosis may later change to PTSD. Adjustment Disorders are negative reactions to any sort of life stressors, as opposed to a trauma. In this case, Jamal has indeed experienced exposure to an extreme stressor meeting the diagnostic definition of trauma, and his reactions conform to the specific constellation symptoms characteristic of Acute Stress Disorder and PTSD, which go beyond the general criteria set for Adjustment Disorder.

To wrap up the diagnosis, Jamal's trauma and other psychosocial stressors are emphasized on Axis IV, and on Axis V his functioning is represented by GAF scores indicating good functioning in all areas prior to the traumatic event, changing to moderate symptoms causing moderately serious difficulty at present. The information on these axes is consistent with the Axis I diagnosis of Acute Stress Disorder as presented in this case.

CASE CONCEPTUALIZATION

When Jamal Malik came in to the Government Community Services Center of Mumbai, his intake counselor collected as much information as possible about the symptoms and situations leading to his referral. Included among the intake materials were a thorough history, client report, the reports of his brother and referring Center for Spiritual Enlightenment staff, counselor observations, and written psychological assessments.

Based on the intake, Jamal's counselor developed diagnostic impressions, describing his presenting concerns as Acute Stress Disorder (ASD). A case conceptualization next was developed.

At the Government Community Services Center of Mumbai, Brief Solution-Focused Counseling is used. The Center employs this particular model because it is believed to be an efficient and effective method of providing services, and outcome studies suggest the approach can be successful with a range of presenting problems (de Jong & Berg, 2002; MacDonald, 1994). Whereas the purpose of diagnostic impressions is to *describe* the client's concerns, the goal of case conceptualization as it is applied to Brief Solution-Focused Counseling is to better *understand* and clinically *organize* the person's experiences (Neukrug & Schwitzer, 2006). It helps the counselor determine the circumstances leading to Jamal's Acute Stress Disorder, and the factors maintaining his presenting concerns. In turn, case conceptualization sets the stage for treatment planning. Treatment planning then provides a road map that plots out how the counselor and client expect to move from presenting concerns to positive outcomes (Seligman, 1993, p. 157)—helping Jamal Malik return to his previous level of functioning.

Generally speaking, when forming a theoretically based case conceptualization, the clinician applies a purist counseling theory, an integration of two or more theories, an eclectic mix of theories that focuses extensively on diagnosis, history, and etiology; by comparison, when forming a solution-focused case conceptualization, the counselor applies an eclectic combination of solution-focused, or solution-creating tactics to his or her immediate understanding of the client and engages quickly in identifying and reaching goals (Berg, 1994; de Shazer & Dolan, 2007; Gingerich & Eisengart, 2000).

Jamal's counselor used the Inverted Pyramid Method of case conceptualization because this method is especially designed to help clinicians more easily form their conceptual pictures of their clients' needs (Neukrug & Schwitzer, 2006; Schwitzer, 1996, 1997). Generally speaking, when the method is used with a theory-based

conceptual model, there are four steps: Problem Identification, Thematic Groupings, Theoretical Inferences, and Narrowed Inferences. However, when the Brief Solution-Focused Counseling model is applied, only the first two steps are needed: Problem Identification and Thematic Grouping. From a solution-focused perspective, it is these two steps that focus attention on what clients want and need and what concerns will be explored and resolved (Bertolino & O'Hanlon, 2002). Brief solution-focused counselors make carefully thought-out professional clinical decisions at Steps 1 and 2 of the pyramid; they are sure to have a rational framework for their decisions rather than implementing techniques and approaches at random (Lazarus, Beutler, & Norcross, 1992; Norcross & Beutler, 2008). Jamal Malik's counselor's solution-focused clinical thinking can be seen in Figure 8.2.

Step 1: Problem Identification. The first step is Problem Identification. Aspects of the presenting problem (thoughts, feelings, behaviors, physiological features), additional areas of concern besides the presenting concern, family and developmental history, in-session observations, clinical inquiries (medical problems, medications, past counseling, substance use, suicidality), and psychological assessments (problem checklists, personality inventories, mental status exam, specific clinical measures) all may contribute information at Step 1. The counselor "casts a wide net" in order to build Step 1 as exhaustively as possible (Neukrug & Schwitzer, 2006, p. 202). As can be seen in Figure 8.2, the counselor identified Jamal Malik's recent traumatic events (game show and police capture), his various presenting symptoms (dissociations, avoidance, etc.), additional environmental and situational obstacles (poverty, living on street, etc.), as well as positive relationships (with brother) and supports (spiritual center). The counselor attempted to go beyond just the presenting symptoms in order to be as descriptive as he could.

The counselor first grouped together all of Jamal's cognitive concerns connected to dissociation, derealization, nightmares, all of Jamal's

Figure 8.2   Jamal Malik's Inverted Pyramid Case Conceptualization Summary: Brief Solution-Focused Counseling Emphasizing Cognitive Behavioral Interventions With Adolescents

1. IDENTIFY AND LIST CLIENT CONCERNS

Recent capture by police
History of being orphan
Recent torture by police
History of living in severe poverty
Recent injury
Fear of serious damage or death
Previously seen in spiritual center
Millionaire game show winner
Primary important relationship is
   with brother

Dissociation, feeling "in a daze"
Derealization, world seems "unreal"
Nightmares
History of homelessness on streets
Avoiding topic of game show experience
Avoiding places (police station, jail)
Sleep disruption

2. ORGANIZE CONCERNS INTO LOGICAL THEMATIC GROUPINGS

1. Problematic posttraumatic cognitive, affective,
   physiological, and behavioral symptoms
2. Cognitive, affective, physiological, and behavioral
   challenges resulting from the environmental
   problems of poverty, homelessness

**3. THEORETICAL INFERENCES: ATTACH THEMATIC
GROUPINGS TO INFERRED AREAS OF DIFFICULTY**

**4. NARROWED INFERENCES: SUICIDALITY
AND DEEPER DIFFICULTIES**

behavioral concerns connected to avoiding anxiety-producing people, places, and topics reminiscent of the trauma, and all of Jamal's physiological symptoms of anxiety and post-trauma, into the theme "problematic posttraumatic cognitive, affective, physiological, and behavioral symptoms." The counselor next formed an additional category comprising all of Jamal's environmental problems connected to being an orphan and in poverty: "cognitive, affective, physiological, and behavioral challenges resulting from the environmental problems of poverty and homelessness." The counselor selected the Clinical Targets Approach to organize Jamal's concerns from a Solution-Focused Counseling perspective on the basis that he planned to emphasize cognitive and behavioral interventions that he believed would lead to good solutions with adolescents such as Jamal (Vernon, 2009).

With this two-step conceptualization completed, the client information in Step 1 leads to logical-intuitive groupings on the basis of common denominators in Step 2, and the counselor is ready to engage the client in planning and implementing Brief Solution-Focused Counseling.

Treatment Planning

At this point, Jamal Malik's clinician at the Government Community Services Center of Mumbai has collected all available information about the problems that have been of concern to him and the referring counselor. Based upon this information, the counselor developed a five-axis *DSM-IV-TR* diagnosis and then, using the "inverted pyramid" (Neukrug & Schwitzer, 2006; Schwitzer, 1996, 1997), formulated a working clinical *explanation* of Jamal's difficulties and their etiology that we called the *case conceptualization.* This in turn, guides us to the next critical step in our clinical work called the *treatment plan,* the primary purpose of which is to map out a logical and goal-oriented strategy for making positive changes in the client's life. In essence, the treatment plan is a *road map "*for

reducing or eliminating disruptive symptoms that are impeding the client's ability to reach positive mental health outcomes" (Neukrug & Schwitzer, 2006, p. 225). As such, it is the cornerstone of our work with not only Jamal Malik, but with all clients who present with disturbing and disruptive symptoms and/or posttraumatic patterns (Jongsma & Peterson, 2006; Jongsma et al., 2003a, 2003b; Seligman, 1993, 1998, 2004).

A comprehensive treatment plan must integrate all of the information from the biopsychosocial interview, diagnosis, and case conceptualization into a coherent plan of action. This *plan* comprises four main components, which include (1) a behavioral definition of the problem(s), (2) the selection of achievable goals, (3) the determination of treatment modes, and (4) the documentation of how change will be measured. The *behavioral definition of the problem(s)* consolidates the results of the case conceptualization into a concise hierarchical list of problems and concerns that will be the focus of treatment. The *selection of achievable goals* refers to assessing and prioritizing the client's concerns into a *hierarchy of urgency* that also takes into account the client's motivation for change, level of dysfunction, and real-world influences on his or her problems. The *determination of treatment modes* refers to selection of the specific interventions, which are matched to the uniqueness of the client and to his or her goals and clearly tied to a particular theoretical orientation (Neukrug & Schwitzer, 2006). Finally, the clinician must establish how change will be measured, based upon a number of factors, including client records and self-report of change, in-session observations by the clinician, clinician ratings, results of standardized evaluations such as the Beck Depression Inventory-II (Beck & Steer, 1990) or a family functioning questionnaire, pre-post treatment comparisons, and reports by other treating professionals.

The four-step method discussed above can be seen in Figure 6.1 (p. 109) and is outlined below for the case of Jamal Malik, followed by his specific treatment plan.

Step 1: Behavioral Definition of Problems. The first step in solution-focused treatment planning is to carefully review the case conceptualization, paying particular attention to the results of Step 2 (Thematic Groupings), Step 3 (Theoretical Inferences), and Step 4 (Narrowed Inferences). The identified clinical themes reflect the core areas of concern and distress for the client, while the theoretical and narrowed inferences offer clinical speculation as to their origins. In the case of Jamal, there are three primary areas of concern. The first, "problematic posttraumatic cognitive, affective, physiological, and behavioral symptoms," refers to Jamal's fear of serious damage or death; sleep disruption; dissociation or feeling "in a daze"; derealization in which the world seems "unreal"; nightmares; and avoiding people, places, and the topic of the game show experience. The second, "environmental problems," refers to his history of being an orphan, homelessness, and severe poverty. These symptoms and stresses are consistent with the diagnosis of Acute Stress Disorder (APA, 2000a; Bradley, Greene, Russ, Dutra, & Westen, 2001; Brunello et al., 2001; Bryant et al., 2008; Kessler et al., 1994; Kessler et al., 1995).

Step 2: Identify and Articulate Goals for Change. The second step is the selection of achievable goals, which is based upon a number of factors, including the most pressing or urgent behavioral, emotional, and interpersonal concerns and symptoms as identified by the client and clinician, the willingness and ability of the client to work on those particular goals, and the realistic (real-world) achievability of those goals (Neukrug & Schwitzer, 2006). At this stage of treatment planning, it is important to recognize that not all of the client's problems can be addressed at once, so we focus initially on those that cause the greatest distress and impairment. New goals can be created as old ones are achieved. In the case of Jamal, the goals are divided into two prominent areas. The first, "problematic posttraumatic cognitive, affective, physiological and behavioral symptoms,"

requires that we help Jamal to verbalize an understanding of how the symptoms of ASD develop, to reduce the negative impact that the traumatic event had on his life, to develop and implement effective coping skills, and to recall the traumatic event without becoming overwhelmed with stressful feelings or dissociating. The second, "environmental problems," requires that we help Jamal to understand the relationship between the conditions in which he grew up and his current psychological and behavioral functioning as well as use his game show winnings to improve the quality of his life.

Step 3: Describe Therapeutic Interventions. This is perhaps the most critical step in the treatment planning process because the clinician must now integrate information from a number of sources, including the case conceptualization, the delineation of the client's problems and goals, and the treatment literature, paying particular attention to *empirically supported treatment* (EST) and *evidence-based practice* (EBP). In essence, the clinician must align his or her treatment approach with scientific evidence from the fields of counseling and psychotherapy. Wampold (2001) identifies two types of evidence-based counseling research: studies that demonstrate "absolute efficacy," that is, the fact that counseling and psychotherapy work, and those that demonstrate "relative efficacy," that is, the fact that certain theoretical/technical approaches work best for certain clients with particular problems (Psychoanalysis, Gestalt Therapy, Cognitive Behavior Therapy, Brief Solution-Focused Therapy, Cognitive Therapy, Dialectical Behavior Therapy, Person-Centered Therapy, Expressive/Creative Therapies, Interpersonal Therapy, and Feminist Therapy); and when delivered through specific treatment modalities (individual, group, and family counseling).

In the case of Jamal, we have decided to use Brief Solution-Focused Therapy (De Jong & Berg, 2002; de Shazer & Dolan, 2007; Gingerich & Eisengart, 2000; Gutterman, 2006), emphasizing cognitive interventions with adolescents (Corcoran & Stephenson, 2000; Hopson & Kim, 2005; Lines, 2002; Vernon, 2009). This counseling approach is "pragmatic, anti-deterministic and future oriented [and as such] offers optimism, and hope about the ability of the client to change" (Neukrug, 2011, p. 426). It de-emphasizes psychopathology and the past, and instead focuses on the client's strengths, resources, and skills in order to generate solutions to the problems and concerns. Forward-looking and quickly moving, Solution-Focused Therapy's basic assumptions include that change is constant and inevitable, clients have the inherent skills and abilities to change, small steps lead to big changes, exceptions to problems do occur and can be used for change, and the future is both created and negotiable; as well as the simple axioms "if it ain't broke, don't fix it," "if it works, do more of it" and "if it's not working, do something different" (Neukrug, 2011).

We view Brief Solution-Focused Therapy as being particularly useful in Jamal's case due to its emphasis on change, the future, and tapping into the client's resources and skills. Additionally, solution-focused treatment is fast-moving, makes use of creative techniques (art, play, and narrative) with children and adolescents, and relies on challenging, strength-based questioning that can be highly engaging with adolescents. Specific techniques for his symptoms include education and orientation to Brief-Solution Focused Treatment, goal setting with regard to Acute Stress Disorder symptoms, "scaling" of his posttraumatic symptoms to provide context and perspective as well as a starting point for change and then ongoing scaling to gauge improvement, use of the miracle question to help him begin to cognitively process the possibility of change, externalizing the symptoms by using solution talk and creating hypothetical solutions, identifying and complimenting Jamal on past and current use of skills to solve problems and amplification of previously successful strategies for self-care; using preferred-goal, evaluative, coping, exception-seeking, and solution-focused questions; and psychiatric referral for possible psychopharmacotherapy, and relaxation training. Specific techniques for his environmental problems include referral to a financial planner and a real estate agent.

Step 4: Provide Outcome Measures of Change. This last step in treatment planning requires that we specify how change will be measured and indicate the extent to which progress has been made toward realizing these goals (Neukrug & Schwitzer, 2006). The counselor has considerable flexibility in this phase and may choose from a number of objective domains (psychological tests and measures of self-esteem, depression, psychosis, interpersonal relationship, anxiety, etc.), quasi-objective measures (the *DSM-IV-TR's* Axis V GAF scale; prepost clinician, client, and psychiatric ratings), and subjective ratings (client self-report, clinician's in-session observations). In Jamal's case, we have implemented a number of these, including pre-post measures on the Clinician-Administered PTSD Scale for Children and Adolescents (Newman et al., 2004), post-only measures of GAF functioning in the mild range (>70), and clinician-observed and client report of reduction in affective, cognitive, physiological, and behavioral symptoms of ASD, effective wealth management, and improved living circumstances.

The completed treatment plan is now developed through which the counselor and Jamal will work through the traumatic experience and reverse the circumstances of his poverty and homelessness. The treatment plan appears below and is summarized in Table 8.2.

TREATMENT PLAN

Client: Jamal Malik

Service Provider: Government Community Services Center of Mumbai

BEHAVIORAL DEFINITION OF PROBLEMS:

1. Problematic posttraumatic cognitive, affective, physiological, and behavioral symptoms—Fear of serious damage or death, sleep disruption, dissociation, or feeling "in a daze," derealization in which the world seems "unreal," nightmares and avoiding people, places, and topic of the game show experience

2. Environmental problems—History of being an orphan, homelessness, severe poverty

GOALS FOR CHANGE:

1. Problematic posttraumatic cognitive, affective, physiological, and behavioral symptoms

   - Verbalize an understanding of how the symptoms of ASD develop
   - Reduce the negative impact that the traumatic event had on life
   - Develop and implement effective coping skills
   - Recall the traumatic event without becoming overwhelmed with stressful feelings or dissociating

2. Environmental problems

   - Understand the relationship between growing up in poverty and his current beliefs, behaviors, and emotions
   - Use his game show winnings to improve the quality of his life

THERAPEUTIC INTERVENTIONS:

A short-to-moderate-term course (3–4 months) of individual Brief Solution-Focused Counseling supplemented with psychopharmacotherapy and relaxation training

1. Problematic posttraumatic cognitive, affective, physiological, and behavioral symptoms

   - Education and orientation to brief solution-focused treatment
   - Goal setting with regard to ASD symptoms
   - "Scaling" of posttraumatic symptoms to provide context and perspective as well as a starting point for change
   - Ongoing scaling to gauge improvement
   - Use of the miracle question to help begin to cognitively process the possibility of change
   - Externalizing the symptoms by using solution talk and creating hypothetical solutions
   - Identifying and complimenting past and current use of skills to solve problems
   - Amplification of previously successful strategies for self-care
   - Using preferred-goal, evaluative, coping, exception-seeking, and solution-focused questions
   - Psychiatric referral for possible psychopharmacotherapy
   - Relaxation training involving deep breathing, progressive muscle work, and guided imagery

(Continued)

(Continued)

  2. Environmental problems
     • Referral to a financial planner and a real estate agent

OUTCOME MEASURES OF CHANGE:

Alleviation of symptoms of posttraumatic stress and reversal of circumstances of his poverty and homelessness as measured by:

  • Pre-post measures on the Clinician-Administered PTSD Scale for Children and Adolescents (CAPS-CA)
  • Post-only measure of GAF functioning in the mild range (>70)
  • Clinician-observed reduction in affective, cognitive, physiological, and behavioral symptoms of ASD
  • Client reports of reduction in affective, cognitive, physiological, and behavioral symptoms of ASD
  • Physician report of medication compliance
  • Effective wealth management and improved living circumstances

Table 8.2 Jamal Malik's Treatment Plan Summary: Brief Solution-Focused Counseling Emphasizing Cognitive Behavioral Interventions With Adolescents

Goals for Change	Therapeutic Interventions	Outcome Measures of Change
Problematic posttraumatic cognitive, affective, physiological, and behavioral symptoms

Verbalize an understanding of how the symptoms of ASD develop

Reduce the negative impact that the traumatic event had on life

Develop and implement effective coping skills

Recall the traumatic event without becoming overwhelmed with stressful feelings or dissociating

Environmental problems

Use his game show winnings to improve the quality of his life | Problematic posttraumatic cognitive, affective, physiological, and behavioral symptoms

Education and orientation to brief-solution focused treatment

Goal setting with regard to posttraumatic stress disorder symptoms

"Scaling" of posttraumatic symptoms to provide context and perspective as well as a starting point for change

Ongoing scaling to gauge improvement

Use of the miracle question to help begin to cognitively process the possibility of change

Externalizing the symptoms by using solution talk and creating hypothetical solutions

Identifying and complimenting past and current use of skills to solve problems | Alleviation of symptoms of posttraumatic stress and reversal of circumstances of his poverty and homelessness as measured by:

Pre-post measures on the Clinician-Administered PTSD Scale for Children and Adolescents (CAPS-CA)

Post-only measure of GAF functioning in the mild range (>70)

Clinician-observed reduction in affective, cognitive, physiological, and behavioral symptoms of posttraumatic stress disorder

Client reports of reduction in affective, cognitive, physiological, and behavioral symptoms of posttraumatic stress disorder |

Goals for Change	Therapeutic Interventions	Outcome Measures of Change
	Amplification of previously successful strategies for self-care	Physician report of medication compliance
	Use preferred-goal, evaluative, coping, exception-seeking, and solution-focused questions	Effective wealth management and improved living circumstances
	Psychiatric referral for possible psychopharmacotherapy	
	Relaxation training involving deep breathing, progressive muscle work, and guided imagery	
	Environmental problems	
	Referral to a financial planner and a real estate agent	

CASE 8.3 *JUNO'S* JUNO MacGUFF

INTRODUCING THE CHARACTER

Juno MacGuff, a 16-year-old junior at Dancing Elk High School, is the central character in the Academy Award–winning film *Juno* (Reitman, 2007) about a Minnesota teenager and the poignant, occasionally humorous challenges she confronts over the course of her unplanned and unwanted pregnancy. Lauded by some critics as a feminist anthem and described by others as a powerful forum for the prolife/prochoice debate, *Juno* clearly stirred the hearts of millions and won box-office acclaim. Perhaps the sentiments of the film writer, Diablo Cody, best capture her creation. She noted, "You can look at it as a film that celebrates life and celebrates childbirth, or you can look at it as a film about a liberated young girl who makes a choice to continue being liberated . . . or you can look it as some kind of twisted love story, you know, a meditation on maturity." Our professional counseling view of Juno's character, including some of our own conjectures about her early years, is described in the following basic case summary and diagnostic impressions.

Meet the Client

You can assess the client in action by viewing clips of Juno's video material at the following websites:

- http://xfinitytv.comcast.net/movies/Juno/139277/715137535/Pregnancy-Test/videos?cmpid=FCST_rdrct Pregnancy test
- http://www.youtube.com/watch?v=K0SKf0K3bxg Juno trailer
- http://www.fancast.com/movies/Juno/139277/607007527/-Juno-%3A-Hallway-Confrontation/videos Hallway confrontation with Bleeker

BASIC CASE SUMMARY

Identifying Information. At the time of her first interview 7 months ago, Juno MacGuff was a 16-year-old white female who resides with her father and stepmother in Minnetonka, Minnesota, and is a junior at Dancing Elk High School. She appeared healthy, appropriately dressed for her age and context, and is of modest height, fair-skinned, and sandy-haired. She very recently revealed to her parents that she was about 2 months pregnant, but to date shows no obvious physical signs that she is pregnant.

Presenting Concern. Upon learning of their daughter's pregnancy 7 months ago, Mr. and Mrs. MacGuff immediately made an appointment for their daughter at the Minnetonka Family Services Center in order to help her decide on the best course of action as well as to provide her with a therapeutic outlet that they believed would be necessary over the coming months. The parents appeared very concerned for and supportive of Juno, but also appeared notably distressed regarding their circumstance, and according to her mother, "the devastating effect that this pregnancy is going to have on all of us." Although Juno sat relatively quietly throughout this meeting, she asserted that "I think I'm old enough to make an important decision affecting my own life."

Background, Family Information, and Relevant History. Juno was born in Minnetonka, Minnesota, the only child of the MacGuffs. At birth and throughout early childhood, Juno experienced health problems, including cardiac and respiratory difficulties that resulted in numerous hospitalizations. According to her father's report, Juno's parents often quarreled about their daughter's care and the resulting tension led to irretrievable marital stress and a divorce that occurred when Juno was 5 years old. By that time, Juno's father had initiated a relationship with one of his daughter's nurses at Minnetonka Regional Hospital. The couple married soon after his divorce was final. Juno's mother left town and has had only sporadic contact with the family for years (such as sending her daughter an annual "Valentine's Day cactus" in February).

By the time Juno entered third grade, her health had stabilized and she experienced normally expected, successful psychosocial development. Early written reports describe her at this time as a "vibrant, self-assured, and sociable child" who seemed to have grown immeasurably from the medical adversities that marked her earlier years. She was voted "most popular" by her elementary school peers and, by her report, eagerly moved on to Minnetonka Middle School. There, Juno's social integration was very positive and the older students regarded her as considerably more mature than her peers. She was invited to be involved in the student government and helped to establish charity efforts for the disenfranchised American Indians in the community. Juno was also described as a "fierce defender" of those whom she believed were being unfairly treated within the school and led Minnetonka Middle School's first-ever rally against bullying. Throughout her middle school years, Juno enjoyed a very close relationship with her father and moderately close relationship with her stepmother, Bren, who she regarded as "an adult who I could usually relate to."

Near the end of middle school, Juno applied for a competitive slot at Dancing Elk High School, which had a Social Justice program that was very attractive to her. By her description, much to her surprise, although not surprising to her parents, Juno was accepted after the first round. Juno described her first 2 years of high school as "the best in my life." She had a satisfying number of friends, was active on the school newspaper, and participated in several community-awareness drives. She was described in an interview with a *Twin City Gazette* reporter as "a promising, highly intelligent, funny, and extraordinarily wise young woman who is a leader in her school community." As she describes the experience, on the night of the release of the interview in the newspaper, Juno and a few of her friends gathered at the gymnasium to celebrate. After the event, she and her best friend and confidant, Paulie Bleeker, had their own private celebration and in recounting that night, Juno noted, "One thing led to another and got out of hand, and before I knew it, we had had sex." Three weeks later, Juno was pregnant.

Juno reported that during the initial 2 months of pregnancy, she confided only in a few close peers. At 2 months, Juno sought the support of her parents, attended a family session here at the Minnetonka Family Services Center, and consulted her pastor. She also attempted to visit her biological mother; however, she was unsuccessful in locating her. Although not inclined to return to counseling, Juno did so for two additional meetings at the request of her parents, but held firmly that "I'm really doing okay, it's just a real big decision, and I'm not sure what the right thing to do is."

The outcome was that Juno made a determination to continue her pregnancy and pursue placing the baby for adoption. As she describes it, upon recommendation of her best friend, Juno put an ad in the local *Penny Saver* to see if anyone would be interested in adopting her child should she decide to carry to term. She was fortunate to find a young couple, the Lorings, who were very interested in pursuing adoption. However, shortly before the birth of Juno's child, Mr. Loring left his wife in order to pursue his music career. Three days after her 17th birthday, Juno gave birth to a healthy boy and immediately placed him in the hands of Mrs. Loring who, along with her parents and Paulie, had been in the hospital throughout her labor and delivery.

Goals for Counseling and Course of Therapy to Date. Seven months ago, Juno participated at the Center in one family session and two individual meetings, which primarily were supportive in nature. At present she has returned for a follow-up, the primary goal of which is to determine remaining needs for counseling during her postpregnancy and postadoption adjustment. Juno arrived with her parents for the follow-up, which included a 30-minute family meeting and a 30-minute individual session. During the family meeting she appeared quiet and subdued. By comparison, in the individual session, she appeared animated and enthusiastic. Near the end of the individual session, she commented: "I think my parents are more upset than I am . . . I have my whole life ahead of me and I don't see the need to look back."

Diagnostic Impressions

Axis I. V61.20 Parent-Child Relational Problem

Axis II. V71.09 No Diagnosis or Condition on Axis II

Axis III. Recent child-birth

Axis IV. Problem with primary support group—Recent loss of child to adoption

Problem with primary support group—Stresses of parent-daughter dynamics during adolescent pregnancy and loss of child to adoption

Axis V. GAF = 78 (at time of initial intake)

GAF = 88 (at present)

DISCUSSION OF DIAGNOSTIC IMPRESSIONS

Juno MacGuff came into the Minnetonka Family Services Center because her parents made an appointment after learning of her teenage pregnancy. As she was presented in this case, Juno appeared to be a high-functioning adolescent girl who did not present any clinically significant signs of distress or impairment. Still, her parents were concerned that she receive the support and consultation of a counseling professional with a focus on her pregnancy and its effects and consequences.

Along with all the various diagnosable disorders, a multiaxial diagnosis also lists Other Conditions That May Be a Focus of Clinical Attention. The client concerns contained in this section (appearing at the end of the *DSM-IV-TR*, following all of the diagnosable disorders) are not diagnosable mental disorders according to the *DSM* classification system; instead, they are client problems or issues that may be a focus of treatment when the individual is not experiencing any clinically significant symptoms of distress or impairment, or they are client problems that are a focus of counseling but not a part of the individual's diagnosable mental disorder. Specifically, Relational Problems, Occupational Problems, Academic Problems, Identity Problems, Religious or Spiritual Problem, and Phase of Life Problems all are included under Other Conditions That May Be a Focus of Clinical Attention. They are listed on Axis I of a multiaxial diagnosis. In our professional counseling view, Juno's experiences were in this category.

Differential diagnoses might include any diagnosable Axis I Mental Disorder or Axis II Personality Disorder; however, no prominent, clinically significant difficulties are present. We therefore only consider Other Conditions That May Be a Focus of Clinical Attention. For example, Phase of Life Problem might be listed if Juno's primary counseling focus was on changes in life circumstances due to her pregnancy, Identity Problem if Juno's primary counseling focus was on challenges to her psychosocial identity development resulting from her pregnancy, or Religious or Spiritual Problem if the focus was primarily on faith-based questions or doubts pertaining to decisions about a course of action. Adolescents and young adults commonly experience such concerns, and they often are an important focus of clinical attention (Evans, Forney, & Guido-DiBrito, 1998). However, as this case was written, Juno's primary purpose for counseling was to address interactions with her parents in the context of her pregnancy—rather than other problems.

To finish the diagnosis, Juno's pregnancy is listed on Axis III because it carries with it numerous physical and physiological challenges, her current stressors are emphasized on Axis IV, and on Axis V her functioning is represented by GAF scores indicating that initially she experienced some transient, mild, and expectable reactions to the stresses of unexpected pregnancy, resolving to good functioning and the absence of concerns beyond everyday problems at the present time. The information on these axes is consistent with the Axis I diagnosis portrayed by Juno in this case.

CASE CONCEPTUALIZATION

When Juno and her family first came into the Minnetonka Family Services Center, the counselor fully explored their reasons for coming in and Juno's collateral experiences and concerns. The counselor first used this information to develop diagnostic impressions. Juno's concerns were described as a Parent-Child Relational Problem with psychosocial stressors of teen pregnancy and loss of the child to adoption. Next, the counselor developed a case conceptualization. Whereas the purpose of diagnostic impressions is to *describe* the client's concerns, the goal of case conceptualization is to better *understand* and clinically *explain* the person's experiences (Neukrug & Schwitzer, 2006). It helps the counselor understand the nature of Juno's reason for counseling. In turn, case conceptualization sets the stage for treatment planning. Treatment planning then provides a road map that plots out how the counselor and client expect to move from presenting concerns to positive outcomes (Seligman, 1993, p. 157)— helping Juno better adjust to her relational dynamics with her father and stepmother, and perhaps address her recent pregnancy experiences.

When forming a case conceptualization, the clinician applies a purist counseling theory, an integration of two or more theories, an eclectic mix of theories, or a solution-focused combination of tactics to his or her understanding of the client. In this case, Juno's counselor based her conceptualization on a purist theory, Person-Centered Therapy. The counselor selected this approach because it is the primary counseling method used at the Minnetonka Family Services Center when the clinician believes the client has the capabilities to use the therapeutic experience to gain self-understanding, improve self-direction, make his or her own constructive changes, and act effectively and productively, and when facilitating the client's own self-directed adjustment seems to be a desired outcome (Rogers, 1986)— as in the case of Juno, who apparently is self-directed, achieving, and has natural talents and resources.

The counselor used the Inverted Pyramid Method of case conceptualization because this method is especially designed to help clinicians more easily form their conceptual pictures of their clients' needs (Neukrug & Schwitzer, 2006; Schwitzer, 1996, 1997). The method has four steps: Problem Identification, Thematic Groupings, Theoretical Inferences, and Narrowed Inferences. The counselor's clinical thinking can be seen in Figure 8.3.

Step 1: Problem Identification. The first step is Problem Identification. Aspects of the presenting problem (thoughts, feelings, behaviors, physiological features), additional areas of concern besides the presenting concern, family and developmental history, in-session observations, clinical inquiries (medical problems, medications, past counseling, substance use, suicidality), and psychological assessments (problem checklists, personality inventories, mental status exam, specific clinical measures) all may contribute information at Step 1. The counselor "casts a wide net" in order to build Step 1 as exhaustively as possible (Neukrug & Schwitzer, 2006, p. 202). As can be seen in Figure 8.3, the counselor identified Juno's primary life concerns (pregnancy, adoption, etc.); main reasons for counseling associated with parental relationship (communication difficulties, lack of supportive confident, etc.); all of the important family

dynamic factors (divorce, remarriage, absent mother, etc.); and additional life issues (romantic relationship, adolescent adjustment) at Step 1. The counselor attempted to go beyond just listing "pregnancy" as the main reason for referral and to be as complete as she could.

Step 2: Thematic Groupings. The second step is Thematic Groupings. The clinician organizes all of the exhaustive client information found in Step 1 into just a few intuitive-logical clinical groups, categories, or themes, on the basis of sensible common denominators (Neukrug & Schwitzer, 2006). Four different ways of forming the Step 2 theme groups can be used: Descriptive-Diagnosis Approach, Clinical Targets Approach, Areas of Dysfunction Approach, and Intrapsychic Approach. As can be seen in Figure 8.3, Juno's counselor selected the Areas of Dysfunction Approach. This approach sorts together all of the Step 1 information into "areas of dysfunction according to important life situations, life themes, or life roles and skills" (Neukrug & Schwitzer, 2006, p. 205).

The counselor grouped together (a) Juno's ongoing family dynamics into a theme of "background stresses of being a high-functioning adolescent in a challenging blended family"; (b) her recent pregnancy factors into a theme of "pregnancy, adoption, and boyfriend stresses"; and (c) dealing with parental communication, confidence, etc. into a theme of "stresses from parental reactions regarding pregnancy and adoption." Her conceptual work at Step 2 gave the counselor a way to begin organizing Juno's areas of functioning and areas of concern more clearly and meaningfully.

So far, at Steps 1 and 2, the counselor has used her clinical assessment skills and her clinical judgment to begin meaningfully understanding Juno's needs. Now, at Steps 3 and 4, she applies the theoretical approach she has selected. She begins making theoretical inferences to interpret and explain the processes or underlying Juno's concerns as they are seen in Steps 1 and 2.

Step 3: Theoretical Inferences. At Step 3, concepts from the counselor's selected theory, Person-Centered Therapy, are applied to explain the experiences maintaining Juno's present challenges. The counselor tentatively matches the theme groups in Step 2 with this theoretical approach. In other words, the symptom constellations in Step 2, which were distilled from the symptoms in Step 1, now are combined using theory to show what are believed to be the underlying causes or psychological etiology of Juno's current needs (Neukrug & Schwitzer, 2006; Schwitzer, 2006, 2007).

According to Person-Centered Therapy, individuals are capable of self-understanding and self-direction. Further, under the correct conditions, individuals progressively experience greater self-realization, fulfillment, autonomy, self-determination, and self-perfection as their lives progress, in a process referred to as the actualizing tendency (Broadley, 1999). The needed conditions are empathy, accurate understanding, and positive regard from the important others in our lives (Bohart & Greenberg, 1997; Rogers, 1961, 1977). In other words, under these conditions, individuals move forward toward their own self-fulfillment across the life span (Thorne, 2002). Conversely, according to the theory, lack of empathy, accurate understanding, and positive regard from the important others in our lives can disrupt or derail forward actualizing movement and result in maladjustment (Broadley, 1999; Rogers, 1961, 1977).

As can be seen in Figure 8.3, when the counselor applied these Person-Centered Therapy concepts, she explained at Step 3 that the various issues noted in Step 1 (the current pregnancy-related parent relationship issues, family factors, etc.), which can be understood to be themes of (a) background family stresses and (b) parental reaction stresses regarding (c) pregnancy issues (Step 2), together comprise a situation in which Juno is experiencing "Lack of conditions of worth by parents." According to Person-Centered Therapy inferences, lacking these conditions of worth is Juno's central focus. The theme appears on Figure 8.3.

Step 4: Narrowed Inferences. At Step 4, the clinician's selected theory continues to be used to address still-deeper issues when they exist (Schwitzer, 2006, 2007). At this step, "still-deeper, more encompassing, or more central, causal themes" are formed (Neukrug & Schwitzer, 2006, p. 207). Continuing to apply Person-Centered Therapy concepts at Step 4, Juno's counselor presented the deeper implication of Juno's lack of conditions of self-worth from her parents, specifically, the possibility of Impeded Actualization. The counselor infers that improving Juno's experience of conditions of worth (positive regard, accurate empathy, etc.) is needed in order to further her adolescent progress toward self-actualization.

When all four steps are completed, the client information in Step 1 leads to logical-intuitive groupings on the basis of common denominators in Step 2, the groupings then are explained using theory at Step 3, and then, finally, at Step 4, further deeper explanations are made. From start to finish, the thoughts, feelings, behaviors, and physiological features in the topmost portions are connected on down the pyramid into deepest dynamics.

The completed pyramid now is used to plan treatment, in which the counselor will engage Juno with congruence, unconditional positive regard, and accurate empathy to promote her directional process of self-actualizing.

TREATMENT PLANNING

At this point, Juno's clinician at the Minnetonka Family Services Center has collected all available information about the issues that have been of concern to Juno and those around her who performed her assessment. Based upon this information, the counselor developed a five-axis *DSM-IV-TR* diagnosis and then, using the "inverted pyramid" (Neukrug & Schwitzer, 2006; Schwitzer, 1996, 1997), formulated a working clinical *explanation* of Juno's difficulties and their etiology that we called the *case conceptualization.* This, in turn, guides us to the

Figure 8.3 Juno's Inverted Pyramid Case Conceptualization Summary: Person-Centered Counseling

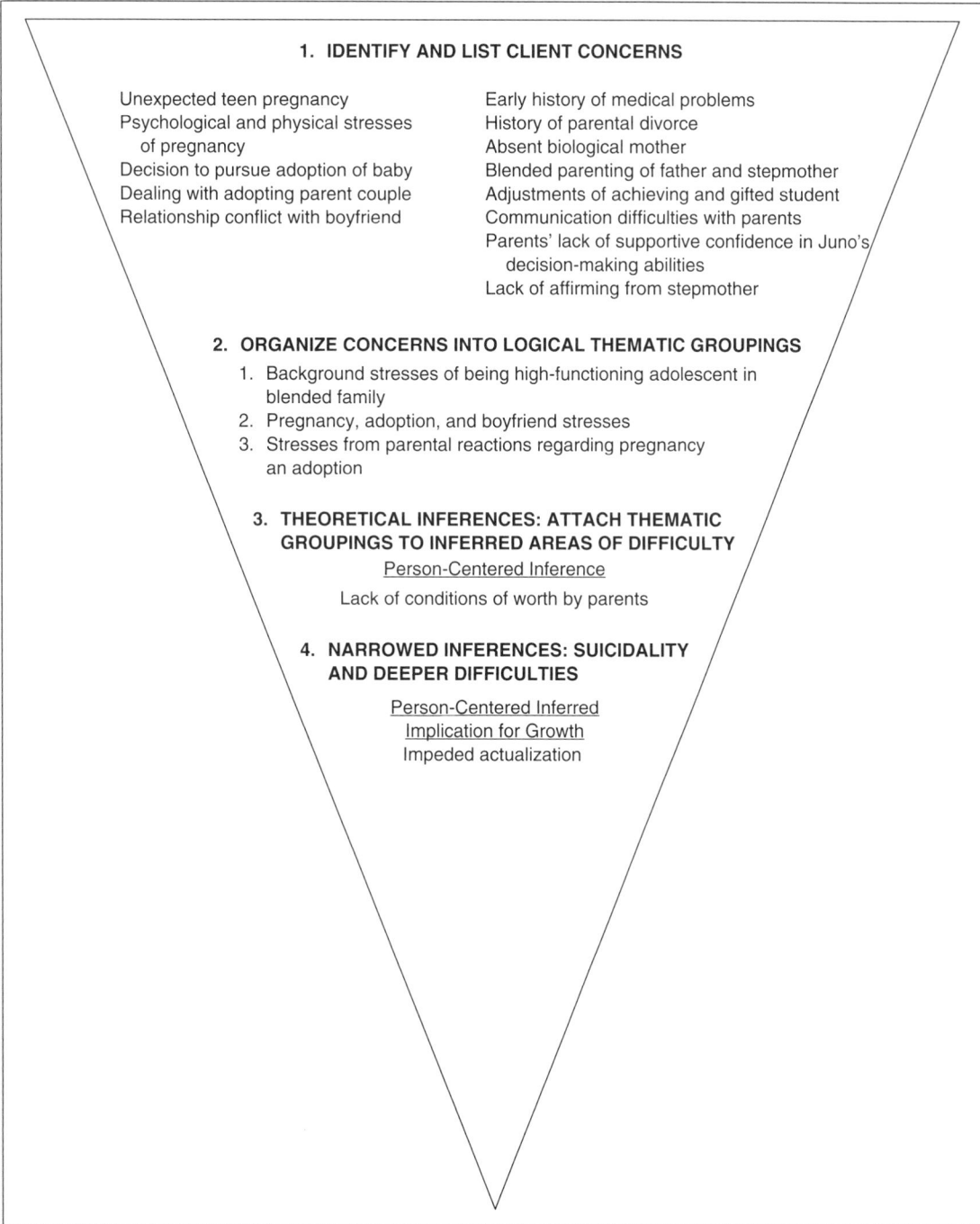

1. **IDENTIFY AND LIST CLIENT CONCERNS**

Unexpected teen pregnancy
Psychological and physical stresses
  of pregnancy
Decision to pursue adoption of baby
Dealing with adopting parent couple
Relationship conflict with boyfriend

Early history of medical problems
History of parental divorce
Absent biological mother
Blended parenting of father and stepmother
Adjustments of achieving and gifted student
Communication difficulties with parents
Parents' lack of supportive confidence in Juno's
  decision-making abilities
Lack of affirming from stepmother

2. **ORGANIZE CONCERNS INTO LOGICAL THEMATIC GROUPINGS**

   1. Background stresses of being high-functioning adolescent in
      blended family
   2. Pregnancy, adoption, and boyfriend stresses
   3. Stresses from parental reactions regarding pregnancy
      an adoption

3. **THEORETICAL INFERENCES: ATTACH THEMATIC
   GROUPINGS TO INFERRED AREAS OF DIFFICULTY**

   Person-Centered Inference

   Lack of conditions of worth by parents

4. **NARROWED INFERENCES: SUICIDALITY
   AND DEEPER DIFFICULTIES**

   Person-Centered Inferred
   Implication for Growth
   Impeded actualization

next critical step in our clinical work, called the *treatment plan,* the primary purpose of which is to map out a logical and goal-oriented strategy for making positive changes in the client's life. In essence, the treatment plan is a road map *"for reducing or eliminating disruptive symptoms that are impeding the client's ability to reach positive mental health outcomes"* (Neukrug & Schwitzer, 2006, p. 225). As such, it is the cornerstone of our work with not only Juno, but with all clients who present important counseling issues (Jongsma & Peterson, 2006; Jongsma et al., 2003a, 2003b; Seligman, 1993, 1998, 2004).

A comprehensive treatment plan must integrate all of the information from the biopsychosocial interview, diagnosis, and case conceptualization into a coherent plan of action. This *plan* comprises four main components, which include (1) a behavioral definition of the problem(s), (2) the selection of achievable goals, (3) the determination of treatment modes, and (4) the documentation of how change will be measured. The *behavioral definition of the problem(s)* consolidates the results of the case conceptualization into a concise hierarchical list of problems and concerns that will be the focus of treatment. The *selection of achievable goals* refers to assessing and prioritizing the client's concerns into a *hierarchy of urgency* that also takes into account the client's motivation for change, level of dysfunction, and real-world influences on his or her problems. The *determination of treatment modes* refers to selection of the specific interventions, which are matched to the uniqueness of the client and to the client's goals and clearly tied to a particular theoretical orientation (Neukrug & Schwitzer, 2006). Finally, the clinician must establish how change will be measured, based upon a number of factors, including client records and self-report of change, in-session observations by the clinician, clinician ratings, results of standardized evaluations such as the Beck Depression Inventory-II (Beck, Steer & Brown, 1996) or a family functioning questionnaire, pre-post treatment comparisons, and reports by other treating professionals.

The four-step method discussed above can be seen in Figure 6.1 (p. 109) and is outlined below for the case of Juno MacGuff, followed by her specific treatment plan.

Step 1: Behavioral Definition of Problems. The first step in treatment planning is to carefully review the case conceptualization, paying particular attention to the results of Step 2 (Thematic Groupings), Step 3 (Theoretical Inferences), and Step 4 (Narrowed Inferences). The identified clinical themes reflect the core areas of concern and distress for the client, while the theoretical and narrowed inferences offer clinical speculation as to their origins. In the case of Juno, there are three primary areas of concern. The first, "background stresses of being high-functioning adolescent in blended family," refers to her difficulties adjusting to her parent's divorce, the absence of her biological mother, and conflictual relationship with her stepmother. The second, "pregnancy, adoption and boyfriend stress," refers to her attempts to cope with her unexpected pregnancy, its accompanying physical and psychological stressors, the pressure of the adoption process, and the tensions with her boyfriend in relation to all of these issues. The third, "stresses from parental reaction regarding pregnancy and adoption," refers to communication difficulties with her parents, lack of affirmation by her stepmother (in spite of being an intellectually gifted adolescent), and their lack of support of her decision-making abilities. These symptoms and stresses are consistent with the diagnosis of Parent-Child Relational Problem on Axis I, and the physical reality of pregnancy on Axis III (APA, 2000a; Leitch, 1998; Miller, Benson, & Galbraith, 2000).

Step 2: Identify and Articulate Goals for Change. The second step is the selection of achievable goals, which is based upon a number of factors, including the most pressing or urgent behavioral, emotional, and interpersonal concerns and symptoms as identified by the client and clinician, the willingness and ability of the client to work on those particular goals, and the realistic (real-world) achievability of those goals (Neukrug & Schwitzer, 2006). At this stage of treatment planning, it is important to recognize that not all of the client's issues can be addressed at once, so we focus initially on those that cause the greatest distress and impairment. New goals can be created as old ones are achieved. In the case of Juno, the goals are divided into three prominent clusters. The first, "background stresses of being high-functioning adolescent in blended family," requires that we help Juno to recognize and express thoughts and feelings about her parents' divorce, address and resolve feelings of loss of her biological mother, express conflictual feelings about her stepmother, identify abandonment issues and their relationship to ongoing family stress, connect thoughts and feelings about divorce with behaviors outside of the family, and validate her intellectual capacities. The second, "pregnancy, adoption and boyfriend stress," requires that we help Juno to address conflictual thoughts and feelings regarding adoption, identify the physical, emotional, and behavioral stresses related to pregnancy, develop strategies for communicating with her boyfriend about the adoption plans, and improve her ability to discuss the pregnancy with peers. The last, "stresses from parental reaction regarding pregnancy and adoption," requires that we improve overall parent-child communications, explore, understand, and resolve conflictual relations with her stepmother, and assist her parents to recognize and support Juno's competencies and decision-making skills.

Step 3: Describe Therapeutic Interventions. This is perhaps the most critical step in the treatment planning process because the clinician must now integrate information from a number of sources, including the case conceptualization, the delineation of the client's problems and goals, and the treatment literature, paying particular attention to *empirically supported treatment* (EST) and *evidence-based practice* (EBP). In essence, the clinician must align his or her treatment approach with scientific evidence from the fields of counseling and psychotherapy. Wampold (2001) iden-

tifies two types of evidence-based counseling research: studies that demonstrate "absolute efficacy," that is, the fact that counseling and psychotherapy work, and those that demonstrate "relative efficacy," that is, the fact that certain theoretical/technical approaches work best for certain clients with particular problems (Psychoanalysis, Gestalt Therapy, Cognitive Behavior Therapy, Brief Solution-Focused Therapy, Cognitive Therapy, Dialectical Behavior Therapy, Person-Centered Therapy, Expressive/Creative Therapies, Interpersonal Therapy, and Feminist Therapy); and when delivered through specific treatment modalities (individual, group, and family counseling).

In the case of Juno, we have decided to use Person-Centered Counseling (Bohart & Greenberg, 1997; Broadley, 1999; Carkhuff, 2000; Raskin & Rogers, 2000; Rogers, 1961, 1977) due to its humanistic emphasis on each person's inherent capacity for self-determination, growth, and actualization. Given Juno's intelligence, self-awareness, and decision-making competence, the therapeutic conditions of unconditional positive regard, genuineness, empathy, and congruence would help her and her family to work through the stresses of her pregnancy as well as those related to their blended family. Additionally, the nondirective nature of client-centered counseling would facilitate Juno's self-determination as well as help her parents value her more deeply as an emerging young adult. The highly supportive nature of this type of counseling has been found to be highly effective with teens (Lemoire & Chen, 2005; Taffel, 2005) and useful around issues related to pregnancy (McBride & Glenapp, 2000). Specific techniques for Juno will include exploration of feelings about her parents' divorce and maternal abandonment, postpregnancy family and career planning, and improving parent-child communication.

Step 4: Provide Outcome Measures of Change. This last step in treatment planning requires that we specify how change will be measured and indicate the extent to which progress has been made toward realizing these goals (Neukrug & Schwitzer, 2006). The counselor has considerable flexibility in this phase and may choose from a number of objective domains (psychological tests and measures of self-esteem, depression, psychosis, interpersonal relationship, anxiety, etc.), quasi-objective measures (the *DSM-IV-TR's* Axis V GAF scale; pre-post clinician, client, and psychiatric ratings), and subjective ratings (client self-report, clinician's in-session observations). In Juno's case, we have implemented a number of these, including client and family self-report of improved functioning and communication and pre-post improvement on the Family Adaptability and Cohesion Evaluation Scale-FACES III (Olson & Gorall, 2003).

The completed treatment plan is now developed through which the counselor, Juno, and her family will begin their shared work of improving their relationships with each other, helping both Juno and her parents to cope effectively with her pregnancy and plans for adoption as well as assist Juno in the grieving process. Juno's treatment plan is as follows and is summarized in Table 8.3.

TREATMENT PLAN

Client: Juno MacGuff

Service Provider: Minnetonka Family Services Center

BEHAVIORAL DEFINITION OF PROBLEMS:

1. Background stresses of being high-functioning adolescent in blended family—Difficulties adjusting to her parents' divorce, the absence of her biological mother, and conflictual relationship with her stepmother

2. Pregnancy, adoption, and boyfriend stress—Attempts to cope with her unexpected pregnancy, accompanying physical and psychological stressors, the pressure of the adoption process, and the tensions with her boyfriend in relation to these issues

3. Stresses from parental reaction regarding pregnancy and adoption—Communication difficulties with her parents, lack of affirmation by her stepmother, lack of parental support of her decision-making abilities

GOALS FOR CHANGE:

1. Background stresses of being high-functioning adolescent in blended family

   - Explore and resolve thoughts and feelings about parents' divorce
   - Alleviate feelings of loss of biological mother
   - Resolve conflictual feelings about stepmother
   - Reconcile abandonment issues and their relation to family stress
   - Connect thoughts and feelings about divorce with behavior outside of the family
   - Validate intellectual capacities and otherwise high level of functioning

2. Pregnancy, adoption, and boyfriend stress

   - Resolve conflictual feelings and thoughts regarding adoption
   - Decrease the physical, emotional, and behavioral stresses related to being pregnant
   - Improve communicating with boyfriend about plans for adoption
   - Improve ability to discuss pregnancy and adoption plans with peers

3. Stresses from parental reaction regarding pregnancy and adoption

- Improve overall parent-child communication
- Explore, understand, and resolve conflictual relationship with stepmother
- Enhance parents' perceptions of their daughter's competencies and problem-solving skills

THERAPEUTIC INTERVENTIONS:

A short-term course of individual person-centered counseling and family counseling (2–3 months) supplemented with teen pregnancy psychoeducational group support

1. Background stresses of being high-functioning adolescent in blended family

- Support clear and open communications between family members
- Explore the changes in roles, boundaries, and communication and expression of affection in blended families
- Address the loss issues related to divorce and remarriage
- Promote balance of independence and reliance on nuclear family
- Bibliotherapy around stepfamily issues

2. Pregnancy, adoption, and boyfriend stress

- Acknowledge feelings of loss with regard to adoption
- Develop and enhance self-care skills for managing pregnancy
- Encourage open and clear communication between client and boyfriend around pregnancy and adoption
- Support and encourage regular medical visits
- Incorporate peer support into individual counseling
- Referral to support group for pregnant teens
- Support post-pregnancy educational and career planning

3. Stresses from parental reaction regarding pregnancy and adoption

- Improve overall family communication skills through family counseling
- Address conflictual parent feelings regarding pregnancy
- Decrease parental reactivity to daughter's behavior
- Assist parents in their understanding of teen pregnancy

OUTCOME MEASURES OF CHANGE:

The development of congruence between her ideal and actual self, improved self-esteem, greater capacity for understanding and expression of feelings, and the development of healthy attitudes toward pregnancy and adoption within the context of open and effective communications within and outside of the family will be measured by:

- Pre-post comparisons of effective family communications within session
- Parents' reports of reduced stress and improved overall relationships within the home
- Improved pre-post scores of overall family adjustment and communication on the Family Adaptability and Cohesion Evaluation Scales IV (FACES IV) Questionnaire
- Client self-reported awareness of ability to express feelings of grief and loss
- Client and boyfriend self-report and clinical observations of open and ongoing discussions about the pregnancy and adoption plan
- Post-only evidence of clear educational and career planning

Table 8.3   Juno's Treatment Plan Summary: Person-Centered Counseling

Goals for Change	Therapeutic Interventions	Outcome Measures of Change
Background stresses of being high-functioning adolescent in blended family	Background stresses of being high-functioning adolescent in blended family	The development of congruence between her ideal and actual self, improved self-esteem, greater capacity for understanding and expression of feelings, and the development of healthy attitudes toward pregnancy and adoption within the context of open and effective communications within and outside of the family will be measured by:
Explore and resolve thoughts and feelings about parents' divorce	Support clear and open communications between family members	
Alleviate feelings of loss of biological mother	Explore the changes in roles, boundaries, and communication and expression of affection in blended families	
Resolve conflictual feelings about stepmother	Address the loss issues related to divorce and remarriage	Pre-post comparisons of effective family communications within session
Reconcile abandonment issues and their relation to family stress	Promote balance of independence and reliance on nuclear family	Parents' reports of reduced stress and improved overall relationships within the home
Connect thoughts and feelings about divorce with behavior outside of the family	Bibliotherapy around stepfamily issues	
	Pregnancy, adoption, and boyfriend stress	Improved pre-post scores of overall family adjustment and communication on the FACES IV inventory
Validate intellectual capacities and otherwise high level of functioning	Acknowledge feelings of loss with regard to adoption	
Pregnancy, adoption, and boyfriend stress	Develop and enhance self-care skills for managing pregnancy	Client self-reported awareness of ability to express feelings of grief and loss
Resolve conflictual feelings and thoughts regarding adoption	Encourage open and clear communication between client and boyfriend around pregnancy and adoption	
Decrease the physical, emotional, and behavioral stresses related to being pregnant	Support and encourage regular medical visits	Client and boyfriend self-report and clinical observations of open and ongoing discussions about the pregnancy and adoption plan
	Incorporate peer support into individual counseling	
Improve communicating with boyfriend about plans for adoption	Referral to support group for pregnant teens	
Improve ability to discuss pregnancy and adoption plans with peers	Support post-pregnancy educational and career planning	Post-only evidence of clear educational and career planning
Stresses from parental reaction regarding pregnancy and adoption	Stresses from parental reaction regarding pregnancy and adoption	
Improve overall parent-child communication	Improve overall family communication skills through family counseling	
Explore, understand, and resolve conflictual relationship with stepmother	Address conflictual parent feelings regarding pregnancy	
	Decrease parental reactivity to daughter's behavior	
Enhance parents' perceptions of their daughter's competencies and problem-solving skills	Assist parents in their understanding of teen pregnancy	

CASE 8.4 *THE BREAKFAST CLUB'S* CLAIRE

INTRODUCING THE CHARACTER

Claire Standish is the main female character in the coming-of-age movie *The Breakfast Club* (Hughes, 1985). Although Hollywood had a history of ensemble movies, *The Breakfast Club* was one of the first to feature a cast of adolescents—who, in this case, became known as the "Brat Pack," which was loosely modeled after the "Rat Pack" of the 1950s and 1960s. The film takes place over an 8-hour period during the weekend detention of an improbable group of teenagers, featuring Claire Standish, "the Princess," Brian, "the Brain," Andy, "the Athlete," Allison, "the Basket Case," and John Bender, "the Criminal." Over the course of the day they are forced to spend with one another, the five students—each representing a different familiar faction commonly found among American high schools' varied and divided social demography—come to learn about each other, to question the rigid stereotypes that divide them, and to gain a deeper awareness of themselves. In so doing, they unite as a singular and powerful emerging group of young adults who hopefully will go on to question and challenge the prevailing biases and misconceptions about the adolescent in society. Building on our impressions of Claire's character portrayal, the following basic case summary and diagnostic impressions present symptoms we believe she may have been experiencing in the areas of eating-related concerns, substance use, and impulse control.

Meet the Client

You can assess the client in action by viewing clips of Claire Standish's video material at the following websites:

- http://www.youtube.com/watch?v=dkX 8J-FKndE Movie trailer
- http://www.youtube.com/watch?v=mgd UBSDwL9g Claire steps out of her comfort zone
- http://www.youtube.com/watch?v=jsZkk qLDFmg videos Bender (the criminal) mocks Claire

BASIC CASE SUMMARY

Identifying Information. Claire Standish is a 17-year-old female senior at Shermer High School in Shermer, Illinois, who resides with her parents in a socioeconomically upper-class suburb of Chicago. Claire was referred to this independent practice, Great Lakes Clinical Associates of Chicago, following concerns raised by her school counselor. She was brought in by her father.

She was dressed appropriately, with obvious meticulous attention to peer-group fashion conventions regarding hair, makeup, and dress. She appeared the appropriate weight for her height.

Claire is highly accomplished with above-average academic grades and PSAT scores as well as social successes, including student council president, honor council representative, prom committee, and prom queen candidate. According to referral notes, she maintained good discipline and performance until several weeks ago; then, on March 24, 1984, she served 1 day of in-school Saturday detention for skipping school to go shopping with friends. As a result of the attention focused on her behavior leading up to, during, and following her detention, several additional behavioral concerns were raised.

Presenting Concern. Claire came to her school counselor's attention on several occasions following her 1-day detention. On the first occasion, a school security guard identified Claire as one of several students repeatedly found smoking marijuana under the football field bleachers during lunch breaks. A school janitor confirmed that he had suspected from odors and debris he found that she had also smoked marijuana in the school building during her Saturday detention. Because there was no definitive evidence, a note was made in her school records, and Claire was found in the cafeteria as assigned during subsequent lunch periods.

On the next occasion, the same security guard reported that she had overheard Claire vomiting in the girls' bathroom on several occasions; however Claire denied this as well as any health problems. When consulting with her father, the school counselor learned that the father also had heard her vomiting in the bathroom at home, but "assumed that's what girls do when they are 17, right?"

The father also noted that he thought she seemed overly preoccupied with her eyebrows and eyelashes and arm hair, which all seemed to be becoming sparse. Again he said his perception was that "that's what teenage girls do."

Background, Family Information, and Relevant History. Claire has one older brother, an adult who has graduated college and is an architect who lives in urban Chicago. Her father is a highly successful physician who is chief of radiology at Sherman Hospital in Elgin. Her mother does not work outside the home; she participates in a large number of charitable efforts throughout the Midwest region. Regarding medical histories, her mother has been in treatment as an outpatient and inpatient for alcohol abuse and prescription-drug dependence on an ongoing basis over the past 10 years. Both parents are highly recognized patrons of the arts and humanitarian efforts and perceived to be community leaders.

Regarding school history, reports indicate that Claire has been consistently recognized for her above-average academic performance, leadership in school, and extracurricular organized activities, social success among her peers, and skill as both a gymnast and cheerleader, throughout her elementary, middle school, and high school years. It is unclear whether Claire's presenting concerns have been present for some time but overlooked, or alternatively, have emerged only in the past year.

Problem and Counseling History. Claire has been seen three times with the goals of conducting an extended assessment and establishing a therapeutic alliance. She appeared quite resistant during the initial meeting, with a special concern that her parents would have access to her records. A working agreement was established among Claire and her father that although her attendance at counseling sessions will be reported to her father, no information about session contents will be shared without Claire's permission (within the "normal" limits of confidentiality). Claire also is aware that suspension from school might result should she not pursue counseling as agreed. Her concerns appear in three areas.

First, Claire admits to regular marijuana use during and immediately after school. She reports that her use began only recently, in March, but admits that she is aware her use has resulted in late papers and missed homework. At the same time, she has said that "it doesn't really matter, because my teachers always give me a break." She is aware that she risks school suspension at this late point in her school career and responds that "I'm coming to counseling, and they'll leave me alone." She also admits she has begun associating with unfamiliar boys of peer age and boys in their early 20s "so I can bum some pot. All you have to do is flirt a little to go home with a few free joints!"

Second, when queried about being suspected of vomiting regularly at home and in the school bathroom, Claire at first was silent. Later, apparently feeling greater trust, admitted that she vomits after eating to avoid weight gain "maybe once every week or two." By her report, she also occasionally ("I don't know, maybe once a month") steals her mother's laxatives for use to prevent weight gain. When confronted about these behaviors, Claire explained that "this way I can eat all I want sometimes and keep my nice body. And you know what, when my body looks nice in my clothes and I'm kind of extra thin, I feel hotter and better than any of my friends. I know I'm going to win prom queen and staying nice and thin is why. Plus I just feel better. So it's not really a problem. I know what I'm doing."

Third, although Claire denies recognizing any problems associated with pulling her eyelashes, eyebrows, or arm hair, she did readily admit to pulling out hair and said that she "needs the relief sometimes after dealing with my mom, especially when she's been at the club drinking." She characterized these behaviors as "only when I feel like it, they're under total control and I don't want to talk about them anymore. Besides, thin eyebrows look great." By observation, she appears to have very few eyelashes and on one occasion, an exposed arm appeared to display areas bare of hair that were not the result of cosmetic attention.

Claire has agreed to participate in ongoing sessions at least through the end of her high school year.

Goals for Counseling and Course of Therapy to Date. The primary goals at this point are to clarify diagnostic impressions; maintain and increase client motivation for change; and determine a treatment plan appropriate for the 6 weeks remaining in the school year or, alternatively, solicit the client's agreement to continue counseling through the summer until the start of college. An associated goal is obtain Claire's permission for the clinician to obtain her father's at-home observations of her eating and compensatory weight management and hair-pulling behaviors. Treatment modalities may include individual, family, and/or group interventions.

Diagnostic Impressions

Axis I.   305.20 Cannabis Abuse

307.50 Eating Disorder Not Otherwise Specified

312.39 Trichotillomania

Axis II.   V71.09 No Diagnosis or Condition on Axis II

Axis III.   None

Axis IV.   Problems with primary support group—Alcohol dependence of mother, estrangement of parents, neglect of child by parents

Axis V.   GAF = 61 (estimated at intake)

GAF = 81 (highest level past year as estimated at intake)

DISCUSSION OF DIAGNOSTIC IMPRESSIONS

Claire was referred to a private practitioner at the Great Lakes Clinical Associates of Chicago by her school counselor, who was worried about several domains of Claire's functioning. Claire's school counselor believed that she may have been experiencing concerns found in each of these three areas: substance use, eating-related concerns, and impulse control.

Each section of the *DSM-IV-TR* classification system contains a group of diagnoses that share qualitatively similar symptoms or features. For instance, the Substance-Related Disorders section contains all of the Substance-Use Disorders (Dependence and Abuse) and Substance-Induced Disorders (Intoxication, Withdrawal, and substance-induced disruptions in mood, sleep, and sexual function); the Eating Disorders section contains three diagnoses that all are characterized by severe disturbances in eating, weight management, and body perceptions (Anorexia, Bulimia, and Eating Disorders Not Otherwise Specified); and the Impulse-Control Disorders Not Elsewhere Classified section contains clinical problems all featuring a person's failure to resist a harmful impulse, drive, or temptation (e.g., Kleptomania, Pyromania, and Pathological Gambling).

The counselor's first concern pertained to Claire's substance use. On several occasions she was suspected of smoking marijuana on school grounds, which led to disciplinary notes in her school records and could lead to further disciplinary actions. Her use continued even after her knowledge that she was under special scrutiny following a day of in-school suspension. In other words, her marijuana use comprises a maladaptive pattern in which she continues smoking despite her knowledge of negative consequences at school and potentially in other areas of her life such as social and family relationships. In such cases the diagnosis is Substance Abuse, and more exactly, Cannabis Abuse.

Cannabis Dependence might be a reasonable differential consideration; however, Claire's use pattern meets the criteria for the less advanced diagnosis, abuse, rather than the more advanced diagnosis, dependence. Another differential consideration is whether Claire is engaged in nonproblematic experimental or social or recreational use of marijuana, which would not require a diagnosis; however, her use meets the criteria for a maladaptive pattern of substance-related behavior resulting in negative life consequences (Inaba & Cohen, 2000)—namely, recurrent use leading to problems with major role obligations at school—and therefore warrants a diagnosis indicating clinical significance.

The counselor's second concern pertained to Claire's eating and weight-management behaviors. On several occasions, she was overheard vomiting at home as well as in the girl's bathroom on a day that she was not ill with a gastrointestinal problem. Claire also admitted in her sessions that she vomits for weight management a few times a month. Likewise, she admitted to occasionally using her mother's laxatives for weight management. Further, in her session she described an overly close relationship between her overall feelings about herself and her perceptions of her body and appearance. The primary symptoms are recurrent, inappropriate behavior to compensate for eating in order to prevent weight gain, occurring less frequently than twice weekly, without any report of binge-eating, and with self-evaluation unduly influenced by body considerations. In such cases, the diagnosis is Eating Disorders Not Otherwise Specified.

Eating Disorders Not Otherwise Specified (sometimes also referred to as subthreshhold eating disorders because eating and compensatory symptoms, although clinically significant, fall below the thresholds of the frequency and duration criteria for anorexia and bulimia) are, by far, the most commonly seen eating disorders among adolescent girls and young adult women (Schwitzer, Rodriguez, Thomas, & Salimi, 2001; Schwitzer , Hatfield et al., 2008). Correspondingly, clinicians should vigilantly assess for, rather than overlook, signs of these subthreshhold eating concerns among their young women clients. Although Bulimia Nervosa might be a reasonable differential diagnostic consideration, Claire does not report any binge eating behaviors, or frequent enough purging behaviors, to meet the criteria for bulimia.

The counselor's third concern pertained to Claire's behavioral pattern of recurrently pulling out her eyelashes, eyebrows, and arm hair. In her sessions, Claire reported feeling increasing tension that was relieved once she engaged in hair pulling. The hair loss in her eyelashes and eyebrows was noticeable. Having very few lashes left and bare spots on her arms suggests clinical significance. In such cases, the diagnosis is Trichotillomania, an Impulse-Control Disorder Not Otherwise Specified. Regarding differential diagnoses, temporary periods of hair pulling earlier in childhood may be benign and warrant no diagnosis at all. Alternatively, Obsessive-Compulsive Disorder, which is one of the Anxiety Disorders, might be considered because this diagnosis is defined partly by repetitive behaviors. However, Claire's behaviors occurred after childhood, in adolescence, and appear to be recurrent and clinically significant rather than temporary and benign; further, her behaviors are not in response to characteristic obsessions, as required for Obsessive-Compulsive Disorder.

On Axis I, since there are multiple diagnoses, the diagnosis that is the primary reason for the referral was listed first, followed by the other diagnoses in order of clinical importance. To round out the diagnosis, Claire's family stressors are emphasized on Axis IV, and on Axis V her functioning is represented by GAF scores ranging from a recent period of good functioning with only normally expected, transient, everyday reactions and concerns, to the current period of mild symptoms causing some difficulty in school and social functioning that led to her referral. The information on these axes is consistent with the diagnoses listed on Axis I.

CASE CONCEPTUALIZATION

When Claire Standish visited the Great Lakes Clinical Associates of Chicago, the counselor's first task was to collect detailed clinical information about the situation leading to Claire's appointment. The counselor first used this information to develop diagnostic impressions. Her concerns were described by Cannabis Abuse, Eating Disorder Not Otherwise Specified, and Trichotillomania. Next, the counselor developed a case conceptualization. Whereas the purpose of diagnostic impressions is to *describe* the client's concerns, the goal of case conceptualization is to better *understand* and clinically *explain* the person's experiences (Neukrug & Schwitzer, 2006). It helps the counselor understand the conditions leading up to Claire's three presenting concerns and the conditions keeping them going. In turn, case conceptualization sets the stage for treatment planning. Treatment planning then provides a road map that plots out how the counselor and client expect to move from presenting concerns to positive outcomes (Seligman, 1993, p. 157)—helping Claire better control her cannabis abuse, eating and weight management, and hair-pulling.

When forming a case conceptualization, the clinician applies a purist counseling theory, an integration of two or more theories, an eclectic mix of theories, or a solution-focused combination of tactics to his or her understanding of the client. In this case, Claire's counselor based her conceptualization on a purist theory, Brief Contemporary Psychodynamic Psychotherapy. Various contemporary psychodynamic models are available, such as Ego Psychology, Objects-Relations Therapy, Kohut's Self-Psychology, and similar post- or neoanalytic models. Claire's counselor based her conceptualization on Kohut's Self-Psychology. She selected this approach because she found evidence that the model can be especially useful for the conceptualization of late adolescent and young adult clinical situations such as Claire's (Patton & Robbins, 1982; Robbins, 1989; Schwitzer, 1997, 2005). Brief contemporary psychodynamic therapies also are the approaches of choice at the Great Lakes practice.

The counselor used the Inverted Pyramid Method of case conceptualization because this method is especially designed to help clinicians more easily form their conceptual pictures of their clients' needs (Neukrug & Schwitzer, 2006; Schwitzer, 1996, 1997). The method has four steps: Problem Identification, Thematic Groupings, Theoretical Inferences, and Narrowed Inferences. The counselor's clinical thinking can be seen in Figure 8.4.

Step 1: Problem Identification. The first step is Problem Identification. Aspects of the presenting problem (thoughts, feelings, behaviors, physiological features), additional areas of concern besides the presenting concern, family and developmental history, in-session observations, clinical inquiries (medical problems, medications, past counseling, substance use, suicidality), and psychological assessments (problem checklists, personality inventories, mental status exam, specific clinical measures) all may contribute information at Step 1. The counselor "casts a wide net" in order to build Step 1 as exhaustively as possible (Neukrug & Schwitzer,

2006, p. 202). As can be seen in Figure 8.4, the counselor identified all of the information pertaining to Claire's current concerns—details describing her problems with marijuana use, purging, and hair-pulling. She also identified all of the information she could gather pertaining to Claire's family dynamics, her high school adjustment, strengths and talents, and other important psychosocial information. The counselor went beyond just the main reason for referral to describe Claire's situation as fully as possible.

Step 2: Thematic Groupings. The second step is Thematic Groupings. The clinician organizes all of the exhaustive client information found in Step 1 into just a few intuitive-logical clinical groups, categories, or themes on the basis of sensible common denominators (Neukrug & Schwitzer, 2006). Four different ways of forming the Step 2 theme groups can be used: Descriptive-Diagnosis Approach, Clinical Targets Approach, Areas of Dysfunction Approach, and Intrapsychic Approach. As can be seen in Figure 8.4, Claire's counselor selected the Areas of Dysfunction Approach. This approach sorts together all of the Step 1 information into "areas of dysfunction according to important life situations, life themes, or life roles and skills" (Neukrug & Schwitzer, 2006, p. 205).

Interestingly, the counselor distilled all of the information collected at Step 1 into just two overarching themes at Step 2: (a) Historically, successful high-achieving, high-socioeconomic-status female student; and (b) in recent adolescence, engaging in multiple problematic "acting out" behaviors, including marijuana use, purging for weight control, and eye-hair pulling. In other words, she grouped all of Claire's strengths, family information, and background material into the first theme, and all of the details of her three current clinical concerns into the second theme. The counselor believed this distillation allowed her to begin more clearly thinking about Claire and her needs.

Step 3: Theoretical Inferences. At Step 3, concepts from the counselor's selected theory, Kohut's Self-Psychology, are applied to explain the dynamics causing and maintaining Claire's problematic thoughts, feelings, behaviors, and physiological responses. The counselor tentatively matches the theme groups in Step 2 with this theoretical approach. In other words, the symptom constellations in Step 2, which were distilled from the symptoms in Step 1, now are combined using theory to show what is believed to be the psychological etiology of Claire's current needs (Neukrug & Schwitzer, 2006; Schwitzer, 2006, 2007).

According to Kohut's Self-Psychology (Kohut, 1971, 1977, 1984), infants, children, and adolescents require specific dynamics in their relationships with their parents or primary caregivers. Specifically, parents must provide "mirroring," "idealization," and "mentorship." When provided adequately, these lead to healthy development of the self, including three different lines of development (Grandiose, Idealized Self-Image, and Twinship). When the psychodynamic parenting requirements are unmet or insufficient, the person can grow up to develop ways of covering over the inadequacies, depressed mood, anxieties, or other psychological deficiencies that form as a consequence. These ways of covering over fragile self-development are called Defensive Maneuvers and Compensatory Actions. In this way, client symptoms are reinterpreted as ways of coping.

As can be seen in Figure 8.4, when Claire's counselor applied these concepts to Claire's situation; she inferred at Step 3 that Claire's three clinical problems were methods of coping with problems in her self-development stemming from absent or emotionally absent parents (Patton & Robbins, 1982; Schwitzer, 1997, 2005). Specifically, following the theory, the counselor inferred: (a) use of marijuana and eye-hair pulling were Defensive Maneuvers to cover over defects in self-development; and (b) use of purging via vomiting and laxatives to maintain thinness were Compensatory Actions to compensate for defects in self-development.

Step 4: Narrowed Inferences. At Step 4, the clinician's selected theory continues to be used to address still-deeper issues when they exist

(Schwitzer, 2006, 2007). At this step, "still-deeper, more encompassing, or more central, causal themes" are formed (Neukrug & Schwitzer, 2006, p. 207). Continuing to apply Self Psychology concepts at Step 4, Claire's counselor presented a single, deepest, most-fundamental explanation of Claire's needs, namely, that she is experiencing: Defects in the Grandiose Line of Development due to Insufficient Mirroring by her parents. (In other words, due to lack of psychological mirroring, at a very deep psychological level Claire is unsure whether she is competent and worthy as an emerging adult; in turn, she is covering the feelings of doubt, low mood, and anxiety that she has about herself by using marijuana to lift her mood, pulling her hair for tension relief, and driving to be especially thin to feel good about herself).

When all four steps are completed, the client information in Step 1 leads to logical-intuitive groupings on the basis of common denominators in Step 2, the groupings then are explained using theory at Step 3, and then, finally, at Step 4, further deeper explanations are made. From start to finish, the thoughts, feelings, behaviors, and physiological features in the topmost portions are connected on down the pyramid into deepest dynamics. The completed pyramid now is used to plan treatment, where the counselor will work with Claire in brief psychotherapy.

TREATMENT PLANNING

At this point, Claire's clinician at the Great Lakes Clinical Associates of Chicago has collected all available information about the problems that have been of concern to her and her school. Based upon this information, the counselor developed a five-axis *DSM-IV-TR* diagnosis and then, using the "inverted pyramid" (Neukrug & Schwitzer, 2006; Schwitzer, 1996, 1997), formulated a working clinical *explanation* of Claire's difficulties and their etiology that we called the *case conceptualization*. This, in turn, guides us to the next critical step in our

clinical work, called the *treatment plan,* the primary purpose of which is to map out a logical and goal-oriented strategy for making positive changes in the client's life. In essence, the treatment plan is a road map "for reducing or eliminating disruptive symptoms that are impeding the client's ability to reach positive mental health outcomes" (Neukrug & Schwitzer, 2006, p. 225). As such, it is the cornerstone of our work with not only Claire, but with all clients who present with disturbing or disruptive symptoms (Jongsma & Peterson, 2006; Jongsma, Peterson, & McInnis, 2003a, 2003b; Seligman, 1993, 1998, 2004).

A comprehensive treatment plan must integrate all of the information from the biopsychosocial interview, diagnosis, and case conceptualization into a coherent plan of action. This *plan* comprises four main components, which include (1) a behavioral definition of the problem(s), (2) the selection of achievable goals, (3) the determination of treatment modes, and (4) the documentation of how change will be measured. The *behavioral definition of the problem(s)* consolidates the results of the case conceptualization into a concise hierarchical list of problems and concerns that will be the focus of treatment. The *selection of achievable goals* refers to assessing and prioritizing the client's concerns into a *hierarchy of urgency* that also takes into account the client's motivation for change, level of dysfunction, and real-world influences on his or her problems. The *determination of treatment modes* refers to selection of the specific interventions, which are matched to the uniqueness of the client and to his or her goals and clearly tied to a particular theoretical orientation (Neukrug & Schwitzer, 2006). Finally, the clinician must establish how change will be measured, based upon a number of factors, including client records and self-report of change, in-session observations by the clinician, clinician ratings, results of standardized evaluations such as the Beck Anxiety Inventory-II (Beck, Steer, & Brown, 1996) or a family functioning questionnaire, pre-post treatment comparisons, and reports by other treating professionals.

Figure 8.4 Claire's Inverted Pyramid Case Conceptualization Summary: Brief Contemporary Psychodynamic Psychotherapy (Kohut's Self-Psychology)

1. IDENTIFY AND LIST CLIENT CONCERNS

Above-average grades
Above-average PSAT scores
Student activities leader
Student government leader
Cheerleader
Gymnast
Prom queen candidate
Highly successful father and brother
Frequently absent father
Socially successful mother
Prescription dependence of
   mother
Alcohol abuse of mother
Emotionally absent mother

Vomits to purge as weight control
Uses mother's laxatives to purge
Self-image associated with body
Self-image associated with thinness
Skipped day of school for shopping
One-day in-school Saturday detention
Suspected and admitted recently
   begun problematic marijuana use
Smokes marijuana at school
Has missed homework assignments due to use
Has begun "hanging around" unfamiliar boys due to use
Sparse eyelashes and eyebrows
Admits eye-hair pulling for stress relief
Pulls hairs to feel calm and in control

2. ORGANIZE CONCERNS INTO LOGICAL THEMATIC GROUPINGS

1. Historically, successful, high-achieving high-SES female student
2. In recent adolescence, engaging in multiple problematic "acting out" behaviors, including marijuana use, purging for weight control, and eye-hair pulling

3. THEORETICAL INFERENCES: ATTACH THEMATIC GROUPINGS TO INFERRED AREAS OF DIFFICULTY

Brief Contemporary Psychodynamic Approach:
Kohut's Self-Psychology

Inferred Difficulties in Self-Function

1. Use of marijuana and eye-hair-pulling as Defensive Maneuvers to cover over defects in self-development
2. Use of purging via vomiting and laxatives to maintain thinness as Compensatory Action to compensate for defects in self-development

4. NARROWED INFERENCES: SUICIDALITY AND DEEPER DIFFICULTIES

Brief Contemporary Psychodynamic Approach:
Kohut's Self-Psychology

Deeper Inferences of Difficulties in Self-Function

Defects in Grandiose Line of Development due to Insufficient Mirroring by parents (Due to lack of psychological mirroring, unsure whether she is competent and worthy as an emerging adult; she is covering associated feelings of doubt, low mood, anxiety with marijuana use, hair pulling, drive for thinness)

The four-step method discussed above can be seen in Figure 6.1 (p. 109) and is outlined below for the case of Claire, followed by her specific treatment plan.

Step 1: Behavioral Definition of Problems. The first step in treatment planning is to carefully review the case conceptualization, paying particular attention to the results of Step 2 (Thematic Groupings), Step 3 (Theoretical Inferences) and Step 4 (Narrowed Inferences). The identified clinical themes reflect the core areas of concern and distress for the client, while the theoretical and narrowed inferences offer clinical speculation as to their origins. In the case of Claire, there is one primary area of concern, "multiple problematic 'acting-out' behaviors, including marijuana use, purging for weight control, and eye-hair pulling." This array of symptoms refers to smoking marijuana at school and missing homework assignments and hanging around unfamiliar boys due to marijuana use. It also refers to pulling her eye-hair for stress control and to feel calm and in control, vomiting to purge as weight control, using her mother's laxatives to purge, and self-image. These symptoms are consistent with a diagnosis of Cannabis Abuse, Eating Disorder NOS, and Trichotillomania (APA, 2000a; Budney, Hughes, Moore, & Vandrey, 2004; Flessner, Conolea, Woods, Franklin, & Keuthen, 2008; Keel, Heatherton, Dorer, Joiner, & Zalta, 2006; National Institute on Drug Abuse, 2008; Stein, Christiansen, & Hollander, 1999).

Step 2: Identify and Articulate Goals for Change. The second step is the selection of achievable goals, which is based upon a number of factors, including the most pressing or urgent behavioral, emotional, and interpersonal concerns and symptoms as identified by the client and clinician, the willingness and ability of the client to work on those particular goals, and the realistic (real-world) achievability of those goals (Neukrug & Schwitzer, 2006). At this stage of treatment planning, it is important to recognize that not all of the client's problems can be addressed at once, so we focus initially on those that cause the greatest distress and impairment. New goals can be created as old ones are achieved. In the case

of Claire, the goals flow from her pattern of acting out behavior that includes cannabis abuse, purging, and trichotillomania.

With regard to her cannabis abuse, the goals are to maintain abstinence from marijuana use, to reduce the level of personal and family stress related to marijuana use, and to develop coping/self-regulation skills necessary to remain abstinent. With regard to the symptoms of Claire's eating disorder, the goals are to terminate the pattern of eating/purging behavior, to help her develop awareness of the relationship between stress and purging, to assist her in changing the definition of "self" that does not include weight, and to restructure the distorted thoughts that maintain this behavior and to restore her normal eating/elimination patterns. With regard to her trichotillomania, we will help Claire to recognize the relationship between stress and hair pulling, to eliminate the hair pulling behavior, and to replace the hair-pulling behavior with adaptive responses to stress. All of these goals are consistent with helping Claire to develop a clear and valued sense of self, in spite of the emotional neglect she has experienced in her family.

Step 3: Describe Therapeutic Interventions. This is perhaps the most critical step in the treatment planning process because the clinician must now integrate information from a number of sources, including the case conceptualization, the delineation of the client's problems and goals, and the treatment literature, paying particular attention to *empirically supported treatment* (EST) and *evidence-based practice* (EBP). In essence, the clinician must align his or her treatment approach with scientific evidence from the fields of counseling and psychotherapy. Wampold (2001) identifies two types of evidence-based counseling research: studies that demonstrate "absolute efficacy," that is, the fact that counseling and psychotherapy work, and those that demonstrate "relative efficacy," that is, the fact that certain theoretical/technical approaches work best for certain clients with particular problems (Psychoanalysis, Gestalt Therapy, Cognitive Behavior Therapy, Brief Solution-Focused Therapy, Cognitive Therapy, Dialectical Behavior Therapy, Person-Centered Therapy, Expressive/Creative

Therapies, Interpersonal Therapy, and Feminist Therapy); and when delivered through specific treatment modalities (individual, group, and family counseling).

In the case of Claire, we have decided to use a Brief Contemporary Approach based upon Heinz Kohut's Self-Psychology (Kohut, 1971, 1977, 1984). According to Kohut, we all have specific needs that must be met if we are going to achieve a healthy sense of self; these include the need to feel special (recognition), the need to believe that parents are strong, capable, and self-assured (idealizing parents), and the need to be like others and to belong (twinship) (Neukrug, 2011). Parents who possessed these qualities and were capable of nurturing the child's sense of importance were considered "good enough parents" whom the child would internalize as a guidance system of sorts. Children who were not valued developed poor self-esteem and a sense of worthlessness. Additionally, if parents were emotionally unavailable or punitive, the child would internalize them as negative parts of his or her own sense of self. Without the mirroring of people who regarded the child in positive ways, he or she would grow up to feel unwanted and as an outsider. Based upon this model, the role of the therapist is to be a good-enough parent substitute who values the client and provides a "corrective emotional experience" in which a positive sense of self can be developed. Kohut divided the therapeutic work into two phases: the empathic mirroring phase (understanding) and the interpretation phase (explaining) (Bachar, 1998). In the case of eating disorders, and other conditions in which the client is attempting to regulate states of inner tension along with his or her self-image (substance use and hair-pulling), the therapeutic relationship can re-establish confidence in the "capacity of close human relationships [rather than substances and dysfunctional behaviors] to calm and mitigate dysphoric moods and build a positive self image" (Bachar, 1998, p. 152).

Specific techniques drawn from this theoretical model as applied to Claire will include using empathic attunement in order to understand and acknowledge Claire's unique perspective on her problems and to confirm her inner reality, to allow an unfolding of the various self-objects that Claire has internalized, to help her understand the relationship between early family experiences and her current ways of perceiving herself, to facilitate a valuing mirroring of Claire, analyze her defenses and resistance against the emergence of new versions of herself, and perhaps most importantly, reflect pride in Claire and her accomplishments.

Step 4: Provide Outcome Measures of Change. This last step in treatment planning requires that we specify how change will be measured and indicate the extent to which progress has been made toward realizing these goals (Neukrug & Schwitzer, 2006). The counselor has considerable flexibility in this phase and may choose from a number of objective domains (psychological tests and measures of self-esteem, depression, psychosis, interpersonal relationship, anxiety, etc.), quasi-objective measures (the *DSM-IV-TR's* Axis V GAF scale; pre-post clinician, client, and psychiatric ratings), and subjective ratings (client self-report, clinician's in-session observations). In Claire's case, we have implemented a number of these, including pre-post measures on the Eating Disorder Inventory-III (Garner, Olmsted, & Polivy, 1983), pre-post measures on the Milwaukee Inventory for Styles of Trichotillomania–Child Version (Flessner et al., 2007), pre-post measures on the Marijuana Screening Inventory (Alexander, 2003), post-only measures of GAF functioning in the "normal" range (>85), client self-reported awareness of and ability to regulate mood and behavior without acting out, clinician-observed improvement in self-object awareness and self-image, and client and parent report of improved relationships.

The completed treatment plan is now developed through which the counselor and Claire will begin their shared work of enhancing her self-image and eliminating the symptoms of her eating disorder, cannabis abuse, and trichotillomania. Claire's treatment plan appears below and a summary can be found in Table 8.4.

TREATMENT PLAN

Client: Claire Standish

Service Provider: Great Lakes Clinical Associates of Chicago

BEHAVIORAL DEFINITION OF PROBLEMS**:**

1. Multiple problematic "acting-out" behaviors—Smoking marijuana at school, missing home-work assignments, and hanging around unfamiliar boys due to marijuana use, pulling eye-hair for stress control and to feel calm and in control, vomiting to purge as weight control, using mother's laxatives to purge, and self-image problems associated with body and thinness

GOALS FOR CHANGE:

1. Multiple problematic acting-out behaviors

   With regard to cannabis abuse

   - Maintain abstinence from marijuana use
   - Reduce level of personal and family stress related to marijuana
   - Develop coping/self-regulation skills necessary to remain abstinent

   With regard to the eating disorder

   - Terminate the pattern of eating/purging behavior
   - Develop awareness of the relationship between stress and purging
   - Assist in changing the definition of "self" to one that does not include weight
   - Restructure the distorted thoughts that maintain this behavior
   - Restore normal eating/elimination patterns

   With regard to trichotillomania

   - Recognize the relationship between stress and hair pulling
   - Eliminate hair pulling behavior and with adaptive responses to stress

THERAPEUTIC INTERVENTIONS:

A short-to-moderate-term course (4–6 months) of Brief Contemporary Psychodynamic Psychotherapy supplemented with group counseling

1. Multiple problematic "acting-out" behaviors

   - Using empathic attunement to understand and acknowledge unique perspective and to confirm inner reality
   - Allow an unfolding of the various internalized self-objects
   - Help understand the relationship between early family experiences and current ways of perceiving herself
   - Facilitate a valuing mirroring
   - Analyze defenses and resistance against the emergence of new versions of self
   - Reflect pride in accomplishments and herself
   - Supportive group counseling

(Continued)

(Continued)

OUTCOME MEASURES OF CHANGE:

An elimination of acting-out behaviors and improved overall functioning at home and at school as measured by:

- Pre-post measure on the Eating Disorder Inventory-III
- Pre-post measures on the Milwaukee Inventory for Styles of Trichotillomania–Child Version
- Pre-post measures on the Marijuana Screening Inventory
- Post-only measures of GAF functioning in the normal range (>85)
- Client self-reported awareness of and ability to regulate mood and behavior
- Clinician-observed improvement in self-object awareness and self-image
- Client and parent report of improved relationships

Table 8.4 Claire's Treatment Plan Summary: Brief Contemporary Psychodynamic Psychotherapy (Kohut's Self-Psychology)

Goals for Change	Therapeutic Interventions	Outcome Measures of Change
Multiple problematic acting-out behaviors	Multiple problematic acting-out behaviors	An elimination of acting-out behaviors and improved overall functioning at home and at school as measured by:
With regard to cannabis abuse	Using empathic attunement to understand and acknowledge unique perspective and to confirm inner reality	Pre-post measure on the Eating Disorder Inventory-III
Maintain abstinence from marijuana use		
Reduce level of personal and family stress related to marijuana	Allow an unfolding of the various internalized self-objects	Pre-post measures on the Milwaukee Inventory for Styles of Trichotillomania–Child Version
Develop coping/self-regulation skills necessary to remain abstinent.	Help understand the relationship between early family experiences and current ways of perceiving herself	Pre-post measures on the Marijuana Screening Inventory
With regard to the eating disorder		
Terminate the pattern of eating/purging behavior	Facilitate a valuing mirroring	Post-only measures of GAF functioning in the normal range (>85)
Develop awareness of the relationship between stress and purging	Analyze defenses and resistance against the emergence of new versions of self	Client self-reported awareness of and ability to regulate mood and behavior
Assist in changing the definition of "self" to one that does not include weight		
Restructure the distorted thoughts that maintain this behavior	Reflect pride in accomplishments and herself	Clinician-observed improvement in self-object awareness and self-image
Restore normal eating/elimination patterns.	Supportive group counseling	Client and parent report of improved relationships
With regard to trichotillomania		
Recognize the relationship between stress and hair-pulling		
Eliminate hair-pulling behavior with adaptive responses to stress		

CASE 8.5 *WICKED'S* ELPHABA

INTRODUCING THE CHARACTER

Elphaba Thropp is the central character in Gregory Maguire's 1995 revisionist fictional biography of a character in L. Frank Baum's *The Wonderful Wizard of Oz* (1900), titled *Wicked: The Life and Times of the Wicked Witch of the West.* In 2007, it was adapted into a Broadway musical. The story follows Elphaba (later to become the Wicked Witch), from childhood in the Land of Oz through her high school and young adult years as a student at Shiz University.

The story opens with a focus on Elphaba's mother Melena, who is seduced by a traveling salesman (later to become the Wizard of Oz) with a vile of emerald passion potion called *Green 29*. As a result, Elphaba, who is born out of wedlock and with green skin, is rejected by both the salesman and by Melena's husband, who quickly realizes that the child is not his. Ridiculed and ostracized, Elphaba spends her childhood largely devoid of peer interaction, among the animals of the farm and woods. Upon entering Shiz University, Elphaba meets Galinda (later to become Glinda, the Good Witch of the North) who unlike herself is a self-confident, popular, and upwardly mobile teen. In spite of their class differences, Galinda befriends her. Through the relationship between Elphaba and Galinda, political and racial tensions of the seemingly idyllic Land of Oz are revealed, and Elphaba, as an activist, gains approval, power, and a deeper understanding of her femininity. Ultimately, Elphaba must depart from Oz and "defy gravity" in order to break the bonds, both inner and outer, that tether her.

Expanding on what is known about the Elphaba character, the following basic case summary and diagnostic impressions fill in more of our own details about Elphaba and describe areas of dysfunction we believe she has been confronting since childhood and now in young adulthood, stemming from her dysfunctional preoccupation with the physical anomaly of green skin and its impact on her young adult transition to college life.

Meet the Client

You can assess the client in action by viewing clips of Elphaba Thropp's video material at the following websites:

- http://www.youtube.com/watch?v= 7P4QvtyZhoo Introduction to musical
- http://www.youtube.com/watch?v=F4PC KL2vvhs&feature=PlayList&p=DF92D0B F970495A4&index=15 Elphaba
- http://www.youtube.com/watch?v=3A2Q4 7Y8XHM&feature=PlayList&p=DF92D0BF 970495A4&index=13 *Wicked* discussed on the View

BASIC CASE SUMMARY

Identifying Information. Elphaba Thropp is a 22-year-old emeraldine (green-skinned) female who is an honors graduate student at Shiz University, where she is taking a double major in animal studies and social justice. She lives on campus with her roommate, Galinda, with whom she shares a close friendship and together with whom she also shows her works in the school's primate laboratory. She is a tall, slender, and striking woman whose oddly green skin is accentuated by her jet black hair and piercing brown eyes. She attests to a nondenominational spirituality.

Presenting Concern. Elphaba was court ordered to counseling following an arrest for attempting to, in her words, "liberate the downtrodden animals" from the University laboratory. The counselor at the detention center noted that, "The client's anger, hostility, and seeming sense of persecution place her and others around her at risk." Elphaba was indignant over the counselor's suggestion, angrily claiming that "I was just doing what was right."

Background, Family Information, and Relevant History. Elphaba was born in Emerald County, Oz, the older of two children born to different fathers. As she discovered during late childhood, Elphaba's biological father was a traveling salesman who had visited town and her mother for only one night. Elphaba was born with a highly rare skin condition (Emeraldia Pigmentosa) affecting pigmentation over her entire body and resulting in an emerald green hue. Otherwise, her birth was uncomplicated and her developmental milestones were attained within expectable limits. Elphaba attended Oz Elementary and Middle School where, in spite of her advanced intelligence and academic skills, she felt as if "I never fit in . . . they made fun of me and couldn't get past my skin color." Elphaba reports the she was "mercilessly bullied" throughout her middle school years, but realized upon entering Emerald County High School, which was far from her home, that her wit, intelligence, and keen sense of justice (and injustice) garnered her a degree of popularity. During high school, she was active in the social justice movement aimed at liberating laboratory animals and fighting discrimination of the Munchkins, a group of genetic dwarfs. Elphaba had numerous encounters with school administration during her tenure at Emerald High due to her outspokenness. Elphaba was close to those in the social club as well as to a few select friends. She retained a tenuous connection with her mother and always felt "a strange distance from my father." Because her sister, born several years after Elphaba, was favored by the father for her "lily white skin," Elphaba resented her.

Elphaba accepted a full academic scholarship to Shiz University, where soon after her arrival, she once again became active in campus politics, the school newspaper, *The Shiz Tornado,* and was elected president of the student body as a sophomore. Galinda, a woman she initially viewed as self-important, superficial, and unsafe, quickly proved her loyalty and the two became fast friends. During her senior year, Elphaba took up the cause of resisting the oppression by the Wizard of Oz, a tyrannical despot who was bent on turning dissenters into voiceless animals. Although popular and successful, she was highly preoccupied with her green skin color. In contrast to the positive reactions of those around her, she focused almost singularly on her skin color and

grew increasingly resentful, distrustful, angry, and outspoken. During an episode of poppy intoxication, she broke into the school laboratory and released all the animals. She was subsequently arrested and referred to counseling.

Problem and Counseling History. Elphaba made it clear from the outset that the counseling was "just another form of mind control" by the Wizard, and that she saw it as an infringement on her constitutional rights. She asserted that "if I didn't have green skin I wouldn't be here." Elphaba sat rigidly throughout the interview with her legs tightly crossed and her foot bouncing dramatically. She maintained intense eye contact, scowling at times as she asserted her indignation over having to come to counseling against her will. Although articulate, oriented, and capable of retrieving both recent and remote details, Elphaba voiced suspiciousness regarding the counselor's intent, suggested that he might be part of the conspiracy and a pawn of the Wizard, and that she had to carefully guard herself. Elphaba's mood was somewhat blunted, her affect staid, and her words carefully chosen. Elphaba denied experiencing depression either currently or in the past, sensory disturbance, or troubling thoughts. Elphaba indicated that she had never been in counseling and wanted to "keep that record clean" because "with green skin, I'll need every advantage I can get after I graduate."

Goals for Counseling and Course of Therapy to Date. As of this writing, Elphaba was seen for two extended assessment sessions that included biopsychosocial and clinical interviews as well as the administration of standardized personality inventories (MMPI-2, 16PF), Projective Drawings, and Incomplete Sentences. A follow-up session was planned during which time the results of the assessment are to be shared with Elphaba and a treatment plan developed that incorporates both the counselor's concerns for her and the issues that she might regard as important to address. It is anticipated that Elphaba will be highly resistant to therapeutic intervention; however, given that participation is mandated, she will at the very least have to attend counseling for a minimum of 3 months. During that period, the counselor would like to address Elphaba's anger and more thoroughly assess her antisocial behaviors.

Diagnostic Impressions

Axis I.   300.7 Body Dysmorphic Disorder

Axis II.   Antisocial Personality Features

Axis III. Emeraldia Pigmentosa

Axis IV.   Problems with primary support group—History of parental rejection

              Problems related to the social environment—History of discrimination

Axis V.   GAF = 70 (At admission)

              GAF = 80 (Highest level past year)

DISCUSSION OF DIAGNOSTIC IMPRESSIONS

As we presented her, Elphaba was court-ordered to attend counseling. Her detention center counselor detected in her attitude and behavior a sense of being persecuted. In fact, Elphaba's history indicated an exaggerated preoccupation with the medical condition, Emeraldia Pigmentosa, that affected her skin with greenish pigmentation (and one aspect of her preoccupation was feeling persecuted because of the condition). Elphaba reported no other problems with mood, thoughts, or behavior besides preoccupation with her slight skin defect (keeping in mind that she was defensive about self-disclosure in the mandated counseling session).

Each section of the *DSM-IV-TR* classification system contains a group of diagnoses that share qualitatively similar symptoms or features. The common feature shared by all of the diagnoses contained in the Axis I category, Somatoform Disorders, is the experience of physical or bodily symptoms that suggest a medical problem, but for which there is not a full medical explanation (Pain Disorder and Hypochondriasis are two examples). Expanding on Elphaba's character, we detailed a distressing preoccupation with the physical anomaly of green skin that was impairing her adjustment. This kind of client presentation suggests a diagnosis of Body Dysmorphic Disorder.

When this diagnosis is made, it indicates that the client is preoccupied with an imagined defect in appearance—or, if a slight physical anomaly is noticeable, the person's concerned reactions are "markedly excessive" (APA, 2000a, p. 510), and cause clinically significant distress or impairment in important areas of functioning such as work, school, or social domains. This disorder is relatively common in medical settings, especially dermatology and cosmetic surgery settings, and sometimes is referred to as beauty hypochondria (Phillips, 2005).

One differential consideration regarding this Axis I diagnosis is whether Elphaba is experiencing a normally expected concern about her appearance, given her skin condition, rather than any diagnosable mental disorder at all. However, because her preoccupation is so consuming and has impaired her functioning in school, social, and other areas, a diagnosis is warranted to indicate clinical significance. Another differential consideration might be Delusional Disorder, Somatic Type; however, her skin anomaly, though less florid than she believes, is real and not a delusion.

On Axis II, problematic personality features and defenses can be listed even when they do not reflect a diagnosable Personality Disorder, particularly if these personality characteristics are important to understanding the client's functioning and are maladaptive for the person. We provided the notation, Antisocial Personality

Features, to describe Elphaba's offensive actions, which were disruptive to people and property, and therefore have some features of "disregard for, and violation of, the rights of others "(APA, 2000a, p. 685).

To complete the diagnosis, Elphaba's medical condition, Emeraldia Pigmentosa *(sic)* is listed on Axis III, her important social pressures are emphasized on Axis IV, and on Axis V her functioning is represented by GAF scores ranging from a recent period of good functioning with only normally expected, transient, everyday reactions and concerns, to the current period of mild symptoms causing some difficulty in school and social functioning that led to her referral. The information on these axes is consistent with the information on Axes I and II.

CASE CONCEPTUALIZATION

When Elphaba arrived at counseling, the counselor collected as much information as possible about the problematic situation Elphaba presented. The counselor first used this information to develop diagnostic impressions. Her concerns were described by Body Dysmorphic Behavior along with Antisocial Personality Features. Next, the counselor developed a case conceptualization. Whereas the purpose of diagnostic impressions is to *describe* the client's concerns, the goal of case conceptualization is to better *understand* and clinically *explain* the person's experiences (Neukrug & Schwitzer, 2006). It helps the counselor understand the etiology leading to Elphaba's Body Dysmorphic Disorder and the factors maintaining the concern. In turn, case conceptualization sets the stage for treatment planning. Treatment planning then provides a road map that plots out how the counselor and client expect to move from presenting concerns to positive outcomes (Seligman, 1993, p. 157)—helping Elphaba reduce or eliminate her problematic perceptions about herself and her reactions toward others.

When forming a case conceptualization, the clinician applies a purist counseling theory, an integration of two or more theories, an eclectic mix of theories, or a solution-focused combination of tactics to his or her understanding of the client. In this case, Elphaba's counselor based her conceptualization on a purist theory, Cognitive Behavior Therapy. She selected this approach based on her knowledge of current outcome research with clients experiencing Body Dysmorphic Disorder, and related personality factors and other symptoms (Critchfield & Smith-Benjamin, 2006; Livesley, 2007; Looper & Kirmayer, 2002). Cognitive Behavior Therapy also is consistent with this counselor's professional therapeutic viewpoint.

The counselor used the Inverted Pyramid Method of case conceptualization because it is especially designed to help clinicians more easily form their conceptual pictures of their clients' needs (Neukrug & Schwitzer, 2006; Schwitzer, 1996, 1997). The method has four steps: Problem Identification, Thematic Groupings, Theoretical Inferences, and Narrowed Inferences. The counselor's clinical thinking can be seen in Figure 8.5.

Step 1: Problem Identification. The first step is Problem Identification. Aspects of the presenting problem (thoughts, feelings, behaviors, physiological features), additional areas of concern besides the presenting concern, family and developmental history, in-session observations, clinical inquiries (medical problems, medications, past counseling, substance use, suicidality), and psychological assessments (problem checklists, personality inventories, mental status exam, specific clinical measures) all may contribute information at Step 1. The counselor "casts a wide net" in order to build Step 1 as exhaustively as possible (Neukrug & Schwitzer, 2006, p. 202). As can be seen in Figure 8.5, the counselor identified Elphaba's current primary concerns (anger, hostility, resentment, etc.); related concerns (poppy intoxication, freeing animals while intoxicated, etc.); and past concerns (history of being bullied, etc.) at Step 1. She attempted to go beyond just listing the main reason for referral and to be as complete as she could.

Step 2: Thematic Groupings. The second step is Thematic Groupings. The clinician organizes all of the exhaustive client information found in Step 1 into just a few intuitive-logical clinical groups, categories, or themes, on the basis of sensible common denominators (Neukrug & Schwitzer, 2006). Four different ways of forming the Step 2 theme groups can be used: Descriptive-Diagnosis Approach, Clinical Targets Approach, Areas of Dysfunction Approach, and Intrapsychic Approach. As can be seen in the figure, Elphaba's counselor selected the Areas of Dysfunction Approach. This approach sorts together all of the Step 1 information into "areas of dysfunction according to important life situations, life themes, or life roles and skills" (Neukrug & Schwitzer, 2006, p. 205).

The counselor grouped together (a) her growing-up experiences, history of being bullied, developmental history of her absent, ethnically different father into the theme, "history of negative experiences due to green skin"; (b) her anger, hostility, and antisocial features into the theme, "angry, hostile, fearful reactions to other people"; and (c) her illegal behaviors and use of intoxication into the theme "difficulty managing feelings of injustice." Her conceptual work at Step 2 gave the counselor a way to begin understanding and explaining Elphaba's areas of functioning and areas of concern more clearly, deeply, and meaningfully.

So far, at Steps 1 and 2, the counselor has used her clinical assessment skills and her clinical judgment to begin meaningfully understanding Elphaba's needs. Now, at Steps 3 and 4, she applies the theoretical approach she has selected. She begins making theoretical inferences to interpret and explain the processes or roots underlying Elphaba's concerns as they are seen in Steps 1 and 2.

Step 3: Theoretical Inferences. At Step 3, concepts from the counselor's selected theory, Cognitive Behavior Therapy, are applied to explain the experiences causing, and the mechanisms maintaining, Elphaba's problematic thoughts, feelings, and behaviors. The counselor tentatively matches the theme groups in Step 2

with this theoretical approach. In other words, the symptom constellations in Step 2, which were distilled from the symptoms in Step 1, now are combined using theory to show what are believed to be the underlying causes or psychological etiology of Elphaba's current needs (Neukrug & Schwitzer, 2006; Schwitzer, 2006, 2007).

According to Cognitive Behavior Therapy (Beck, 1995; 2005; Ellis, 1994; Ellis & MacLaren, 2005), irrational thinking, faulty beliefs, or other forms of cognitive errors lead individuals to engage in problematic behaviors and to experience negative moods and attitudes. As can be seen in Figure 8.5, when the counselor applied these cognitive-behavior therapy concepts, she explained at Step 3 that the various issues noted in Step 1 (hostility, history of bullying, etc.), which can be understood to be themes of (a) a history of negative experiences, (b) angry and fearful reactions to others, and (c) difficulty managing reactions to perceived injustices (Step 2), are rooted in or caused by several types of cognitive errors (magnification, overgeneralization, and absolutist thinking) and inaccurate, problem behavioral responses (reacting hostilely before others can be unfair and mistreating, and acting on injustice without concern for consequences). These are detailed on Figure 8.5.

Step 4: Narrowed Inferences. At Step 4, the clinician's selected theory continues to be used to address still-deeper issues when they exist (Schwitzer, 2006, 2007). At this step, "still-deeper, more encompassing, or more central, causal themes" are formed (Neukrug & Schwitzer, 2006, p. 207). Continuing to apply Cognitive Behavior Therapy concepts at Step 4, Elphaba's counselor presented a single, deepest, most-fundamental cognitive error that she believed to be most explanatory and causal regarding Elphaba's reasons for referral: the deepest irrational belief that "people must always treat me unfairly because of my pigmentation and I am helpless to change this." When all four steps are completed, the client information in Step 1 leads to logical-intuitive groupings on the basis of

Figure 8.5   Elphaba's Inverted Pyramid Case Conceptualization Summary: Cognitive Behavior Therapy

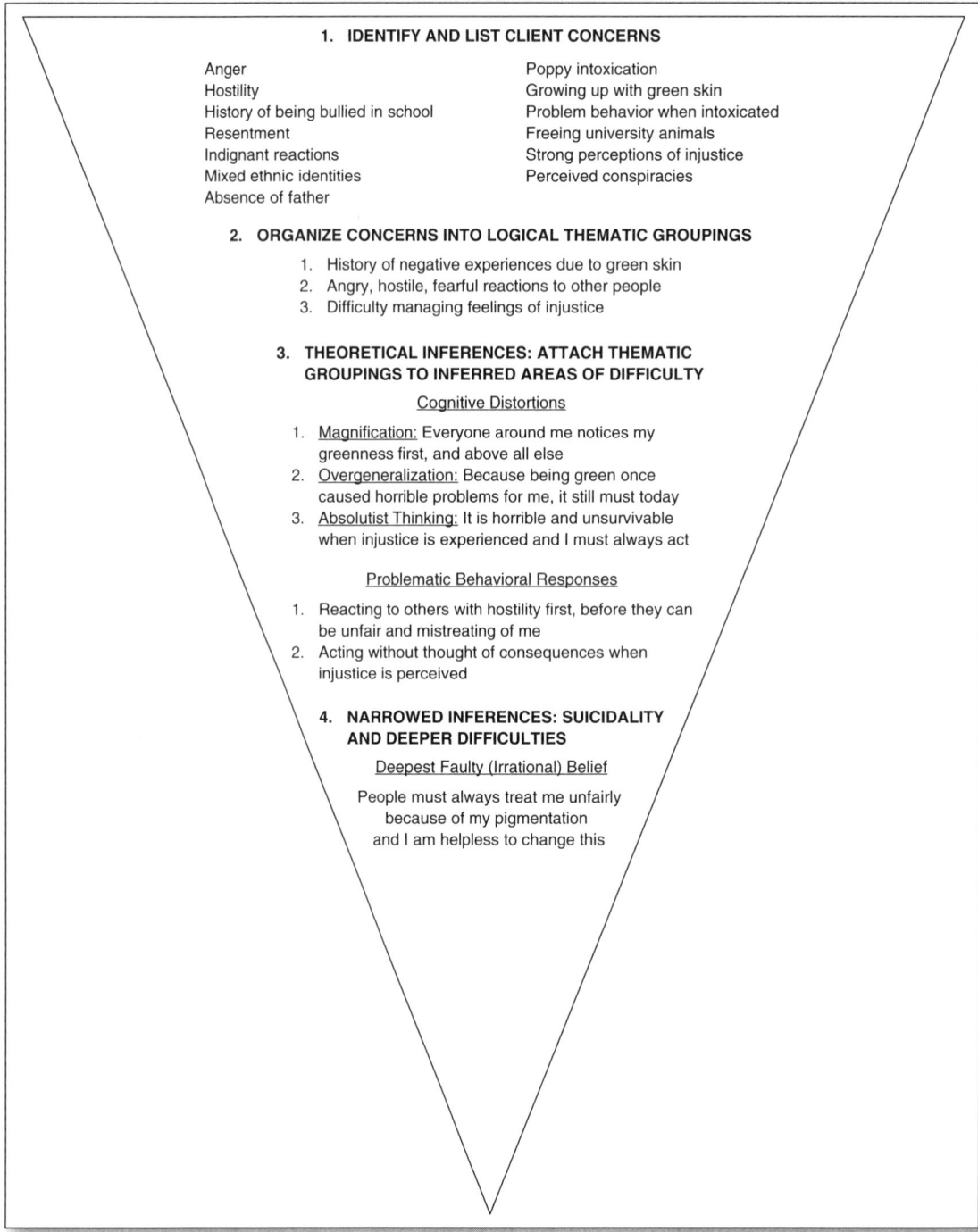

1. IDENTIFY AND LIST CLIENT CONCERNS

Anger
Hostility
History of being bullied in school
Resentment
Indignant reactions
Mixed ethnic identities
Absence of father

Poppy intoxication
Growing up with green skin
Problem behavior when intoxicated
Freeing university animals
Strong perceptions of injustice
Perceived conspiracies

2. ORGANIZE CONCERNS INTO LOGICAL THEMATIC GROUPINGS

1. History of negative experiences due to green skin
2. Angry, hostile, fearful reactions to other people
3. Difficulty managing feelings of injustice

3. THEORETICAL INFERENCES: ATTACH THEMATIC GROUPINGS TO INFERRED AREAS OF DIFFICULTY

Cognitive Distortions

1. Magnification: Everyone around me notices my greenness first, and above all else
2. Overgeneralization: Because being green once caused horrible problems for me, it still must today
3. Absolutist Thinking: It is horrible and unsurvivable when injustice is experienced and I must always act

Problematic Behavioral Responses

1. Reacting to others with hostility first, before they can be unfair and mistreating of me
2. Acting without thought of consequences when injustice is perceived

4. NARROWED INFERENCES: SUICIDALITY AND DEEPER DIFFICULTIES

Deepest Faulty (Irrational) Belief

People must always treat me unfairly
because of my pigmentation
and I am helpless to change this

common denominators in Step 2, the groupings then are explained using theory at Step 3, and then, finally, at Step 4, further deeper explanations are made. From start to finish, the thoughts, feelings, behaviors, and physiological features in the topmost portions are connected on down the pyramid into deepest dynamics.

The completed pyramid now is used to plan treatment, in which the counselor and Elphaba will confront her cognitive distortions, problematic behavioral responses, and deep faulty belief.

TREATMENT PLANNING

At this point, Elphaba's clinician at the Oz Community Mental Health Center (OCMHC) has collected all available information about the problems that have been of concern and led to her referral. Based upon this information, the counselor developed a five-axis *DSM-IV-TR* diagnosis and then, using the "inverted pyramid" (Neukrug & Schwitzer, 2006; Schwitzer, 1996, 1997), formulated a working clinical *explanation* of Elphaba's difficulties and their etiology that we called the *case conceptualization.* This, in turn, guides us to the next critical step in our clinical work, called the *treatment plan,* the primary purpose of which is to map out a logical and goal-oriented strategy for making positive changes in the client's life. In essence, the treatment plan is a road map *"for reducing or eliminating disruptive symptoms that are impeding the client's ability to reach positive mental health outcomes"* (Neukrug & Schwitzer, 2006, p. 225). As such, it is the cornerstone of our work with not only Elphaba, but with all clients who present with Body Dysmorphic Disorder and Antisocial Personality Features (Jongsma & Peterson, 2006; Jongsma et al., 2003a, 2003b; Seligman, 1993, 1998, 2004).

A comprehensive treatment plan must integrate all of the information from the biopsychosocial interview, diagnosis, and case conceptualization into a coherent plan of action. This *plan* comprises four main components, which include (1) a behavioral definition of the problem(s), (2) the selection of achievable goals,

(3) the determination of treatment modes, and (4) the documentation of how change will be measured. The *behavioral definition of the problem(s)* consolidates the results of the case conceptualization into a concise hierarchical list of problems and concerns that will be the focus of treatment. The *selection of achievable goals* refers to assessing and prioritizing the client's concerns into a *hierarchy of urgency* that also takes into account the client's motivation for change, level of dysfunction, and real-world influences on his or her problems. The *determination of treatment modes* refers to selection of the specific interventions, which are matched to the uniqueness of the client and to his or her goals and clearly tied to a particular theoretical orientation (Neukrug & Schwitzer, 2006). Finally, the clinician must establish how change will be measured, based upon a number of factors, including client records and self-report of change, in-session observations by the clinician, clinician ratings, results of standardized evaluations such as the Beck Depression Inventory-II (Beck et al., 1996) or a family functioning questionnaire, pre-post treatment comparisons, and reports by other treating professionals.

The four-step method discussed above can be seen in Figure 6.1 (p. 109) and is outlined below for the case of Elphaba Thropp, followed by her specific treatment plan.

Step 1: Behavioral Definition of Problems. The first step in treatment planning is to carefully review the case conceptualization, paying particular attention to the results of Step 2 (Thematic Groupings), Step 3 (Theoretical Inferences) and Step 4 (Narrowed Inferences). The identified clinical themes reflect the core areas of concern and distress for the client, while the theoretical and narrowed inferences offer clinical speculation as to their origins. In the case of Elphaba, there are three primary areas of concern. The first, "history of negative experiences due to green skin," refers to the negative feelings and thoughts about herself and others related to growing up with green skin and the sense of mixed ethnic/racial identity. The second, "angry, hostile, fearful reactions to other people," refers to her anger, hostility, indignant reactions, and resentment of others throughout her life and continuing into the present. The third, "difficulty managing feelings of injustice," refers to her perceptions of conspiracies, antisocial acts such as freeing the clinic animals, and feelings of righteous indignation. These symptoms and stresses are consistent with the diagnosis of Body Dysmorphic Disorder and Antisocial Personality Features (APA, 2000a; Critchfield & Smith-Benjamin, 2006; Livesley, 2007; Looper & Kirmayer, 2002; Phillips, McElroy, Keck, Pope, & Hudson, 1993).

Step 2: Identify and Articulate Goals for Change. The second step is the selection of achievable goals, which is based upon a number of factors, including the most pressing or urgent behavioral, emotional, and interpersonal concerns and symptoms as identified by the client and clinician, the willingness and ability of the client to work on those particular goals, and the realistic (real-world) achievability of those goals (Neukrug & Schwitzer, 2006). At this stage, of treatment planning, it is important to recognize that not all of the client's problems can be addressed at once, so we focus initially on those that cause the greatest distress and impairment. New goals can be created as old ones are achieved. In the case of Elphaba, the goals are divided into three prominent areas. The first, "history of negative experiences due to green skin," requires that we help Elphaba to resolve her negative feelings and thoughts about herself and her green skin as well as reconcile conflicts within her sense of racial and ethnic identity. The second, "angry, hostile, fearful reactions to other people," requires that we help Elphaba to resolve negative perceptions of and reactions to other people, and understand the relationship between her negative feelings and thoughts about herself and toward others. The third, "difficulty managing feelings of injustice," requires that we help Elphaba to develop an understanding of the relationship between her feelings of injustice and her antisocial behavior and to eliminate her conspiratorial thoughts and antisocial behavior.

Step 3: Describe Therapeutic Interventions. This is perhaps the most critical step in the treatment planning process because the clinician must now integrate information from a number of sources, including the case conceptualization, the delineation of the client's problems and goals, and the treatment literature, paying particular attention to *empirically supported treatment* (EST) and *evidence-based practice* (EBP). In essence, the clinician must align his or her treatment approach with scientific evidence from the fields of counseling and psychotherapy. Wampold (2001) identifies two types of evidence-based counseling research: studies that demonstrate "absolute efficacy," that is, the fact that counseling and psychotherapy work, and those that demonstrate "relative efficacy," that is, the fact that certain theoretical/technical approaches work best for certain clients with particular problems (Psychoanalysis, Gestalt Therapy, Cognitive Behavior Therapy, Brief Solution-Focused Therapy, Cognitive Therapy, Dialectical Behavior Therapy, Person-Centered Therapy, Expressive/Creative Therapies, Interpersonal Therapy, and Feminist Therapy); and when delivered through specific treatment modalities (individual, group, and family counseling).

In the case of Elphaba, we have decided to use Cognitive Behavior Therapy (Beck, 1995, 2005; Ellis, 1994; Ellis & MacLaren, 2005), which has been found to be highly effective in counseling and psychotherapy with adults who experience the symptoms of Body Dysmorphic Disorder (Butters & Cash, 1987; Looper & Kirmayer, 2002; Rosen, Reiter, & Orosan, 1995). The approach relies on a variety of cognitive techniques (reframing, challenging irrational thoughts, and cognitive restructuring) and behavioral techniques (reinforcement for and shaping of adaptive behavior, extinction of maladaptive behaviors, systematic desensitization, and exposure with response prevention) (Ball et al., 2006; Frank et al., 2005; Milkowitz, 2008). Elphaba's long-standing and deeply ingrained issues and problems will be addressed through a variety of techniques that have been found to be effective with a range of personality disorders (Critchfield & Smith-Benjamin, 2006; Livesley, 2007; Looper & Kirmayer, 2002), while her additional emotional, behavioral, and cognitive symptoms will be addressed through group Gestalt Therapy, which relies on a variety of empathetic, directive, and confrontational techniques (the use of "I" language, dream work, bringing together parts of self, and taking responsibility)

(Gaffney, 2006a, 2006b; Neukrug, 2011; Polster & Polster, 1999). In Elphaba's case, some of the techniques will include identifying and changing negative thoughts about her skin and identifying anger triggers

Step 4: Provide Outcome Measures of Change. This last step in treatment planning requires that we specify how change will be measured and indicate the extent to which progress has been made toward realizing these goals (Neukrug & Schwitzer, 2006). The counselor has considerable flexibility in this phase and may choose from a number of objective domains (psychological tests and measures of self-esteem, depression, psychosis, interpersonal relationship, anxiety, etc.), quasi-objective measures (the *DSM-IV-TR's* Axis V GAF scale; pre-post

clinician, client, and psychiatric ratings), and subjective ratings (client self-report, clinician's in-session observations). In Elphaba's case, we have implemented a number of these, including a pre-post measure on the Body Image Disturbance questionnaire (Cash, Phillips, Santos, & Hrabosky, 2004) and Clinical Anger Scale (Snell, Gum, Shuck, Mosley, & Hite, 1995), post measures of GAF functioning in the normal range (>85), client acceptance of herself and her skin and no arrests for antisocial acts for a period of 1 year.

The completed treatment plan is now developed through which the counselor and Elphaba will modify the way she thinks about herself, others, and the world, and help her to channel her many skills into prosocial directions. The treatment plan is described below and summarized in Table 8.5.

TREATMENT PLAN

Client: Elphaba Thropp

Service Provider: Oz Community Mental Health Center (OCMHC)

BEHAVIORAL DEFINITION OF PROBLEMS:

1. History of negative experiences due to green skin—Negative feelings and thoughts about herself and others related to growing up with green skin, and the sense of mixed ethnic/racial identity

2. Angry, hostile, fearful reactions to other people—Anger, hostility, indignant reactions, and resentment of others throughout her life and continuing into the present

3. Difficulty managing feelings of injustice—Feelings of righteous indignation, perceptions of conspiracies, and antisocial acts such as freeing the clinic animals

GOALS FOR CHANGE:

1. History of negative experiences due to green skin

   - Resolve negative feelings and thoughts about herself and her green skin
   - Reconcile conflicts within her sense of racial/ethnic identity

2. Angry, hostile, fearful reactions to other people

   - Resolve negative perceptions of and reactions to other people
   - Understand the relationship between her negative feelings about herself and toward others
   - Eliminate use of Poppies to regulate mood states

(Continued)

(Continued)

3. Difficulty managing feelings of injustice

- Develop understanding of the relationship between her feelings of injustice and her anti-social behavior
- Eliminate thoughts of conspiracies
- Eliminate antisocial behavior

THERAPEUTIC INTERVENTIONS:

A moderate-term course of individual cognitive behavior and group Gestalt counseling (6–9 months)

1. History of negative experiences due to green skin

- Identify and change automatic negative thoughts about her skin
- Substituting negative thoughts with positive statements about her appearance
- Response prevention to inhibit compulsive checking of her skin in reflective surfaces
- Developing alternate beliefs about her appearance

2. Angry, hostile, fearful reactions to people

- Identify situations, thoughts, and feelings that trigger anger
- Learn anger-management techniques in context of self-calming strategies
- Identify and change automatic negative thoughts about people
- Substitute negative thoughts about people with positive statements
- Verbalize an understanding of the benefits to self and others of empathy and sensitivity to others' beliefs and needs
- Implement relapse-prevention plan for anger management

3. Difficulty managing feelings of injustice

- Identify and understand origin of "injustice schema" in early family relationships and social experiences
- Use "empty chair" technique to dialogue with perpetrators of perceived injustice
- Gestalt "dream work" around injustice

OUTCOME MEASURES OF CHANGE:

The resolution of her conflictual relationship with herself and others, elimination of antisocial thoughts, feelings, and actions, and overall improved adjustment and functioning in her daily life as measured by:

- Client report of improved self-image absent preoccupation with her green skin
- Pre-post improvement of functioning as measured by the Body Image Disturbance Questionnaire
- Pre-post improvement on the Clinical Anger Scale (CAS)
- Post measures of GAF functioning in the normal (>85) range
- Absence of arrests for antisocial behavior and illegal acts for a period of 1 year
- Clinician observation of improved self-image and reduced anger toward self and others

Table 8.5   Elphaba's Treatment Plan Summary: Cognitive Behavior Therapy

Goals for Change	Therapeutic Interventions	Outcome Measures of Change
History of negative experiences due to green skin	History of negative experiences due to green skin	The resolution of her conflictual relationship with herself and others, elimination of antisocial thoughts, feelings, and actions, and overall improved adjustment and functioning in her daily life as measured by:
Resolve negative feelings and thoughts about herself and her green skin	Identify and change automatic negative thoughts about her skin	
Reconcile conflicts within her sense of racial/ethnic identity	Substituting negative thoughts with positive statements about her appearance	Client report of improved self-image absent preoccupation with her green skin
Angry, hostile, fearful reactions to other people	Response prevention to inhibit compulsive checking of her skin in reflective surfaces	
Resolve negative perceptions of and reactions to other people	Developing alternate beliefs about her appearance	Pre-post improvement of functioning as measured by the Body Image Disturbance Questionnaire
Understand the relationship between her negative feelings about herself and toward others	Angry, hostile, fearful reactions to other people	Pre-post improvement on the Clinical Anger Scale (CAS)
Eliminate use of Poppies to regulate mood states	Identify situations, thoughts, and feelings that trigger anger	Post measures of GAF functioning in the normal (>85) range
Difficulty managing feelings of injustice	Learn anger-management techniques in context of self-calming strategies	Absence of arrests for antisocial behavior and illegal acts for a period of 1 year
Develop understanding of the relationship between her feelings of injustice and her antisocial behavior	Identify and change automatic negative thoughts about people	Clinician observation of improved self-image and reduced anger toward self and others
Eliminate thoughts of conspiracies	Substitute negative thoughts about people with positive statements	
Eliminate antisocial behavior	Verbalize an understanding of the benefits to self and others of empathy and sensitivity to others' beliefs and needs	
	Implement relapse-prevention plan for anger management	
	Difficulty managing feelings of injustice	
	Identify and understand origin of "injustice schema" in early family relationships and social experiences	
	Use "empty chair" technique to dialogue with perpetrators of perceived injustice	
	Gestalt "dream work" around injustice	

FOLLOW-UP: DIAGNOSIS, CASE CONCEPTUALIZATION, AND TREATMENT PLANNING THEMES—CHAPTER SUMMARY

This chapter presented a compelling clinical caseload comprising adolescents, Edward Cullen, Jamal, Juno, and Claire, along with a young adult, Elphaba. The caseload had a gender balance of three female clients and two males. Among the caseload's diversity were three American clients; one international person, Jamal, of Mumbai, India; and Elphaba, from the Land of Oz. Upper, middle, and very low socioeconomic statuses were represented by this group of clients. The clients all were presented as having heterosexual identities.

One of the clients, Jamal, was referred to the local Government Community Services Center, and Juno was seen at Minnetonka's local Family Services Center. One client, Edward, was referred to counseling by his school counselor, and another, Elphaba, was court mandated to seek treatment.

Among the adolescent and young adult concerns presented by our clients making up this chapter's caseload, Edward sought assistant for difficulties characterized diagnostically as recurrent episodes of Major Depressive Disorder, along with dependent personality features; Jamal required assistance with Acute Stress Disorder; and Elphaba was dealing with Body Dysmorphic Disorder, along with Antisocial Personality Features. Whereas Claire addressed three different diagnostic concerns related to cannabis abuse, eating problems, and hair-pulling (trichotillomania), Juno presented counseling issues related to teen pregnancy but no clear-cut diagnosable mental health problems.

Looking at the counseling theories represented, their counselors formed case conceptualizations and then treatment plans based on Person-Centered Counseling, Brief Contemporary Psychodynamic Psychotherapy, and Cognitive Behavior Therapy—along with a psychotherapeutic integration of Cognitive Behavior Therapy and Interpersonal Psychotherapy, and an application of Brief Solution-Focused Counseling emphasizing cognitive behavioral interventions with adolescents.

In their treatment plans, these clients' counselors expressed hopes that their clients would achieve such outcomes as developing self-affirming self-attitudes, decreased dependence, and improved mood and functioning (Edward); alleviation of symptoms of posttraumatic stress and reversal of poverty circumstances (Jamal); development of congruence between ideal and actual self, healthy attitudes, and open and effective communication (Juno); elimination of acting-out behaviors and improved overall functioning at home and at school (Claire); and resolution of conflictual relationship with self and others, and antisocial dynamics (Elphaba).

STUDY QUESTIONS AND LEARNING ACTIVITIES

Based on your understanding of this chapter's cases, consider and respond to these Study Questions and Learning Activities:

1. This caseload is a compelling one.

   a. If you were assigned this group of clients, what would be your initial reactions to their individual characteristics and differences? Working with adolescents, late adolescents, and young adults? Their reasons for referral?

   b. What would you identify as your greatest strengths for assisting these five clients? Your areas of greatest need for growth?

2. In their Basic Case Summaries, this chapter's counselors focused on their clients' earlier developmental and family experiences, presenting concerns, assessment of current distress and areas and life roles in which they were experiencing difficulties, client strengths, and hopes for change. There was an emphasis on Edward's earlier and recent developmental history, and the patterns and severity of his mood symptoms; the recent traumatic events

Jamal experienced and their consequences; Juno's recent issues surrounding her pregnancy in the context of her earlier and ongoing developmental and family experiences and changes; Claire's various recent concerns, also in the context of her ongoing and current developmental and family experiences and dynamics; and for Elphaba, medical information about her "pigmentosa" as well as the negative effects of her problematic behaviors on campus and in the local community.

a. Keeping in mind that the initial counseling meeting, screening session, or intake interview usually requires the counselor to balance rapport and trust-building, on one hand, and assessment and information-gathering, on the other hand, what would you identify as your greatest strengths when engaging these five clients in the counseling process, and gathering the clinical information needed to conceptualize and plan for their counseling process? Your areas of greatest need for growth?

b. Looking at the five Basic Case Summaries, how does this type of clinical writing differ from your everyday thinking and conversation about adolescents and young adults? What are your levels of comfort, skill, and experience with this type of professional writing? What steps can you take to further develop or improve these skills?

c. What suggestions would you have for one of more of the counselors in this chapter regarding missing, overlooked, or underemphasized—or overemphasized—information gathered and reported in the Basic Case Summaries? What would you like to have known more about? What methods could be used—clinical interview questions, observations, psychological measures, or other means—to find the additional information you would seek?

3. This chapter illustrated *DSM-IV-TR* diagnoses found in the following sections: Mood Disorders; Anxiety Disorders; Substance-Related Disorders; Somatoform Disorders; Eating Disorders; Impulse Control Disorders Not Elsewhere Classified; and Personality Disorders—plus Other Conditions That May Be a Focus of Clinical Attention.

a. How familiar are you with these sections of the *DSM-IV-TR?* What is your comfort level using the *DSM-IV-TR* to explore these sets of concerns? Which of these groups of disorders are likely to be most important to you in the practicum, internship, residency, or professional practice settings in which you hope to work?

b. What are your attitudes, reactions, or thoughts concerning diagnosis of childhood disorders? Concerning the diagnosis of behavioral consequences of problematic substance use? Concerning diagnosing life-long patterns characterized as personality disorders? How can you further explore or develop your professional attitudes about diagnosis of these types of concerns?

c. What will be your next steps in gaining greater comfort and skills at diagnosis of the attention-deficit and disruptive behavior disorders of childhood? Substance use and substance-induced disorders? Personality disorders?

d. What are your attitudes, reactions, or thoughts concerning use of Axis IV to record psychosocial and environmental stressors (such as Jamal's economic and housing problems of extreme poverty and homelessness) and Axis V to record general medical problems (such as Elphaba's "Emeraldia Pigmentosa" [sic])? What will be your next steps in gaining greater comfort and skills with these axes?

e. Among this group of clients, Axis V Global Assessment of Functioning (GAF) scores ranged from 50 (Edward's serious symptoms) to 78 (Juno's transient and expectable reactions). What are your attitudes, reactions, or thoughts concerning use of Axis V GAF scores to estimate the client's overall level of functioning? Do you agree with the counselors' estimates found in this chapter? What will be your next steps in gaining greater comfort and skills estimating Axis V GAF scores?

4. This chapter's cases included three examples of case conceptualization and treatment planning using purist counselor theories, one example of psychotherapeutic integration, and one application of brief solution-focused counseling.

a. What is your level of familiarity with the various counseling theories illustrated in this chapter: Cognitive Behavior Therapy? Interpersonal Psychotherapy? Brief Solution-Focused Counseling (Emphasizing Cognitive Behavioral Interventions With Adolescents)? Person-Centered Counseling? Brief Contemporary Psychodynamic Psychotherapy? What do you believe are their relative strengths and weaknesses? For which individuals do they seem to be a good match? For what types of client concerns do they seem to be potentially effective? What do the evidence and discussions found in the current literature say about this?

b. Which of these theories seem to be a good fit with your own attitudes and skills? Which interest you the most?

c. To learn more, review the resources and references cited in the chapter, interview a practicing counselor who uses these theories in his or her everyday work, seek clinical supervision from a supervisor experienced with the approach, enroll in a special topics class, or look for continuing education workshops and conference presentations covering these approaches.

d. What are your thoughts, reactions, and comfort level integrating multiple psychotherapeutic approaches to address the needs of your clients? Which theories are you most likely, or least likely, to consider integrating into your approach? How will you decide when, with whom, and in what ways, to integrate multiple approaches? To consider and learn more about integrating approaches such as Cognitive Behavior Therapy and Interpersonal Therapy, interview a practicing counselor who uses an integration of these theories in his or her everyday work, seek clinical supervision from a supervisor experienced with psychotherapeutic integration of these theories, or seek other professional consultations and learning opportunities.

e. What are your thoughts, reactions, and comfort level employing a Brief Solution-Focused Approach to address the needs of your clients? What knowledge or skills will you need to be an effective Brief Solution-Focused Counselor?

f. How will you decide when, with whom, and in what ways to employ Brief Solution-Focused Approaches? To consider and learn more about solution-focused counseling strategies, interview a practicing counselor who uses a solution focus in his or her everyday work, seek clinical supervision from a supervisor experienced with solution-focused counseling, or seek other professional consultations and learning opportunities.

5. The case conceptualizations found in this chapter began with casting a wide net for client concerns and dynamics, next forming intuitive-logical groupings to begin better understanding the clients' presentations, and then applying counseling theories to make clinical inferences about the clients' situations.

a. How does this type of professional clinical thinking differ from your everyday thinking, conversation, and analysis about people? What are your levels of comfort, skill, and experience with this type of clinical thinking? What steps can you take to further develop or improve your conceptualizing skills?

b. What are your thoughts, reactions, and critique of the ways these counselors grouped together: Edward's severe depression symptoms and personality features? Jamal's cognitive, affective, physiological, and behavioral posttraumatic symptoms and environmental challenges? Juno's adolescent background stresses, pregnancy-related stresses, and stresses from parental reactions? Claire's successful developmental history and current multiple "acting-out" problems? Elphaba's negative history, angry reactions to other people, and difficulty with feelings of injustice? Do you agree with each of these thematic groupings? How might you have organized these differently, more usefully, or more effectively?

c. What are your thoughts and reactions pertaining to the ways the counselors applied the various theoretical approaches in order to explain, make inferences about, and prepare for treatment planning with, these clients? What were your reactions to the counselors' presentations of: Edward's negative cognitive distortions (Cognitive Behavior Therapy) and habitual learned response pattern (Interpersonal Psychotherapy)? Juno's lack of conditions of self-worth impeding her actualization? Claire's adopting problematic behaviors as defenses and compensations for insufficient psychological parental mirroring (Kohut's Self-Psychology)? Elphaba's magnification, overgeneralization, problematic behavioral responses, and deeper faulty belief (also Cognitive Behavior Therapy)? Do you agree with the ways the counselor used the various theories with these clients? How might you have applied the theories differently, more usefully, or more effectively?

6. A fully developed treatment plan was presented for each of the individuals comprising this chapter's caseload. The treatment plans provide goals for change, interventions, and outcome measures.

   a. How does this type of clinical writing, thinking, and preparation for the professional counseling process differ from your everyday approach to engaging in helpful relationships with people? What are your levels of comfort, skill, and experience with this type of professional writing, thinking, and preparation? What steps can you take to further develop or improve your treatment planning skills for the types of practicum, internship, residency, or work settings that are of most interest to you?

   b. This chapter's treatment plans first list goals for change for each "client" character, next apply the selected counseling theory to clearly state the interventions and approaches to be used, and finally identify ways to measure the expected changes. What are your thoughts, reactions, and critique of the ways this chapter's counselors prepared Edward's, Jamal's, Juno's, Claire's, and Elphaba's treatment plans? What interests you most about these plans? What raises questions for you?

   c. What are your thoughts and reactions pertaining to the cognitive behavioral (Edward and Elphaba) and interpersonal psychotherapeutic work (Edward), solution-focused cognitive behavioral strategies (Jamal), person-centered practices (Juno), and contemporary psychodynamic techniques (Claire) outlined as interventions? With which are you most familiar? Least familiar? Unfamiliar? Which will you select to learn more about through further reading, clinical supervision, or other professional development? Alternatively, which do not seem to be close fits with your own preferred approach?

   d. These clients' counselors' used counselor observation, client report, change scores on psychological measures and the GAF, behavioral reports, and other means to measure outcomes. As you review the outcome measures found on Edward's, Jamal's, Juno's, Claire's, and Elphaba's treatment plans, consider these questions: Do the measures seem realistic and accomplishable? Are they concrete and specific enough to indicate change? Are they sensitive to the needs of the client? Which of these measures will become a regular part of your own repertoire, which might you decline to use, and what additional measures might you add to your own list? What new skills and competencies might you need to develop in order to effectively report on your own clients' outcomes?

7. Now, working independently, with a partner, or in a small group, select your own "client" from among the pop culture world of Troubled Youth in Film and on Stage. Develop your own narrative about the client's arrival at counseling. Then, prepare a fully completed Basic Case Summary, Diagnostic Impressions, Case Conceptualization, and Treatment Plan!

9

ANIMATED CHARACTERS

The Cases of Cleveland Brown,
Jessie, Tinkerbell, Smithers, and Belle

PREVIEW: POPULAR CULTURE THEMES

In this section, you will meet a group of characters who share the unique pedigree of being animated. Although they vary in age, race, sexual orientation, and, of course, life circumstances, they are all fantasy characters created, at least ostensibly, for child audiences, but in reality have appeal to all age groups. Some of them have come from television while others have their origins in film; however, when taken together they offer a fascinating array of individuals.

As a group, these characters demonstrate the very powerful way in which popular culture bridges the gap between nonfiction and fantasy as well as between entertainment and serious story-telling. This type of analysis is particularly important in light of the ongoing controversy over the value and potentially destructive effect of cartoons on viewers, particularly younger ones. It has been argued that cartoons are a diminutive and debased form of entertainment that perpetuate gender stereotyping, racism, and violence (Abel, 1995; Levinson, 1975; McCauley, Woods, Coolidge, & Kulick,1983; Swan, 1995; Thompson & Zerbino, 1995), and that they are a medium that distorts children's moral development by modeling the demonization of the "other" (Fouts, Callan, & Piasentin, 2006). Further, given the liberal use of pejorative terms like "daffy," "loony," and "crazy," it has been asserted that cartoons sow the seeds for stigmatization of the mentally ill through negative vocabulary and character depictions (Wilson, Nairn, Coverdale, & Panapa, 2000). In contrast to these arguments, it has been suggested that "cartoons also contain prosocial messages, provide an opportunity for shared narratives and tap into timeless truths often found in myth and folklore" (Rubin, 2008, p. 229).

With regard to the specific characters in this section, Cleveland Brown had his origins as the mousey neighbor of the Griffins in Seth McFarland's brash and satirical Fox Broadcasting Company's cartoon *Family Guy*. Too big and rich a character to survive as second-string, Cleveland left the familiar confines of Quahog to star in his own show called *The Cleveland Show.* In our presentation, Cleveland Brown struggles with Dysthymic Disorder, Alcohol Abuse, and Erectile Dysfunction. Jessie is the feisty cowgirl toy and costar of the blockbuster films *Toy Story*

2 and *Toy Story 3,* and as depicted in these films, part of the fictional vintage children's television show *Woody's Roundup.* Beyond film. Jessie has become popular as a real toy in the marketplace. In our presentation, Jessie struggles with Reactive Attachment Disorder. Tinkerbell, or Momma Pixie as we refer to her in this book, is the sidekick of the perennial Disney child character Peter Pan. She has flown far from Neverland and her role in the Hollywood film to star in contemporary animated and musical versions of the original story, and has also been made and remade into a toy. In our presentation, Tinkerbell struggles with a Schizoaffective Disorder and Borderline Personality Features. Waylon Smithers is the tormented nice guy/whipping boy of his employer Montgomery Burns on the long-running Fox Broadcasting Company's not-really-for-children cartoon *The Simpsons.* In our presentation, Waylon Smithers struggles with Identity Problems. And finally, there is Belle, whom we call Belle Beastly, star of the classic tale *Beauty and the Beast.* Although now best known through her incarnation in Disney's movie of the same title, Belle has actually been around for well over a century since first appearing in literature, and later on stage, television, lunchboxes, and in the Ice Capades. In our presentation, Belle struggles with Social Phobia and Avoidant Personality Features. This unlikely cast of characters brought to life in virtually every venue of popular culture seems, on the surface, to have been created for little more than our entertainment. They dance, sing, tell jokes, come from exotic places, and even bear the brunt, at times, of caustic humor. In essence, they do just what we expect of animated characters. However, as you will see in this section, each one of these fictional and fantasy characters experiences very real and compelling stories. They struggle to convince themselves and each other that they matter and that their pain and suffering are very real. Each, in his or her own way, struggles to be acknowledged and validated. Although they are both young and older, each one of them has experienced loss, has fantasies of being complete or whole, and suffers at the hands of demons, both from within and outside of themselves. Cleveland Brown, Jessie, Tinkerbell, Waylon Smithers, and Belle will provide you with the opportunity to explore "very real" clinical issues.

APPROACHES TO LEARNING

As you learn about this group of characters, pay attention to:

- Whether these cartoon characters perpetuate destructive stereotypes or contain useful stories for clinical development, or both.
- How closely the details of their "fictional" life stories and symptom presentations match your current understanding of psychopathology.
- The way that the stories of Cleveland Brown, Waylon Smithers, and Belle Beastly realistically reflect issues of race, sexual orientation, and gender in the clinical population.
- How your understanding of the various theories of normative development and psychopathology help you to appreciate these characters' treatment needs.

CASE 9.1   *THE CLEVELAND SHOW'S* CLEVELAND

INTRODUCING THE CHARACTER

Cleveland Brown stars in *The Cleveland Show,* the recent spin-off of Fox TV's irreverent animated television smash hit *Family Guy.* Although some writers have cautioned that aspects of Cleveland's portrayal seem to incorporate negative *Amos and Andy* sorts of historically stereotypical portrayals of race, other critics have more positively characterized Cleveland and his show as an interesting effort to expand the representation of African American characters and their issues as seen on television and especially on animated television. We believe Cleveland's character has enough depth and richness to be an engaging popular culture figure that raises important and challenging clinical and social questions.

On *Family Guy,* Cleveland Brown is the gentle, patient, pleasant-natured African American neighbor of the Griffin family. The butt of jokes because of his perennial smile and the unflappable good nature it represents, Cleveland is taken advantage of by neighbors and friends. One neighbor in particular, Leonard Quagmire, has an affair with Cleveland's wife, Loretta. While still reeling from his wife's infidelity, Cleveland's home in Quahog is accidentally destroyed by his neighbor, Peter.

Although the house destruction is a running gag on *Family* Guy, this time it is Cleveland's last straw. He divorces his wife, Loretta, takes custody of his son, Cleveland, Jr., leaves his former life behind, and sets off to restart and reclaim his life in his childhood town of Stoolbend. On the way to his childhood home, Cleveland has a chance encounter in Virginia with his high school sweetheart, Donna Tubbs. Their romance is rekindled, and Donna decides to rearrange her own life by marrying Cleveland. Cleveland, Cleveland, Jr., Donna, and her two children, Roberta, age 16, and Rallo, age 5, all relocate to Stoolbend, where Cleveland leaves his old occupation as a deli operator behind and begins a new career installing TV cable. Naturally, Cleveland brings many of his dynamics and concerns with him to the new setting. Using *The Cleveland Show* as our starting point, the following basic case summary and diagnostic impressions explore our view of several possible clinically significant patterns that are evident, pertaining to mood, substance use, sexual dysfunction, and family relationship problems.

Meet the Client

You can assess the client in action by viewing clips of Cleveland Brown's video material at the following websites:

- http://www.youtube.com/watch?v=sT-sNBKpDEo *The Cleveland Show* trailer
- http://www.youtube.com/watch?v=HHXZ-UMLY60 Welcome to Stoolbend
- http://www.imdb.com/title/tt1195935/videogallery/content_type-Full%20 Episode This link provides access to full episodes of *The Cleveland Show*

BASIC CASE SUMMARY

Identifying Information. Cleveland Brown is a 42-year-old African American man who recently relocated to Stoolbend, Virginia. Mr. Brown currently lives in a blended family comprising his biological son, Cleveland, Jr., age 14; wife, Donna, to whom he has been married for about 1 year (following a divorce from his first wife and mother of Cleveland, Jr.); and Donna Brown's two children from a previous marriage, Roberta, age 16, and Rallo, age 5. Mr. Brown is employed as a cable TV installation professional. He was dressed and appeared appropriate during the interview and was an open and engaged participant in the session. It is notable that Mr. Brown appears considerably overweight for his height.

Presenting Concern. Mr. Brown was self-referred to the Stoolbend, Family Enrichment Center, having set an appointment after a casual conversation with a staff member while installing cable in the Center's multimedia room. During his social conversation, Mr. Brown seems to have acknowledged to himself that he was experiencing several concerns that have been causing him distress and dysfunction for an extended time period, including chronic symptoms of low mood; chronic problematic use of alcohol; recently, recurrent sexual performance concerns;

and recently, stresses associated with remarriage and establishing a blended stepfamily. He described his self-acknowledgment by saying he thought his problems were "normal when you make a big change like mine, but I guess it's my turn to get what I need and to finally be happy."

Background, Family Information, and Relevant History. Cleveland Brown was born in Stoolbend, Virginia, the older of two children to LeVar "Freight Train" Brown, whom he described as "a local high school football legend and adult alcoholic" and for whom Mr. Brown did not identify an occupation, and Cookie, a kindly woman and "wonderful mom" who Cleveland reports worked in the home. Mr. Brown's parents divorced during his early childhood. Based on his report in the session, while growing up, Mr. Brown knew little of his father other than his legendary prowess on the football field and notoriety for romantic pursuits; and often was disappointed by his father, who promised but never followed through with weekend visits. Mr. Brown grew up in a very close relationship with his mother, whom he says he "idolized." Mr. Brown often expressed sadness to his mother about not having any contact with his older brothers, Germaine and Gerald, who were, unbeknownst to him, his father's children from an extramarital affair.

During his elementary and middle school years, Mr. Brown remembers that he was occasionally taunted and bullied because he was overweight and uncommonly good natured. Because of his reticence and passivity, Mr. Brown's teachers thought he might have a developmental disability; however, subsequent psychological and educational evaluation during the fifth grade revealed that he was functioning well within the "average range of overall abilities." Mr. Brown believes that his teachers, who were almost exclusively white, may have reached their faulty conclusion partly on the basis of his race. Mr. Brown's early high school years were marked by continued occasional taunting, particularly by the "school

jocks" who found it easy to embarrass him. However, when Mr. Brown demonstrated athletic prowess on the baseball field, he quickly earned the respect of his peers and began to develop a positive reputation. By the time Mr. Brown was in his junior year of high school, he had trimmed down, focused his sights on a business career, and was voted "Most Popular" in the graduating class of the Stoolbend Senior High School.

Soon after graduation from high school, Mr. Brown met Donna Tubbs whom he dated for several years and planned to marry; however, his father re-emerged and moved the family to a small town in Massachusetts called Quahog. There, Mr. Brown found employment, first as an auctioneer and then as the owner of a small delicatessen. About this time, Mr. Brown sustained a blow to the head in a construction accident, which resulted in his current slow speech pattern. He and his wife, Loretta, had one child, Cleveland, Jr., who experienced a number of developmental challenges, some of which manifested in the form of increased appetite and obesity.

Over the course of the next 15 years, Mr. Brown settled into what he thought was a very comfortable and rewarding lifestyle; however, Loretta emerged as a domineering and unavailable spouse, and, unbeknownst to him, had an affair that lasted for 10 years. Soon after discovering the infidelity, Mr. Brown confronted his wife, who confirmed the allegations. Soon after, Mr. Brown filed for divorce. As a result, Mr. Brown decided to "return to my roots and start over." On the way to Virginia, Mr. Brown met Donna, his first girlfriend, who decided to return to Stoolbend with him. Mr. Brown and Donna, along with Cleveland, Jr. and Donna's two children resettled in Stoolbend; and 2 years after returning to Stoolbend, the couple married.

Since living in Stoolbend, Mr. Brown has been working as a TV cable installer and identifies a "small but dedicated group of friends," including his best friend, "Bear," with whom he "shares a drink" after work. However and more recently, Mr. Brown and his wife Donna have been experiencing an escalation in marital conflict triggered by their different perspectives on how to raise the three children who often quarrel among themselves. Mrs. Brown has accused her husband of excessive drinking and believes that he might even be having an affair; however, he adamantly denies this. He also reports that he has been diagnosed with Borderline Hypertension. Fearing that Mrs. Brown is becoming increasingly disenchanted with their marriage, Mr. Brown says that his casual conversation with one of this Center's staff members catalyzed his self-acknowledgment of difficulties and subsequent help-seeking.

Problem and Counseling History. Mr. Brown has been seen twice for evaluation, including one intake session accompanied by his wife, Donna, and their three children, Roberta, age 16, Cleveland, Jr., age 14, and Rallo, age 5. Mr. Brown sat nervously during the family session and appeared to have difficulty expressing himself amidst the loud and rapid conversation of the members of his family. As the interview progressed, Mr. Brown grew increasingly withdrawn and passive, which escalated his wife's irritable responses and led her to say, for example, "See that's what he does . . . he just goes into his own world . . . he's just like his father." At that point, Mr. Brown angrily responded: "You know how devoted I've been to your kids, so how dare you compare me to that lying cheating man who called himself my father." At one point during their angry interchange, the precocious 5-year-old, Rallo, stood on a chair and said, "Daddy drinks, daddy drinks, mommy even thinks he stinks." As the family departed the session, Mr. Brown whispered to the therapist, "This is exactly what happened when I went to therapy with my first wife, and look what happened to that marriage." He turned and walked away dejected.

During the individual follow-up session, Mr. Brown appeared more hopeful. He was open, expressive, and engaging. Although he declined to have the family participate in further meeting,

he reported that after the first meeting, Mrs. Brown apologized and expressed support for his continued counseling. Based on one family meeting and one individual intake session, Cleveland Brown's concerns appear in four areas:

First, Mr. Brown presents a chronic history throughout adulthood of moderately depressed mood. He reports that "for as long as I can remember," he has experienced low mood many days of the week and "certainly most of the time." He also describes feeling "not too much energy a lot of the time" and "not very confident about myself." He describes often seeing himself as "just plain not good enough." Until his recent self-acknowledgment, he seems to have seen little hope of improvement. It is likely that his overeating and alcohol use may be associated with his low mood. At the same time, his scores on the Beck Depression Inventory-II were only moderately elevated, he denies any suicidal ideation or persistent thoughts of death and dying, and reports that he still enjoys aspects of his life and that "sometimes, some days, I really feel happy and I know what that should feel like." His chronic mood concerns appear to precede his recent divorce, relocation, and remarriage and similarly precede his blow to the head earlier in adulthood.

Second, although Mr. Brown denies any negative effects of his alcohol use, his use pattern might be clinically significant. His wife has expressed strong dissatisfaction with his everyday after-work drinking and accuses him of avoiding early evening parenting duties and of being drunk at times in front of his family. Mr. Brown believes that because he does not experience hangovers or "almost never misses work" due to his alcohol use, and because "it's the same it's been for years," that his use is not problematic; however, he expressed motivation to "make Donna happy" by examining his drinking.

Third, Mr. Brown indicated in written intake materials that he has been experiencing occasional but recurring sexual function problems over the past year. He has been hesitant to discuss this issue in further detail during the interview but did acknowledge that "with all the family stuff going on, who wouldn't have a little male trouble?" His written responses suggest that this concern emerged shortly after establishing his new blended household. He was willing to admit that being aware that his stepson, Rally, frequently "storms into the bedroom" has "worked on my nerves a little bit in bed."

Fourth, overall, Mr. Brown appears to be confronting normally expected stresses associated with remarriage that entailed a geographic relocation and three children. Although normally expected, these issues appear to be exacerbating his low mood and perhaps his alcohol use, and may be contributing to his sexual dysfunction.

Goals for Counseling and Course of Therapy to Date. Mr. Brown has been seen twice for intake and assessment with the goals of evaluation and treatment planning. He is motivated for ongoing individual therapy to address his concerns. A summary and diagnostic report will be sent to his workplace-provided managed-care company, Virginia Care, seeking coverage for treatment.

Diagnostic Impressions

Axis I.   300.4 Dysthymic Disorder, Early Onset

305.00 Alcohol Abuse

307.72 Male Erectile Disorder, Acquired Type, Situational Type, Due to Psychological Factors

V61.10 Partner Relational Problem

V61.20 Parent-Child Relational Problem

Axis II.   Dependent Personality Disorder Features

Axis III.   Borderline Hypertension

Axis IV.   Problems with primary support group—Recent divorce, recent remarriage, recent discord with stepfamily

Problem related to social environment—Recent geographic relocation

Axis V.   GAF = 60 (at intake)

GAF = 73 (highest level past year)

DISCUSSION OF DIAGNOSTIC IMPRESSIONS

Cleveland Brown set up a counseling appointment at the Stoolbend Family Enrichment Center on his own volition, as he was worried about several domains his everyday adjustment. He had been experiencing clinically significant concerns in each these three areas: mood, substance use, and sexual function. He was also experiencing several significant life stressors.

Each section of the *DSM-IV-TR* classification system contains a group of diagnoses that share qualitatively similar symptoms or features. For instance, the Mood Disorders section contains all of the disorders associated with a disturbance in mood (including depressive disorders and bipolar disorders); the Substance-Related Disorders section contains all of the Substance-Use Disorders (Dependence and Abuse) and Substance-Induced Disorders (Intoxication, Withdrawal, and substance-induced disruptions in mood, sleep, and sexual function); and the Sexual and Gender Identity Disorders section contains clinical problems all featuring a person's difficulties in the area of sexuality (including Sexual Dysfunctions, Paraphilias, and Gender Identity Disorders).

Cleveland Brown's first concern pertained to his mood; he reported having experienced low mood for many years. He also described low self-esteem and, until his interest in counseling, a sense of hopelessness that his situation could improve, reported overeating and fatigue. However, he denied any suicidal ideation or thoughts with themes of death; his mood is positively reactive to life events, he experiences and recognizes periods of nondepressed mood, and his depression does not appear severe. Scores on the BDI-II indicated moderate depressive symptoms. Taken together, Cleveland described a long-term experience of moderately depressed mood and related symptoms that do not meet the criteria for a Major Depressive Disorder. In his case, there is no evidence that his mood disturbance is due to the direct consequences of a general medication condition such as hypothyroidism or a negative reaction to a life event, which would otherwise suggest an Adjustment Disorder With Depressed Mood (he reports his depression preceded his life stressors). Taken together, this pattern of symptoms and concerns suggests the diagnosis of Dysthymia.

A differential diagnosis that might be considered is Alcohol-Induced Mood Disorder With Depressive Features. However, according to Cleveland's report, the onset of his low mood likely preceded his problematic alcohol use, and apparently is not the direct result of intoxication, withdrawal, or prolonged use. These factors suggest a primary mood disorder rather than one that is substance-induced.

Cleveland Brown's second concern pertained to his alcohol use. He is experiencing marital discord and has failed to fulfill parental responsibilities as a result of his regular pattern of weekday alcohol use—and he has been drunk in front of his family without intending to do so. He has continued his drinking despite his awareness of these ongoing problematic consequences. In turn, the diagnosis is Substance Abuse and, more specifically, Alcohol Abuse.

Alcohol Dependence might be a reasonable differential consideration; however, Mr. Brown's use pattern meets the criteria for the less advanced diagnosis, abuse, rather than the more advanced diagnosis, dependence. Another differential consideration is whether Cleveland Brown is engaged in nonproblematic social or recreational drinking, which would not require a diagnosis; however, his use meets the criteria for a maladaptive pattern of substance-related behavior resulting in negative life consequences (Inaba & Cohen, 2000)—namely, recurrent use leading to problems with major role obligations at home—and therefore warrants a diagnosis indicating clinical significance.

Cleveland Brown's third concern pertained to his sexual function. He eventually was able to disclose to his counselor that he had been experiencing a recurrent inability to attain an erection when desired, and at other times, maintain an adequate erection through completion of sexual activity. This pattern had persisted for an extended period of time, ever since beginning life in his new household. He attributed his sexual disturbance to the stresses of entering a new marriage and new family of children as well as the practical stress of children sometimes interrupting his and his wife's sexual activity. In the absence of any evidence of a general medical condition or another diagnosable mental disorder causing his sexual symptoms, the diagnosis is Male Erectile Disorder. The onset is subtyped, Acquired Type (compared with Lifelong Type), the context is subtyped Situational (compared with Generalized), and the etiology is specified as Due to Psychological Factors (compared with a combination of psychological and other sorts of factors).

As with Cleveland's mood, one differential consideration is Alcohol-Induced Sexual Dysfunction With Impaired Arousal. However, there is no evidence from the history that his sexual dysfunction developed within a month of his alcohol intoxication, or any physical exam or lab evidence to support this etiology.

Next, along with all the various diagnosable disorders, a multiaxial diagnosis also may list Other Conditions That May Be a Focus of Clinical Attention. The client concerns contained in this section (appearing at the end of the *Diagnostic and Statistical Manual of Mental Disorders, Fourth Edition, Text Revision* [*DSM-IV-TR*], following all of the diagnosable disorders), are nondiagnosable mental disorders according to the *DSM* classification system; instead, they are client problems or issues that are a focus of concern and/or treatment. We decided to list Partner Relational Problem and Parent-Child Relational Problem. Although these two concerns are associated with Cleveland's diagnosable substance use and sexual dysfunction, we believed they were of enough clinical importance to warrant clinical attention during counseling and to merit inclusion on Axis I.

Finally, on Axis II, problematic personality features and defenses can be listed even when they do not reflect a diagnosable Personality Disorder, if these personality characteristics are important to understanding the client's functioning and are maladaptive for the person. We provided the notation, Dependent Personality Features, to describe Cleveland Brown's pattern of an overly submissive general attitude and excessively deferential behaviors in his intimate relationship and other interpersonal relationships, which have some maladaptive qualities associated with "a self-perception of being unable to function adequately without the help of others" (APA, 2000a, p. 721).

To wrap up the diagnosis, Cleveland's medical condition, Borderline Hypertension, is listed on Axis III, his important social pressures are emphasized on Axis IV, and on Axis V his functioning is represented by Global Assessment of Functioning (GAF) scores ranging from a recent period of good functioning with only normally expected, transient, everyday reactions and concerns, to the current period of moderate symptoms causing moderate difficulties in social and other areas, which led to his counseling appointment.

The information on these axes is consistent with the information on Axes I and II.

CASE CONCEPTUALIZATION

When Cleveland Brown arrived at the Stoolbend Family Enrichment Center, his assigned counselor collected as much information as possible about the symptoms and situations leading to Cleveland's decision to seek assistance. Included among the intake materials were a thorough history, client report, counselor observations, and meetings involving Cleveland Brown's new family. Based on the intake, Mr. Brown's counselor developed diagnostic impressions, describing his presenting concerns as falling into several categories, including dysthymic mood, alcohol abuse, sexual dysfunction, and various relational concerns (including dependent features). A case conceptualization next was developed. Whereas the purpose of diagnostic impressions is to *describe* the client's concerns, the goal of case conceptualization is to better *understand* and clinically *explain* the person's experiences (Neukrug & Schwitzer, 2006). It helps the counselor understand the etiology leading to, and the factors sustaining, Mr. Brown's depressive disorder, substance use, sexual dysfunction, and interpersonal and personality features. In turn, case conceptualization sets the stage for treatment planning. Treatment planning then provides a road map that plots out how the counselor and client expect to move from presenting concerns to positive outcomes (Seligman, 1993, p. 157)— helping Mr. Brown to improve his mood, change his alcohol use, restore his sexual function, and improve his family relationships.

When forming a case conceptualization, the clinician applies a purist counseling theory, an integration of two or more theories, an eclectic mix of theories, or a solution-focused combination of tactics, to his or her understanding of the client. In this case, Mr. Brown's counselor based his conceptualization on psychotherapeutic integration of two theories (Corey, 2009). Psychotherapists very commonly integrate more than one theoretical approach in order to form a conceptualization and treatment plan that will be as efficient and effective as possible for meeting the client's needs (Dattilo & Norcross, 2006; Norcross & Beutler, 2008). In other words, counselors use the psychotherapeutic integration method attempt to flexibly tailor their clinical efforts to "the unique needs and contexts of the individual client" (Norcross & Beutler, 2008, p. 485). Like other counselors using integration, Mr. Brown's clinician chose this method because he had not found one individual theory that was comprehensive enough, by itself, to address all of the "complexities," "range of client types," and "specific problems" seen among his everyday caseload (Corey, 2009, p. 450). Further, Cleveland Brown's counselor was aware of literature suggesting that an integration of approaches sometimes is particularly responsive to the needs of clients from ethnically diverse backgrounds (Corey, 2009; Ivey, Ivey, D'Andrea, & Simek-Morgan, 2005).

Specifically, Cleveland Brown's counselor selected an integration of (a) Schema-Focused Cognitive Behavior Therapy and (b) Interpersonal Psychotherapy. He selected this approach based on Mr. Brown's presentation of intrapersonal mood concerns along with relationship patterns and interpersonal personality features and associated problematic behaviors, and his knowledge of current outcome research with clients experiencing these types of concerns (Critchfield & Smith-Benjamin, 2006; Fochtmann & Gelenberg, 2005; Hollon, Thase, & Markowitz, 2002; Livesley, 2007; Westen & Morrison, 2001). According to the research, cognitive therapy's focus on family schema as well as interpersonal psychotherapy's focus on family-of-origin characterological conflicts and habitual response patterns often is indicated for adults with a combinations of concerns such as Mr. Brown's. His counselor is comfortable theoretically integrating these approaches.

The counselor used the Inverted Pyramid Method of case conceptualization because this method is especially designed to help clinicians more easily form their conceptual pictures of

their clients' needs (Neukrug & Schwitzer, 2006; Schwitzer, 1996, 1997). The method has four steps: Problem Identification, Thematic Groupings, Theoretical Inferences, and Narrowed Inferences. The counselor's clinical thinking can be seen in Figure 9.1.

Step 1: Problem Identification. The first step is Problem Identification. Aspects of the presenting problem (thoughts, feelings, behaviors, physiological features), additional areas of concern besides the presenting concern, family and developmental history, in-session observations, clinical inquiries (medical problems, medications, past counseling, substance use, suicidality), and psychological assessments (problem checklists, personality inventories, mental status exam, specific clinical measures) all may contribute information at Step 1. The counselor "casts a wide net" in order to build Step 1 as exhaustively as possible (Neukrug & Schwitzer, 2006, p. 202). As can be seen in the figure, the counselor identified Cleveland Brown's primary mood concerns (moderate depression and associated low self-esteem); current family adjustment concerns (associated with his new marriage and family roles); current auxiliary concerns (alcohol and sexual function problems); and important family-of-origin, developmental, and past concerns (father and mother dynamics, school experiences). He attempted to go beyond just the current events leading to Mr. Brown's decision to seek counseling in order to be descriptive as he could.

Step 2: Thematic Groupings. The second step is Thematic Groupings. The clinician organizes all of the exhaustive client information found in Step 1 into just a few intuitive-logical clinical groups, categories, or themes, on the basis of sensible common denominators (Neukrug & Schwitzer, 2006). Four different ways of forming the Step 2 theme groups can be used: Descriptive-Diagnosis Approach, Clinical Targets Approach, Areas of Dysfunction Approach, and Intrapsychic Approach. As can be seen in the figure, Cleveland Brown's counselor selected the Areas of

Dysfunction Approach. This approach sorts together all of the Step 1 information into "areas of dysfunction according to important life situations, life themes, or life roles and skills" (Neukrug & Schwitzer, 2006, p. 205).

The counselor grouped together Mr. Brown's (a) chronic symptoms of moderate depression and low self-esteem, (b) current adjustment difficulties (family relationships and conflicts), and (c) two associated concerns (with alcohol and sexual function). His conceptual work at Step 2 gave the counselor a way to begin understanding and explaining Cleveland Brown's many concerns as a narrower list of a few clear, meaningful areas of negative functioning.

So far, at Steps 1 and 2, the counselor has used his clinical assessment skills and his clinical judgment to begin critically understanding Mr. Brown's needs. Now, at Steps 3 and 4, he applies the theoretical approach he has selected. He begins making theoretical inferences to explain the factors leading to Cleveland's issues as they are seen in Steps 1 and 2.

Step 3: Theoretical Inferences. At Step 3, concepts from the counselor's theoretical integration of two approaches—Schema-Focused Cognitive Behavior Therapy and Interpersonal Psychotherapy—are applied to explain the experiences causing, and the mechanisms maintaining, Cleveland Brown's problematic thoughts, feelings, and behaviors. The counselor tentatively matches the theme groups in Step 2 with this theoretical approach. In other words, the symptom constellations in Step 2, which were distilled from the symptoms in Step 1, now are combined using theory to show what are believed to be the underlying causes or psychological etiology of Cleveland Brown's current needs (Neukrug & Schwitzer, 2006; Schwitzer, 2006, 2007).

A combination of approaches was used. First, generally speaking, according to Cognitive Behavior Therapy (Beck, 1995, 2005; Ellis, 1994; Ellis & MacLaren, 2005), irrational thinking, faulty beliefs, or other forms of cognitive errors lead individuals to engage in problematic behaviors and to experience negative moods and attitudes. More specifically, when the cognitive behavioral approach, Schema-Focused Cognitive Therapy is used, there is an emphasis on identifying jointly held core beliefs that emerge in families (Dattilo, 2001, 2005, 2006). According to the approach, these jointly held core beliefs—or family schema—often have a strong influence on individual family members' thoughts, feelings, and behaviors. In the case of individuals experiencing depression and low self-esteem, schema learned in one's family of origin is believed to cause attitudes and feelings of self-devaluing, weakness, inadequacy, or inability to fill major life roles (Beck, 1995, 2005; Dattilo, 2001, 2005, 2006). As can be seen in Figure 9.1, Mr. Brown's counselor presented two such distorted core beliefs: (a) "I am not good enough as a husband, father, or man" and (b) "I do not deserve to be happy."

Second, Interpersonal Psychotherapy was applied. This second approach was thought to complement the schema already identified as a source of Mr. Brown's concerns. According to Interpersonal Psychotherapy, problematic, repetitive, rule-bound communication and transactional patterns in a person's family of origin can be the source of many long-standing young and adult intrapersonal personality dynamics and problematic interpersonal relationship behaviors (Teyber, 1992; Wenar, 1990). According to the theory, family transactional patterns are highly emotionally charged and powerful, and occur repetitively. Correspondingly, "These repetitive patterns of family interaction, roles, and relationships are internalized and become the foundation of our sense of self and the social world" (Teyber, 1992, p. 13). More specifically, conflictual, disapproving, rejecting, or ambivalent parental and family interpersonal responses cause the cognitive and emotional strain that leads to problematic interpersonal behaviors (Wenar, 1990). As also can be seen in Figure 9.1, when the counselor applied these interpersonal psychotherapy concepts, he additionally explained at Step 3 that the various Step 1 issues, which can be understood in Step 2 to be themes of chronic, current adjustment, and recent associated problems, were rooted in repetitive, negative family transactional patterns: (a) negative, undermining, rejecting transactional patterns with Mr. Brown's father, and (b) compensating and protecting, but undermining, transactional patterns with his mother.

Step 4: Narrowed Inferences. At Step 4, the clinician's selected theory continues to be used to address still-deeper issues when they exist (Schwitzer, 2006, 2007). At this step, "still-deeper, more encompassing, or more central, causal themes" are formed (Neukrug & Schwitzer, 2006, p. 207). Mr. Brown's counselor continued to use the psychotherapeutic integration of two approaches.

First, continuing to apply Schema-Focused Cognitive Therapy concepts at Step 4, Mr. Brown's counselor presented a single, deepest, most-fundamental faulty family schema that he believed to be most explanatory and causal regarding his combination of presenting problems: the shared family core belief that "My father is the only man in the family who is powerful and has prowess and therefore I can never become a powerful adult man." Second, continuing to apply Interpersonal Psychotherapy, the counselor presented a single, most deeply rooted characterological conflict and habitual response pattern: Due to repeated undermining and rejecting transactions with his father, and compensating emotionally overprotecting transactions with his mother, Mr. Brown must cover his anxieties about failing as a man by being overly dependent and compliant with his wife, children, and friends; and cover over his low mood and disappointments with alcohol and good-naturedness. These two narrowed inferences, together, form the basis for understanding the etiology and maintenance of Mr. Brown's combination of difficulties.

When all four steps are completed, the client information in Step 1 leads to logical-intuitive groupings on the basis of common denominators in Step 2, the groupings then are explained using

theory at Step 3, and then, finally, at Step 4, further deeper explanations are made. From start to finish, the thoughts, feelings, behaviors, and physiological features in the topmost portions are connected on down the pyramid into deepest dynamics.

TREATMENT PLANNING

At this point, Cleveland's clinician at the Stoolbend Family Enrichment Center has collected all available information about the problems that have been of concern to him. Based upon this information, the counselor developed a five-axis *DSM-IV-TR* diagnosis and then, using the "inverted pyramid" (Neukrug & Schwitzer, 2006; Schwitzer, 1996, 1997), formulated a working clinical *explanation* of Cleveland's difficulties and their etiology that we call the *case conceptualization.* This, in turn, guides us to the next critical step in our clinical work, called the *treatment plan,* the primary purpose of which is to map out a logical and goal-oriented strategy for making positive changes in the client's life. In essence, the treatment plan is a road map "for reducing or eliminating disruptive symptoms that are impeding the client's ability to reach positive mental health outcomes" (Neukrug & Schwitzer, 2006, p. 225). As such, it is the cornerstone of our work with not only Cleveland, but with all clients who present with disruptive symptoms and/or personality patterns (Jongsma & Peterson, 2006; Jongsma, Peterson, & McInnis, 2003a, 2003b; Seligman, 1993, 1998, 2004).

A comprehensive treatment plan must integrate all of the information from the biopsychosocial interview, diagnosis, and case conceptualization into a coherent plan of action. This *plan* comprises four main components, which include (1) a behavioral definition of the problem(s), (2) the selection of achievable goals, (3) the determination of treatment modes, and (4) the documentation of how change will be measured. The *behavioral definition of the problem(s)* consolidates the results of the case

Figure 9.1   Cleveland Brown's Inverted Pyramid Case Conceptualization: Psychotherapeutic Integration of Schema-Focused Cognitive Behavior Therapy and Interpersonal Psychotherapy

1.   IDENTIFY AND LIST CLIENT CONCERNS

History of alcoholic father
History of "football legend" father
History of "high sexual prowess" father
Father's affair
Idolized mother
Two distant half-brothers by affair
Domineering first wife
First wife's infidelity
Failed first marriage
Blow to head
Geographic relocation
Marriage adjustment
Blended family and parenting adjustment
Marital stress and conflict over child-rearing
Relational stress with stepchildren

Race-based academic misassessment
Childhood taunting and bullying
Childhood overweight
Characterized as "overly good natured"
Daily after-work alcohol use
Accused of missing parental duties
Alcohol use causing marital conflict
Recent sexual dysfunction maintaining erection
Anxiety about stepson barging in on sexual activity
Chronic, long-standing moderately low mood
Domineering first wife
Chronic low self-confidence

2.   ORGANIZE CONCERNS INTO LOGICAL THEMATIC GROUPINGS

1.   Chronic concerns: Moderate depression and low self-esteem
2.   Current adjustment concerns: Family adjustment, relationship conflicts, and interpersonal stresses
3.   Recent associated concerns: Alcohol use and sexual function problems

3.   THEORETICAL INFERENCES: ATTACH THEMATIC GROUPINGS TO INFERRED AREAS OF DIFFICULTY

Psychotherapeutic Integration

Schema-Focused Cognitive Behavior Therapy
1.   Distorted core beliefs: I am not good enough as a husband, as a father, or as a man
2.   I do not deserve to be happy

Interpersonal Psychotherapy
Repetitive negative family transactional patterns:
1.   Negative, undermining, rejecting transactional patterns with father
2.   Compensating and protecting, but undermining transactional patterns with mother

4.   NARROWED INFERENCES: SUICIDALITY AND DEEPER DIFFICULTIES

Psychotherapeutic Integration

Schema-Focused Cognitive Behavior Therapy
Fundamental Faulty Family Schema
My father is the only man in the family who is powerful and has prowess and therefore I can never become a powerful adult man

Interpersonal Psychotherapy
Characterological Conflict and Habitual Response Pattern
Due to repeated undermining and rejecting transactions with compensating emotionally overprotecting transactions with mother, Cleveland must cover his anxieties about failing as a man by being overly dependent and compliant with wife, children, friends; and cover his low mood and disappointment with alcohol and good-naturedness

conceptualization into a concise hierarchical list of problems and concerns that will be the focus of treatment. The *selection of achievable goals* refers to assessing and prioritizing the client's concerns into a *hierarchy of urgency* that also takes into account the client's motivation for change, level of dysfunction, and real-world influences on his or her problems. The *determination of treatment modes* refers to selection of the specific interventions, which are matched to the uniqueness of the client and to his or her goals and clearly tied to a particular theoretical orientation (Neukrug & Schwitzer, 2006). Finally, the clinician must establish how change will be measured, based upon a number of factors, including client records and self-report of change, in-session observations by the clinician, clinician ratings, results of standardized evaluations such as the Beck Anxiety Inventory (Beck & Steer, 1990) or a family functioning questionnaire, pre-post treatment comparisons, and reports by other treating professionals.

The four-step method discussed above can be seen in Figure 6.1 (p. 109) and is outlined below for the case of Mr. Brown, followed by his specific treatment plan.

Step 1: Behavioral Definition of Problems. The first step in treatment planning is to carefully review the case conceptualization, paying particular attention to the results of Step 2 (Thematic Groupings), Step 3 (Theoretical Inferences), and Step 4 (Narrowed Inferences). The identified clinical themes reflect the core areas of concern and distress for the client, while the theoretical and narrowed inferences offer clinical speculation as to their origins. In the case of Mr. Brown, there are three primary areas of concern. The first, "chronic concerns," refers to his long-standing moderately low mood, self-confidence, self-esteem, and hopes of happiness. The second, "current adjustment concerns," refers to his abdication of parental duties and responsibilities, relationship conflicts in and outside of marriage, marital stress over child rearing, and relational stress with his stepchildren. The third, "recent associated concerns," refers to his alcohol use to minimize emotional stress and sexual functioning problems. These symptoms and stresses are consistent with the diagnosis of Dysthymic Disorder, Early Onset; Alcohol Abuse; Male Erectile Disorder, Acquired Type, Situational Type Due to Psychological Factors; Partner Relational Problem; Parent-Child Relational Problem; Dependent Personality Features (APA, 2000a; Critchfield & Smith-Benjamin, 2006; Dobson, 1989; Grant et al., 2006; Hollon et al., 2002; Livesley, 2007; Leiblum, 2006; O'Farrell & Fals-Stewart, 2003; Winger, Woods, & Hoffman, 2004).

Step 2: Identify and Articulate Goals for Change. The second step is the selection of achievable goals, which is based upon a number of factors, including the most pressing or urgent behavioral, emotional, and interpersonal concerns and symptoms as identified by the client and clinician, the willingness and ability of the client to work on those particular goals, and the realistic (real-world) achievability of those goals (Neukrug & Schwitzer, 2006). At this stage of treatment planning, it is important to recognize that not all of the client's problems can be addressed at once, so we focus initially on those that cause the greatest distress and impairment. New goals can be created as old ones are achieved. In the case of Mr. Brown, the goals are divided into three prominent areas. The first, "chronic concerns," requires that we help Mr. Brown to understand how his mood, self-esteem, and coping strategies are related to family-of-origin experiences with his parents, examine his life experiences that confirm and refute these maladaptive schema, and modify these schema accordingly. The second, "current adjustment concerns," requires that we help Mr. Brown to understand the bases of his passive-dependent personality style, identify family-of-origin issues that contribute to this overall interpersonal schema, and modify his parental and marital perceptions, roles, and behavior. The third, "recent associated concerns," requires that we help Mr. Brown to recognize, understand and correct the faulty schema that contribute to his alcohol and sexual performance difficulties, and in so doing, help him to become satisfied and secure in his relationships within and outside of the home.

Step 3: Describe Therapeutic Interventions. This is perhaps the most critical step in the treatment planning process because the clinician must now integrate information from a number of sources, including the case conceptualization, the delineation of the client's problems and goals, and the treatment literature, paying particular attention to *empirically supported treatment* (EST) and *evidence-based practice* (EBP). In essence, the clinician must align his or her treatment approach with scientific evidence from the fields of counseling and psychotherapy. Wampold (2001) identifies two types of evidence-based counseling research: studies that demonstrate "absolute efficacy," that is, the fact that counseling and psychotherapy work, and those that demonstrate "relative efficacy," that is, the fact that certain theoretical/technical approaches work best for certain clients with particular problems (Psychoanalysis, Gestalt Therapy, Cognitive Behavior Therapy, Brief Solution-Focused Therapy, Cognitive Therapy, Dialectical Behavior Therapy, Person-Centered Therapy, Expressive/Creative Therapies, Interpersonal Therapy, and Feminist Therapy); and when delivered through specific treatment modalities (individual, group, and family counseling). In the case of Cleveland Brown, we have decided to use a two-pronged or integrated approach to therapy. This is comprised of Interpersonal Therapy, which has been found to be effective with clients struggling with depression and maladaptive interpersonal behaviors centered on early unhealthy and conflictual relationships (APA, 2000b; Depression Guideline Panel, 1993; Klerman & Weissman, 1993; Weissman, Markowitz, & Klerman, 2000). This approach relies upon an eclectic mix of techniques to help clients to understand and resolve conflicting and self-limiting thoughts, feelings, and behaviors as well as interpersonal deficits in their adult life that have origin in early as well as ongoing family roles, conflicts, and losses. Specific techniques for Mr. Brown that are drawn from these approaches include providing empathy and support for the expression of painful feelings, challenging self and

relational attributions that undermine the development of a positive and mature self-image, and encouragement in the expression of conflictual parental messages and their impact on problematic behaviors. The clinician will also use Schema-Focused Therapy (Dattilo, 2001, 2005, 2006; Young, Klosko, & Weishart, 2003), which is a variant of Cognitive Therapy (Beck, 1997) and is based on the premise that people form schemas, or mental representations, perceptions, and expectations about themselves, and relationships and their roles within them, based upon early life experiences, and in particular their family-of-origin ties. The therapist's goal is to help clients recognize, understand, and modify these schema. It has been found effective in helping clients to gain self-understanding, improved relational functioning, and mature and flexible role expectations and behaviors (Hoffart, Verslund, & Sexton, 2002; Young, 1990; Young et al., 2003). Specific techniques that are drawn from this approach include educating Cleveland about the nature of cognitive schema, assisting him to identify schema-based triggers for avoidance of parental and marital responsibilities, and encouraging and shaping effective parenting skills. Once these interventions have been employed, the counselor and Cleveland can address his "recent associated symptoms" by identifying triggers for alcohol use and sexual dysfunction and then providing opportunities for corrective experiences in individual, marital, and family counseling.

Step 4: Provide Outcome Measures of Change. This last step in treatment planning requires that we specify how change will be measured and indicate the extent to which progress has been made toward realizing these goals (Neukrug & Schwitzer, 2006). The counselor has considerable flexibility in this phase and may choose from a number of objective domains (psychological tests and measures of self-esteem, depression, psychosis, interpersonal relationship, anxiety, etc.), quasi-objective measures (the *DSM-IV-TR's* Axis V GAF scale; pre-post clinician, client, and psychiatric ratings), and subjective ratings (client self-report, clinician's in-session observations). In Mr. Brown's case, we have implemented a number of these including pre-post measure on the Beck Depression Inventory-II

(Beck, Steer, & Brown, 1996) and Alcohol Use Inventory (Horn, Wanberg, & Foster, 1990), post measures of GAF functioning in the mild range (>70), clinician-observed replacement of maladaptive cognitive schema with adaptive beliefs about self, relationships, and family functioning, client and spouse report of reduced alcohol use as a coping strategy, client and spouse reported improvement in marital and sexual relationship.

The completed treatment plan is now developed through which the counselor and Cleveland (along with his wife and family) will begin their shared work of modifying his cognitive schema with regard to himself and intimate relationships, improving his overall mood, interpersonal and family functioning, and optimizing his coping skills. Cleveland Brown's treatment plan follows, and is summarized in Table 9.1.

TREATMENT PLAN

Client: Cleveland Brown

Service Provider: Stoolbend Family Enrichment Center

BEHAVIORAL DEFINITION OF PROBLEMS:

1. Chronic concerns—Long-standing moderately low mood, self-confidence, self-esteem, and hopes of happiness

2. Current adjustment concerns—Abdication of parental duties and responsibilities, relationship conflicts in and outside of marriage, marital stress over child-rearing, and relational stress with his stepchildren

3. Recent associated concerns—Alcohol use to minimize emotional stress and sexual functioning problems

GOALS FOR CHANGE:

1. Chronic concerns

   - Understand how mood and self-esteem issues as well as maladaptive coping strategies are related to family of origin-based "early maladaptive schema"
   - Examine life experiences that confirm and refute the thoughts, feelings, and behaviors that flow from maladaptive schema
   - Modify interpersonal and personal schema in order to develop adaptive coping strategies, self-regulation skills, and interpersonal relational behavior

2. Current adjustment concerns

   - Understand the basis of passive-dependent personality style in family of origin and early life circumstances with (protective) mother and (caustic/rejecting) father
   - Identify family of origin bases for maladaptive self-, parent-, and martial-role behaviors
   - Modify parental- and marital-role expectations and behaviors in order to achieve optimal functioning in these roles

3. Recent associated concerns

   - Recognize the relationship between alcohol use, family conflict, and parental-/marital-role stress

(Continued)

(Continued)

- Identify elements of maladaptive cognitive schema that perpetuate alcohol use
- Develop effective coping strategies to eliminate reliance upon alcohol
- Recognize the relationship between erectile dysfunction, family conflict, and parental-/marital-role stress
- Modify self- and marital-role expectations and behaviors in order to achieve optimal sexual functioning

THERAPEUTIC INTERVENTIONS:

A moderate-term course (6–9 months) of integrated individual Interpersonal and Schema-Focused Cognitive Therapy supplemented with couples/family counseling

1. Chronic concerns
   - Psycho-education about the nature of cognitive schema
   - Identifying schema-based triggers for poor self-image, passive-dependent relational style, and avoidance of parental and marital responsibilities
   - Providing support and empathy for expression of painful feelings and negative self-beliefs stemming from relationship with parents
   - Challenging self and relational attributions that undermine development of a positive and mature self-image

2. Current adjustment concerns
   - Encourage expression of conflictual, disapproving, rejecting, or ambivalent parental messages and their impact on problematic interpersonal behaviors
   - Identify and gently refute maladaptive assumptions underlying gender and relational roles and behavior
   - Identify the effect of faulty schema on communication patterns within marital counseling
   - Encourage and shape effective parenting through teaching, role-play, and structured exercises within family counseling

3. Recent associated concerns
   - Identify maladaptive nature of alcohol use as a coping strategy
   - Verbalize the triggers at home and at work for drinking
   - Build alternative stress-relief and coping strategies, including meditation, relaxation, and exercise
   - Implement and role-play relapse-prevention strategies
   - Identify family-of-origin factors that undermine sexual fulfillment and sexual performance
   - Referral to a qualified sex therapist for enhancement of sexual communication skills

OUTCOME MEASURES OF CHANGE:

The development of healthy, positive, and self-affirming attitudes toward himself, improved marital functioning, responsible parental behavior, decreased dependence upon alcohol for coping as measured by:

- Pre-post measures on the Beck Depression Inventory-II
- Pre-post measures on the Alcohol Use Inventory
- Post-only measures of GAF functioning in the mild range (>70)
- Client and spouse self-report of increased involvement in day-to-day domestic and child-care responsibilities
- Clinician-observed replacement of maladaptive cognitive schema with adaptive beliefs about self, relationships, and family functioning
- Client-reported elimination of negative self-talk and negative interpretations of experiences
- Client and spouse report of reduced use of alcohol as a coping strategy

Table 9.1   Cleveland Brown's Treatment Plan Summary: Psychotherapeutic Integration of Schema-Focused Cognitive Therapy and Interpersonal Therapy

Goals for Change	Therapeutic Interventions	Outcome Measures of Change
Chronic Concerns Understand how mood and self-esteem issues as well as maladaptive coping strategies are related to family of origin-based "early maladaptive schema" Examine life experiences that confirm and refute the thoughts, feelings, and behaviors that flow from maladaptive schema Modify interpersonal and personal schema in order to develop adaptive coping strategies, self-regulation skills, and interpersonal relational behavior Current adjustment concerns Understand the basis of passive-dependent personality style in family-of-origin and early life circumstances with (protective) mother and (caustic/rejecting) father Identify family of origin bases for maladaptive self-, parent-, and martial-role behaviors Modify parental- and marital-role expectations and behaviors in order to achieve optimal functioning in these roles Recent associated concerns Recognize the relationship between alcohol use, family conflict, and parental-/marital-role stress Identify elements of maladaptive cognitive schema that perpetuate alcohol use Develop effective coping strategies to eliminate reliance upon alcohol Recognize the relationship between erectile dysfunction, family conflict, and parental-/marital-role stress Modify self- and marital-role expectations and behaviors in order to achieve optimal sexual functioning	Chronic Concerns Psychoeducation about the nature of cognitive schema Identifying schema-based triggers for poor self-image, passive-dependent relational style, and avoidance of parental and marital responsibilities Providing support and empathy for expression of painful feelings and negative self-beliefs stemming from relationship with parents Challenging self- and relational attributions that undermine development of a positive and mature self-image Current adjustment concerns Encourage expression of conflictual, disapproving, rejecting, or ambivalent parental messages and their impact on problematic interpersonal behaviors Identify and gently refute maladaptive assumptions underlying gender and relational roles and behavior Identify the effect of faulty schema on communication patterns within marital counseling Encourage and shape effective parenting through teaching, role-play, and structured exercises within family counseling Recent associated concerns Identify maladaptive nature of alcohol use as a coping strategy Verbalize the triggers at home and at work for drinking Build alternative stress-relief and coping strategies, including meditation, relaxation, and exercise Implement and role-play relapse-prevention strategies Identify family-of-origin factors that undermine sexual fulfillment and sexual performance Referral to a qualified sex therapist for enhancement of sexual communication skills	The development of healthy, positive, and self-affirming attitudes toward himself, improved marital functioning, responsible parental behavior, decreased dependence upon alcohol for coping as measured by: Pre-post measures on the Beck Depression Inventory-II Pre-post measures on the Alcohol Use Inventory Post-only measures of GAF functioning in the mild range (>70) Client and spouse self-report of increased involvement in day-to-day domestic and child-care responsibilities Clinician-observed replacement of maladaptive cognitive schema with adaptive beliefs about self, relationships, and family functioning Client-reported elimination of negative self-talk and negative interpretations of experiences Client and spouse report of reduced use of alcohol as a coping strategy

CASE 9.2 *TOY STORY'S* JESSIE

INTRODUCING THE CHARACTER

Jessie is one of the main characters in the Pixar/Disney animated blockbuster movie *Toy Story 2* (Plotkin, Jackson, & Lasseter, 1999). In the story, Jessie is a cowgirl doll modeled after the fictitious cowgirl character in a 1960s children's western TV show called *Woody's Roundup*. The story centers on a band of toys who are going to be sold to a Japanese toy museum, and their efforts to undermine that sale and remain together. As the story unfolds, we learn that Jessie, once a favored toy to her owner, was abandoned when the girl grew out of her interest in childhood play things. Jessie was subsequently purchased by Al of Al's Toy Barn, who was in the process of collecting a full set of toys that were marketed in conjunction with the *Woody's Roundup* television show. As *Toy Story 2* unfolds, the pain of Jessie's abandonment becomes obvious to the other toys, and especially to Woody, who is also struggling to remain in the favor of his boy owner, Andy. As the toys work together to overcome the differences that divide them, they ultimately rally to liberate themselves, and in the process, stage a last minute rescue of Jessie and provide her once again with connection, attachment, and a sense of being loved.

Jessie's is a poignant story of abandonment, loss, and reconnection. Using her experiences in *Toy Story 2* as our building blocks, in the following basic case summary and diagnostic impressions, we reinvent Jessie in order to illustrate Reactive Attachment Disorder.

Meet the Client

You can assess the client in action by viewing clips of Jessie's video material at the following website:

- http://www.youtube.com/watch?v=px0j1EHF8Y0 Jessie tells the story of her abandonment

BASIC CASE SUMMARY

Identifying Information. Jessie, who refuses to use her last name because "It reminds me of them" (her foster parents), is an 11-year-old white preteen who has, for the last 3 months, been living at the Storyland Home for Girls. She has displayed increasingly disturbing asocial behavior at this facility, which has led to her spending increasing time alone, "shying away" from staff, and watching other peer residents with what was described as a "cold aloofness." In appearance, she can be described as a wiry, energetic, and wide-eyed red-haired waif. She has her own room at the facility because of her wary behavior and unwillingness to interact with the other residents.

Presenting Concerns. Jessie was referred for counseling by the disciplinary dean at the Storyland School due to escalating concerns about her highly ambivalent reactions to staff and peers.

Background, Family Information, and Relevant History. Jessie was born in Muskegon, Wisconsin, the youngest and unexpected third child to parents who were both under 20 years old. Jessie's mother and father were both raised in the Wisconsin Foster Care System after being abandoned at birth; her father was in recovery for alcohol abuse. When Jessie was born, her parents were living in a one-bedroom apartment over a grocery store in downtown Muskegon, were receiving government support, and had recently placed Jessie's older brother for adoption.

Jessie was born 5 weeks premature and presented a significant challenge to her young parents, who were referred to, but did not take advantage of, pre- and postnatal social services resources. As a result, Jessie received poor postnatal care and was often left in the company of her parents' friends, where she was also neglected. When Jessie was 1 year old, she was removed from her parents' care and placed with a private foster family who hoped to adopt her; however, when those plans fell through, Jessie was moved into a foster-care facility where she remained until 4 years of age. By that time, Jessie was already showing signs of disrupted attachment, including resisting the attentions of her foster parents, avoiding her foster parents' soothing touch or comforting remarks, hiding from foster siblings in the home, and carefully watching babysitters before responding. She also began a habit of sometimes leaving the home and telling strangers that she was lost. Invariably, she would be returned to the foster home. In spite of her troubled history, Jessie was once again adopted at age 6 by an ostensibly loving and older couple who convinced the state that they had ample financial and psychological resources to provide for the girl's needs. However, Jessie was harassed by the biological child of this couple and when she began running away from their care at age 8 she had already displayed a pattern of seeming to indiscriminately approach strangers on the sidewalk as if she was closely familiar to them.

When one of these "strangers" turned out to be a state care worker, Jessie was immediately removed from this couple's care and placed with a middle-aged couple who had successfully raised their own children and who had been foster parents for 15 years. In that home, Jessie appeared to thrive and slowly began to trust her new parents. Although she tested limits, attempted to run away from home, aggressed toward them, and challenged their patience and experience, the couple's commitment to the 9-year-old seemed to be having a positive effect on her. By the time Jessie was enrolled in Storyland Middle School she, at least outwardly, appeared ready to enter into a new social world. She was placed in a small classroom with a teacher who had been extensively trained in providing for the educational and emotional needs of troubled children, and Jessie seemed to trust this woman, at least as much as she had ever trusted anyone before. She formed very tentative bonds with several classmates, mostly other troubled children, joined the school's Martial Arts Program, and was referred to the school guidance department for possible inclusion in group and individual therapy.

Problem and Counseling History. Jessie was referred by the Storyland facility to Creative Counseling Consultants where she was seen for three sessions separated by a week in time. She was a very charming and superficially endearing child who was playfully dressed in what appeared to be a cowgirl outfit and indicated that "this reminds me of that movie cartoon character who lost her parents and was looking for a family." Ironically, much of Jessie's creative play, whether it was art, storytelling, clay modeling, or dollhouse activities, centered on themes of disrupted families, abuse of children, and retaliatory behavior against parents. Jessie's affect during this disturbing play was quite flat as she recounted incidents in several of the foster and adoptive placements that "make me feel so angry and sad." The results were a very highly destructive element to her play in that she would angrily erase, destroy, or negate her various creations, followed by a tantrum and withdrawal to a corner of the room. She resisted supportive and compassionate gestures by the evaluator and made it quite clear that "I don't like you and I'm only doing this because they made me." At such moments, her body stiffened, her face reddened, and she quickly withdrew and stared off into space for minutes at a time.

Jessie spoke dispassionately about the various families with whom she had lived over the years and noted that "if they really loved me they would have kept me . . . I hate them all so much." She angrily added that "they all thought that if they just sent me to a shrink, that I could be fixed . . . like some sort of broken toy." When asked about her current living situation at the Storyland Home for Girls, she quickly shot back with, "Oh yeah, they're nice enough people, but I don't think they're going to keep me and maybe they're just using me to get money from the state like everybody else." Nevertheless, Jessie acknowledged that staff at the facility seemed different from previous foster or adoptive parents but that "I'm going to keep a really close eye on them and if they make one wrong move that's it." Jessie denied having difficulty with her anger, trusting people, or feeling safe, but reluctantly agreed to return to counseling.

Goals for Counseling and Course of Therapy to Date. Jessie has been seen for three sessions, and conjointly receives facilitative care at the Storyland home. It is recommended that she continue to participate in intensive therapeutic experiences as outlined in the attached treatment plan.

Diagnostic Impressions

Axis I.   313.89 Reactive Attachment Disorder of Infancy or Early Childhood, Inhibited Type

Axis II.   V71.09 No Diagnosis on Axis II

Axis III.   None

Axis IV.   Problems with primary support group—Removal from the home, removal from multiple foster placements, social problems in current residential facility

Axis V.   GAF = 54 (current)

GAF = 54 (highest level past year by estimation)

DISCUSSION OF DIAGNOSTIC IMPRESSIONS

Jessie was referred for counseling by her school's disciplinary dean because the faculty was concerned about her lack of appropriate sociability at the Storyland Home for Girls. She appeared highly ambivalent about receiving the affections and professional support of staff, shied away from other residents, and seemed warily watchful of others. Her behaviors were of enough concern for her to be assigned a single room at the foster care facility to assist with her transition there.

The Disorders Usually First Diagnosed in Infancy, Childhood, or Adolescence is a wide-reaching section of the *DSM-IV-TR* and is organized into many groupings of disorders that all share the feature of occurring early in the life cycle. The last grouping to appear in this section is titled "Other Disorders of Infancy, Childhood, or Adolescence." This section contains such problems as Separation Anxiety Disorder, Selective Mutism, and Reactive Attachment Disorder.

Using Jessie the Cowgirl's story as our starting point, in this case example we presented an 11-year-old girl named Jessie whose background history included repeated changes in primary caregivers: She began life before age 1 in the Wisconsin Foster Care System, lived in several homes where adoption was attempted, moved among various foster families, and currently is residing in a foster-care group home. As early as age 4, she engaged in disrupted interpersonal behaviors: She persistently declined to respond in developmentally appropriate ways to social and supportive advances by adoptive and foster parents and families and others. She avoided their responses, resisted comforting, and was watchful of babysitters and others. At the same time, she developed a pattern of overapproach to strangers and was indiscriminate in her social advances toward adults she did not know.

A logical presumption made by social service workers and counseling staff was that Jessie's history of social relatedness problems was a consequence of her disturbed early social experiences characterized by removal from her parents around age 1, followed by repeated disruptions in care. Jessie's situation in this case suggests a diagnosis of Reactive Attachment Disorder of Infancy or Early Childhood. Most of her behaviors center on failure to "initiate or respond in a developmentally appropriate way to social interactions" (APA, 2000a, p. 130) and therefore the subtype is Inhibited Type.

One set of differential considerations might be Autistic Disorder, Asperger's Disorder, and the other Pervasive Developmental Disorders based partly upon impaired social interaction. However, these diagnoses generally require not only disrupted formation of developmentally appropriate social attachment, but also patterns of restricted, repetitive, or stereotypical behaviors, which Jessie did not demonstrate. Generally speaking, these other disorders also are characterized by developmental disruptions in social communication in the context of normally expected, supportive family or social environments—whereas an essential feature of Reactive Attachment Disorder is a history of pathogenic care (disregard for the child's psychoemotional needs or physical needs, or repeated changes in primary caregiver) such as Jessie experienced.

To finish the diagnosis, Jessie's critical psychosocial stressors associated with her primary supports are emphasized on Axis IV, and on Axis V her functioning is represented by GAF scores indicating moderately serious symptoms causing significant difficulties in social and other functioning, which has been stable across two time points. The information on these axes is consistent with the Axis I diagnosis describing Jessie's situation.

CASE CONCEPTUALIZATION

When Jessie was referred to counseling, the first step was to take part in an intake and evaluation session. The intake counselor collected as much information as possible about the problematic situations in school and outside of school that led to Jessie's referral. The counselor first used this information to develop diagnostic impressions. Jessie's concerns were described by Reactive Attachment Disorder. Next, the counselor developed a case conceptualization. Whereas the purpose of diagnostic impressions is to *describe* the client's concerns, the goal of case conceptualization is to better *understand* and clinically *explain* the person's experiences (Neukrug & Schwitzer, 2006). It helps the counselor understand the etiology leading to Jessie's presenting concerns and the factors maintaining these needs. In turn, case conceptualization sets the stage for treatment planning. Treatment planning then provides a road map that plots out how the counselor and client expect to move from presenting concerns to positive outcomes (Seligman, 1993, p. 157)—helping increase Jessie's successful, normally expected, developmentally appropriate attachments in relationships with adults and peers.

When forming a case conceptualization, the clinician applies a purist counseling theory, an integration of two or more theories, an eclectic mix of theories or a solution-focused combination of tactics, to his or her understanding of the client. In this case, Jessie's counselor based her conceptualization on a purist theory applicable to the behavioral needs of child clients: Theraplay. She selected this approach based on her knowledge of current outcome research and the best-practice literature pertaining to child clients dealing with disorders of infancy and childhood (Kazdin & Weisz, 2003; Mowder, Rubinson, & Yasik, 2009). The Theraplay conceptual approach also is consistent with this counselor's professional therapeutic viewpoint.

The counselor used the Inverted Pyramid Method of case conceptualization because this method is especially designed to help clinicians more easily form their conceptual pictures of their clients' needs (Neukrug & Schwitzer, 2006; Schwitzer, 1996, 1997). The method has four steps: Problem Identification, Thematic Groupings, Theoretical Inferences, and Narrowed Inferences. The counselor's clinical thinking can be seen in Figure 9.2.

Step 1: Problem Identification. The first step is Problem Identification. Aspects of the presenting problem (thoughts, feelings, behaviors, physiological features), additional areas of concern besides the presenting concern, family and developmental history, in-session observations, clinical inquiries (medical problems, medications, past counseling, substance use, suicidality), and psychological assessments (problem checklists, personality inventories, mental status exam, specific clinical measures) all may contribute information at Step 1. The counselor "casts a wide net" in order to build Step 1 as exhaustively as possible (Neukrug & Schwitzer, 2006, p. 202). As can be seen in Figure 9.2, the counselor thoroughly noted not just all of Jessie's poor relationship behaviors and related difficulties at school and at home—but also as much important information as she could find regarding Jessie's earlier developmental experiences, childhood life transitions, environmental factors, and medical notes. The counselor attempted to go beyond just listing the main behaviors causing the referral and to be as complete as she could.

Step 2: Thematic Groupings. The second step is Thematic Groupings. The clinician organizes all of the exhaustive client information found in Step 1 into just a few intuitive-logical clinical groups, categories, or themes, on the basis of sensible common denominators (Neukrug & Schwitzer, 2006). Four different ways of forming the Step 2 theme groups can be used: Descriptive-Diagnosis Approach, Clinical Targets Approach, Areas of Dysfunction Approach, and Intrapsychic Approach. As can be seen in Figure 9.2, Jessie's counselor selected the Descriptive-Diagnosis Approach. This approach sorts together all of the various Step 1 information about the client's adjustment, development, distress, or dysfunction "to show larger clinical problems as reflected through a diagnosis" (Neukrug & Schwitzer, 2006, p. 205).

In this case, the counselor formed just a single theme by grouping together all of Jessie's behavioral, cognitive, and affective challenges comprising Reactive Attachment Disorder—occurring since an early age and throughout family changes, foster arrangements, adoptions, and further transitions—into one clear, logical grouping. The counselor's conceptual work at Step 2 gave her a way to begin thinking about Jessie's functioning and concerns more insightfully.

So far, at Steps 1 and 2, the counselor has used her clinical assessment skills and her clinical judgment to begin critically understanding

Jessie's presentation. Now, at Steps 3 and 4, she applies the theoretical approach she has selected. She begins making theoretical inferences to explain the factors leading to Jessie's issues as they are seen in Steps 1 and 2.

Step 3: Theoretical Inferences. At Step 3, concepts from the counselor's selected theory, Theraplay, are applied to explain the experiences causing, and the mechanisms maintaining, Jessie's problematic behaviors. The counselor tentatively matches the theme groups in Step 2 with this theoretical approach. In other words, the symptom constellations in Step 2, which were distilled from the symptoms in Step 1, now are combined using theory to show what are believed to be the underlying causes or psychological etiology of Jessie's current needs (Neukrug & Schwitzer, 2006; Schwitzer, 2006, 2007).

Theraplay is based on the assumption that relationships "modeled on healthy interaction between parents their children" can lead to enhanced "attachment, self-esteem, trust, and joyful engagement" (Koller & Booth, 1997, p. 204). According to the theory, when these types of relationships occur successfully in the family, they lead to healthy, normally expected child attachments and capacities for relationships. Alternatively, according to the model, the absence of these types of ideal experiences in the family can lead to relational and other types of developmental difficulties. Correspondingly, using the approach, therapeutic relationships involving counselors, parents, or primary caretakers and a child who is in need are constructed via the Theraplay treatment method. The relationships, modeled on healthy parent-child interactions, emphasize several relational dimensions: structure and limits, challenge, intrusion and engagement, and nurture (Jernberg & Booth, 1999; Jenberg & Jernberg, 1993). These therapeutic activities are expected to remediate and remedy problems in the attachment process that lead to children's intrapersonal and interpersonal difficulties (Jernberg & Jernberg, 1993).

As can be seen in Figure 9.2, when the counselor applied these concepts to her conceptualization of Jessie's presentation, she made the following theoretical inference at Step 3: Jessie missed out on access to models of healthy interaction between parents and children from pre-age-1 years onward.

Step 4: Narrowed Inferences. At Step 4, the clinician's selected theory continues to be used to address still-deeper issues when they exist (Schwitzer, 2006, 2007). At this step, "still-deeper, more encompassing, or more central, causal themes" are formed (Neukrug & Schwitzer, 2006, p. 207). Continuing to apply Theraplay concepts at Step 4, Jessie's counselor presented a single, most-fundamental construct that she inferred to be most explanatory and causal regarding Jessie's reasons for referral: Jessie required but did receive exposure to healthy experiences of relationship structure and limits, challenges, intrusion and engagement, and nurture (see Figure 9.2). When all four steps are completed, the client information in Step 1 leads to logical-intuitive groupings on the basis of common denominators in Step 2, the groupings then are explained using theory at Step 3, and then, finally, at Step 4, further deeper explanations are made. From start to finish, the thoughts, feelings, behaviors, and physiological features in the topmost portions are connected on down the pyramid into deepest dynamics.

The completed pyramid now is used to plan treatment to assist Jessie in multiple psychosocial systems.

TREATMENT PLANNING

At this point, Jessie's clinician at Creative Counseling Consultants has collected all available information about the problems that have been of concern to her and her school. Based upon this information, the counselor developed a five-axis *DSM-IV-TR* diagnosis and then, using the "inverted pyramid" (Neukrug &

Schwitzer, 2006; Schwitzer, 1996, 1997), formulated a working clinical *explanation* of Jessie's difficulties and their etiology that we called the *case conceptualization.* This, in turn, guides us to the next critical step in our clinical work, called the *treatment plan,* the primary purpose of which is to map out a logical and goal-oriented strategy for making positive changes in the client's life. In essence, the treatment plan is a road map "for reducing or eliminating disruptive symptoms that are impeding the client's ability to reach positive mental health outcomes" (Neukrug & Schwitzer, 2006, p. 225). As such, it is the cornerstone of our work with not only Jessie, but with all clients who present with disturbing and disruptive symptoms and/or personality patterns (Jongsma & Peterson, 2006; Jongsma et al., 2003a, 2003b; Seligman, 1993, 1998, 2004).

A comprehensive treatment plan must integrate all of the information from the biopsychosocial interview, diagnosis, and case conceptualization into a coherent plan of action. This *plan* comprises four main components, which include (1) a behavioral definition of the problem(s), (2) the selection of achievable goals, (3) the determination of treatment modes, and (4) the documentation of how change will be measured. The *behavioral definition of the problem(s)* consolidates the results of the case conceptualization into a concise hierarchical list of problems and concerns that will be the focus of treatment. The *selection of achievable goals* refers to assessing and prioritizing the client's concerns into a *hierarchy of urgency* that also takes into account the client's motivation for change, level of dysfunction, and real-world influences on his or her problems. The *determination of treatment modes* refers to selection of the specific interventions, which are matched to the uniqueness of the client and to his or her goals and clearly tied to a particular theoretical orientation (Neukrug & Schwitzer, 2006). Finally, the clinician must establish how change will be measured, based upon a number of factors, including client records and self-report of change, in-session observations by the clinician, clinician ratings,

Figure 9.2 Jessie's Inverted Pyramid Case Conceptualization Summary: Theraplay

1. IDENTIFY AND LIST CLIENT CONCERNS

Biological parents were both abandoned at birth and raised in foster care themselves

Biological father in alcohol recovery

Economically impoverished parents

Hiding, avoidant, wary throughout placements, settings, and developmental time periods

Increasingly aggressive or hostile reactions to others

Destructive aspects of play

Adopted but harassed by sibling at elementary age

Later fostered by current foster family

Early child foster care hiding from others

Early child foster care avoided touch of others

Early child foster care suspicious and wary of others

Older brother given for adoption

Born biologically premature

Poor access to prenatal and postnatal health care

Removed to foster family at age 1

Relocated to foster group home at ages 1–4

Feels "sad and angry"

2. ORGANIZE CONCERNS INTO LOGICAL THEMATIC GROUPINGS

Reactive Attachment Disorder of Infancy or Childhood: negative, avoiding, wary, suspicious with adults and peers—occurring since an early infant age and in reaction to a history of poor very early parenting relationships; early and subsequent foster family care, foster facility care; adopted care; and current foster care

3. THEORETICAL INFERENCES: ATTACH THEMATIC GROUPINGS TO INFERRED AREAS OF DIFFICULTY

Theraplay Inference

Jessie missed out on access to models of healthy interaction between parents and children from age 1 onward

4. NARROWED INFERENCES: SUICIDALITY AND DEEPER DIFFICULTIES

Deeper Theraplay Inference

Jessie required but did not receive exposure to healthy experiences of: relationship structure and limits; challenges; intrusion versus engagement; and nurture results of standardized evaluations such as the Beck Anxiety Inventory (Beck & Steer, 1990) or a family functioning questionnaire, pre-post treatment comparisons, and reports by other treating professionals.

The four-step method discussed above can be seen in Figure 6.1 (p. 109) and is outlined below for the case of Jessie, followed by her specific treatment plan.

Step 1: Behavioral Definition of Problems. The first step in treatment planning is to carefully review the case conceptualization, paying particular attention to the results of Step 2 (Thematic Groupings), Step 3 (Theoretical Inferences), and Step 4 (Narrowed Inferences). The identified clinical themes reflect the core areas of concern and distress for the client, while the theoretical and narrowed inferences offer clinical speculation as to their origins. In the case of Jessie, there is one overarching area of concern. "Reactive attachment disorder of infancy or early childhood" refers to her increasingly aggressive and hostile reactions toward others, destructive play, feelings of sadness along with anger and hatred toward caretakers. These symptoms and stresses are consistent with the diagnosis of Reactive Attachment Disorder of Infancy or Early Childhood, Inhibited Type (APA, 2000a; Hersen & Ammerman, 2000; Lieberman & Pawl, 1990; Parritz & Troy, 2011; Zeanah & Boris, 2005; Zero to Three Association, 2005).

Step 2: Identify and Articulate Goals for Change. The second step is the selection of achievable goals, which is based upon a number of factors, including the most pressing or urgent behavioral, emotional, and interpersonal concerns and symptoms as identified by the client and clinician, the willingness and ability of the client to work on those particular goals, and the realistic (real-world) achievability of those goals (Neukrug & Schwitzer, 2006). At this stage of treatment planning, it is important to recognize that not all of the client's problems can be addressed at once, so we focus initially on those that cause the

greatest distress and impairment. New goals can be created as old ones are achieved. In the case of Jessie, all of the goals are related to her primary problem, "reactive attachment disorder of infancy and early childhood." This complex developmental challenge requires that we help Jessie to resolve the impediments to forming healthy attachments, to establish and maintain a bond with her primary caregivers, to help her maintain appropriate boundaries with others, and to tolerate absences from her primary caregivers without excessive anxiety and behavioral/emotional dyscontrol.

Step 3: Describe Therapeutic Interventions. This is perhaps the most critical step in the treatment planning process because the clinician must now integrate information from a number of sources, including the case conceptualization, the delineation of the client's problems and goals, and the treatment literature, paying particular attention to *empirically supported treatment* (EST) and *evidence-based practice* (EBP). In essence, the clinician must align his or her treatment approach with scientific evidence from the fields of counseling and psychotherapy. Wampold (2001) identifies two types of evidence-based counseling research: studies that demonstrate "absolute efficacy," that is, the fact that counseling and psychotherapy work, and those that demonstrate "relative efficacy," that is, the fact that certain theoretical/technical approaches work best for certain clients with particular problems (Psychoanalysis, Gestalt Therapy, Cognitive Behavior Therapy, Brief Solution-Focused Therapy, Cognitive Therapy, Dialectical Behavior Therapy, Person-Centered Therapy, Expressive/Creative Therapies, Interpersonal Therapy, and Feminist Therapy); and when delivered through specific treatment modalities (individual, group, and family counseling).

In the case of Jessie, we have decided to use a multimodal treatment strategy as "specific interventions proposed for clinical disturbances or disorders of attachment have included individual psychotherapy for the child and/or caregiver, parent training with emphasis on developmental expectations and sensitive responsiveness, family therapy or caregiver/child dyadic therapy" (Zeanah & Boris, 2005, p. 365).

Developmental Play Therapy (Brody, 1999) is based on six basic premises: (1) a child who experiences herself as touched develops a sense of self; (2) in order for a child to experience herself touched, a capable adult must touch her; (3) in order to be a Toucher, the adult must first be willing to learn to be the one Touched; (4) in order to feel touched, a child has to allow herself to be touched; (5) a child feels seen first through touch; (6) to provide the relationship the child needs to feel touched, the adult controls the activities that take place within the Developmental Play Therapy session. Together, Jessie and the therapist will safely explore their relationship through the use of highly structured touch-based activities, including the "Slippery Hand Game," the "Hills and Valley Game," the "Knock at the Door Game," "Cradling," and the "Portrait Game." Each of these intimate contact activities will help Jessie to develop trust in the therapist and physical touch.

The therapist will also incorporate elements of Theraplay (Jernberg, 1979) into Jessie's treatment, which unlike Developmental Play Therapy incorporates the parents in the training. Theraplay is a "playful, engaging, short-term treatment method that is intimate, physical, focused and fun" (Jernberg & Booth, 1999, p. 3). In Theraplay, parents are included in treatment, first as observers and then as co-therapists, with the ultimate goal being to enhance the physical and emotional bond between caregiver and child through the use of structured assessment called the Marshak Interaction Method (Jernberg, Booth, Koller, & Allert, 1991) and a series of play-based activities that are structured, engaging, nurturing, and challenging.

Finally, the therapist will use elements of Parent-Child Interaction Therapy (Hembree-Kigin & McNeil, 1995), which, although developed for use with children younger than Jessie, has been found effective in reducing disruptive behavior (Eyberg, Nelson, & Boggs, 2008; Timmer, Ware, Urquiza, & Zebell, 2010). This intervention relies on teaching parents/caregivers effective and positive parenting skills both interactively in the clinic and at home through the use of assignments.

Step 4: Provide Outcome Measures of Change. This last step in treatment planning requires that we specify how change will be measured and indicate the extent to which progress has been made toward realizing these goals (Neukrug & Schwitzer, 2006). The counselor has considerable flexibility in this phase and may choose from a number of objective domains (psychological tests and measures of self-esteem, depression, psychosis, interpersonal relationship, anxiety, etc.), quasi-objective measures (the *DSM-IV-TR's* Axis V GAF scale; pre-post clinician, client, and psychiatric ratings), and subjective ratings (client self-report, clinician's in-session observations). In Jessie's case, we have implemented a number of these including sustained post-only measures of GAF functioning in the mild range (>70), client self-report of friendly and pro-social relationships with peers at school, parent reported improvement in quality of attachment (increased affection and parent attention-seeking), and pre-post improvement on the Attachment Q-Sort (Van IJzendoorn, Vereijken, Bakermans-Kranenburg, & Riksen-Walraven, 2004).

The completed treatment plan is now developed through which the counselor, Jessie, and her caretakers can develop mutually rewarding bonds of affection; it appears below and is summarized in Table 9.2.

TREATMENT PLAN

Client: Jessie

Service Provider: Creative Counseling Consultants

BEHAVIORAL DEFINITION OF PROBLEMS:

1. Reactive attachment disorder of infancy or early childhood—Increasingly aggressive and hostile reactions toward others, destructive play, feelings of sadness along with anger and hatred toward caretakers

GOALS FOR CHANGE:

1. Reactive attachment disorder of infancy or early childhood

   • Resolve the impediments to forming healthy attachments
   • Establish and maintain a bond with her primary caregivers
   • Help her maintain appropriate boundaries with others
   • Tolerate absences from her primary caregivers without excessive anxiety and emotional/ behavioral dyscontrol

THERAPEUTIC INTERVENTIONS:

A moderate- to long-term course of multimodal treatment (9–12 months), including Developmental Play Therapy, Theraplay, and Parent-Child Interaction Therapy

1. Reactive attachment disorder of infancy or early childhood

   • Elements of Developmental Play Therapy
   • Elements of Theraplay
   • Elements of Parent-Child Interaction Therapy

OUTCOME MEASURES OF CHANGE:

Improved quality of caregiver/client attachment and reduction in aggressive behaviors both at home and in school as measured by:

   • Sustained post-only measures of GAF functioning in the mild range (>70)
   • Client self-report of friendly and pro-social relationships with peers and teachers at school
   • Parent reported improvement in quality of attachment (increased affection and parent attention-seeking)
   • Clinician-observed improvement in parent-client relationship and client-attachment behaviors
   • Pre-post improvement on the Attachment Q-Sort

Table 9.2 Jessie's Treatment Plan Summary: Theraplay

Goals for Change	Therapeutic Interventions	Outcome Measures of Change
Reactive attachment disorder of infancy or early childhood	Reactive attachment disorder of infancy or early childhood	Improved quality of caregiver/ client attachment and reduction in aggressive behaviors both at home and in school as measured by:
Resolve the impediments to forming healthy attachments	Elements of Developmental Play Therapy	Sustained post-only measures of GAF functioning in the mild range (>70)
Establish and maintain a bond with her primary caregivers	Elements of Theraplay	
Help her maintain appropriate boundaries with others	Elements of Parent-Child Interaction Therapy	Client self-report of friendly and pro-social relationships with peers and teachers at school
Tolerate absences from her primary caregivers without excessive anxiety and emotional/behavioral dyscontrol		Parent reported improvement in quality of attachment (increased affection and parent attention-seeking)
		Clinician-observed improvement in parent-client relationship and client-attachment behaviors
		Pre-post improvement on the Attachment Q-Sort

CASE 9.3 *PETER PAN'S* TINKERBELL

INTRODUCING THE CHARACTER

Tinkerbell is a pixie in J. M. Barrie's fantasy tale *Peter and Wendy* (1911), which was later made into the *Peter Pan* films by Disney (Geronimi & Jackson, 1953; Hogan, 2003). She is both companion and guardian of the story's protagonist Peter Pan, and unbeknownst to him, an unrequited lover.

The story of Peter Pan, the perennially youthful leader of the Lost Boys and nemesis of Captain Hook, begins in London, where Peter has traveled to retrieve his shadow from the bedroom of Wendy Darling. Awakening with a fright, Wendy meets Peter for the first time and is immediately attracted to his playfulness, fearlessness, and spirit of adventure. She, along with

her siblings Michael and John, follow Peter back to Never Land where she meets the Lost Boys and Captain Hook and his deadly band of pirates. Wendy also meets Tinkerbell, a pixie who, unknown to Peter, falls deeply in love with him. Inventive, clever, and impish, Tinkerbell is very possessive of Peter and immediately jealous of his growing affections for Wendy. A muse who enjoys the arts, Tinkerbell is determined to thwart the budding romance. However, because of her diminutive size, Tinkerbell is capable of expressing only one emotion at a time and vacilates between giddy glee, vengeful rage, painful guilt, and moments of deep despair. In spite of her powers and abilities, Tinkerbell is ultimately no match for the life-sized and more well-rounded Wendy Darling. The story of Peter Pan is a timeless comedy, adventure, and passion play with something for audiences of all ages.

Peter Pan's pixie, Tinkerbell, experiences prominent changes in mood, delusional ideas about winning Peter's love, and notions about pixie dust and flying that might be seen as hallucinations outside of Never Land. As follows, using her experiences as our jumping-off point, in the following basic case summary and diagnostic impressions we recreate Tinkerbell in order to illustrate one example of the Schizophrenic and Other Psychotic Disorders.

Meet the Client

You can assess the client in action by viewing clips of Tinkerbell's video material at the following websites:

- http://www.youtube.com/watch?v= A4XuWT7n-aw&feature=related Internal struggle with various emotions
- http://www.youtube.com/watch?v=Y3k8 nto5Sgl&feature=related Shows her jealous nature
- http://www.youtube.com/watch?v=WtEv 3ktX30I&feature=related Her creative, mischievous side

Basic Case Summary

Identifying Information. Ms. Tinker Bell is a 45-year-old owner of the Never Land Foster Home, an institution she single-handedly built and operates. Her diminutive size, owing to a congenital growth condition and deceptively youthful appearance, has given her the nickname of Momma Pixie among the generations of orphaned boys whom she has taken into her care. She is an outspoken advocate for her charges whom she has lovingly come to call "my lost boys."

Presenting Concern. Ms. Bell was referred to the Never Land Community Mental Health Center out of concern by the chairman of the Never

Land Foster Home Board of Directors, Charles Smee, III. In a phone interview, Mr. Smee noted that although Ms. Bell has been an invaluable asset to the community, she seems to "be acting out of the ordinary." He said he has been getting increasing reports of her expressing very odd statements and beliefs about magic potions, pixie dust, spells, and being able to fly. He said she seems focused on finding what she calls "love spells." Out of respect, Ms. Bell came to the intake appointment, but vociferously denied anything unusual, although she did admit that she has been feeling very depressed lately and has been looking for a cure that will make her feel better and also bring her the love of her life.

Background, Family Information and Relevant History. Ms. Bell was born at Never Land General Hospital, where she was abandoned soon after birth by her parents who were reportedly incapable of caring for a "special needs child." Although they received counseling and the offer of unlimited state resources, Mr. and Mrs. Bell believed that their daughter, because of her translucent skin and diminutive size, was "an aberration."

Ms. Bell was raised in the Never Land foster-care system where she was the subject of ongoing ridicule as well as verbal and physical abuse by the other children. Ms. Bell excelled in academics and tinkering (and hence, her nickname Tinker), but showed an early interest in the occult and believed that she had the ability to cast spells with a homemade substance she called "pixie dust." She was evaluated by several psychiatrists over the course of her childhood and early adolescence, who could never quite agree on a diagnosis, but suspected an underlying psychotic process. She also experienced periods of depressed mood during which she ruminated about suicide and themes of death.

With intensive support that included psychiatric medication, individual psychotherapeutic support, and group support, she was able to progress through her school years. During her senior year of high school, Ms. Bell did a psychology internship at the Never Land Outreach Clinic and believed at that time that she had found her calling. It was at the clinic that Ms. Bell met Peter Pan, a spry and waif-like boy who, like her, was abandoned at birth. She became fascinated by Peter and his seeming ability to ignore the demands of both the real and adult world in favor of a rich fantasy life that included the delusion that he could fly and was being persecuted by a one-armed pirate named Hook. To the exclusion of her work and peer relations, Ms. Bell spent most of her time at the Outreach Center Library researching material that would help her better understand Mr. Pan. Being an accomplished tinkerer, Ms. Bell devised numerous exotic contraptions that she believed had the power to read minds and connect with other people's souls. She also claimed to have built a virtual sensory device that created the illusion of flight.

Around age 20, Ms. Bell experienced what was described as a "setback" that constituted a deterioration in her ability to manage her mood and everyday functioning. In her thinking and conversation, she seemed to easily become derailed. She held closely to her romantic delusion about winning Mr. Pan's love with a potion. Following what appeared to be a several months-long gradual decline, she was no longer able to successfully complete her work due to intruding hallucinations and bizarre ideas. She was seen on intake by a community counselor and was then admitted to the psychiatric unit of the Never Land General Hospital, where she was treated with antipsychotic medication, electroconvulsive therapy to improve her mood, and psychological counseling. By the time of her discharge 2 months later, Ms. Bell was considered to be recovered with continued reliance on medication and outpatient supportive counseling for chronic mental illness. Eventually, she even was able to procure a license as a foster facility administrator. It was through her work with the state and her compassion for children that Ms. Bell was referred the most difficult and challenging boys in Never Land. It was her hope that she could "help my lost boys to find the home that everyone deserves." However, she continued to occasionally experience passing thoughts of developing ways to attract her love interest, Peter; other strange ideas she could not eliminate; and sometimes, periods of depression.

Problem and Counseling History. When she was seen for the current intake session, Ms. Bell's small stature and odd pinkish skin did indeed give a pixielike impression to the evaluator. She was dwarfed in size by the chair in which she sat uncomfortably and from which she angrily darted at times when the conversation turned to her "delusion" about Mr. Pan. Ms. Bell raged when describing his interest in another woman by the name of Wendy Darling, and vowed that she would "do whatever it takes to rid Never Land of that beast of a girl." When asked about her relationship history, Ms. Bell receded into the chair and cried for minutes at a time. The intensity of her labile affect and implausibility of her stories suggested that, as was noted by her coworker, that Ms. Bell might indeed be a danger to both herself and to Mr. Pan. Ms. Bell was reluctant to talk about her 5-year experience at the residential facility and asserted that "no one has the right to know about my past except me." Evident on Ms. Bell's forearms was a series of parallel cuts that she acknowledged inflicting upon herself and that the evaluator later found out was a component of a self-mutilation ritual that she had been engaging in for the last 5 years. Given the severity of her presenting symptomology, Ms. Bell was detained and referred to the Crisis Treatment Center at Never Land Regional Psychiatric Hospital.

Goals for Counseling and Course of Therapy to Date. At the time of this report, Ms. Bell was not able to convince the evaluation team at Never Land Regional that she was capable of caring for herself as well as not be a danger to herself or others. She was being referred for a comprehensive neuropsychiatric assessment by the multidisciplinary team at Regional, which was charged with developing a comprehensive treatment plan that would assess her multitude of needs. Ms. Bell was noted to have said, "Just because I'm an orphaned pixie doesn't mean I can't help other people or myself."

Diagnostic Impressions

Axis I.   295.7 Schizoaffective Disorder

Axis II.   Borderline Personality Disorder Features

Axis III. Pixiated Growth

Axis IV. Problems with primary support group—Estrangement by parent, stresses of foster care

Axis V.   GAF = 30 (at admission)

GAF = 62 (highest level past year)

GAF = 72 (highest level recorded with medication)

DISCUSSION OF DIAGNOSTIC IMPRESSIONS

Ms. Tinker Bell was referred to the Never Land Community Mental Health Center by peers who were concerned that she was behaving out of the ordinary. In the interview, Ms. Bell described bizarre ideas pertaining to her ability to prepare magic potions, love spells, and a concoction she called "pixie dust," as well as a specific romantic delusion about winning love by using her magic abilities. She described a tactile hallucination of flying. In addition to these psychotic features, Ms. Bell also described depressed mood and cried notably during the interview. A review of records showed a history of both psychotic symptoms (flying hallucinations, romantic delusions, and bizarre ideas about magic and potions) and Major Depressive Episode symptoms (low mood disrupting everyday functioning, diminished ability to think and concentrate, and feelings of worthlessness).

The *DSM-IV-TR* section, Schizophrenic and Other Psychotic Disorders, contains a variety of mental disorders featuring delusions, prominent hallucinations, disorganized speech, disorganized behavior, or catatonic behavior. Included in this section are schizophrenic disorders (Schizophrenia, Schizophreniform Disorder, and Schizoaffective Disorder), Delusional Disorder (Erotomanic, Jealous, Grandiose, Persecutory, Somatic, and Mixed) and several other psychotic disorders (Brief Psychotic Disorder, Shared Psychotic Disorder, and psychotic disorders that are due to substance use or a medical problem). These disorders are listed on Axis I.

Ms. Bell presented a complex combination of depressive mood symptoms, together with the predominant psychotic symptoms of Schizophrenia, suggesting a diagnosis of Schizoaffective Disorder. Because she presented a history of depressive episodes but no manic or mixed episodes, the subtype is Depressive Type. The criteria for Schizoaffective Disorder, Depressive Type, have several components. First, there must be an extended period in which the client experiences the symptoms of a Major Depressive Episode (depressed mood or loss of interest and pleasure, together with characteristic disruptions in weight or sleep or energy, plus feelings of worthlessness or thoughts of death) at the very same time as she is experiencing the predominant psychotic symptoms of Schizophrenia (delusions, hallucinations). Second, the client must experience delusions or hallucinations for at least 2 weeks in the absence of prominent Major Depressive symptoms; however, third, the person must experience prominent mood symptoms during most of the disorder's duration.

Correspondingly, Ms. Bell's presenting concerns, interview information, and history provided evidence of an uninterrupted period of dysfunction during which she experienced the mood symptoms of a Major Depressive Episode at the same time as her flying hallucinations and delusions about magic—including time spans (we assume of at least 2 weeks according to her history) during which her mood symptoms were mostly absent but her hallucinations and delusions were still prominent, and with the additional note, that even during time spans when her hallucinations and delusions seemed less prominent, she did still have depressive symptoms.

Schizoaffective Disorder is a challenging diagnosis. Several differential diagnoses might be considered. There must be no evidence that the client's or patient's symptoms are the direct consequence of a general medical condition (e.g., Psychotic Disorder Due to a General Medical Disorder or Delirium Due to a General Medical Condition) or substance use (e.g., Substance-Induced Psychotic Disorder or Substance-Induced Delirium). There must be diagnosable mood symptoms concurrently with the active phase of the schizophrenic symptoms (otherwise the more appropriate diagnosis might be Schizophrenia). Conversely, the psychotic features must not be limited only to periods during mood episodes (which would suggest a Mood Disorder, Severe with Psychotic Features). One suggested resource for new clinicians is Noll's *The Encyclopedia of Schizophrenia and Other Psychotic Disorders* (2007). Based on our clinical evidence, Ms. Bell's history best matched the complex criteria for Schizoaffective Disorder.

On Axis II, problematic personality features and defenses can be listed even when they do not reflect a diagnosable Personality Disorder, if these personality characteristics are important to understanding the client's functioning and are maladaptive for the person. We provided the notation, Borderline Personality Disorder Features, to describe Ms. Bell's pattern of frantic efforts to win love, relationship intensity, and self-cutting behavior—which suggested a maladaptive pattern of instability in interpersonal relationships and self-image, and impulsivity. Although the

Axis I diagnosis described accounted for much of her behavior, we took the step of noting personality features on Axis II because they seemed clinically important and we recognized they could be easily overlooked in light of Ms. Bell's more florid schizophrenic symptoms.

To round out the diagnosis, Ms. Bell's pixiated growth *(sic)* is listed on Axis III, her history of family and social stressors are emphasized on Axis IV, and on Axis V her functioning is represented by GAF scores indicating very serious current problems in functioning (including behavior influenced by delusions and hallucinations) as well as information that, in the recent past, Ms. Bell has had a period of only mild symptoms and, with medication, functioned during other periods with only transient symptoms and stress reactions. The information on these axes is consistent with the Axis I and Axis II diagnoses describing Ms. Bell's patterns.

CASE CONCEPTUALIZATION

Upon Ms. Bell's referral to the Never Land Community Mental Health Center, her intake counselor conducted a thorough, detailed evaluation interview. The intake evaluation comprised a thorough history, client report, the reports of Ms. Bell's colleagues who had made the referral, counselor observations, and written psychological assessments. Based on the intake, Ms. Bell's psychotherapist developed diagnostic impressions, describing her presenting concerns as Schizoaffective Disorder, along with features of Borderline Personality Disorder. A case conceptualization next was developed.

At the Never Land Community Mental Health Center, Solution-Focused Counseling is used. The Center employs a solution-focused model because it is believed to be an efficient and effective method of providing services, and outcome studies suggest the approach can be successful with a range of presenting problems (De Jong & Berg, 2002; MacDonald, 1994). Whereas the purpose of diagnostic impressions is to *describe* the client's concerns, the goal of case conceptualization as it is applied to Solution-Focused Counseling is to better *understand* and clinically *organize* the person's experiences (Neukrug & Schwitzer, 2006). It helps the counselor determine the circumstances leading to Ms. Bell's Schizoaffective Disorder and personality features, and the factors maintaining her presenting concerns. In turn, case conceptualization sets the stage for treatment planning. Treatment planning then provides a road map that plots out how the counselor and client expect to move from presenting concerns to positive outcomes (Seligman, 1993, p. 157)—helping Ms. Bell return to an adequate level of functioning.

Generally speaking, when forming a theoretically based case conceptualization, the clinician applies a purist counseling theory, an integration of two or more theories, an eclectic mix of theories that focuses extensively on diagnosis, history, and etiology; by comparison, when forming a solution-focused case conceptualization, the counselor applies an eclectic combination of solution-focused, or solution-creating, tactics to his or her immediate understanding of the client and engages quickly in identifying and reaching goals (Berg, 1994; de Shazer & Dolan, 2007; Gingerich & Eisengart, 2000).

Ms. Bell's counselor used the Inverted Pyramid Method of case conceptualization because this method is especially designed to help clinicians more easily form their conceptual pictures of their clients' needs (Neukrug & Schwitzer, 2006; Schwitzer, 1996, 1997). Generally speaking, when the method is used with a theory-based conceptual model, there are four steps: Problem Identification, Thematic Groupings, Theoretical Inferences, and Narrowed Inferences. However, when the Brief Solution-Focused Counseling model is applied, only the first two steps are needed: Problem Identification and Thematic Grouping. From a solution-focused perspective, it is these two steps that focus attention on what clients want and need and what concerns will be explored and resolved (Bertolino & O'Hanlon, 2002). Brief solution-focused counselors make carefully thought-out professional clinical decisions at Steps 1 and 2 of the

pyramid; they are sure to have a rational framework for their decisions, rather than pulling techniques and approaches at random (Lazarus, Beutler, & Norcross, 1992; Norcross & Beutler, 2008). Ms. Bell's counselor's solution-focused clinical thinking can be seen in Figure 9.3.

Step 1: Problem Identification. The first step is Problem Identification. Aspects of the presenting problem (thoughts, feelings, behaviors, physiological features), additional areas of concern besides the presenting concern, family and developmental history, in-session observations, clinical inquiries (medical problems, medications, past counseling, substance use, suicidality), and psychological assessments (problem checklists, personality inventories, mental status exam, specific clinical measures) all may contribute information at Step 1. The counselor "casts a wide net" in order to build Step 1 as exhaustively as possible (Neukrug & Schwitzer, 2006, p. 202). As can be seen in Figure 9.3, the counselor identified Ms. Bell's current as well as past symptoms of depression (low mood, crying, poor thinking and concentration, etc.), current as well as past psychotic symptoms (bizarre ideation, delusions, tactile flying hallucinations, etc.), information about her romantic relationship behaviors (frantic efforts to win love, self-cutting, etc.), details of her treatment history, as well as a medical note about her growth disorder and a listing of her strength running her boys' home. The counselor attempted to go beyond just the presenting symptoms in order to be descriptive as she could.

Step 2: Thematic Groupings. The second step is Thematic Groupings. The clinician organizes all of the exhaustive client information found in Step 1 into just a few intuitive-logical clinical groups, categories, or themes, on the basis of sensible common denominators (Neukrug & Schwitzer, 2006). Four different ways of forming the Step 2 theme groups can be used: Descriptive-Diagnosis Approach, Clinical Targets Approach, Areas of Dysfunction Approach, and Intrapsychic Approach. As can be seen in the figure,

Ms. Bell's counselor selected the Clinical Targets Approach. This approach sorts together all of the Step 1 information "according to the basic division of behavior, thoughts, feelings, and physiology" (Neukrug & Schwitzer, 2006, p. 205).

The counselor grouped together: (a) all of Ms. Bell's historical and current negative thoughts and feelings associated with depression resulting in distress, dysfunction, and psychiatric treatment; (b) all of Ms. Bell's historical and current psychotic thoughts and perceptions associated with schizophrenic disorders resulting in distress, dysfunction, and psychiatric treatment; and (c) all of Ms. Bell's historic and current impulsive, troublesome relationship and interpersonal behaviors associated with borderline personality resulting in distress and dysfunction. The counselor selected the Clinical Targets Approach to organize Ms. Bell's concerns from a Solution-Focused Counseling perspective on the rational basis that she planned to emphasize cognitive and dialectical behavioral interventions that she believed would lead to good solutions with individuals such as Ms. Bell (Feigenbaum, 2007; McGurk, Twamley, Spitzer, McHugo, & Mueser, 2007; Pfammatter, Junghan, & Brenner, 2006).

With this two-step conceptualization completed, the client information in Step 1 leads to logical-intuitive groupings on the basis of common denominators in Step 2, and the counselor is ready to engage the client in Solution-Focused Counseling.

TREATMENT PLANNING

At this point, Ms. Bell's clinician at the Never Land Community Mental Health Center has collected all available information about the problems that have been of concern to her and the psychiatric team that performed her assessment. Based upon this information, the counselor developed a five-axis *DSM-IV-TR* diagnosis and then, using the "inverted pyramid" (Neukrug & Schwitzer, 2006; Schwitzer, 1996, 1997), formulated a working clinical *explanation* of

Ms. Bell's difficulties and their etiology that we called the *case conceptualization.* This, in turn, guides us to the next critical step in our clinical work, called the *treatment plan,* the primary purpose of which is to map out a logical and goal-oriented strategy for making positive changes in the client's life. In essence, the treatment plan is a road map "for reducing or eliminating disruptive symptoms that are impeding the client's ability to reach positive mental health outcomes" (Neukrug & Schwitzer, 2006, p. 225). As such, it is the cornerstone of our work with not only Ms. Bell, but with all clients who present with disturbing and disruptive symptoms and/or personality patterns (Jongsma & Peterson, 2006; Jongsma et al., 2003a, 2003b; Seligman, 1993, 1998, 2004).

A comprehensive treatment plan must integrate all of the information from the biopsychosocial interview, diagnosis, and case conceptualization into a coherent plan of action. This *plan* comprises four main components, which include (1) a behavioral definition of the problem(s), (2) the selection of achievable goals, (3) the determination of treatment modes, and (4) the documentation of how change will be measured. The *behavioral definition of the problem(s)* consolidates the results of the case conceptualization into a concise hierarchical list of problems and concerns that will be the focus of treatment. The *selection of achievable goals* refers to assessing and prioritizing the client's concerns into a *hierarchy of urgency* that also takes into account the client's motivation for change, level of dysfunction, and real-world influences on his or her problems. The *determination of treatment modes* refers to selection of the specific interventions, which are matched to the uniqueness of the client and to his or her goals and clearly tied to a particular theoretical orientation (Neukrug & Schwitzer, 2006). Finally, the clinician must establish how change will be measured, based upon a number of factors, including client records and self-report of change, in-session observations by the clinician, clinician ratings, results of standardized evaluations such as the Beck Anxiety Inventory

Figure 9.3   Ms. Bell's Inverted Pyramid Case Conceptualization Summary: Solution-Focused
Counseling Emphasizing Cognitive Interventions and Dialectical Behavioral Interventions

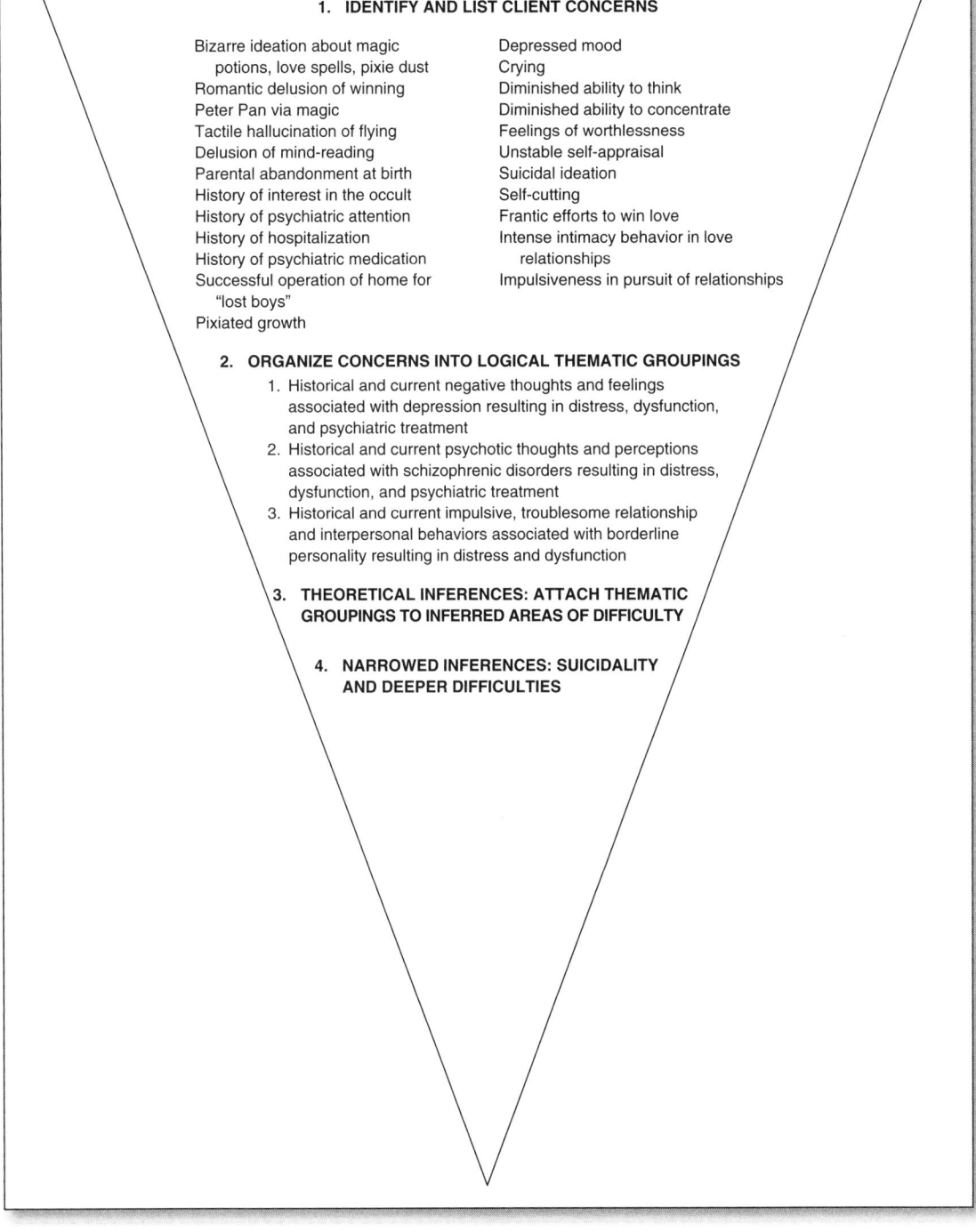

1. **IDENTIFY AND LIST CLIENT CONCERNS**

Bizarre ideation about magic
    potions, love spells, pixie dust
Romantic delusion of winning
Peter Pan via magic
Tactile hallucination of flying
Delusion of mind-reading
Parental abandonment at birth
History of interest in the occult
History of psychiatric attention
History of hospitalization
History of psychiatric medication
Successful operation of home for
    "lost boys"
Pixiated growth

Depressed mood
Crying
Diminished ability to think
Diminished ability to concentrate
Feelings of worthlessness
Unstable self-appraisal
Suicidal ideation
Self-cutting
Frantic efforts to win love
Intense intimacy behavior in love
    relationships
Impulsiveness in pursuit of relationships

2. **ORGANIZE CONCERNS INTO LOGICAL THEMATIC GROUPINGS**

    1. Historical and current negative thoughts and feelings
        associated with depression resulting in distress, dysfunction,
        and psychiatric treatment
    2. Historical and current psychotic thoughts and perceptions
        associated with schizophrenic disorders resulting in distress,
        dysfunction, and psychiatric treatment
    3. Historical and current impulsive, troublesome relationship
        and interpersonal behaviors associated with borderline
        personality resulting in distress and dysfunction

3. **THEORETICAL INFERENCES: ATTACH THEMATIC
    GROUPINGS TO INFERRED AREAS OF DIFFICULTY**

4. **NARROWED INFERENCES: SUICIDALITY
    AND DEEPER DIFFICULTIES**

(Beck & Steer, 1990) or a family functioning questionnaire, pre-post treatment comparisons, and reports by other treating professionals.

The four-step method discussed above can be seen in Figure 6.1 (p. 109) and is outlined below for the case of Ms. Bell, followed by her specific treatment plan.

Step 1: Behavioral Definition of Problems. The first step in solution-focused treatment planning is to carefully review the case conceptualization, paying particular attention to the results of Step 2 (Thematic Groupings). The identified clinical themes reflect the core areas of concern and distress for the client. In the case of Ms. Bell, there are three primary areas of concern. The first, "historical and current negative thoughts and feelings associated with depression," refers to her depressed mood, crying, feelings of worth-lessness, diminished ability to think and concen-trate, unstable self-appraisal, and suicidal ideation. The second, "historical and current psychotic thoughts and perceptions associated with schizoaffective disorder," refers to her bizarre ideation about magic potions, romantic delusion of winning Peter Pan via magic, her tactile hallucination of flying, and her delusion of mind-reading. The third, "historical and cur-rent impulsive and troublesome relationship and interpersonal behaviors associated with border-line personality," refers to her frantic efforts to win his love, self-cutting, intense intimacy behavior in love relationships, and impulsive-ness in pursuit of relationships and suicidal ide-ation. These symptoms and stresses are consistent with the diagnosis of Schizoaffective Disorder and Borderline Personality Features (APA, 2000a; Krabbandam & Aleman, 2003; Linehan, Heard & Armstrong, 1993; Livesley, 2007; Pfammatter et al., 2006).

Step 2: Identify and Articulate Goals for Change. The second step is the selection of achievable goals, which is based upon a number of factors, including the most pressing or urgent behavioral, emotional, and interpersonal concerns and symp-toms as identified by the client and clinician, the

willingness and ability of the client to work on those particular goals, and the realistic (real-world) achievability of those goals (Neukrug & Schwitzer, 2006). At this stage of treatment plan-ning, it is important to recognize that not all of the client's problems can be addressed at once, so we focus initially on those that cause the greatest distress and impairment. New goals can be created as old ones are achieved. In the case of Ms. Bell, the goals are divided into three prominent areas. The first, "historical and cur-rent negative thoughts and feelings associated with depression," requires that we assist Ms. Bell to understand the basis for her depression; to identify its cognitive, behavioral, emotional, and physiological triggers; to recognize her strengths and problem-solving skills, to implement problem-solving strategies to avoid depressive outcome, to learn and implement relapse preven-tion strategies, and to develop positive, life-affirming activities and a supportive social network. The second, "historical and current psy-chotic thoughts and perceptions associated with schizoaffective disorder," requires that we help Ms. Bell to control (or eliminate) her active psy-chotic symptoms through medication compli-ance, to distinguish between hallucinations/delusions and reality, improve her social skills and problem-solving, to empower her to make positive and healthy changes in her life, and to increase her goal-directed behaviors. The third, "historical and current impulsive, and trouble-some relationship and interpersonal behaviors associated with borderline personality," requires that we assist her to enhance her abil-ity to accurately label and express feelings, to understand and eliminate dangerous and impulsive behavior, to reduce the frequency of her suicidal ideation and behavior by recogniz-ing its relationship to depressive and angry states, and to decrease dependence on others to meet her own needs while building confidence and assertiveness.

Step 3: Describe Therapeutic Interventions. This is perhaps the most critical step in the treatment planning process because the clinician must now integrate information from a number of sources, including the case conceptualization, the delineation of the client's problems and goals, and the treatment literature, paying particular attention to *empirically supported treatment* (EST) and *evidence-based practice* (EBP). In essence, the clinician must align his or her treatment approach with scientific evidence from the fields of counseling and psychotherapy. Wampold (2001) identifies two types of evidence-based counseling research: studies that demonstrate "absolute efficacy," that is, the fact that counseling and psychotherapy work, and those that demonstrate "relative efficacy," that is, the fact that certain theoretical/technical approaches work best for certain clients with particular problems (Psychoanalysis, Gestalt Therapy, Cognitive Behavior Therapy, Brief Solution-Focused Therapy, Cognitive Therapy, Dialectical Behavior Therapy, Person-Centered Therapy, Expressive/Creative Therapies, Interpersonal Therapy, and Feminist Therapy); and when delivered through specific treatment modalities (individual, group, and family counseling).

In the case of Ms. Bell, we have decided to primarily use Brief Solution-Focused Therapy (De Jong & Berg, 2002; de Shazer & Dolan, 2007; Gingerich & Eisengart, 2000; Gutterman, 2006). We will supplement it with elements of both Cognitive Therapy (Beck, 1997) and Dialectical Behavior Therapy (Binks et al., 2009; Feigenbaum, 2007; Linehan et al., 1993). Solution-focused counseling is "pragmatic, anti-deterministic and future oriented [and as such] offers optimism, and hope about the ability of the client to change" (Neukrug, 2011, p. 426). It de-emphasizes psychopathology and the past, and instead focuses on the client's strengths, resources, and skills in order to generate solutions to the client's problems and concerns. Forward-looking and quickly moving, Solution-Focused Therapy's basic assumptions are that change is constant and inevitable, clients have the inherent skills and abilities to change, small steps lead to big changes, exceptions to problems do occur and can be used for change, and the

future is both created and negotiable—as well as simple axioms such as "if it ain't broke, don't fix it," "if it works, do more of it," and "if it's not working, do something different" (Neukrug, 2011).

We view Brief Solution-Focused Therapy as being particularly useful in Ms. Bell's case due to its positivistic emphasis on change, the future, and tapping into the client resources and skills. Rather than delve too deeply into her personality structure, it makes more clinical sense to strengthen her overall coping skills. This approach, which, in addition, focuses on empowerment, hope, and the strengthening of support networks, has been found to be particularly useful in case management with clients coping with persistent mental health issues (Greene et al., 2006). Specific techniques for Ms. Bell include asking a series of "miracle questions" to assess goals for change, and using preferred-goal, evaluative, coping, exception-seeking, and solution-focused questions; "scaling" her depressive feelings to provide context and perspective as well as a starting point for change; identifying and complimenting her use of skills; amplification of previously successful strategies for self-care; reframing her mood problems as the result of a chronic condition; identifying triggers for depressive thoughts; challenging and then reframing them; and finally, psychiatric referral.

Once Ms. Bell has been stabilized through the use of medication, we will also implement elements of both Cognitive Therapy and Dialectical Behavior Therapy (DBT). DBT relies on a combination of methods (cognitive behavior modification, mindfulness training, transference work, and dialectics), which target the "common factors" of personality disorder treatment (therapeutic structure, relationships) (Livesley, 2007) and the deficits that are specific to borderline conditions. Specific techniques for Ms. Bell will include identification of and desensitization (imaginal and in vivo) to cognitive triggers of behavioral, emotional, and physiological stress that precipitates psychotic thoughts, identification and refutation of irrational (and delusional) thoughts about the relationship with Peter Pan, cognitive restructuring and reframing of thoughts related to valuing and devaluing of self and others, and relaxation, including deep muscle work, breathing, and imagery.

In conjunction with DBT, we will use elements of Cognitive Therapy in order to restructure the way she thinks about herself and relationships. Specific techniques drawn from this approach will include identifying cognitive triggers for feelings of abandonment and their relationship to suicidal thoughts and feelings, and cognitive challenging and restructuring and reframing thoughts that give rise to distorted perceptions in relationships.

Step 4: Provide Outcome Measures of Change. This last step in treatment planning requires that we specify how change will be measured and indicate the extent to which progress has been made toward realizing these goals (Neukrug & Schwitzer, 2006). The counselor has considerable flexibility in this phase and may choose from a number of objective domains

(psychological tests and measures of self-esteem, depression, psychosis, interpersonal relationship, anxiety, etc.), quasi-objective measures (the *DSM-IV-TR's* Axis V GAF scale; pre-post clinician, client, and psychiatric ratings), and subjective ratings (client self-report, clinician's in-session observations). In Ms. Bell's case, we have implemented a number of these, including pre-post measures on the Beck Depression Inventory-II, post-only measures of GAF functioning in the mild range (>70), client self-reported elimination of obsessive preoccupation with Peter Pan, clinician-observed and client-reported improvement in mood, and physician-reported compliance with psychopharmacotherapy.

The completed treatment plan is now developed through which the counselor and Ms. Bell will begin their shared work of enhancing her overall coping and adaptive skills, including her physical and mental health. Ms. Bell's treatment plan is as follows and is summarized in Table 9.3.

TREATMENT PLAN

Client: Ms. Tinker Bell

Service Provider: Never Land Community Mental Health Center

BEHAVIORAL DEFINITION OF PROBLEMS:

1. Historical and current negative thoughts and feelings associated with depression resulting in distress, dysfunction, and psychiatric treatment—Depressed mood, crying, feelings of worthlessness, diminished ability to think and concentrate, unstable self-appraisal, and suicidal ideation

2. Historical and current psychotic thoughts and perceptions associated with Schizoaffective Disorder—Bizarre ideation about magic potions, romantic delusion of winning Peter Pan via magic, tactile hallucination of flying, and delusion of mind-reading

3. Historical and current impulsive and troublesome relationship and interpersonal behaviors associated with borderline personality—Frantic efforts to win love, self-cutting, intense intimacy behavior in love relationships, impulsiveness in pursuit of relationships, and suicidal ideation

GOALS FOR CHANGE:

1. Historical and current negative thoughts and feelings associated with depression
    *   Understand the basis for her depression
    *   Identify its cognitive, behavioral, emotional, and physiological triggers
    *   Recognize her strengths and problem-solving skills
    *   Implement problem-solving strategies to avoid depressive outcome
    *   Learn and implement relapse prevention strategies
    *   Develop positive, life-affirming interests, activities, and a supportive social network

2. Historical and current psychotic thoughts and perceptions associated with Schizoaffective Disorder
    *   Control (or eliminate) active psychotic symptoms through medication compliance
    *   Distinguish between hallucinations/delusions and reality
    *   Improve social skills and problem-solving
    *   Empowerment to make positive and healthy life changes in her life
    *   Increase goal-directed behaviors

3. Historical and current impulsive and troublesome relationship and interpersonal behaviors associated with borderline personality
    *   Enhance ability to accurately label and express feelings
    *   Understand and eliminate dangerous and impulsive behavior
    *   Reduce the frequency of suicidal ideation and behavior by recognizing its relationship to depressive and angry states
    *   To decrease dependence on others to meet own needs while building confidence and assertiveness

THERAPEUTIC INTERVENTIONS:

A moderate- to long-term course (6–9 months) of Solution-Focused Therapy supplemented with Cognitive and Dialectical Behavior Interventions; and both inpatient hospitalization and psychopharmacotherapy

1. Historical and current negative thoughts and feelings associated with depression resulting in distress, dysfunction, and psychiatric treatment
    *   Asking a series of "miracle questions" to assess goals for change
    *   Using preferred-goal, evaluative, coping, exception-seeking, and solution-focused questions centered on depression and effective coping with it
    *   "Scaling" depressive feelings to provide context and perspective as well as a starting point for change
    *   Identifying and complimenting use of self-affirming and positive problem-identification and problem-solving skills
    *   Amplification of previously successful strategies for mood improvement

(Continued)

(Continued)
- Reframing mood problems as the result of a chronic condition
- Identifying triggers for depressive thoughts, and challenging and then reframing them
- Referral for psychopharmacological intervention for depression

2. Historical and current psychotic thoughts and perceptions associated with Schizoaffective Disorder

- Identification of and cognitive desensitization (imaginal and in vivo) to triggers of behavioral, emotional, and physiological stress that precipitate psychotic thoughts and behaviors
- Identification and refutation of irrational (and delusional) thoughts about the relationship with Peter
- Referral for psychopharmacological intervention for psychotherapy

3. Historical and current impulsive and troublesome relationship and interpersonal behaviors associated with borderline personality

- Identifying cognitive triggers for feelings of abandonment and their relationship to suicidal thoughts and feelings
- Identify and then challenge, restructure, and reframe thoughts that give rise to distorted perceptions in relationships
- Cognitive restructuring and reframing of thoughts related to valuing and devaluing of self and others

OUTCOME MEASURES OF CHANGE:

The reinforcement and strengthening of already-present coping skills and alleviation of depression through appropriate medical care as measured by:

- Pre-post measures on the Beck Depression Inventory-II
- Post-only measures of GAF functioning in the mild range (>70)
- Clinician-observed and client-reported improvement in mood
- Client-reported and clinician-observed elimination of psychotic thoughts
- Physician-reported compliance with psychopharmacotherapy

Table 9.3   Ms. Bell's Treatment Plan Summary: Solution-Focused Counseling Emphasizing Cognitive Interventions and Dialectical Behavioral Interventions

Goals for Change	Therapeutic Interventions	Outcome Measures of Change
Historical and current negative thoughts and feelings associated with depression	Historical and current negative thoughts and feelings associated with depression resulting in distress, dysfunction, and psychiatric treatment	The reinforcement and strengthening of already-present coping skills and alleviation of depression through appropriate medical care as measured by:
Understand the basis for her depression	Asking a series of "miracle questions" to assess goals for change	Pre-post measures on the Beck Depression Inventory-II
Identify its cognitive, behavioral, emotional, and physiological triggers	Using preferred-goal, evaluative, coping, exception-seeking, and solution-focused questions centered on depression and effective coping with it	Post-only measures of GAF functioning in the mild range (>70)
Recognize her strengths and problem-solving skills	"Scaling" depressive feelings to provide context and perspective as well as a starting point for change	Clinician-observed and client-reported improvement in mood
Implement problem-solving strategies to avoid depressive outcome	Identifying and complimenting use of self-affirming and positive problem-identification and problem-solving skills	Client-reported and clinician observed elimination of psychotic thoughts
Learn and implement relapse prevention strategies	Amplification of previously successful strategies for mood improvement	Physician-reported compliance with psychopharmacotherapy
Develop positive, life-affirming interests, activities, and a supportive social network	Reframing mood problems as the result of a chronic condition	
Historical and current psychotic thoughts and perceptions associated with Schizoaffective Disorder	Identifying triggers for depressive thoughts, challenging and then reframing them	
Control (or eliminate) active psychotic symptoms through medication compliance	Referral for psychopharmacological intervention for depression	
Distinguish between hallucinations/delusions and reality	Historical and current psychotic thoughts and perceptions associated with Schizoaffective Disorder	
Improve social skills and problem-solving	Identification of and cognitive desensitization (imaginal and in vivo) to triggers of behavioral, emotional, and physiological stress that precipitate psychotic thoughts and behaviors	
Empowerment to make positive and healthy life changes in her life	Identification and refutation of irrational (and delusional) thoughts about the relationship with Peter	
Increase goal-directed behaviors	Referral for psychopharmacological intervention for psychotherapy	

(Continued)

Table 9.3 (Continued)

Goals for Change	Therapeutic Interventions	Outcome Measures of Change
Historical and current impulsive and troublesome relationship and interpersonal behaviors associated with borderline personality	Historical and current impulsive and troublesome relationship and interpersonal behaviors associated with borderline personality	
Enhance ability to accurately label and express feelings	Identifying cognitive triggers for feelings of abandonment and their relationship to suicidal thoughts and feelings	
Identify the triggers that lead to vacillation between idealizing and devaluing self and others	Identify and then challenge, restructure, and reframe thoughts that give rise to distorted perceptions in relationships	
Understand and eliminate dangerous and impulsive behavior	Cognitive restructuring and reframing of thoughts related to valuing and devaluing of self and others	
Recognize and control use of sex to manipulate others		
Become comfortable with own sexuality		
Reduce the frequency of suicidal ideation and behavior by recognizing its relationship to depressive and angry states		
Decrease dependence on others to meet own needs while building confidence and assertiveness		

CASE 9.4 *THE SIMPSONS'* WAYLON SMITHERS

INTRODUCING THE CHARACTER

Waylon Smithers, Jr., is an animated character and one of the "regular" cast members of the long-running Fox network's cartoon for adults *The Simpsons*. The show, which recently entered its fourth decade, is a comedy and parody that takes a satirical look at American society and Western cultural values.

Waylon Smithers, Jr., is the personal assistant to Mr. Montgomery Burns, the chief executive officer (CEO) of the Springfield Nuclear Power Plant. Cast as Mr. Burns's selfless, self-effacing, and dedicated assistant, Smithers, as he is referred to on the show, is a gay man who has not let his sexual identity become known to others on the show. He secretly fantasizes about sexual trysts with his boss and even has a pop-up screen saver on his computer that contains a naked image of Mr. Burns that says "Hello Smithers, you're quite good at turning me on." Smithers is often the butt of jokes by others at the power plant, most notoriously Homer Simpson, who has long suspected Smithers of being gay. Smithers continually ingratiates himself to Mr. Burns—a deeply narcissistic and sadistic employer and person who may at some level know of Smithers's interest in him and who takes advantage of him at all turns. The following basic case summary and diagnostic impressions present our portrayal of Smithers's recent counseling session as a result of troubles at work.

Meet the Client

You can assess the client in action by viewing clips of Waylon Smithers's video material at the following websites:

- http://www.youtube.com/watch?v= QW6DTVK4aCk Smithers loves Mr. Burns
- http://www.dailymotion.com/video/ x7mjqk_the-simpsons-homers-brain_ shortfilms Smithers and Burns perform brain surgery
- http://www.dailymotion.com/video/ x7mjf0_the-simpsons-homer-gets-hired_ shortfilms Smithers and Burns hire Homer

---

BASIC CASE SUMMARY

Identifying Information. Waylon Smithers, Jr., is a 38-year-old European American male of Norwegian desent who has been working as an executive assistant at the Springfield Nuclear Power Plant for the last 20 years. He presented himself as a well-groomed professional who prides himself on his personal appearance and presentation of self.

Presenting Concern. Mr. Smithers was referred to the Springfield Counseling Center by the employee assistance program (EAP) coordinator at the Springfield Nuclear Power Plant following a physical altercation with a fellow employee, Homer Simpson. According to Mr. Smithers, Mr. Simpson had "goaded and provoked me to rage by circulating a Valentine's card with a picture of me and Mr. Burns on it." Mr. Smithers added, "People at work can't appreciate the profound respect I have for Mr. Burns and somehow think this means that I'm in love with him . . . how preposterous that is."

Background, Family Information, and Relevant History. Mr. Smithers was born into an intact family in which he was the only child. Reports indicate that his parents, Mrs. and Mr. Waylon Smithers, Sr., of the city of Springfield (the U. S. state in which Springfield is located was missing from the paperwork provided), had been attempting to have a child for a number of years and were ecstatic over finally conceiving. As a child, Mr. Smithers was showered with love, affection, and attention.

Waylon Smithers, Jr., indicated that he grew up loving and admiring his parents and particularly his father, who was employed as an executive at the nearby Shelbyville Nuclear Power Plant. Waylon Smithers, Jr., excelled academically at Springfield Elementary and Middle Schools, where he was recognized for his keen sense of social awareness and deep sense of responsibility. He described his high school years as far more challenging: Mr. Smithers remembers often being singled out for what was regarded as a preference for intellectual and aesthetic activities rather than athletic or other stereotypical teenage boy pursuits. He dated only sporadically during high school and was far more comfortable in the role of friend and confidant with girls than he was in that of boyfriend.

Upon high school graduation, Mr. Smithers was admitted to the highly competitive Executive Management Studies program at Springfield School of Business, where he impressed both faculty and peers with his planning, organizational, and aesthetic skills, which garnered him numerous awards in both local and state competitions within the industry. It was while organizing a trade show at the Springfield Development Council that Mr. Smithers was approached by Montgomery

Burns, the owner and CEO of the town's nuclear power plant. Mr. Smithers was immediately attracted to the powerful yet seemingly kind and generous demeanor of Mr. Burns and immediately accepted the position as his executive assistant. Already in his mid-20s at that point, Mr. Smithers had only sporadically dated and chose to "devote my life and my energies to this fabulous man." Although Mr. Smithers's mother was appreciative of this wonderful opportunity for her son, she cautioned him against "surrendering your life and everything important to you for any person." Nevertheless, Mr. Smithers said he "did just that" and "dedicated my energies, time, and passion to providing Mr. Burns with the most comfortable and efficient organization possible."

Mr. Smithers noted one particularly significant event: One evening after a highly successful company function that Mr. Smithers had orchestrated, Mr. Burns, after having perhaps a bit too much to drink, hugged his loyal employee and whispered "I don't know what I would ever do without you." In looking back, Mr. Smithers recalled that as "a pivotal moment in our blossoming relationship." He began to fantasize about his boss, often spent long periods in sexual daydreams, and was even purported by his fellow employees to have a nude and seductive desktop picture of Mr. Burns on his computer. Mr. Smithers adamantly denied this and began to experience anger and resentment toward those who "thought my feelings for him were anything less than those of an admiring son." One day, while eating in the employee cafeteria, Mr. Smithers overheard a fellow employee, Homer Simpson, say, "That Smithers is really a gay duck . . . I think he and Mr. Burns should just run off and get hitched."

Problem and Counseling History. Due to the mandatory nature of his referral to the Springfield Counseling Center, Mr. Smithers was understandably perturbed and commented, "This is a witch hunt. . . . Am I here because they think I'm gay? . . . I should probably lodge

a discrimination lawsuit." Clearly agitated and visibly distressed, Mr. Smithers reluctantly entered the counselor's office and presented as a very nicely dressed, well-groomed, thin man of average height. He sat rigidly and tensely in his chair throughout the interview offering very terse, and at times, sarcastic comments to the interviewer. Visibly distressed when queried about his relationship with his employer, Mr. Smithers nevertheless relaxed somewhat as the conversation unfolded. He regarded Mr. Burns as a benevolent father figure, and particularly so in light of his earlier admiration of his own father during the very important and formative years of his childhood and adolescence. When gently queried about others' comments and speculative observations about his sexual orientation, Mr. Smithers took a deep breath, sat back in the overstuffed chair, and wondered aloud "If I was gay, would it really change anything in my life?" "Why are people that interested . . . maybe they're just jealous of my relationship with Mr. Burns." Mr. Smithers noted that he had a "crush" on his high school P.E. coach, but "could certainly never say anything to anyone about it." With regard to the altercation in the staff lounge, Mr. Smithers said, "It has always been dumbasses like Homer Simpson who have made it hard for me to just be who I am. Why can't people just leave others alone?" He denied any previous history of violent or aggressive behavior and in looking back at the incident, added, "It really shocked me that I went after him, but he just pushed me way too far."

Goals for Counseling and Course of Therapy to Date. The Springfield Executive EAP Program allows for three evaluative sessions prior to certifying an existing need for counseling. Mr. Smithers agreed to attend the two subsequent sessions and to participate in a routine psychological evaluation that includes the MMPI-2, Beck Depression Inventory II, California Personality Inventory, and the Ned Flanders Inventory of Attitudes.

Diagnostic Impressions

Axis I.   393.82 Identity Problem

Axis II.   V71.09 No Diagnosis

Axis III.   None

Axis IV.   Occupational problem—Discord with coworkers

Axis V.   GAF = 71 (current)

GAF = 81 (highest level past year)

DISCUSSION OF
DIAGNOSTIC IMPRESSIONS

Mr. Smithers came into the Springfield Counseling Center on EAP referral because of an altercation with another employee at work. He appeared to be a well-functioning adult who did not present any clinically significant signs of distress or impairment. Still, the EAP coordinator was concerned that he participate in meetings with a counseling professional with a focus on personal issues contributing to the workplace difficulties he was experiencing.

Along with all the various diagnosable disorders, a multiaxial diagnosis also lists "Other Conditions That May Be a Focus of Clinical Attention." The client concerns contained in this section (appearing at the end of the *DSM-IV-TR,* following all of the diagnosable disorders) are not diagnosable mental disorders according to the *DSM* classification system; instead, they are client problems or issues that are the focus of treatment when the individual is not experiencing any diagnosable disorder at all, or they are client problems that are a focus of counseling but not a part of the individual's diagnosable mental disorder. For example, Bereavement, Relational Problems, Occupational Problems, Academic Problems, Religious or Spiritual Problem, and Phase of Life Problems all are included under Other Conditions That May Be a Focus of Clinical Attention. They are listed on Axis I of a multiaxial diagnosis. In our professional counseling view, Smithers's experiences fall within this category.

Differential diagnoses might include any diagnosable Axis I mental disorder or Axis II Personality Disorder; however, no prominent, clinically significant difficulties were present. Another consideration is the specific category of Other Conditions That May Be a Focus of Clinical Attention to be selected. We selected Identity Problem. This category applies when the focus of counseling will be on multiple identity issues including, for example, career, patterns of friendships and interpersonal relationships, sexual orientation, sexual behavior, and other aspects of self-identity. A different selection of Other Conditions That May Be a Focus of Clinical Attention might be considered. For example, Occupational Problem might be a compelling category if the counseling focus were to be more narrowly on job dissatisfaction and career decisions. However, as this case was written, clinical attention is likely to be focused most compellingly on the ways in which aspects of Smithers's identity are interfering with his functioning in the work setting and elsewhere. In fact, sexual orientation–based problems in the workplace have been described as a factor influencing individuals' mental health (Herek, 1995). We believed that listing Identity Problem on

Axis I, and his discord with coworkers on Axis IV, best described and communicated about Smithers's reason for referral.

To complete the diagnosis, Smithers's occupational stressor, discord with workers, is emphasized on Axis IV, and on Axis V his functioning is represented by GAF scores indicating that although at present he is experiencing some transient, expectable reactions to the stresses of his identity problems in the workplace context, within the recent past he has demonstrated good functioning and the absence of concerns beyond everyday problems. The information on these axes is consistent with the Axis I diagnosis portrayed by Smithers in this case.

CASE CONCEPTUALIZATION

When Smithers made his first required visit to the Springfield Counseling Center, he and his counselor met for an intake appointment during which she collected detailed assessment information. The counselor first used this information to develop diagnostic impressions. Smithers's presenting concerns were described as comprising an Identity Problem with workplace discord as a stressor. Next, the counselor developed a case conceptualization. Whereas the purpose of diagnostic impressions is to *describe* the client's concerns, the goal of case conceptualization is to better *understand* and clinically *explain* the person's experiences (Neukrug & Schwitzer, 2006). It helps the counselor understand the origins of Smithers's difficulties and the factors maintaining them. In turn, case conceptualization sets the stage for treatment planning. Treatment planning then provides a road map that plots out how the counselor and client expect to move from presenting concerns to positive outcomes (Seligman, 1993, p. 157).

When forming a case conceptualization, the clinician applies a purist counseling theory, an integration of two or more theories, an eclectic mix of theories, or a solution-focused combination of tactics, to his or her understanding of the client. In this case, Smithers's counselor based her conceptualization on a purist theory, Person-Centered Therapy. The counselor selected this approach because it is the primary counseling method used at the Springfield Counseling Center when the clinician believes the client will benefit most from a therapeutic experience centering on gains in self-understanding, improvement in self-direction, and constructive growth in intrapersonal and interpersonal identity (Rogers, 1986)—as in the case of Smithers, who presented with an Identity Problem affecting his work life.

The counselor used the Inverted Pyramid Method of case conceptualization because this method is especially designed to help clinicians more easily form their conceptual pictures of their clients' needs (Neukrug & Schwitzer, 2006; Schwitzer, 1996, 1997). The method has four steps: Problem Identification, Thematic Groupings, Theoretical Inferences, and Narrowed Inferences. The counselor's clinical thinking can be seen in Figure 9.4.

Step 1: Problem Identification. The first step is Problem Identification. Aspects of the presenting problem (thoughts, feelings, behaviors, physiological features), additional areas of concern besides the presenting concern, family and developmental history, in-session observations, clinical inquiries (medical problems, medications, past counseling, substance use, suicidality), and psychological assessments (problem checklists, personality inventories, mental status exam, specific clinical measures) all may contribute information at Step 1. The counselor "casts a wide net" in order to build Step 1 as exhaustively as possible (Neukrug & Schwitzer, 2006, p. 202). As can be seen in Figure 9.4, the counselor identified at Step 1 all of Smithers's main reasons for his employee referral (physical altercation at work, taunting at work about being gay, etc.); information about his thoughts and feelings in relation to his employer, suggestive of a sexual identity question (describes as a "profound attraction," "blossoming relationship," etc.); information about his intrapersonal thoughts and feelings about self-identity (denies gay sexual identity despite evidence, etc.); and relevant history ("crush" on gym teacher, antagonism, etc.). The counselor went beyond just listing "workplace altercation" as the main reason for referral and was as complete as she could be about the present and relevant past, and Smithers's wider needs.

Step 2: Thematic Groupings. The second step is Thematic Groupings. The clinician organizes all of the exhaustive client information found in Step 1 into just a few intuitive-logical clinical groups, categories, or themes, on the basis of sensible common denominators (Neukrug & Schwitzer, 2006). Four different ways of forming the Step 2 theme groups can be used: Descriptive-Diagnosis Approach, Clinical Targets Approach, Areas of Dysfunction Approach, and Intrapsychic Approach. As can be seen in Figure 9.4, Smithers's counselor selected the Descriptive-Diagnosis Approach. This approach sorts together all of the various Step 1 information about the client's adjustment, development, distress, or dysfunction "to show larger clinical problems as reflected through a diagnosis" (Neukrug & Schwitzer, 2006, p. 205).

The counselor grouped together all of Smithers's various issues, concerns, and dynamics—including his workplace difficulties, relational dynamics, intrapersonal themes, and so on—into one straightforward descriptive-diagnostic theme: Identity Problem centering on sexual orientation, sexual behavior, patterns of interpersonal relationships (including those of the workplace), and self-identity. The counselor's conceptual work at Step 2 gave her a way to think about Smithers's functioning and concerns more insightfully.

So far, at Steps 1 and 2, the counselor has used her clinical assessment skills and her clinical judgment to begin critically understanding Smithers's needs. Now, at Steps 3 and 4, she applies the theoretical approach she has selected. She begins making theoretical inferences to explain the factors leading to Smithers's issues as they are seen in Steps 1 and 2.

Step 3: Theoretical Inferences. At Step 3, concepts from the counselor's selected theory, Person-Centered Therapy, are applied to explain the experiences leading to, and maintaining, Smithers's present issues. The counselor tentatively matches the theme groups in Step 2 with this theoretical approach. In other words, the symptom constellations in Step 2, which were distilled from the symptoms in Step 1 is now are combined using theory to show what is believed to be the underlying etiology of Smithers's current needs (Neukrug & Schwitzer, 2006; Schwitzer, 2006, 2007).

According to Person-Centered Therapy, individuals are capable of self-understanding and self-direction. Further, under the correct conditions, individuals progressively experience greater self-realization, fulfillment, autonomy, self-determination, and self-perfection as their lives progress, in a process referred to as the actualizing tendency (Broadley, 1999). The needed conditions are empathy, accurate understanding, and positive regard from the important others in our lives (Bohart & Greenberg, 1997; Rogers, 1961, 1977). In other words, under these conditions, individuals move forward toward their own self-fulfillment across the life span (Thorne, 2002). On the other hand, according to the theory, lack of empathy, accurate understanding, and positive regard from important others in our lives can disrupt or derail forward actualizing movement and result in maladjustment (Broadley, 1999; Rogers, 1961, 1977).

As can be seen in Figure 9.4, when the counselor applied these Person-Centered Therapy concepts, she explained at Step 3 that the various issues noted in Step 1 (workplace discord, taunting, idealized father, high school antagonism, self-denial and self-doubt, etc.), which can be characterized as a theme of Identity Problem centering on sexual orientation and interpersonal patterns (Step 2), together comprise a situation in which Smithers has in the past, and is at the present, experiencing a "history of perceived and actual lack of conditions of worth by important others."

According to Person-Centered Therapy inferences, lacking these conditions of worth is a central focus of Smithers's life developmental process. Further, it was important for the counselor to include in the theme, "actual" as well as "perceived" lack of positive interpersonal conditions: although the model operates on the assumption that clients can understand and address the core conditions in their lives causing distress, when working with diverse clients it must be recognized that sometimes cultural norms, or negative social pressures, can interfere with this (Cain, 2008). The theme appears on Figure 9.4.

Step 4: Narrowed Inferences. At Step 4, the clinician's selected theory continues to be used to address still-deeper issues when they exist (Schwitzer, 2006, 2007). At this step, "still-deeper, more encompassing, or more central, causal themes" are formed (Neukrug & Schwitzer, 2006, p. 207). Continuing to apply Person-Centered Therapy concepts at Step 4, Smithers's counselor presented the deeper implication of his lack of conditions impeded actualization. The counselor is inferring that improving Smithers's experience of conditions of worth (positive regard, accurate empathy, etc.) is needed in order to further his progress toward self-actualization.

Further, the counselor borrows from Minority Sexual Orientation Identity Development models (Evans & Levine, 1990; Meyer & Schwitzer, 1999) to infer that Smithers has been impeded from progressing through the sequential stages of identity development common among gay men and lesbians. These stages include (Meyer & Schwitzer, 1999): Recognizing a Difference, Reflective Observations, Internalizing Reflective Observations, Self-Identifying, Coming Into Proximity, Networking, and Connecting. These developmental concepts are compatible and can be helpful when applying the Person-Centered Theory to minority sexual orientation client's self-actualization because they emphasize "an increasing realization and

acceptance" of one's sexual orientation (p. 51), clarifying and shifting to more positive feelings about one's self-identity, and more frequent and closer involvement with a gay community, which provides conditions of worth (Evans & Levine, 1990).

When all four steps are completed, the client information in Step 1 leads to logical-intuitive groupings on the basis of common denominators in Step 2, the groupings then are explained using theory at Step 3, and then, finally, at Step 4, further deeper explanations are made. From start to finish, the thoughts, feelings, behaviors, and physiological features in the topmost portions are connected on down the pyramid into deepest dynamics.

The completed pyramid now is used to plan treatment, in which the counselor will engage Smithers with congruence, unconditional positive regard, and accurate empathy to promote his increased sense of self-worth, process of self-actualization, and resolution of his identity development.

TREATMENT PLANNING

At this point, Smithers' clinician at the Springfield Counseling Center has collected all available information about the problems that have been of concern. Based upon this information, the counselor developed a five-axis *DSM-IV-TR* diagnosis and then, using the "inverted pyramid" (Neukrug & Schwitzer, 2006; Schwitzer, 1996, 1997), formulated a working clinical *explanation* of Smithers's difficulties and their etiology that we called the *case conceptualization.* This, in turn, guides us to the next critical step in our clinical work, called the *treatment plan,* the primary purpose of which is to map out a logical and goal-oriented strategy for making positive changes in the client's life. In essence, the treatment plan is a road map "for reducing or eliminating disruptive symptoms that are impeding the client's ability to reach positive

Figure 9.4   Waylon Smithers's Inverted Pyramid Case Conceptualization Summary: Person-Centered Counseling

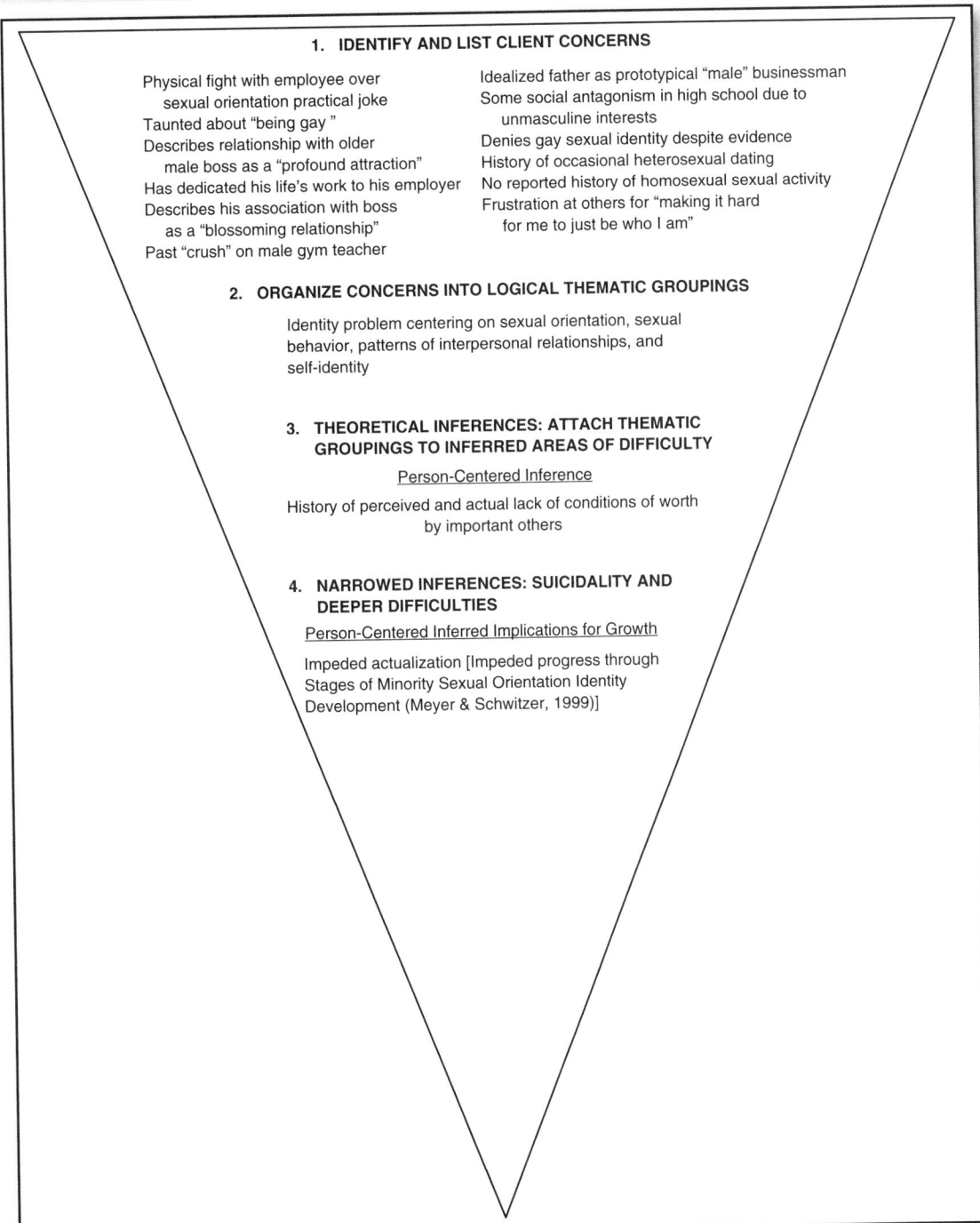

1. IDENTIFY AND LIST CLIENT CONCERNS

Physical fight with employee over sexual orientation practical joke

Taunted about "being gay "

Describes relationship with older male boss as a "profound attraction"

Has dedicated his life's work to his employer

Describes his association with boss as a "blossoming relationship"

Past "crush" on male gym teacher

Idealized father as prototypical "male" businessman

Some social antagonism in high school due to unmasculine interests

Denies gay sexual identity despite evidence

History of occasional heterosexual dating

No reported history of homosexual sexual activity

Frustration at others for "making it hard for me to just be who I am"

2. ORGANIZE CONCERNS INTO LOGICAL THEMATIC GROUPINGS

Identity problem centering on sexual orientation, sexual behavior, patterns of interpersonal relationships, and self-identity

3. THEORETICAL INFERENCES: ATTACH THEMATIC GROUPINGS TO INFERRED AREAS OF DIFFICULTY

Person-Centered Inference

History of perceived and actual lack of conditions of worth by important others

4. NARROWED INFERENCES: SUICIDALITY AND DEEPER DIFFICULTIES

Person-Centered Inferred Implications for Growth

Impeded actualization [Impeded progress through Stages of Minority Sexual Orientation Identity Development (Meyer & Schwitzer, 1999)]

mental health outcomes" (Neukrug & Schwitzer, 2006, p. 225). As such, it is the cornerstone of our work with not only Waylon Smithers, but with all clients who present with concerns (Jongsma & Peterson, 2006; Jongsma et al., 2003a, 2003b; Seligman, 1993, 1998, 2004).

A comprehensive treatment plan must integrate all of the information from the biopsychosocial interview, diagnosis, and case conceptualization into a coherent plan of action. This *plan* comprises four main components, which include (1) a behavioral definition of the problem(s), (2) the selection of achievable goals, (3) the determination of treatment modes, and (4) the documentation of how change will be measured. The *behavioral definition of the problem(s)* consolidates the results of the case conceptualization into a concise hierarchical list of problems and concerns that will be the focus of treatment. The *selection of achievable goals* refers to assessing and prioritizing the client's concerns into a *hierarchy of urgency* that also takes into account the client's motivation for change, level of dysfunction, and real-world influences on his or her problems. The *determination of treatment modes* refers to selection of the specific interventions, which are matched to the uniqueness of the client and to his or her goals and clearly tied to a particular theoretical orientation (Neukrug & Schwitzer, 2006). Finally, the clinician must establish how change will be measured, based upon a number of factors, including client records and self-report of change, in-session observations by the clinician, clinician ratings, results of standardized evaluations such as the Beck Anxiety Inventory (Beck & Steer, 1990) or a family functioning questionnaire, pre-post treatment comparisons, and reports by other treating professionals.

The four-step method discussed above can be seen in Figure 6.1 (p. 109) and is outlined below for the case of Smithers, followed by his specific treatment plan.

Step 1: Behavioral Definition of Problems. The first step in treatment planning is to carefully review the case conceptualization, paying particular attention to the results of Step 2 (Thematic Groupings), Step 3 (Theoretical Inferences), and Step 4 (Narrowed Inferences). The identified clinical themes reflect the core areas of concern and distress for the client, while the theoretical and narrowed inferences offer clinical speculation as to their origins. In the case of Smithers, there is one primary areas of concern, "identity problem," which refers to his internal and external conflicts regarding his sexual orientation. His symptoms and stresses are consistent with the diagnosis of Identity Problem (APA, 2000a; Bieschke, Perez, & DeBord, 2007; Fontaine & Hammond, 1996; Meyer & Schwitzer, 1999; Ometo & Kurtzman, 2006).

Step 2: Identify and Articulate Goals for Change. The second step is the selection of achievable goals, which is based upon a number of factors, including the most pressing or urgent behavioral, emotional, and interpersonal concerns and symptoms as identified by the client and clinician, the willingness and ability of the client to work on those particular goals, and the realistic (real-world) achievability of those goals (Neukrug & Schwitzer, 2006). At this stage of treatment planning, it is important to recognize that not all of the client's problems can be addressed at once, so we focus initially on those that cause the greatest distress and impairment. New goals can be created as old ones are achieved. In the case of Smithers, the goals center around his primary "identity problem," which requires that we help him to understand the impact of societal heterosexism in his identity development, to develop self-acceptance and a positive sense of identity, as well as to be able to make a comfortable choice in pursuing a healthy and satisfying intimate relationship.

Step 3: Describe Therapeutic Interventions. This is perhaps the most critical step in the treatment planning process because the clinician must now integrate information from a number of sources, including the case conceptualization, the delineation of the client's problems and goals, and the treatment literature, paying particular attention to *empirically supported treatment* (EST) and *evidence-based practice* (EBP). In essence, the clinician must align his or her treatment approach with scientific evidence from the fields of counseling and psychotherapy. Wampold (2001) identifies two types of evidence-based counseling research: studies that demonstrate "absolute efficacy," that is, the fact that counseling and psychotherapy work, and those that demonstrate "relative efficacy," that is, the fact that certain theoretical/technical approaches work best for certain clients with particular problems (Psychoanalysis, Gestalt Therapy, Cognitive Behavior Therapy, Brief Solution-Focused Therapy, Cognitive Therapy, Dialectical Behavior Therapy, Person-Centered Therapy, Expressive/Creative Therapies, Interpersonal Therapy, and Feminist Therapy); and when delivered through specific treatment modalities (individual, group, and family counseling). In the case of Smithers, we have decided to use Person-Centered Counseling (Bohart & Greenberg, 1997; Broadley, 1999; Carkhuff, 2000; Raskin & Rogers, 2000; Rogers, 1961, 1977) due to its humanistic emphasis on each person's inherent capacity for self-determination, growth, and actualization. Given Smithers's intrapersonal and interpersonal conflicts surrounding his sexual identity, the therapeutic conditions of unconditional positive regard, genuineness, empathy, and congruence would help him to understand and work through his issues related to his identity struggles. Additionally, the nondirective nature of Client-Centered Counseling would facilitate Smithers's overall life satisfaction and interpersonal relationships, and in particular, the one with his boss (and secret love interest), Mr. Burns. The highly supportive nature of this type of counseling with clients struggling with identity issues, and in particular sexual identity concerns, will

assist Smithers in making sense of conflicting sexual feelings and thoughts, strengthening his sense of empowerment, and overall life satisfaction (Fontaine & Hammond, 1996; Savage, Harley, & Nowak, 2005). Specific techniques for Smithers will include supporting him in describing the fear, anger, anxiety, and distress over confusion related to his sexual identity, recognition of heteronormative societal pressures, identifying and expressing homoerotic thoughts, feelings, and fantasies, and group support.

Step 4: Provide Outcome Measures of Change. This last step in treatment planning requires that we specify how change will be measured and indicate the extent to which progress has been made toward realizing these goals (Neukrug & Schwitzer, 2006). The counselor has considerable flexibility in this phase and may choose from a number of objective domains (psychological tests and measures of self-esteem, depression, psychosis, interpersonal relationship, anxiety, etc.), quasi-objective measures (the *DSM-IV-TR's* Axis V GAF scale; pre-post clinician, client, and psychiatric ratings), and subjective ratings (client self-report, clinician's in-session observations). In Smithers's case, we have implemented a number of these, including pre-post measures on the Beck Depression Inventory-II (1996), post-only scores on the Sexual Identity Scale (Stern, Barack, & Gould, 1987), client report of improvement in overall self and life satisfaction, clinician observation of improved overall mood and outlook, and client-reported interest in exploring an intimate relationship.

The completed treatment plan is now developed through which the counselor and Waylon Smithers will work toward improving his overall self-image, eliminating conflicts in his sexual identity, and pursuing satisfying intimate relationships. Smithers's treatment plan appears below and a summary can be found in Table 9.4.

TREATMENT PLAN

Client: Waylon Smithers

Service Provider: Springfield Counseling Center

BEHAVIORAL DEFINITION OF PROBLEMS:

1. Identity problem—Physical fights with coworker over sexual-orientation practical joke, worried about and angry at coworkers for thinking he is gay, taunted by coworkers for being gay, denial of gay identity despite evidence, secretive crush on male employer, sole dedication to his employer, frustration at others for "making it hard for me to just be who I am"

GOALS FOR CHANGE:

1. Identity Problem

   - Recognize and resolve conflicted thoughts and feelings regarding sexual identity
   - Understand the impact of societal heterosexism in his identity development
   - Develop a non pathology-based understanding of homosexuality
   - Develop a positive sense of identity, including but not limited to sexual orientation
   - Establish an accurate representation of the lives and lifestyles of homosexual men
   - Develop self-acceptance, positive self-regard, and a sense of personal empowerment
   - Make a comfortable choice in pursuing a healthy and satisfying intimate relationship

THERAPEUTIC INTERVENTIONS:

A short- to moderate-term course of individual, client-centered counseling, supplemented with group support

1. Identity Problem

   - Describe fear, anger, anxiety, and distress over confusion related to sexual identity
   - Address pressures of hiding homoerotic thoughts and feelings from self and others
   - Identify sexual experiences, thoughts, and feelings that have been interesting and/or exciting
   - Verbalize understanding of societal heteronormative pressures
   - Role-play disclosure of sexual interests and orientation and identify a trusted person to disclose to
   - Attend support group for people planning to disclose or who have already disclosed their sexual identity

OUTCOME MEASURES OF CHANGE:

The development of congruence between his ideal and actual self, improved self-esteem, greater capacity for understanding and expression of feelings, reconciliation and resolution of his gender identity issues as measured by:

- Post-only scores on the Sexual Identity Scale
- Pre-post measures on the Beck Depression and Beck Anxiety Inventories
- Client report of improvement in overall life satisfaction
- Client report and clinician's observation of gradually increasing comfort over expressing his homosexual thoughts, feelings, and behaviors
- Clinician observation of improved overall mood and outlook
- Client report of improved self-assertion skills at work and related decrease in peer harassment
- Client report of better overall relationships with coworkers

Table 9.4   Waylon Smithers's Treatment Plan Summary: Person-Centered Counseling

Goals for Change	Therapeutic Interventions	Outcome Measures of Change
Identity Problem Recognize and resolve conflicted thoughts and feelings regarding sexual identity Understand the impact of societal heterosexism in his identity development Develop a nonpathology-based understanding of homosexuality Develop a positive sense of identity, including but not limited to sexual orientation Establish an accurate representation of the lives and lifestyles of homosexual men Develop self-acceptance, positive self-regard, and a sense of personal empowerment Make a comfortable choice in pursuing a healthy and satisfying intimate relationship	Identity Problem Describe fear, anger, anxiety, and distress over confusion related to sexual identity Address pressures of hiding homoerotic thoughts and feelings from self and others Identify sexual experiences, thoughts, and feelings that have been interesting and/or exciting Verbalize understanding of societal heteronormative pressures Role-play disclosure of sexual interests and orientation and identify a trusted person to disclose to Attend support group for people planning to disclose, or who have already disclosed their sexual identity	The development of congruence between his ideal and actual self, improved self-esteem, greater capacity for understanding and expression of feelings, reconciliation and resolution of his gender identity issues as measured by: Post-only scores on the Sexual Identity Scale Pre-post measures on the Beck Depression and Beck Anxiety Inventories Client report of improvement in overall life satisfaction Client report and clinician's observation of gradually increasing comfort over expressing his homosexual thoughts, feelings, and behaviors Clinician observation of improved overall mood and outlook Client report of improved self-assertion skills at work and related decrease in peer harassment Client report of better overall relationships with coworkers

CASE 9.5   *BEAUTY AND THE BEAST'S* BELLE

INTRODUCING THE CHARACTER

Belle is a central character in the timeless fairy tale *Beauty and the Beast,* which first appeared in France in the 18th-century as *La Belle et La Bête.* Although now most widely recognized as the Walt Disney animated film of the same name (Trousdale & Wise, 1991), it also has been re-visioned as a Broadway musical.

Disney's popularized version of the tale introduces us to an innocent, unknowing, and gentle girl by the name of Belle who becomes lost in the woods and finds her way to a mountaintop castle, where she is welcomed by magical furniture and pottery. In actuality, the castle is inhabited by the Beast, a horrific and menacing brute who terrorizes a village from his mountaintop castle perch. Unbeknownst to Belle, the furniture, previously castle servants, had been transformed by the same magic spell that turned the Beast, a handsome albeit self-absorbed prince, into a hideous monster. Angrily lamenting the loss of his humanity, the Beast imprisons the girl, hoping to somehow capture her beauty and her art. Initially frightened by his appearance and unwelcoming demeanor, Belle finds her way to the Beast's heart and transforms him through her compassion and love. At the end of the tale, the Beast, by virtue of learning the lessons of the heart, is transformed back into the prince, and with Belle and the house servants "lives happily ever after." It is a timeless tale of the power of love to transform and soften even the most hardened heart, the thin line that separates love and hatred, beauty and ugliness, as well as good and evil.

For us as authors, Belle is one of the most vivid examples of "good" we have identified among many pop culture sources. However, as sometimes occurs among our real-life clients who engage in irrational thinking, in the case summary and diagnostic impressions that follow, we create a scenario in which Belle, despite actually possessing innately good and transformative social and personal qualities, might experience social phobia, characterized by unreasonable fears of being negatively judged, embarrassed, or humiliated by others in social situations.

Meet the Client

You can assess the client in action by viewing clips of Belle's video material at the following websites:

- http://www.youtube.com/watch?v= DGSqt2fD4Xo Movie trailer
- http://www.youtube.com/watch?v= oeoPtz0F2Ck Getting ready to be with Belle

---

BASIC CASE SUMMARY

Identifying Information. Belle Beastly is a 31-year-old white British woman who has been married for several years to Prince Beastly and lives in a socioeconomically upper-class suburb of Manchester, England. She was dressed impeccably in traditional fairy-tale style clothing suited for a heroine. Although she was engaged and appeared motivated during the interview, she spoke hesitantly and sought reassurance and affirmation from the therapist throughout the meeting, and expressed a concern that "her problems probably were just silly" and she hoped the clinician would "just laugh at how trivial she was being."

Presenting Concern. Belle arrived at the Manchester Public Clinic upon the urging of her husband. He encouraged her to attend the session in order to explore what he perceived to be her irrational reticence about being in public. By his report and her self-disclosure, she experienced what they "knew were crazy fears" about "making a darn fool of myself." Her self-doubting concerns led her to avoid major social events such as community balls and cathedral organ recitals and receptions. Her persistent fears and avoidance of major social situations caused her to attend many of these events only with great effort and her ability to endure feelings of anxiety and dread. These issues were beginning to frustrate Prince Beastly, who wished for them to become a more visible, active couple in local society. However, she describes it as "a success" that she is able to attend to minor everyday events like checking out at the grocery store and participating in neighborhood socials and meetings with only mild nervousness or quickly passing self-doubting thoughts.

Background, Family Information, and Relevant History. Belle was born outside of a small mining town in Great Britain, the younger of two girls to uneducated farm workers. Belle's older sister was prized by her father for her striking good looks and musical talent. Belle was unplanned, and was readily made to feel unwanted by her father. Hoping that his second daughter would be every bit as beautiful as his first, Belle's father took every opportunity to belittle his second born in front of her sister as well as friends. Belle's mother was unable to stop her husband's harsh treatment of her daughter, for she too was often berated and belittled by him. When Belle was 12 years of age, her sister, Antigone, moved out of the family home to marry a man she met while on vacation. After the departure of her sister, Belle was left alone in her home and the object of her father's continued undermining comments and unfounded criticism.

Belle's father's emotional abuse escalated when she entered puberty as he then began calling her "filthy and shameful." Internalizing these negative messages, Belle retreated to the world of books and solitude, and began to see herself as less lovable, less accomplished, and less able than her peers. Physically, she downplayed her appearance in spite of her mother's efforts to encourage her daughter to "stand up and be proud of yourself." During her late adolescence, an especially stressful time when she was

required to perform in a school musical event, she briefly refused to attend school or leave the house. In retrospect, Belle remembers that her mother believed that she had "become the self-doubting little girl that my husband saw her as."

At the same time, Belle actually was physically attractive and would have been described in appearance as a "sort of beautiful princess." At school, though persistently fearful of "showing herself" to groups of peers and, especially, students outside of her grade whom she did not know very well, she excelled in psychology and the social sciences. Her empathy skills allowed her to be a peer mentor, where, although hesitant, she excelled in one-on-one helping relationships. At age 19, she happened onto the doorstep of Prince Beastly's castlelike mansion, seeking directions. At the time he was experiencing mood and anger problems of his own; however, Belle's interpersonal helping skills allowed her to begin a friendship, then romance, with Beastly. He and others clearly see in her skills and abilities that she does not.

Problem and Counseling History. Belle remembers feeling "self-conscious around others as far back as I can remember." By her description, she is able to be around others, especially those she does not know very well, only with great effort. She describes "being so afraid I'll embarrass myself. What if I say something stupid? What if they see how crazy I am?" She worries that she will "almost certainly" say something humiliating or do something embarrassing. As a consequence, she primarily avoids any unnecessary social outings. She appeared distressed about the effects of her social fears on her marital relationship.

At the same time, when tested with a mild confrontation by the clinician, she admitted that "Yes, I know I'm overreacting and being unreasonable, but what can I do?" She also is able to rally her resources and engage with others in spite of her symptoms when it is necessary, such as to fulfill an important work-related social role for her husband, or to work on local charity events. In these situations, she says she "just gets on with it" and "gets involved." Further, in her intimate relationship with her husband, and social relationships with her small circle of close friends, she reports that she can easily "be myself" because "well, they already know me." Belle has not sought any previous counseling; however, her primary-care physician provided her with a mild anti-anxiety medication for use as needed. Her physician also has tested and ruled out the presence of hyperthyroidism, and she denies any substance use beyond "occasional red wine on weekends with my husband or at special events."

Goals for Counseling and Course of Therapy to Date. Belle seemed relieved at the end of the interview and agreed to return for ongoing brief, individual counseling to address her presenting problem but volunteered that she would "never be in group therapy." A treatment plan will be developed and followed.

Diagnostic Impressions

Axis I. 300.13 Social Phobia (Social Anxiety Disorder), Generalized

Axis II. Avoidant Personality Disorder Features

Axis III. None

Axis IV. Problem with primary support group—History of discord with father

Axis V. GAF = 68 (estimated at intake)

GAF = 75 (highest level in past year, estimated)

DISCUSSION OF DIAGNOSTIC IMPRESSIONS

Belle came into the Manchester Public Clinic due to persistent fears of being humiliated or embarrassed in front of others, which led her to avoid most social situations and social performance situations. Her fears and avoidance were interfering with her normal routine, such as checking out at the grocery store, and with her ability to fill important roles such as attending major community events like royal balls and recitals. When it was critical that she attend these events, she endured them with extreme anxiety. In spite of their intensity, Belle was aware that her fearful thoughts were unreasonable.

The predominant feature shared by all of the diagnosable disorders found in the Anxiety Disorders section of the *DSM-IV-TR* is the presence of increased arousal, excessive worry, or other signs of anxiety that cause distress or impairment, including panic. Among these are Specific Phobias (characterized by anxiety associated with exposure to a specific feared object or situation, such as an animal or public speaking) and Social Phobia (characterized by anxiety associated with social situations and social performance). These disorders are listed on Axis I. On Axis II, in addition to diagnosable Personality Disorders, prominent maladaptive personality features may be listed when they are clinically important. In our created scenario, Belle presented unreasonable fears of being negatively judged, embarrassed, or humiliated by others in social situations—along with some socially avoidant personality features.

In this case, Belle was experiencing a pattern of avoiding social situations due to an excessive fear of being embarrassed or humiliated, which was interfering with her functioning and her normal routine, and which she realized was excessive and irrational. She has visited a primary-care physician who reported no evidence or the presence of a general medical condition or another mental disorder. These symptoms indicate the presence of Social Phobia. Belle's fears included most of her social situations, so Generalized is specified.

On Axis II, problematic personality features and defenses can be listed even when they do not reflect a diagnosable Personality Disorder, if these personality characteristics are important to understanding the client's functioning and are maladaptive for the person. We provided the notation Avoidant Personality Disorders Features to further describe Belle's pattern of "social inhibition, feelings of inadequacy, and hypersensitivity to negative evaluations" (APA, 2000a, p. 721).

One Axis I, a differential diagnosis might be Generalized Anxiety Disorder, characterized by excessive worry and anxiety about a number of different topic areas. However, Belle's fears and anxiety are confined to being embarrassed in public, the key feature of Social Phobia. One Axis II differential diagnosis might be diagnosable Avoidant Personality Disorder. The additional diagnosis of Avoidant Personality Disorder may be used along with Social Phobia. However, Belle is unrestrained in her intimate relationship with her husband and when she is with her circle of close friends, and successfully completes everyday social tasks and attends neighborhood gatherings and smaller social events with only minor anxiety—indicating a pattern of diagnostically subthreshhold features of a personality disorder.

To complete the diagnosis, an important psychosocial stressor is emphasized on Axis IV, and on Axis V Belle's functioning is represented by GAF scores indicating, at present, mildly serious symptoms that are causing some impairment in social functioning, and in the recent past, functioning characterized by only slight impairment and transient symptoms. The information on these axes is consistent with the diagnostic information on Axes I and II describing Belle as we have pictured her character.

CASE CONCEPTUALIZATION

During Belle's intake meeting at the Manchester Public Clinic, her counselor thoroughly assessed her presenting problems. Based on this assessment, her counselor first developed diagnostic impressions. Belle's presenting problems were described by Social Phobia and Avoidant Personality Features. Next, her counselor formed a case conceptualization. Whereas the purpose of diagnostic impressions is to *describe* the client's concerns, the goal of case conceptualization is to better *understand* and clinically *explain* the person's experiences (Neukrug & Schwitzer, 2006). It helps the counselor understand the etiology leading to Belle's social anxiety avoidance, and the factors maintaining these patterns. In turn, case conceptualization sets the stage for treatment planning. Treatment planning then provides a road map that plots out how the counselor and client expect to move from presenting concerns to positive outcomes (Seligman, 1993, p. 157)—assisting Belle to reduce or eliminate her anxious fears and avoidance.

When forming a case conceptualization, the clinician applies a purist counseling theory, an integration of two or more theories, an eclectic mix of theories, or a solution-focused combination of tactics, to his or her understanding of the client. In this case, Belle's counselor based her conceptualization on a purist theory, Cognitive Behavior Therapy. She selected this approach because the Manchester Public Clinic operates primarily from a cognitive-behavioral viewpoint, she likewise practices primarily from this perspective, and she was aware that current best practices suggest the benefits of a cognitive-behavioral approach when addressing anxiety problems such as Belle's.

The counselor used the Inverted Pyramid Method of case conceptualization because this method is especially designed to help clinicians more easily form their conceptual pictures of their clients' needs (Neukrug & Schwitzer, 2006; Schwitzer, 1996, 1997). The method has four steps: Problem Identification, Thematic Groupings, Theoretical Inferences, and Narrowed

Inferences. The counselor's clinical thinking can be seen in Figure 9.5.

Step 1: Problem Identification. The first step is Problem Identification. Aspects of the presenting problem (thoughts, feelings, behaviors, physiological features), additional areas of concern besides the presenting concern, family and developmental history, in-session observations, clinical inquiries (medical problems, medications, past counseling, substance use, suicidality), and psychological assessments (problem checklists, personality inventories, mental status exam, specific clinical measures) all may contribute information at Step 1. The counselor "casts a wide net" in order to build Step 1 as exhaustively as possible (Neukrug & Schwitzer, 2006, p. 202). As can be seen in Figure 9.5, the counselor identified Belle's primary concerns (avoiding major social events, self-doubting beliefs, etc.); related concerns (minor nervous and anxiety symptoms in other situations); and past concerns (history of shaming and humiliation by father). She attempted to go beyond just the main events that caused Belle difficulties in order to be descriptive as she could.

Step 2: Thematic Groupings. The second step is Thematic Groupings. The clinician organizes all of the exhaustive client information found in Step 1 into just a few intuitive-logical clinical groups, categories, or themes, on the basis of sensible common denominators (Neukrug & Schwitzer, 2006). Four different ways of forming the Step 2 theme groups can be used: Descriptive-Diagnosis Approach, Clinical Targets Approach, Areas of Dysfunction Approach, and Intrapsychic Approach. As can be seen in the figure, Belle's counselor selected the Clinical Targets Approach. This approach sorts together all of the Step 1 information "according to the basic division of behavior, thoughts, feelings, and physiology" (Neukrug & Schwitzer, 2006, p. 205).

The counselor grouped together: (a) Belle's fear of "making a fool of myself," self-doubting beliefs, her problematic thoughts centering around learned messages growing up, and so on,

into the theme "belief in father's unwarranted negative messages"; and (b) her nervousness and feelings of anxiety into a theme about her physiological symptoms of anxiety in social situations, avoiding behavior, past avoiding behavior, and so on into the theme "physiological and affective anxiety reactions, and behavioral avoidance reactions, in interpersonal situations." As per the clinical targets method for Step 2, these two themes capture her problematic thoughts and feelings, behaviors, and physical responses.

So far, at Steps 1 and 2, the counselor has used her clinical assessment skills and her clinical judgment to begin meaningfully understanding Belle's needs. Now, at Steps 3 and 4, she applies the theoretical approach she has selected. She begins making theoretical inferences to interpret and explain the processes or roots underlying Belle's concerns as they are seen in Steps 1 and 2.

Step 3: Theoretical Inferences. At Step 3, concepts from the counselor's selected therapy, Cognitive Behavior Therapy, are applied to explain the experiences causing, and the mechanisms maintaining, Belle's problematic thoughts, feelings, and behaviors. The counselor tentatively matches the theme groups in Step 2 with this theoretical approach. In other words, the symptom constellations in Step 2, which were distilled from the symptoms in Step 1, now are combined using theory to show what are believed to be the underlying causes or psychological etiology of Belle's current needs (Neukrug & Schwitzer, 2006; Schwitzer, 2006, 2007).

According to Cognitive Behavior Therapy (Beck, 1995, 2005; Ellis, 1994; Ellis & MacLaren, 2005), irrational thinking, faulty beliefs, or other forms of cognitive errors lead individuals to engage in problematic behaviors and to experience negative moods and attitudes. As can be seen in Figure 9.5, when the counselor applied these Cognitive Behavior Therapy concepts, she explained at Step 3 that the various issues noted in Step 1 (self-doubt, fear of humiliation, avoiding social situations, anxiety), which can be understood in Step 2 to be themes of (a) self-doubting thoughts and fears of humiliation, and belief in negative messages from father, and (b) anxiety reactions and avoidance, are rooted in or caused by the irrational belief that "social events are awful because people will see the terrible, ridiculous person I am" and the corresponding behavioral consequence of avoiding events that might lead to such negative scrutiny by others. These are presented on Figure 9.5.

Step 4: Narrowed Inferences. At Step 4, the clinician's selected theory continues to be used to address still-deeper issues when they exist (Schwitzer, 2006, 2007). At this step, "still-deeper, more encompassing, or more central, causal themes" are formed (Neukrug & Schwitzer, 2006, p. 207). Continuing to apply Cognitive Behavior Therapy concepts at Step 4, Belle's counselor presented a single, deepest, most-fundamental cognitive error that she believed to be most explanatory and causal regarding Belle's reasons for referral: the deepest irrational belief that "I am as incompetent, unwantable, and unacceptable as my father said I was and I must hide these terrible flaws from those around me." When all four steps are completed, the client information in Step 1 leads to logical-intuitive groupings on the basis of common denominators in Step 2, the groupings then are explained using theory at Step 3, and then, finally, at Step 4, further deeper explanations are made. From start to finish, the thoughts, feelings, behaviors, and physiological features in the topmost portions are connected on down the pyramid into deepest dynamics.

The completed pyramid now is used to plan treatment, through which Belle and her counselor will confront her irrational beliefs and problematic behavioral consequences.

TREATMENT PLANNING

At this point, Belle's clinician at the Manchester Public Clinic has collected all available information about the problems that have been of concern. Based upon this information, the counselor developed a five-axis *DSM-IV-TR* diagnosis and then, using the "inverted pyramid" (Neukrug & Schwitzer, 2006; Schwitzer, 1996, 1997), formulated a working clinical *explanation* of Belle's difficulties and their etiology that we called the *case conceptualization.* This, in turn, guides us to the next critical step in our clinical work, called the *treatment plan,* the primary purpose of which is to map out a logical and goal-oriented strategy for making positive changes in the client's life. In essence, the treatment plan is a road map "for reducing or eliminating disruptive symptoms that are impeding the client's ability to reach positive mental health outcomes" (Neukrug & Schwitzer, 2006, p. 225). As such, it is the cornerstone of our work with not only Belle, but with all clients who present with disruptive symptoms and personality patterns (Jongsma & Peterson, 2006; Jongsma et al., 2003a, 2003b; Seligman, 1993, 1998, 2004).

A comprehensive treatment plan must integrate all of the information from the biopsychosocial interview, diagnosis, and case conceptualization into a coherent plan of action. This *plan* comprises four main components, which include (1) a behavioral definition of the problem(s), (2) the selection of achievable goals, (3) the determination of treatment modes, and (4) the documentation of how change will be measured. The *behavioral definition of the problem(s)* consolidates the results of the case conceptualization into a concise hierarchical list of problems and concerns that will be the focus of treatment. The *selection of achievable goals* refers to assessing and prioritizing the client's concerns into a *hierarchy of urgency* that also takes into account the client's motivation for change, level of dysfunction, and real-world influences on his or her problems. The *determination of treatment modes* refers to selection of the specific interventions, which are matched to the uniqueness of the client and to his or her goals and clearly tied to a particular theoretical orientation (Neukrug & Schwitzer, 2006). Finally, the clinician must establish how change will be measured, based upon a number of factors, including client

Figure 9.5   Belle's Inverted Pyramid Case Conceptualization Summary: Cognitive Behavior Therapy

1. IDENTIFY AND LIST CLIENT CONCERNS

Avoids major social situations due to dread
Endures minor social situations with anxiety
Fear of being negatively judged
Almost all social situations
Avoided going to school at times
Minor nervousness, quickly
   passing doubts in almost all social situations
Feelings of anxiety, physiological signs of stress
Self-conscious except with closest social circle

Fears "making a fool of myself"
Self-doubting thoughts
Fear of being humiliated in almost all social situations
History of being belittled by father
Made to feel unwanted by father
Called "filthy and shameful"
Endured other unfounded criticism

2. ORGANIZE CONCERNS INTO LOGICAL THEMATIC GROUPINGS

1. Self-doubting thoughts and fears of humiliation
2. Belief in father's unwarranted negative messages
3. Anxiety reactions in interpersonal situations
4. Avoidance of social situations

3. THEORETICAL INFERENCES: ATTACH THEMATIC GROUPINGS TO INFERRED AREAS OF DIFFICULTY

Irrational Beliefs

Social events are awful because people in my adult life will see the terrible or ridiculous person I am

Problematic Behavioral Consequence

Avoiding major social events and other opportunities for fear of negative scrutiny by others

4. NARROWED INFERENCES: SUICIDALITY AND DEEPER DIFFICULTIES

Deepest Irrational Belief

I am as incompetent, unwantable, and unacceptable as my father said I was and I must hide these terrible flaws from those around me records and self-report of change, in-session observations by the clinician, clinician ratings, results of standardized evaluations such as the Beck Anxiety Inventory (Beck & Steer, 1990) or a family functioning questionnaire, pre-post treatment comparisons, and reports by other treating professionals.

The four-step method discussed above can be seen in Figure 6.1 (p. 109) and is outlined below for the case of Belle Beastly, followed by her specific treatment plan.

Step 1: Behavioral Definition of Problems. The first step in treatment planning is to carefully review the case conceptualization, paying particular attention to the results of Step 2 (Thematic Groupings), Step 3 (Theoretical Inferences), and Step 4 (Narrowed Inferences). The identified clinical themes reflect the core areas of concern and distress for the client, while the theoretical and narrowed inferences offer clinical speculation as to their origins. In the case of Belle, there are two primary areas of concern. The first, "anxiety in, and avoidance of, social situations, including physiological arousal," refers to her avoidance of and experience of anxiety in most social situations. The second, "belief in her father's unwarranted negative messages, fear of humiliation, fear of being negatively judged, and self-doubting thoughts," refers to her professed "fear of making a fool of myself," painful self-consciousness and severe restriction of her social circles, that are all tied to her history of being belittled by her father. These symptoms and stresses are consistent with the diagnosis of Social Phobia (Generalized) and Avoidant Personality Features (APA, 2000a; Beesdo et al., 2007; Delong & Pollack, 2008; Magee, Eaton, Wittchen, McGonagle, & Kessler, 1996).

Step 2: Identify and Articulate Goals for Change. The second step is the selection of achievable goals, which is based upon a number of factors, including the most pressing or urgent behavioral, emotional, and interpersonal concerns and symptoms as identified by the client and clinician, the willingness and ability of the client to work on those particular goals, and the realistic (real-world) achievability of those goals (Neukrug &

Schwitzer, 2006). At this stage of treatment planning, it is important to recognize that not all of the client's problems can be addressed at once, so we focus initially on those that cause the greatest distress and impairment. New goals can be created as old ones are achieved. In the case of Belle, the goals are divided into two prominent areas. The first, "anxiety in and avoidance of social situations with physiological arousal," requires that we help Belle to understand the components of her anxiety and effectively engage in social situations. The second, "belief in father's unwarranted messages, fear of humiliation and self-doubting thoughts," requires that we help Belle to understand the origin of her self-doubting and improve her self-image.

Step 3: Describe Therapeutic Interventions. This is perhaps the most critical step in the treatment planning process because the clinician must now integrate information from a number of sources, including the case conceptualization, the delineation of the client's problems and goals, and the treatment literature, paying particular attention to *empirically supported treatment* (EST) and *evidence-based practice* (EBP). In essence, the clinician must align his or her treatment approach with scientific evidence from the fields of counseling and psychotherapy. Wampold (2001) identifies two types of evidence-based counseling research: studies that demonstrate "absolute efficacy," that is, the fact that counseling and psychotherapy work, and those that demonstrate "relative efficacy," that is, the fact that certain theoretical/technical approaches work best for certain clients with particular problems (Psychoanalysis, Gestalt Therapy, Cognitive Behavior Therapy, Brief Solution-Focused Therapy, Cognitive Therapy, Dialectical Behavior Therapy, Person-Centered Therapy, Expressive/Creative Therapies, Interpersonal Therapy, and Feminist Therapy); and when delivered through specific treatment modalities (individual, group, and family counseling). In the case of Belle, we have decided to use Cognitive Behavior Therapy (Beck, 1995, 2005; Ellis, 1994; Ellis & MacLaren, 2005), which has been found to be highly effective in counseling and psychotherapy with adults (and adolescents) who experience the symptoms of Social Phobia and Avoidant Personality Features (Delong & Pollack, 2008; Taylor, 1996). The approach relies on a variety of cognitive techniques (reframing, challenging irrational thoughts, and cognitive restructuring) and behavioral techniques (reinforcement for and shaping of adaptive behavior, extinction of maladaptive behaviors, systematic desensitization, exposure with response prevention) (Ball et al., 2006; Frank et al., 2005; Milkowitz, 2008).

Specific techniques for Belle will include the use of imaginal and in vivo exposure and desensitization to social situations along with identification and refutation of irrational thoughts.

Step 4: Provide Outcome Measures of Change. This last step in treatment planning requires that we specify how change will be measured and indicate the extent to which progress has been made toward realizing these goals (Neukrug & Schwitzer, 2006). The counselor has considerable flexibility in this phase and may choose

from a number of objective domains (psychological tests and measures of self-esteem, depression, psychosis, interpersonal relationship, anxiety, etc.), quasi-objective measures (the *DSM-IV-TR's* Axis V GAF scale; pre-post clinician, client, and psychiatric ratings), and subjective ratings (client self-report, clinician's in-session observations). In Belle's case, we have implemented a number of these, including pre-post measure on the Beck Anxiety Inventory, post measures of GAF functioning in the normal range (>85), client self-report of anxiety-free engagement in social situations, counselor-observed and client-reported decrease of negative and increase of positive self-talk.

The completed treatment plan is now developed through which the counselor and Belle will begin their shared work of reducing her anxiety and facilitating her ability to interact socially in not only familiar, but unfamiliar and uncomfortable social situations. The treatment plan is described below and summarized in Table 9.5.

TREATMENT PLAN

Client: Belle Beastly

Service Provider: Manchester Public Clinic

BEHAVIORAL DEFINITION OF PROBLEMS:

1. Anxiety in and avoidance of social situations, including physiological arousal—Endures minor social situations with anxiety, avoids going to school at times, feelings of anxiety and physiological signs of stress, self-conscious except with closest social circle

2. Belief in father's unwarranted negative message, fear of humiliation, and self-doubting thoughts—Fears of "making a fool of myself," fear of being negatively judged

GOALS FOR CHANGE:

1. Anxiety in and avoidance of social situations, including physiological arousal

   - Understand the cognitive, behavioral, and physiological components of anxiety
   - Reduce anxiety in relation to social situations
   - Gradually reduce and eliminate avoidance of social situations

2. Belief in father's unwarranted negative messages, fear of humiliation, and self-doubting thoughts

   - Understand the origin of self-doubt and fear of humiliation
   - Improve self-image

THERAPEUTIC INTERVENTIONS:

A short- to moderate-term course of individual cognitive-behavior counseling (3–6 months)

1. Anxiety in and avoidance of social situations, including physiological arousal

   - Develop a scaling procedure to describe her anxiety in relation to social situation
   - Acquire and practice self-calming techniques, including deep breathing
   - Practice imaginal and in vivo exposure to social situations
   - Identity and refute irrational self-talk with regard to social avoidance
   - Implement relapse prevention strategies for future social situations

2. Belief in father's unwarranted negative messages, fear of humiliation, and self-doubting thoughts

   - Verbalize the relationship between father's unwarranted negative messages and self-doubting thoughts and fear of humiliation
   - Identify and refute irrational self-doubting thoughts and fears of humiliation
   - Replace irrational self-doubting thoughts with positive, self-affirming, and self-empowering thoughts
   - Practice positive affirmations paired with relaxation techniques

OUTCOME MEASURES OF CHANGE:

The development of healthy, positive, and self-affirming attitudes toward herself and the ability to engage with others in social situations as measured by:

- Pre-post measures on the Beck Anxiety Inventory
- Post measures of GAF functioning in the normal range (>85)
- Client self-report of anxiety-free engagement in social situations
- Clinician-observed and client-reported elimination of negative self-talk
- Clinician-observed and client-reported use of positive self-talk

Table 9.5   Belle's Treatment Plan Summary: Cognitive Behavior Therapy

Goals for Change	Therapeutic Interventions	Outcome Measures of Change
Anxiety in and avoidance of social situations, including physiological arousal	Anxiety in and avoidance of social situations, including physiological arousal	The development of healthy, positive, and self-affirming attitudes toward herself and the ability to engage with others in social situations as measured by:
Understand the cognitive, behavioral, and physiological components of anxiety	Develop a scaling procedure to describe her anxiety in relation to social situation	Pre-post measures on the Beck Anxiety Inventory
Reduce anxiety in relation to social situations	Acquire and practice self-calming techniques, including deep breathing	Post measures of GAF functioning in the normal range (>85)
Gradually reduce and eliminate avoidance of social situations	Practice imaginal and in vivo exposure to social situations	Client self-report of anxiety-free engagement in social situations
Belief in father's unwarranted negative messages, fear of humiliation, and self-doubting thoughts	Identity and refute irrational self-talk with regard to social avoidance	Clinician-observed and client-reported elimination of negative self talk
Understand the origin of self-doubt and fear of humiliation	Implement relapse prevention strategies for future social situations	Clinician-observed and client-reported use of positive self-talk
Improve self-image	Belief in father's unwarranted negative messages, fear of humiliation, and self-doubting thoughts	
	Verbalize the relationship between father's unwarranted negative messages and self-doubting thoughts and fear of humiliation	
	Identify and refute irrational self-doubting thoughts and fears of humiliation	
	Replace irrational self-doubting thoughts with positive, self-affirming and self-empowering thoughts	
	Practice positive affirmations paired with relaxation techniques	

FOLLOW-UP: DIAGNOSIS, CASE CONCEPTUALIZATION, AND TREATMENT PLANNING THEMES— CHAPTER SUMMARY

This chapter presented a substantial clinical caseload comprising four adult clients, Cleveland Brown, Tinkerbell, Smithers, and Belle, and a client who is a child, Jessie. The caseload had a gender balance of three female clients and two males. Among the caseload's diversity were one international client, Belle, a white woman from Manchester, England; three Americans, including Cleveland Brown, who is African American, and Smithers and Jessie, who are white; and Tinkerbell, of Never Land. Upper and middle socioeconomic statuses were represented by this group of clients. One of the adults, Smithers, is gay, and the other adults are heterosexual.

Two of the adults were self-referred at the urging of family members: Cleveland Brown sought out a private practice and Belle visited the Manchester Public Clinic. Conversely, Smithers was mandated to the Springfield Counseling Center by his EAP coordinator at work, Tinkerbell was urged by her own agency's board of directors to seek counseling at the Never Land Community Mental Health Center, and Jessie was referred to counseling by her disciplinary dean.

Among the adult concerns presented by our in this chapter's caseload: Cleveland Brown sought assistant for a combination of concerns characterized diagnostically as Dysthymia, Alcohol Abuse, Male Erectile Dysfunction, as well as dependent personality features and relational problems; Tinkerbell required assistance with the challenging problem of Schizoaffective Disorder and borderline personality features; and Belle was experiencing generalized Social Phobia and avoidant personality features. In addition, Smithers presented an identity problem, but no diagnosable mental health problems. Looking at the counseling theories represented, their counselors formed case conceptualizations and then treatment plans based on a psychotherapeutic integration of Schema-Focused Cognitive Therapy and Interpersonal Psychotherapy, Solution-Focused Counseling (emphasizing cognitive and dialectical behavioral interventions), Person-Centered Counseling, and Cognitive Behavior Therapy. The young client, Jessie, was referred for concerns described diagnostically as Reactive Attachment Disorder. Looking at theoretical approach, Jessie's counselor formed a case conceptualization and then treatment plan based on Theraplay.

In their treatment plans, these clients' counselors expressed hopes that their clients would achieve such outcomes as developing self-affirming attitudes, improved marital functioning, responsible parental behavior, and decreased alcohol dependence for coping (Cleveland), improved quality of caregiver/client attachment and reduced aggression (Jessie), strengthening coping skills, and alleviation of depressed mood (Tinkerbell), development of congruence between ideal and actual self, and improved self-esteem (Smithers), and development of positive self-attitudes and ability to engage socially with others (Belle).

STUDY QUESTIONS AND LEARNING ACTIVITIES

Based on your understanding of this chapter's cases, consider and respond to these Study Questions and Learning Activities:

1. This caseload is a substantial one.

   a. If you were assigned this group of clients, what would be your initial reactions to their individual characteristics and differences? Working with both adults and children? Their reasons for referral?
   b. What would you identify as your greatest strengths for assisting these five clients? Your areas of greatest need for growth?

2. In their Basic Case Summaries, this chapter's counselors focused on their clients' earlier developmental and family experiences, presenting concerns, assessment of current distress and areas and life roles in which they were experiencing difficulties, client strengths, and hopes for change. There was an emphasis on Cleveland's family and development history; Jessie's background experiences centering on parental and foster-care dynamics; the historical pattern, severity, and effects of Tinkerbell's schizoaffective difficulties; Smithers's identity questions and interpersonal and intrapersonal attitudes; and Belle's developmental experiences centering on relational factors with her father.

   a. Keeping in mind that the initial counseling meeting, screening session, or intake interview usually requires the counselor to balance rapport and trust-building, on one hand, and assessment and information-gathering, on the other hand, what would you identify as your greatest strengths when engaging these five clients in the counseling process, and gathering the clinical information needed to conceptualize and plan for their counseling process? Your areas of greatest need for growth?
   b. Looking at the five Basic Case Summaries, how does this type of clinical writing differ from your everyday thinking and conversation about people? What are your levels of comfort, skill, and experience, at this type of

professional writing? What steps can you take to further develop or improve these skills?

c. What suggestions would you have for one or more of the counselors in this chapter regarding missing, overlooked, or underemphasized—or overemphasized—information gathered and reported in the Basic Case Summaries? What would you like to have known more about? What methods could be used—clinical interview questions, observations, psychological measures, or other means—to find the additional information you would seek?

3. This chapter illustrated *DSM-IV-TR* diagnoses found in the following sections: Disorders Usually First Diagnosed in Infancy, Childhood, or Adolescence; Schizophrenic and Other Psychotic Disorders; Substance-Related Disorders; Mood Disorders; Anxiety Disorders; Personality Disorders; and Other Conditions That May Be a Focus of Clinical Attention.

a. How familiar are you with these sections of the *DSM-IV-TR?* What is your comfort level using the *DSM-IV-TR* to explore these sets of concerns? Which of these groups of disorders are likely to be most important to you in the practicum, internship, residency, or professional practice settings in which you hope to work?

b. What are your attitudes, reactions, or thoughts concerning diagnosis of childhood disorders? Concerning the diagnosis of behavioral consequences of problematic substance use? Concerning diagnosing lifelong patterns of cognitive difficulties with psychotic and mood symptoms, or with lifelong patterns characterized as personality disorders? Problems with sexual function? Counseling foci like marital and family relational problems, or identity problems? How can you further explore or develop your professional attitudes about diagnosis of these types of concerns?

c. What will be your next steps in gaining greater comfort and skills at diagnosis of the Other Disorders of Infancy, Childhood, or Adolescence? Substance-use disorders? Schizophrenic and psychotic disorders? Mood and anxiety disorders? Sexual dysfunctions? Personality disorders?

d. What are your attitudes, reactions, or thoughts concerning use of Axis IV to record psychosocial and environmental stressors (such as Jessie's removal from the home and foster-care placements) and Axis V to record general medical problems (such as Cleveland Brown's hypertension)? What will be your next steps in gaining greater comfort and skills with these axes?

e. Among this group of clients, Axis V Global Assessment of Functioning (GAF) scores ranged from 30 (Tinkerbell's serious impairment) to 71 (Smithers's transient and expectable symptoms). What are your attitudes, reactions, or thoughts concerning use of Axis V GAF scores to estimate the client's overall level of functioning? Do you agree with the counselors' estimates found in this chapter? What will be your next steps in gaining greater comfort and skills estimating Axis V GAF scores?

4. This chapter's cases included three examples of case conceptualization and treatment planning using purist counselor theories, one example of psychotherapeutic integration, and one application of solution-focused counseling.

a. What is your level of familiarity with the various adult counseling theories illustrated in this chapter: Schema-Focused Cognitive Therapy? Interpersonal Psychotherapy? Solution-Focused Counseling? Person-Centered Counseling? Cognitive Behavior Therapy? What is your level of familiarity with Theraplay, the child-counseling theory illustrated in this chapter? What do you believe are these theories' relative strengths and weaknesses? For which individuals do they seem to be a good match? For what types of client concerns do they seem to be potentially effective? What do the evidence and discussions found in the current literature say about this?

b. Which of these theories seem to be a good fit with your own attitudes and skills? Which interest you the most?

c. To learn more, review the resources and references cited in the chapter, interview a practicing counselor who uses these theories in his or her everyday work, seek clinical supervision from a supervisor experienced with the approach, enroll in a special topics class, or look for continuing education workshops and conference presentations covering these approaches.

d. What are your thoughts, reactions, and comfort level integrating multiple psychotherapeutic approaches to address the needs of your clients? Which theories are you most likely, or least likely, to consider integrating into your approach? How will you decide when, with whom, and in what ways, to integrate multiple approaches? To consider and learn more about integrating approaches such as Schema-Focused Cognitive Therapy and Interpersonal Psychotherapy, interview a practicing counselor who uses an integration of these theories in his or her everyday work, seek clinical supervision from a supervisor experiencing with psychotherapeutic integration of these theories, or seek other professional consultations and learning opportunities.

e. What are your thoughts, reactions, and comfort level employing a brief solution-focused approach to address the needs of your clients? What knowledge or skills will you need to be an effective brief solution-focused counselor?

f. How will you decide when, with whom, and in what ways, to employ brief solution-focused approaches? To consider and learn more about solution-focused counseling strategies, interview a practicing counselor who uses a solution focus in his or her everyday work, seek clinical supervision from a supervisor experienced with solution-focused counseling, or seek other professional consultations and learning opportunities.

5. The case conceptualizations found in this chapter began with casting a wide net for client concerns and dynamics, next formed intuitive-logical groupings to begin better understanding the clients' presentations, and then applied counseling theories to make clinical inferences about the clients' situations.

a. How does this type of professional clinical thinking differ from your everyday thinking, conversation, and analysis about people? What are your levels of comfort, skill, and experience at this type of clinical thinking?

What steps can you take to further develop or improve your conceptualizing skills?

b. What are your thoughts, reactions, and critique of the ways these counselors grouped together: Cleveland Brown's chronic, current adjustment, and recent associated concerns? Jessie's single category, Reactive Attachment Disorder of Infancy or Childhood, and Smithers's single category, Identity Problem? Tinkerbell's historical and current negative thoughts and feelings associated with depression, historical and current psychotic thoughts and feelings associated with schizophrenic disorders, and historical and current troublesome behaviors associated with borderline personality? Belle's self-doubting beliefs and negative messages as well as anxiety reactions and avoidance? Do you agree with each of these thematic groupings? How might you have organized these differently, more usefully, or more effectively?

c. What are your thoughts and reactions pertaining to the ways the counselors applied the various theoretical approaches in order to explain, make inferences about, and prepare for treatment planning with, these clients? What were your reactions to the counselor's presentations of Cleveland Brown's distorted core beliefs and faulty family schema (Schema-Focused Cognitive Behavior Therapy) and negative family transactional patterns, characterological conflict, and habitual responses (Interpersonal Psychotherapy)? The developmental social context of Jessie's Reactive Attachment Disorder symptoms (Theraplay)? The lack of conditions of worth by important others leading to Smithers's impeded actualization (Person-Centered Counseling)? Belle's irrational beliefs and behavioral consequences (Cognitive Behavior Therapy)? Do you agree with the ways the counselor used the various theories with these clients? How might you have applied the theories differently, more usefully, or more effectively?

6. A fully developed treatment plan was presented for each of the individuals comprising this chapter's caseload. The treatment plans provide

goals for change, interventions, and outcome measures.

a. How does this type of clinical writing, thinking, and preparation for the professional counseling process differ from your everyday approach to engaging in helpful relationships with people? What are your levels of comfort, skill, and experience with this type of professional writing, thinking, and preparation? What steps can you take to further develop or improve your treatment planning skills for the types of practicum, internship, residency, or work settings that are of most interest to you?

b. This chapter's treatment plans first list goals for change for each "client" character, next apply the selected counseling theory to clearly state the interventions and approaches to be used, and finally identify ways to measure the expected changes. What are your thoughts, reactions, and critiques of the ways this chapter's counselors prepared Cleveland's, Jessie's, Tinkerbell's, Smithers's, and Belle's treatment plans? What interests you most about these plans? What raises questions for you?

c. What are your thoughts and reactions pertaining to the schema-focused cognitive and interpersonal strategies (Cleveland Brown), Theraplay techniques (Jessie), person-centered practices (Smithers), and cognitive behavioral methods (Belle) outlined as interventions? With which are you most

familiar? Least familiar? Unfamiliar? Which will you select to learn more about through further reading, clinical supervision, or other professional development? Alternatively, which do not seem to be close fits with your own preferred approach?

d. These clients' counselors used counselor observation, client report, change scores on psychological measures and the GAF, behavioral reports, and other means to measure outcomes. As you review the outcome measures found on Cleveland's, Jessie's, Tinkerbell's, Smithers's, and Belle's treatment plans, consider these questions: Do the measures seem realistic and accomplishable? Are they concrete and specific enough to indicate change? Are they sensitive to the needs of the client? Which of these measures will become a regular part of your own repertoire, which might you decline to use, and what additional measures might you add to your own list? What new skills and competencies might you need to develop in order to effectively report on your own clients' outcomes?

7. Now, working independently, with a partner, or in a small group, select your own "client" from among the pop culture world of Animated Characters. Develop your own narrative about the client's arrival at counseling. Then, prepare a fully completed Basic Case Summary, Diagnostic Impressions, Case Conceptualization, and Treatment Plan!

10

ADULTS IN TELEVISION SITCOMS AND DRAMA

The Cases of Jack Bauer, Sophia, George Lopez, Lieutenant Commander Data, and Jack McFarland

PREVIEW: POPULAR CULTURE THEMES

In this section, you will meet a cast of characters who have reached into our living rooms (and hand-held digital devices) directly from the world of television. Each as unique and different from the others as is humanly possible, these characters of television sitcom and drama have richly storied lives and offer us a glimpse into the fundamental struggles of the adult experience. Now that the troubling and angst-ridden years of childhood and adolescence are well behind them, they face challenges that are anchored firmly in the present but that have significant impact on their futures.

This particular group of characters varies considerably in age, race, culture, and sexual identity. It is important to consider how these different contextual features are represented on television. For instance, the depiction of the elderly has evolved from stubbornness, eccentricity, and comical foolishness to respectability, affluence, wisdom, and clever wit (Bell, 1992); however, the full range of diverse characteristics

of this age group has yet to be represented. Similarly, although there is greater diversity in the representation of different racial and ethnic groups in prime-time television, questions remain as to whether the roles and actions of these characters are a fair representation or simply perpetuate stereotypes (Graves, 1999). Although television comedy is clearly designed for laughs, and dramas centering on crime, police, or the legal system titillate, provoke, and shock us, it is important for counselors to consider whether or not the depictions of mental illness are accurate and fair (Hyler, 1988; Hyler, Gabbard, & Schneider, 1991). And finally, although television shows like *Ellen, Will & Grace, Modern Family* & and *Glee* have invited conversations around lesbian, gay, bisexual, and transgender (LGBT) issues (Hart, 2000; Quimby, 2005), here too, we must be careful as counselors and consumers to carefully assess these shows for their potential to misrepresent the homosexual and gay experience as well as to perpetuate prejudicial attitudes.

With regard to the specific characters in this section, Jack Bauer, star of the long-running Fox real-time, action-drama series *24,* has kept audiences riveted to their televisions and on the edge of their seats for 7 years, has won numerous awards, and has challenged us to rethink our beliefs about good and evil. Recently ended, the series promises to film reincarnations, and the character of moral vigilante Jack Bauer has permeated our national consciousness. In our presentation, Jack struggles with Posttraumatic Stress Disorder (PTSD), Bereavement, and Antisocial Personality Features. Through her caustic wit, octogenarian Sophia Petrillo has wrought her brand of truthful terrorism more provincially as one of the stars of television's *The Golden Girls.* Sophia has endeared herself to audiences of all ages by her willingness to share her perceptions of the world as she sees it. In our presentation, Sophia struggles with Dementia of the Alzheimer's Type. George Lopez, star of the largely Hispanic-ensemble television show of the same name, helps us to better understand the Mexican American experience through cleverly crafted one-liners and a glimpse into not-so-middle America with a twist. George Lopez went on to briefly host a late night talk show aptly titled *The George Lopez Show.* In our presentation, George struggles with an Adjustment Disorder and Acculturation Problems. Android Lieutenant Commander Data of the Star Trek franchise's *The Next Generation* perennially wrestles with the same question as Pinocchio and the Velveteen Rabbit—what does it mean to be a "real person"? Originally appearing on all 178 episodes of the acclaimed series, the character of Data has also starred in many of the *Star Trek* movies that followed the ending of the television series. In our presentation, Data struggles with Major Depressive Disorder, Amnestic Disorder, and Identity Problems. And finally, there is Jack McFarland, the way-out-of-the closet costar of the risqué and risk-taking television show *Will and Grace.* Jack's flamboyant character gave us an opportunity to reflect on some very serious issues with a laugh thrown in for good measure. Although the character of Jack ended with the show, he continues to open our eyes to issues of social and sexual justice. In our presentation, Jack struggles with Major Depressive Disorder and Attention-Deficit/Hyperactivity Disorder.

The characters in this section have brought us to our knees in laughter, pushed us to our emotional extremes, and given us opportunities to exercise our imaginations. Sophia Petrillo, Jack McFarland, and George Lopez lead everyday lives, much like those of you and me, and for that reason are relatively easy with which to identify. They neither battle international terrorists nor fly through the galaxy in futuristic spacecraft. That is the province of Counter-Terrorism Unit (CTU) special agent Jack Bauer and Starfleet's Lieutenant Commander Data. Although these characters differ in such fundamental ways, from demography to their television story plots, they also experience very similar internal dramas that are not always funny and that center on mortality, the need for security and safety, the desire for connection—both inside and outside of the family, and answers to basic existential questions such as "Who am I?" "What is the meaning of life?" and "How do I fit into the world?" Jack Bauer, Sophia Petrillo, George Lopez, Lieutenant Commander Data, and Jack McFarland will help you answer many important questions about the human condition and the thin line that separates normalcy and pathology.

APPROACHES TO LEARNING

As you learn about this group of characters, pay attention to:

- How women with counseling problems are presented on TV compared with men.
- The manner in which the plight of older people and those with age-related declines are depicted in popular media.
- Whether or not racial stereotypes pervade or are reinforced in television sitcoms and dramas.
- The difference between the ways that gender, sexuality, and race are portrayed in popular media, and particularly on television, and in your own clinical and personal experience.

CASE 10.1 *24'S* JACK BAUER

INTRODUCING THE CHARACTER

Jack Bauer is the central figure in the 20th Century Fox television action/drama series, *24,* which first aired in 2001. This series was produced collaboratively by Imagine Entertainment, 20th Century Fox Television, Real Time Productions, and Teakwood Lane Productions. It has been directed by numerous individuals, most prominently Jon Cassar and Brad Turner.

Jack Bauer is a highly intelligent, militarily adept, and fiercely loyal patriot who, from the outset of the series, is depicted as a skilled, persistent, and when necessary, brutally aggressive field agent of the CTU. At the start of each season, Bauer and his comrades are presented with a seemingly impossible challenge that involves thwarting both domestic and international terrorist plots. Doing so (in real-time, and hence the title of the series) brings him in direct contact with those who stop at no cost in order to wreak havoc and chaos on organized society and to bring death to as many innocent victims as possible. Although surrounded by a team of highly effective tacticians, technophiles, and warriors, it is Bauer who always seems to be the ultimate point-person in a heart pounding, countdown race to stave off biological, chemical, and nuclear Armageddon.

Over the course of Bauer's relationship with CTU, we see a man capable of seemingly limitless pain tolerance, physical endurance, and capacity to emotionally distance himself from all around him in order to complete his missions. Although revered by his fiercely loyal colleagues and trusted by presidents with the fate of the nation, Bauer is nevertheless persecuted by the "moral majority" who argue that the pursuit of liberty and safeguarding freedom from harm do not justify the use of violence and torture—both of which are powerful social and political issues in today's real world. Thus, he is often a target of the mainstream military and the political Right, and as such, can be truly effective only as a rogue

agent who is ultimately disaffected and disdained by those who rely upon him. He suffers his losses silently, and in spite of ongoing efforts to lead a "normal" life, which includes a relationship with his daughter Kim, he is bitter, alienated, and tragically alone. The following basic case summary and diagnostic impressions describe what we portray as Jack's clinically significant negative reactions to his exposure to traumatic events in which he is subjected to threats of capture, serious injury, and death.

Meet the Client

You can assess the client in action by viewing clips of Jack Bauer's video material at the following websites:

- http://www.hulu.com/watch/994/24-kim-tells-jack-about-chase Kim Bauer tells her father about her boyfriend, Chase
- http://www.youtube.com/watch?v=5CJ8OIDIrj0 A day in the life of Jack Bauer
- http://www.youtube.com/watch?v=kBzwPvaBYWE Jack at work

BASIC CASE SUMMARY

Identifying Information. Jack Bauer is a 43-year-old white male who works as a field agent for a covert governmental paramilitary agency through which he is regularly involved in life-threatening, high-stakes missions. Mr. Bauer was casually attired and unshaven, and appeared visibly fatigued, irritable, and impatient throughout the assessment.

Presenting Concern. Mr. Bauer was mandated to attend counseling by his superior, Bill Buchanan, who was concerned with what he described as his agent's "volatility, emotional exhaustion, and imminent burnout." On further inquiry, Buchanan said he noticed that since his last mission several months ago, Jack Bauer seemed "different." In this context, Mr. Buchanan noted that his agent had begun to drive out of his way to avoid the scene of his last capture and torture, to leave meetings when the capture topic was brought up, seemed less able to rally his subordinates, and instead spends most of his work time in his private office. Buchanan said "I've seen this before. I'll bet he's having nightmares, too, but you'd never get him to admit it!"

By comparison, Mr. Bauer denied that his behavior has changed and indicated that he was "more than capable" of handling job stress, the losses he has experienced in the course of his duties, and that he did not need to "see a shrink!" Noting that exhaustion, physical and emotional stress, exposure to threats, and loss were a routine part of his job description, Mr. Bauer added that he "just needed to rest."

Background, Family Information, and Relevant History. Jack Bauer was born in Santa Monica, California, the older of two children to parents who separated during his early infancy. Mr. Bauer and his brother Graem were raised by their father, Phillip, an industrialist who believed in corporal punishment, absolute obedience to authority, and fostering competitiveness between the siblings, who Mr. Bauer reports did not get along. Mr. Bauer was a highly competitive and successful athlete during his formative years. He described himself as somewhat of a loner who reached out very selectively to others, but only minimally to his father, with whom he had a distant relationship. He had no contact with his mother after the marital dissolution. Following his graduation from the University of California, Los Angeles (UCLA), Mr. Bauer married Terri, with whom he had a daughter, Kim. Prior to completing his master's degree in criminology and law from the University of California, Berkley, Mr. Bauer entered the military. Military records indicate that as a military professional he revealed a cadre of skills and abilities that quickly propelled him through the ranks and into a series of covert affiliations and operations. Success in the field garnered him great respect and the reputation of being a fiercely intelligent, yet lethal combatant who stopped at nothing to accomplish his missions.

Over the past several years, Mr. Bauer has experienced several significant life stressors, including directly witnessing the death of his wife at the hands of a formerly trusted coworker; becoming alienated from his daughter, who, he admits found it impossible to maintain a relationship with him; and developing a growing distrust of anyone around him for fear that he would be betrayed. In the course of his services, Mr. Bauer has also lost numerous colleagues, experienced betrayal, and been confronted by a deep sense of guilt over his inability to save the President of the United States, David Palmer, from assassination. Mr. Bauer has submitted to annual mandatory evaluations by CTU staff psychologists who have consistently recommended, but have never mandated, ongoing counseling.

Problem and Counseling History. From the outset of the meeting, Mr. Bauer made it quite clear that he was not interested in counseling and was only "following orders." He offered little eye contact, spontaneous information, and only the briefest of responses to questions, particularly those aimed at discerning feelings about himself, the job, and the losses he has encountered. Mr. Bauer was oriented in all spheres, seemingly had intact memory for both remote and recent events, and was capable of expressing himself articulately when interested in doing so. His anger at being mandatorily referred was palpable as was his seeming willingness to say whatever needed to be said in order to convince the examiner that he was "alright." At times, he expressed himself through expletives when it seemed that he was not being understood by the examiner. Mr. Bauer described himself as a historically self-reliant individualist who has learned the hard way that it is wise neither to trust nor get close to others.

Mr. Bauer described difficulties falling and remaining asleep, graphic and disruptive dreams in which he failed to protect loved ones from harm, as well as occasional and seemingly random intrusive and similarly themed images during his waking hours. Although he expressed a deep commitment to the importance of his work, he also expressed remorse over the job-related losses, including his wife, Terri, at which time he quickly choked back tears. He did admit that "sometimes I just don't care what the future holds. Who cares about tomorrow when yesterday and today sometimes are so bad?" When the subject of his last mission was introduced, he first said he could not recall anything special about it, and then quickly changed the topic.

Mr. Bauer endorsed no regrets for the multitude of job-related killings he has committed nor did he question the morality of his behavior. However, he wondered aloud if a "normal" relationship with his daughter would ever be possible or if he would ever be able to enjoy a bond with his newly born grandson, Trevor. At that point in the interview, Mr. Bauer's cell phone rang and he indicated the need to quickly depart.

Goals for Counseling and Course of Therapy to Date. In a brief follow-up webcam conversation from an undisclosed location, Mr. Bauer indicated that he was appreciative of the time spent during the interview and that he "got enough out of it to hold me over." He denied having significant bereavement issues or feelings of depression or anxiety, but did express an interest in making his sleep more efficient and eliminating both the nightmares and intrusive memories that "get in the way of doing my job." In that context, he expressed concern that some of his current symptoms could lead to his forcible retirement from active duty.

Mr. Bauer agreed to return for a follow-up interview pending his next assignment, which he hoped would be a domestic one. The primary goals of the follow-up interview will be (a) to confirm clinically significant symptoms of PTSD in the areas of re-experiencing the trauma, avoidance of traumatic stimuli, and increased arousal; and (b) improve Mr. Bauer's motivation for counseling to address these issues and issues and grief and loss.

Diagnostic Impressions

Axis I.   309.81 Posttraumatic Stress Disorder, Chronic

V62.82 Bereavement

Axis II.   Antisocial Personality Disorder Features

Axis III. None

Axis IV. Problems with primary support group—Death of wife, discord with daughter

Occupational problems—Difficult work conditions, severe job stress

Axis V.   GAF = 60 (at evaluation)

GAF = 70 (highest level past year)

DISCUSSION OF DIAGNOSTIC IMPRESSIONS

Jack Bauer was mandated to counseling by his superior based on concerns that he was showing signs of burnout that had become more noticeable since his last paramilitary assignment. His superior officer was concerned that he was avoiding the locations near the scene of his most recent mission as well as his recent mission as a topic of conversation; was having nightmares in which he re-experienced aspects of the mission; and appeared fatigued. Jack Bauer disclosed that he did, in fact, have difficulties maintaining sleep; and had nightmares and, occasionally, waking images of his traumatic experiences. During the interview, he displayed angry outbursts and expressed a lack of aspirations for the future. As discussed in the case, he recently experienced paramilitary capture and torture. Previously he experienced many events during which he, someone for whom he was professionally responsible, or his wife, was in danger or actually killed.

The predominant feature shared by all of the diagnosable conditions found in the Anxiety Disorders section of the *Diagnostic and Statistical Manual of Mental Disorders, Fourth Edition, Text Revision (DSM-IV-TR)* is the presence of increased arousal, excessive worry, or other signs of anxiety that cause distress or impairment, including panic. Among these are Acute Stress Disorder and PTSD, both of which, by definition, occur only in the aftermath of or as a result of a traumatic life event. This case describes what we portray as Jack Bauer's clinically significant negative reactions to his exposure to the traumatic experiences of capture, serious injury, and threat of death.

Mr. Bauer experienced an event characterized by threat to his physical integrity (he was held against his will), subjected to painful torture and physical injury, and threatened with serious physical damage or possibly death. His reactions included horror. These characteristics meet the *DSM-IV-TR* definition of a traumatic event. Following the most recent of these events, he has been re-experiencing the event during nightmares and waking flashbacks. He has been avoiding places (the site near the capture and torture of his most recent mission) reminiscent of the event and avoiding the topic, and he talks about the future without his lost wife in a foreshortened manner. He has signs of anxiety, including sleep disruption and angry outbursts. According to the case timeline, Mr. Bauer's symptoms have been present for several months. These factors indicate a diagnosis

of PTSD. Because symptoms have persisted more than 3 months, the specifier, Chronic, is warranted.

Differential diagnoses might include Acute Stress Disorder and Adjustment Disorder. However, Acute Stress Disorder allows for a maximum duration of symptoms of 1 month, whereas PTSD fits when symptoms have lasted beyond 4 weeks. Whereas Adjustment Disorders are negative reactions to any sort of life stressors, in this case, Mr. Bauer has experienced exposure to multiple extreme stressors meeting the diagnostic definition of trauma, and his reactions conform to the specific constellation of symptoms characteristic of PTSD and Acute Stress Disorder, which go beyond the general criteria set for Adjustment Disorder.

On Axis II, problematic personality disorder features and defenses can be listed even when they do not reflect a diagnosable Personality Disorder, if these personality characteristics are important to understanding the client's functioning and are maladaptive for the person. We provided the notation, Antisocial Personality Disorder Features, to describe aspects of Mr. Bauer's pattern of behavior characterized by "reckless disregard for safety of self" and "disregard for, and violation of, the rights of others" (APA, 2000a, p. 706).

Further, along with all the various diagnosable disorders, a multiaxial diagnosis also lists Other Conditions That May Be a Focus of Clinical Attention. The client concerns contained in this section (appearing at the end of the *DSM-IV-TR,* following all of the diagnosable disorders) are not diagnosable mental disorders according to the *DSM* classification system; instead, they sometimes are client problems that are a focus of counseling but not a part of the individual's diagnosable mental disorder. Mr. Bauer's grief reactions, or Bereavement, are in this category.

To wrap up the diagnosis, Jack Bauer's important family and occupational psychosocial stressors are emphasized on Axis IV, and on Axis V his functioning is represented by GAF scores indicating, at present, moderately serious symptoms that are causing moderate impairment in social and occupational functioning, and earlier in the year, functioning characterized by mild symptoms and some difficulties in social and occupational functioning. The information on these axes is consistent with the diagnostic information on Axes I and II describing Jack Bauer's situation.

CASE CONCEPTUALIZATION

The counselor who met Jack Bauer for his mandated evaluation collected as much information as possible about the problems for which he was referred. Mr. Bauer's counselor first used this information to develop diagnostic impressions. His concerns were described by PTSD and Bereavement, along with Antisocial Personality Features. Next, his counselor developed a case conceptualization. Whereas the purpose of diagnostic impressions is to *describe* the client's concerns, the goal of case conceptualization is to better *understand* and clinically *explain* the person's experiences (Neukrug & Schwitzer, 2006). It helps the counselor understand the etiology leading to Jack Bauer's posttraumatic concerns and the factors maintaining these. In turn, case conceptualization sets the stage for treatment planning. Treatment planning then provides a road map that plots out how the counselor and client expect to move from presenting concerns to positive outcomes (Seligman, 1993, p. 157)—ideally, assisting Jack to reduce or eliminate the problematic trauma reactions and related concerns that led to his referral.

When forming a case conceptualization, the clinician applies a purist counseling theory, an integration of two or more theories, an eclectic mix of theories, or a solution-focused combination of tactics to his or her understanding of the client. In this case, Mr. Bauer's counselor based his conceptualization on a purist theory, Cognitive Behavior Therapy. He selected this approach based on his knowledge of current outcome research with clients experiencing PTSD and related symptoms (Bradley, Greene, Russ, Dutra, & Westen, 2005; Bryant et al., 2008; Foa & Keane, 2000). Cognitive Behavior Therapy also is consistent with this counselor's professional therapeutic viewpoint.

The counselor used the Inverted Pyramid Method of case conceptualization because this method is especially designed to help clinicians more easily form their conceptual pictures of their clients' needs (Neukrug & Schwitzer, 2006; Schwitzer, 1996, 1997). The method has four steps: Problem Identification, Thematic Groupings, Theoretical Inferences, and Narrowed Inferences. The counselor's clinical thinking can be seen in Figure 10.1.

Step 1: Problem Identification. The first step is Problem Identification. Aspects of the presenting problem (thoughts, feelings, behaviors, physiological features), additional areas of concern besides the presenting concern, family and developmental history, in-session observations, clinical inquiries (medical problems, medications, past counseling, substance use, suicidality), and psychological assessments (problem checklists, personality inventories, mental status exam, specific clinical measures) all may contribute information at Step 1. The counselor "casts a wide net" in order to build Step 1 as exhaustively as possible (Neukrug & Schwitzer, 2006, p. 202). As can be seen in Figure 10.1, the counselor collected clinical data about Jack Bauer's trauma events (death of wife, death of colleagues, torture), anxiety symptoms (poor sleep, startle reactions), re-experiencing symptoms (nightmares, etc.), avoiding behaviors, feelings of grief and loss and regret, anger and hostility, suspicion and disregard for others, and history with a strongly authoritarian father. His counselor collected as much detail as possible about Mr. Bauer's posttraumatic symptoms—and went further to assess related concerns such as his antisocial personality features, bereavement, and daughter relationship, as well as relevant history pertaining to his development experiences with his father.

Step 2: Thematic Groupings. The second step is Thematic Groupings. The clinician organizes all of the exhaustive client information found in Step 1 into just a few intuitive-logical clinical groups, categories, or themes, on the basis of sensible common denominators (Neukrug & Schwitzer, 2006). Four different ways of forming the Step 2 theme groups can be used: Descriptive-Diagnosis Approach, Clinical Targets Approach, Areas of Dysfunction Approach, and Intrapsychic Approach. As can be seen in Figure 10.1, Jack Bauer's counselor selected the Descriptive-Diagnosis Approach. This approach sorts together all of the various Step 1 information about the client's adjustment, development, distress, or dysfunction "to show larger clinical problems as reflected through a diagnosis" (Neukrug & Schwitzer, 2006, p. 205).

The counselor grouped together Mr. Bauer's (a) trauma experiences and various symptoms of anxiety, avoidance, and re-experiencing into the theme of "PTSD"; (b) feelings of grief and loss, teariness, and blame and regret regarding his wife's death into the theme of "bereavement"; and (c) his anger, suspicion, alienation, disregard, and violation regarding self and others into the theme, "antisocial thoughts, feelings, and behaviors." His conceptual work at Step 2 gave the counselor a way to begin understanding and thinking about Mr. Bauer's areas of functioning and areas of concern more clearly and meaningfully.

So far, at Steps 1 and 2, the counselor has used his clinical assessment skills and his clinical judgment to begin meaningfully understanding Jack Bauer's needs. Now, at Steps 3 and 4, he applies the theoretical approach he has selected. He begins making theoretical inferences to interpret and explain the processes or roots underlying Jack Bauer's concerns as they are seen in Steps 1 and 2.

Step 3: Theoretical Inferences. At Step 3, concepts from the counselor's selected theory, Cognitive Behavior Therapy, are applied to explain the experiences fueling, and the mechanisms maintaining, Mr. Bauer's problematic thoughts, feelings, and behaviors. The counselor tentatively matches the theme groups in Step 2 with this theoretical approach. In other words, the symptom constellations in Step 2, which were distilled from the symptoms in Step 1, now are combined using theory to show what is believed to be the psychological etiology of Mr. Bauer's current needs (Neukrug & Schwitzer, 2006; Schwitzer, 2006, 2007).

According to Cognitive Behavior Therapy (Beck, 1995, 2005; Ellis, 1994; Ellis & MacLaren, 2005), irrational thinking, faulty beliefs, or other forms of cognitive errors lead individuals to engage in problematic behaviors and to experience negative moods and attitudes. As can be seen in Figure 10.1, when the counselor applied these Cognitive Behavior Therapy concepts, he explained at Step 3 that the various issues noted in Step 1 (witnessing trauma, avoiding and re-experiencing, anxiety, grief feelings, anger and suspicion, etc.), which can be understood to be themes of (a) PTSD, (b) bereavement, and (c) antisocial features (Step 2), are rooted in or caused by a collection of faulty beliefs that it is better to "just live with" these negative symptoms, avoid confronting his traumatic history, and avoid confronting his guilt and grief—and that all people must be regarded with suspicion and attack. These faulty beliefs are fully spelled out in Figure 10.1.

Step 4: Narrowed Inferences. At Step 4, the clinician's selected theory continues to be used to address still-deeper issues when they exist (Schwitzer, 2006, 2007). At this step, "still-deeper, more encompassing, or more central, causal themes" are formed (Neukrug & Schwitzer, 2006, p. 207). Continuing to apply Cognitive Behavior Therapy concepts at Step 4, Mr. Bauer's counselor presented a single, deepest, most-fundamental cognitive error, which he believed to be most explanatory and causal regarding Mr. Bauer's current psychotherapeutic needs: the deepest faulty core belief that "I am a man and therefore responsible to serve and protect with disregard for my own feelings, relationships, or safety—and any other attitude shows

Figure 10.1 Jack Bauer's Inverted Pyramid Case Conceptualization Summary: Cognitive Behavior Therapy

1. IDENTIFY AND LIST CLIENT CONCERNS

Witnessed death of wife
Witnessed death of colleagues
Victim of torture
Victim of additional traumas
Sleep difficulties
Fatigued
Easily startled or angered
Angry/hostile in session
Cursing in session
Avoids trauma in conversation
Inability to recall trauma
Waking flashbacks
Nightmares
Graphic dreams of regret at
  failing to protect

Feelings of grief and loss
Teariness about loss of wife
Self-blame
Anger toward others
Suspicion of others
Alienated from daughter
Reckless disregard for safety of self
Disregard for, violation of, others'
  rights
Highly authoritarian father
Strong sense of duty
Strong competitiveness

2. ORGANIZE CONCERNS INTO LOGICAL THEMATIC GROUPINGS

1. Posttraumatic stress disorder (trauma, re-experiencing, avoiding, anxiety)
2. Bereavement
3. Antisocial thoughts, feelings, and behaviors

3. THEORETICAL INFERENCES: ATTACH THEMATIC GROUPINGS TO INFERRED AREAS OF DIFFICULTY

<u>Faulty Beliefs</u>

1. It is better to just live with the anxiety symptoms,
   re-experiencing of events, and other effects
   than it is to confront my reactions to trauma
2. It is better to avoid thinking about my traumas than
   to confront them
3. It is better to avoid my guilt about putting my
   wife in danger than to confront my grief
4. All other people are potentially dangerous
   so I must be suspicious and ready to attack
   first in all circumstances

4. NARROWED INFERENCES: SUICIDALITY AND DEEPER DIFFICULTIES

<u>Deepest Faulty Core Belief</u>

I learned that I am a man and therefore responsible to serve
  and protect with disregard for my own feelings, relationships,
    or safety. Any other attitude shows unmasculine weakness
      and therefore means I am a complete failure as a man,
        a person, a father and husband, and a professional.

unmasculine weakness and therefore would mean that I am a complete failure as a man, a person, a father and husband, and professional" (see Figure 10.1). When all four steps are completed, the client information in Step 1 leads to logical-intuitive groupings on the basis of common denominators in Step 2, the groupings then are explained using theory at Step 3, and then, finally, at Step 4, further deeper explanations are made. From start to finish, the thoughts, feelings, behaviors, and physiological features in the topmost portions are connected on down the pyramid into deepest dynamics.

The completed pyramid now is used to plan treatment, during which Mr. Bauer and his counselor will attempt to resolve his faulty core beliefs and to improve his overall functioning.

TREATMENT PLANNING

At this point, Mr. Bauer's clinician at the CTU Covert Counseling Center (CTUCCC) has collected all available information about the problems that have been of concern to him and his supervisor. Based upon this information, the counselor developed a five-axis *DSM-IV-TR* diagnosis and then, using the "inverted pyramid" (Neukrug & Schwitzer, 2006; Schwitzer, 1996, 1997), formulated a working clinical *explanation* of Mr. Bauer's difficulties and their etiology that we called the *case conceptualization*. This, in turn, guides us to the next critical step in our clinical work, called the *treatment plan,* the primary purpose of which is to map out a logical and goal-oriented strategy for making positive changes in the client's life. In essence, the treatment plan is a road map "for reducing or eliminating disruptive symptoms that are impeding the client's ability to reach positive mental health outcomes" (Neukrug & Schwitzer, 2006, p. 225). As such, it is the cornerstone of our work with not only Mr. Bauer, but with all clients who present with disturbing and disruptive symptoms and/or personality patterns (Jongsma & Peterson, 2006; Jongsma, Peterson, & McInnis, 2003a, 2003b; Seligman, 1993, 1998, 2004).

A comprehensive treatment plan must integrate all of the information from the biopsychosocial interview, diagnosis, and case conceptualization into a coherent plan of action. This *plan* comprises four main components, which include (2) a behavioral definition of the problem(s), (2) the selection of achievable goals, (3) the determination of treatment modes, and (4) the documentation of how change will be measured. The *behavioral definition of the problem(s)* consolidates the results of the case conceptualization into a concise hierarchical list of problems and concerns that will be the focus of treatment. The *selection of achievable goals* refers to assessing and prioritizing the client's concerns into a *hierarchy of urgency* that also takes into account the client's motivation for change, level of dysfunction, and real-world influences on his or her problems. The *determination of treatment modes* refers to selection of the specific interventions, which are matched to the uniqueness of the client and to his or her goals and clearly tied to a particular theoretical orientation (Neukrug & Schwitzer, 2006). Finally, the clinician must establish how change will be measured, based upon a number of factors including client records and self-report of change, in-session observations by the clinician, clinician ratings, results of standardized evaluations such as the Beck Depression Inventory (Beck, Steer, & Brown, 1996), or a family functioning questionnaire, pre-post treatment comparisons, and reports by other treating professionals.

The four-step method discussed above can be seen in Figure 6.1 (p. 109) and is outlined below for the case of Jack Bauer, followed by his specific treatment plan.

Step 1: Behavioral Definition of Problems. The first step in treatment planning is to carefully review the case conceptualization, paying particular attention to the results of Step 2 (Thematic Groupings), Step 3 (Theoretical Inferences), and Step 4 (Narrowed Inferences). The identified clinical themes reflect the core areas of concern and distress for the client, while the theoretical and narrowed inferences offer clinical speculation as to their origins. In the case of Jack, there are three primary areas of concern. The first, "posttraumatic stress disorder," refers to the psychological effects of torture and witnessing the death of his wife and colleagues, including waking flashbacks, nightmares, avoidance of and general inability to recall trauma-related memories. The second, "bereavement," refers to feelings of grief and loss, teariness about his wife, and self-blame, along with sleep difficulties, fatigue, and being easily startled. The third, "antisocial thoughts, feelings and behaviors," refers to his anger, suspicion, and violence toward others along with his reckless disregard for his and others' safety and rights. These symptoms and stresses are consistent with the diagnosis of PTSD and Antisocial Personality Features and Bereavement (APA, 2000a; Bradley et al., 2005; Critchfield & Smith-Benjamin, 2006).

Step 2: Identify and Articulate Goals for Change. The second step is the selection of achievable goals, which is based upon a number of factors, including the most pressing or urgent behavioral, emotional, and interpersonal concerns and symptoms as identified by the client and clinician, the willingness and ability of the client to work on those particular goals, and the realistic (real-world) achievability of those goals (Neukrug & Schwitzer, 2006). At this stage of treatment planning, it is important to recognize that not all of the client's problems can be addressed at once, so we focus initially on those that cause the greatest distress and impairment. New goals can be created as old ones are achieved. In the case of Mr. Bauer, the goals are divided into three prominent areas. The first, "posttraumatic stress disorder," requires that we help Mr. Bauer to relieve the symptoms of posttraumatic stress and verbalize an understanding of how these symptoms develop. The second, "bereavement," requires that we help him to appropriately grieve his losses and improve his overall daily functioning. The third, "antisocial thoughts, feelings, and behaviors," requires that we help Mr. Bauer to resolve his negative perceptions of and reactions to other people, eliminate his antisocial urges and behavior, and resolve his thoughts about conspiracy theories.

Step 3: Describe Therapeutic Intervention. This is perhaps the most critical step in the treatment planning process because the clinician must now integrate information from a number of sources, including the case conceptualization, the delineation of the client's problems and goals, and the treatment literature, paying particular attention to *empirically supported treatment* (EST) and *evidence-based practice* (EBP). In essence, the clinician must align his or her treatment approach with scientific evidence from the fields of counseling and psychotherapy. Wampold (2001) identifies two types of evidence-based counseling research: studies that demonstrate "absolute efficacy," that is, the fact that counseling and psychotherapy work, and those that demonstrate "relative efficacy," that is, the fact that certain theoretical/technical approaches work best for certain clients with particular problems (Psychoanalysis, Gestalt Therapy, Cognitive Behavior Therapy, Brief Solution-Focused Therapy, Cognitive Therapy, Dialectical Behavior Therapy, Person-Centered Therapy, Expressive/Creative Therapies, Interpersonal Therapy, and Feminist Therapy); and when delivered through specific treatment modalities (individual, group, and family counseling). In the case of Mr. Bauer, we have decided to use Cognitive Behavior Therapy (Beck, 1995, 2005; Ellis, 1994; Ellis & MacLaren, 2005), which has been found to be highly effective in counseling and psychotherapy with adults who experience the symptoms of PTSD (Bradley et al., 2005; Bryant et al., 2008). The approach relies on a variety of cognitive techniques (reframing, challenging irrational thoughts, and cognitive restructuring) and behavioral techniques (reinforcement for and shaping of adaptive behavior, extinction of maladaptive behaviors, systematic desensitization, and exposure with response prevention) (Ball et al., 2006; Frank et al., 2005; Milkowitz, 2008). Additionally, Mr. Bauer will undergo a course of eye movement desensitization and reprocessing (EMDR), which has been found to be particularly useful in addressing the physiological and emotional symptoms of post-traumatic stress (Shapiro, 2002, 2005). Mr. Bauer's grief and loss issues will be addressed through an eclectic variety of empirically supported techniques, including narrative remembering, cognitive restructuring, and group bereavement counseling (Bradley et al., 2005; Bryant et al., 2008; Neimeyer, 2000; Servaty-Seib,

2004; White, 2007), while his antisocial attitudes and behaviors will be addressed through cognitive restructuring.

Step 4: Provide Outcome Measures of Change. This last step in treatment planning requires that we specify how change will be measured and indicate the extent to which progress has been made toward realizing these goals (Neukrug & Schwitzer, 2006). The counselor has considerable flexibility in this phase, and may choose from a number of objective domains (psychological tests and measures of self-esteem, depression, psychosis, interpersonal relationship, anxiety, etc.), quasi-objective measures (the *DSM-IV-TR's* Axis V GAF scale; pre-post clinician, client, and psychiatric ratings), and

subjective ratings (client self-report, clinician's in-session observations). In Mr. Bauer's case, we have implemented a number of these, including pre-post measures on the Clinical Anger Scale (Snell, Gum, Shuck, Mosley, & Hite, 1995), post measures of GAF functioning in the mild range (>70), clinician observation of prosocial attitudes and behavior, and acceptance of losses with reduced guilt over them.

The completed treatment plan is now developed through which the counselor and Mr. Bauer will work through the traumatic loss of his wife and colleagues and develop and implement plans for eliminating his antisocial thoughts, feelings, and behaviors. Jack Bauer's treatment plan follows and is summarized in Table 10.1.

TREATMENT PLAN

Client: Jack Bauer

Service Provider: CTU Covert Counseling Center (CTUCCC)

BEHAVIORAL DEFINITION OF PROBLEMS:

1. PTSD—Psychological effects of torture and witnessing the death of his wife and colleagues, including waking flashbacks, nightmares, avoidance of and inability to recall trauma-related memories

2. Bereavement—Feelings of grief and loss, teariness about his wife and self-blame, along with sleep difficulties, fatigue, and being easily startled

3. Antisocial thoughts, feelings, and actions—Anger, suspicion, and violence toward others along with his reckless disregard for his and others' safety and rights

GOALS FOR CHANGE:

1. PTSD

   - Relieve the symptoms of posttraumatic stress
   - Verbalize an understanding of how the symptoms of PTSD develop

2. Bereavement

   - Appropriately grieve the losses of his wife and colleagues
   - Improvement in overall daily functioning and mood

3. Antisocial thoughts, feelings, and actions

   - Resolve negative perceptions of and reactions to other people
   - Understand the relationship between his negative feelings about herself and toward others
   - Eliminate antisocial behavior
   - Resolve thoughts about conspiracy theories

THERAPEUTIC INTERVENTIONS:

A moderate-term course of individual Cognitive Behavior Therapy, including EMDR along with bereavement counseling (6–9 months)

1. PTSD

   - Participate in imaginal and in vivo exposure with response prevention to elements of traumatic events
   - Practice thought-stopping for unwanted and intrusive recollections
   - Modify irrational thoughts about the trauma and his perceived role
   - Learn skills of EMDR to reduce emotional and physiological reactivity to trauma recollections
   - Participation in trauma-focused group therapy, including relaxation training
   - Discuss and implement relapse strategies for PTSD symptoms

2. Bereavement

   - Understand the stages of bereavement
   - Verbalize feelings and thoughts related to losses
   - Refute irrational beliefs and guilt about his role in the loss
   - Use narrative remembering techniques to maintain healthy connection to lost loved ones
   - Attendance in bereavement group
   - Bibliotherapy for grief and loss issues

3. Antisocial thoughts, feelings, and actions

   - Identify and understand origin of "injustice schema" and its effects on his interpersonal functioning
   - Explore history of antisocial behavior and its effects on his self-image and relationships
   - Plan for restitution to known victims
   - Practice trusting others through disclosure of personal feelings of vulnerabilities

OUTCOME MEASURES OF CHANGE:

The resolution of his posttraumatic stress symptoms, improved overall mood, reconciliation of losses, elimination of antisocial thoughts, feelings, and actions, and overall improved adjustment and functioning in his daily life as measured by:

   - Client report of improved overall daily functioning, including sleep, appetite, and energy level
   - Pre-post improvement on the Clinical Anger Scale (CAS)
   - Post measures of GAF functioning in the mild (>70) range
   - Client report and clinician observation of reduced antisocial thoughts and attitudes
   - Clinician observation and client report of prosocial thoughts and behavior
   - Absence of arrests for antisocial behavior and illegal acts for a period of 1 year
   - Clinician observation of improved mood, accompanied by reduced guilt over losses

Table 10.1   Jack Bauer's Treatment Plan Summary: Cognitive Behavior Therapy

Goals for Change	Therapeutic Interventions	Outcome Measures of Change
PTSD Relieve the symptoms of posttraumatic stress Verbalize an understanding of how the symptoms of PTSD develop Bereavement Appropriately grieve the losses of his wife and colleagues Improvement in overall daily functioning and mood Antisocial thoughts, feelings, and actions Resolve negative perceptions of and reactions to other people Understand the relationship between his negative feelings about himself and toward others Eliminate antisocial behavior Resolve thoughts about conspiracy theories	PTSD Participate in imaginal and in vivo exposure with response prevention to elements of traumatic events Practice thought-stopping for unwanted and intrusive recollections Modify irrational thoughts about the trauma and his perceived role Learn skills of EMDR to reduce emotional and physiological reactivity to trauma recollections Participation in trauma-focused group therapy, including relaxation training Discuss and implement relapse strategies for PTSD symptoms Bereavement Understand the stages of bereavement Verbalize feelings and thoughts related to losses Refute irrational beliefs and guilt about his role in the loss Use narrative remembering techniques to maintain healthy connection to lost loved ones Attendance in bereavement group Bibliotherapy for grief and loss issues Antisocial thoughts, feelings, and actions Identify and understand origin of "injustice schema" and its effects on his interpersonal functioning Explore history of antisocial behavior and its effects on his self-image and relationships Plan for restitution to known victims Practice trusting others through disclosure of personal feelings of vulnerabilities	The resolution of his posttraumatic stress symptoms, improved overall mood, reconciliation of losses, elimination of antisocial thoughts, feelings, and actions, and overall improved adjustment and functioning in his daily life as measured by: Client report of improved overall daily functioning, including sleep, appetite, and energy level Pre-post improvement on the Clinical Anger Scale (CAS) Post measures of GAF functioning in the mild (>70) range Client report and clinician observation of reduced antisocial thoughts and attitudes Clinician observation and client report of prosocial thoughts and behavior Absence of arrests for antisocial behavior and illegal acts for a period of 1 year Clinician observation of improved mood, accompanied by reduced guilt over losses

CASE 10.2   *GOLDEN GIRLS'* SOPHIA PETRILLO

INTRODUCING THE CHARACTER

Sophia Petrillo is the eldest character of the four-woman ensemble cast of NBC's *The Golden Girls,* which aired between 1985 and 1992. Sophia was played by the late actress Estelle Getty. The show was set in Miami Beach, Florida, at the home of Blanche Devereaux, a close friend of Mrs. Petrillo's older daughter, Dorothy, played by the late comic actress Bea Arthur. At the beginning of the series, we meet Sophia, who was forced out of the Shady Pines Retirement Home following a mysterious fire. Later we learn that the fire was caused inadvertently by Sophia and her Shady Pines roommate, who were secretly making s'mores—the hot dessert snack that combines graham crackers, marshmallows, and melted chocolate—on a hotplate. Throughout the series, Sophia was the typically unflappable and perennially caustic "house mother" whose stroke earlier in life "rendered her permanently annoying" according to her daughter, Dorothy. During each episode, Sophia is full of bristling commentary on the plight of women, the importance of traditional family values, and other assorted topics, including love, sex, relationships, and religion. The following basic case summary and diagnostic impressions present our view of Sophia as she begins to experience multiple cognitive deficits later in her life.

Meet the Client

You can assess the client in action by viewing clips of Sophia Petrillo's video material at the following websites:

- http://www.youtube.com/watch?v=HSL0jVe1MkI A day in the life of Sophia
- http://www.youtube.com/watch?v=a4XJszcVt5Q Sophia wants to enter the convent
- http://www.youtube.com/watch?v=FXLcSRoGB38 Sophia stands up

---

BASIC CASE SUMMARY

Identifying Information. Sophia Petrillo is an 85-year-old, widowed Italian American woman who lives with her 63-year-old daughter and two other women, a household group she refers to as the "Golden Girls." Medical reports indicate that Mrs. Petrillo is in good health and of good strength for her age, with no indications of diseases of the central nervous system or other systems; however, she did experience and apparently recover from a stroke several years ago. She presents as a woman of diminutive stature and frail appearance; however, her caustic wit contributes to the impression that she is much larger in stature.

Presenting Concern. Mrs. Petrillo was accompanied to the Greater Miami Counseling Center by her daughter, Dorothy, who was concerned that "Mom has finally lost it." Although Mrs. Petrillo is reportedly capable of taking care of her daily needs, her daughter has noticed that of late, "Mom has been particularly sarcastic, says she can't remember who I am, and walks around the house at night calling out the name of my father." She appears to have forgotten her housemates' names at times. On several occasions, Dorothy found her mother on her knees in the garden planting tomato seeds, which would not otherwise be disturbing; however, it was wintertime, and Mrs. Petrillo was dressed only in her nightgown. Her daughter also reported that Mr. Petrillo no longer seems able to plan meals, follow a recipe, or organize her weekly shopping and other outings. Dorothy reported that Mrs. Petrillo's symptoms had become gradually more noticeable to her and her housemates over "a long while."

Background, Family Information, and Relevant History. Sophia Petrillo was born in Sicily, Italy, the middle of five children to Don and Eleanor. Mrs. Petrillo reportedly was successful in school and enjoyed her studies. She was planning to become a nurse (one of the few vocations open to women in her context) when, instead, at her parents' insistence, she changed plans and prepared to marry her parents' selection of a potential husband. However, deciding at the last minute that "I wasn't going to live somebody else's life," Mrs. Petrillo left her fiance at the altar and came to New York. Within several months she met and married Salvatore Petrillo, who worked by day in a grocery store, but who also is suspected of having some minor involvements with local organized crime.

Over the next several years, Mrs. Petrillo and Salvatore had three children: Dorothy, who along with her husband had one child; Gloria, who briefly married into wealth; and Phil, a devoted husband and father, who, unbeknownst to the family, was cross-dressing. Mrs. Petrillo worked tirelessly to raise her children, particularly after her husband was killed in gang violence. She worked in a number of vocations during her 30s, 40s, and 50s, including at Bloomingdale's in the perfume department, in a neighborhood wine store, as a front desk manager at a Holiday Inn on Staten Island, New York, as well as a substitute teacher in the same school where her Dorothy was working.

Over the years, Mrs. Petrillo had endeared herself to friends and coworkers with her sharp wit, ever-ready smile, and willingness to lend a hand to others in need. All were shocked when shortly after her 65th birthday, Mrs. Petrillo began to experience disturbing and erratic behaviors and the seeming inability to restrain herself from making hurtful and sarcastic comments about other people. These changes were followed soon after by a stroke that left her partially paralyzed on the left side of her body. Her speech, much to the chagrin of her daughter, was left intact.

Soon after the stroke, Mrs. Petrillo was moved to the Shady Pines Nursing Home by her daughter, who was surprised when her mother, after only 6 months in the facility, married fellow resident Max Winestock. When the facility burned to the ground, Mrs. Petrillo was invited to live with Dorothy, who was not able to accommodate Mr. Winestock. He was subsequently transferred to another facility, and over the years, he and Mrs. Petrillo maintained a very cordial (and occasionally sexual) relationship.

As of this writing, Mrs. Petrillo had been comfortably living with her daughter and two other housemates for 2 years and was appreciative of the opportunity to, in her words, "Be with the people I love . . . even though they are a pain in my royal ass if you know what I mean."

Problem and Counseling History. Mrs. Petrillo was accompanied to the intake by her daughter, Dorothy, who had her arm wrapped gently around her mother's shoulder and who escorted her to one of the interviewing chairs. As she sat down, Mrs. Petrillo pushed her daughter's hand away and brusquely said, "I can sit down myself; stop treating me like an old woman." Each time that Dorothy attempted to relate details of her mother's most recent experiences, Mrs. Petrillo interrupted her and announced, "Oh, now you're going to talk for me also."

Mrs. Petrillo was a very animated, articulate, and astutely oriented octogenarian who freely and easily offered information and details about her life, both recent and remote. Placid at times while irritable at others, she proudly proclaimed, "I've lived this long without any help from anyone, and I just need them to know that I'm fine." Mrs. Petrillo denied experiencing the personality and behavioral changes that her daughter noticed, in which regard she said, "I get a little more tired than usual, but I'd like to see if they have half the spirit that I do when they get to be my age . . . with or without a stroke."

Goals for Counseling and Course of Therapy to Date. At the end of the intake session, Mrs. Petrillo was invited to participate in the "Golden Girls Senior Activity Program," which includes social and craft activities, cooking classes, as well as individual and group counseling. Upon hearing this Mrs. Petrillo proclaimed, "Oh, so now you think I'm nuts and want to lock me in this crazy joint . . . no way Jose." She got up from her chair, turned her back, and walked abruptly out of the room. Her daughter agreed to encourage Mrs. Petrillo to return for further assessment and also agreed to participate in an in-home evaluation conducted by a licensed clinical social worker. The primary goals of the follow-up interview and in-home evaluation will be (a) to confirm clinically significant decline in the form of memory loss and other cognitive deficits; and (b) assist the client and her daughter in determining an appropriate plan of action.

Diagnostic Impressions

Axis I. 294.11 Dementia of the Alzheimer's Type, With Behavioral Disturbance, With Late Onset

Axis II. V71.09 No Diagnosis on Axis II

Axis III. History of Stroke (CVA)

Axis IV. Problem with primary support group—Widowed; separated from her current husband

Axis V. GAF = 65 (current)

GAF = 65 (highest level past year)

DISCUSSION OF DIAGNOSTIC IMPRESSIONS

Sophia Petrillo was accompanied to the Greater Miami Counseling Center by her daughter because she was concerned that Sophia was experiencing memory impairment (forgetting her daughter's and her housemates' names) and disturbances in her everyday activities (gardening in a nightgown late on a winter night; failing to follow the steps of a familiar recipe in the kitchen). Her daughter thought Mrs. Petrillo's memory loss and other behavioral changes had developed gradually over time.

The *DSM-IV-TR* section, Delirium, Dementia, Amnestic Disorders, and Other Cognitive Disorders, contains a variety of mental disorders featuring significant deficits in cognitive abilities that signify a clear change from a person's previous level of cognitive functioning. Included are delirium (disturbance in consciousness) due to substance use, a medical problem, or multiple sources; dementia (impairment in memory plus multiple other cognitive deficits) due to various medical etiologies or sources; and amnestic disorders (memory impairments without other cognitive deficits) due to substance use, a medical

problem, or other sources. One of these disorders that is especially important to the everyday practice of counseling professionals who work with older adults in various inpatient and outpatient settings is Dementia of the Alzheimer's Type With Late Onset.

In this case example, Mrs. Petrillo presented multiple cognitive deficits later in her life, manifested by memory impairment in the form of an inability to recall previously learned information, and other deficits in the form of disturbance in executive functioning (such as planning, organizing, and following sequences). The onset of Mrs. Petrillo's cognitive decline was gradual, continuing, and causing impairment in social and other functioning. Although she does have a history of stroke, the current symptoms of cognitive decline were not attributable to the stroke or to any other medical condition or substance use. In such cases the diagnosis is Dementia of the Alzheimer's Type. Mrs. Petrillo's cognitive symptoms were accompanied by behavioral disturbances that were clinically significant, such as gardening on a winter night, and onset was after age 65. Therefore, the specifier is With Behavioral Disturbance and the subtype is With Late Onset.

Distinguishing among physical, cognitive, affective, and behavioral factors influencing changes in older adult clients' functioning requires the counselor's special attention (Schlossberg, 1995). In the case of Dementia of the Alzheimer's Type, perhaps the most important consideration regarding differential diagnoses pertains to etiology: dementias due to a general medical condition, dementias due to substance use, and dementias due to multiple known etiologies might be considered. However, in Mrs. Petrillo's case, there is no evidence from lab tests or physical examinations to suggest any of these causes. Generally speaking, Schizophrenia also might be a differential consideration when considering symptoms of a dementia; however, in Mrs. Petrillo's case, there is no lifelong history at all of Schizophrenia. Alternatively, Major Depressive Disorder may feature impairment in memory, concentration, and thinking—and clinicians are alerted that "particularly in elderly persons, it is often difficult to determine whether cognitive symptoms are better accounted for by a dementia or by a Major Depressive Episode" (APA, 2000a, p. 153). However, in Mrs. Petrillo's case, no other symptoms of a mood disorder were observed or reported, and the nature of, and gradual onset of, symptoms conform to the criteria for Dementia of the Alzheimer's Type.

To finish the diagnosis, Mrs. Petrillo's history of stroke is listed on Axis III, her important family and social stressors are emphasized on Axis IV, and on Axis V her functioning is represented by GAF scores indicating mildly serious symptoms such that although she still is generally functioning fairly well and still has meaningful interpersonal relationships, she also is experiencing some difficulty in social and other areas of functioning. Her scores suggest that her functioning has been in this range for at least the past year. The information on these axes is consistent with the Axis I diagnosis describing Mrs. Petrillo's onset of concerns.

CASE CONCEPTUALIZATION

During Mrs. Petrillo's first visit to the Greater Miami Counseling Center, the intake coordinator obtained present-day and background information about the behaviors and consequences leading Mrs. Petrillo's daughter, at this point, to seek professional consultation. Based on the intake visit, neuropsychological testing, and medical record information, the coordinator developed diagnostic impressions of Alzheimer's type dementia with behavioral disturbance. A case conceptualization next was developed. Whereas the purpose of diagnostic impressions is to *describe* the client's concerns, the goal of case conceptualization is to better *understand* and clinically *explain* the person's experiences (Neukrug & Schwitzer, 2006). In turn, case conceptualization sets the stage for treatment planning. Treatment planning then provides a road map that plots out how the therapy team at the day center and the client expect to move from presenting concerns to positive outcomes (Seligman, 1993, p. 157)— helping Mrs. Petrillo better control the symptoms of Dementia of the Alzheimer's Type, maintain better daily functioning, and continue as much satisfying independent life activity as possible (American Association for Geriatric Psychiatry, 2006).

When forming a case conceptualization, the clinician applies a purist counseling theory, an integration of two or more theories, an eclectic mix of theories, or a solution-focused combination of tactics, to his or her understanding of the client. In this case, the intake coordinator based his conceptualization on psychotherapeutic integration of two theories (Corey, 2009). Psychotherapists very commonly integrate more than one theoretical approach in order to form a conceptualization and treatment plan that will be as efficient and effective as possible for meeting the client's needs (Dattilo & Norcross, 2006; Norcross & Beutler, 2008). In other words, counselors using the psychotherapeutic integration method attempt to flexibly tailor their clinical efforts to "the unique needs and contexts of the individual client" (Norcross & Beutler, 2008, p. 485). Like other counselors using integration, Mrs. Petrillo's clinician chose this method because he had not found one individual theory that was comprehensive enough, by itself, to address all of the "complexities," "range of client types," and "specific problems" seen among his everyday caseload (Corey, 2009, p. 450).

Specifically, the intake coordinator selected an integration of (a) Behavior Therapy and (b) Cognitive Stimulation Therapy. He selected this approach based on Mrs. Petrillo's onset of Alzheimer's type dementia symptoms, and his knowledge of current outcome research with clients experiencing these types of concerns (Anonymous, 2004; Anonymous, 2007). According to the research, Behavior Therapy is one treatment approach indicated when assisting clients to reduce and manage their affective and behavioral symptoms and the consequences of these symptoms for themselves and family members and caretakers (Ayalon, Gunn, Feliciano, & Arean, 2006; Livingston et al., 2005; Spector, Davies, Woods, & Orrell, 2000; Spira & Edelstein, 2006), whereas an integrated approach emphasizing Cognitive Stimulation is indicated to strengthen their cognitive abilities by strengthening memories least affected by dementia, namely, memories of early life (Woods, Spector, Jones, Orrell, & Davies, 1998). The counselor used the Inverted Pyramid Method of case conceptualization because this method is especially designed to help clinicians more easily form their conceptual pictures of their clients' needs (Neukrug & Schwitzer, 2006; Schwitzer, 1996, 1997). The method has four steps: Problem Identification, Thematic Groupings, Theoretical Inferences, and Narrowed Inferences. The counselor's clinical thinking can be seen in Figure 10.2.

Step 1: Problem Identification. The first step is Problem Identification. Aspects of the presenting problem (thoughts, feelings, behaviors, physiological features), additional areas of concern besides the presenting concern, family and developmental history, in-session observations, clinical inquiries (medical problems, medications, past counseling, substance use, suicidality), and psychological assessments (problem checklists, personality inventories, mental status exam, specific clinical measures) all may contribute information at Step 1. The counselor "casts a wide net" in order to build step 1 as exhaustively as possible (Neukrug & Schwitzer,

2006, p. 202). As can be seen in Figure 10.2, the intake coordinator identified not only Mrs. Petrillo's prominent signals of the early onset of Alzheimer's type dementia (irrational behavior, memory losses, reduced planning and organizing abilities, etc.), but also important strengths, events, and other aspects of her previously successful lifetime adjustment—all of which were important to describing her clinical situation.

Step 2: Thematic Groupings. The second step is Thematic Groupings. The clinician organizes all of the exhaustive client information found in Step 1 into just a few intuitive-logical clinical groups, categories, or themes on the basis of sensible common denominators (Neukrug & Schwitzer, 2006). Four different ways of forming the Step 2 theme groups can be used: Descriptive-Diagnosis Approach, Clinical Targets Approach, Areas of Dysfunction Approach, and Intrapsychic Approach. As can be seen in the figure, the intake coordinator selected the Clinical Targets Approach. This approach sorts together all of the Step 1 information "according to the basic division of behavior, thoughts, feelings, and physiology" (Neukrug & Schwitzer, 2006, p. 205). The clinician grouped together: (a) cognitive difficulties (gradual memory loss, gradual confusion, reduced planning and organizing functions), and (b) behavioral and affective difficulties (erratic behaviors and decisions, less able to follow plans, increased sarcastic responses). Mrs. Petrillo's clinician believed that, in her case, the Clinical Targets Approach was most effective bridge between Mrs. Petrillo's various symptoms and the theoretical inferences that would be needed later in his conceptualization pertaining to the early onset of Dementia of the Alzheimer's Type.

So far, at Steps 1 and 2, the intake coordinator has used his clinical assessment skills and his clinical judgment to begin critically understanding Mrs. Petrillo's needs. Now, at Steps 3 and 4, he applies the theoretical approach he has selected. He begins making theoretical inferences to explain the factors leading to Mrs. Petrillo's issues as they are seen in Steps 1 and 2.

Step 3: Theoretical Inferences. At Step 3, concepts from the counselor's theoretical integration of two approaches—Behavior Therapy and Cognitive Stimulation—are applied to the factors causing, and the mechanisms maintaining Mrs. Petrillo's functioning. The counselor tentatively matches the theme groups in Step 2 with this theoretical approach. In other words, the symptom constellations in Step 2, which were distilled from the symptoms in Step 1, now are combined using theory to show what are believed to be the underlying processes or psychological mechanisms of Mrs. Petrillo's current needs (Neukrug & Schwitzer, 2006; Schwitzer, 2006, 2007).

First, Behavior Therapy was applied primarily to clinically thinking through Mrs. Petrillo's needs regarding her behavior and affective responses. As a conceptual approach, Behavior Therapy focuses closely on describing and understanding what behaviors (including affective responses) are occurring, when and how they are occurring, what the antecedents and consequences (i.e., what leads to the behavior and what results from the behavior) of the behaviors are—and in turn, what may be altered or changed in the behavioral chain to improve these responses; in other words, the model focuses conceptually on the specific factors influencing and resulting from current behaviors, and methods of modifying these factors (Lazarus, 2005, 2008; Martell, 2007; Wolpe, 1990). In the more specific situation of clients experiencing the onset of Alzheimer's type dementia, the conceptual focus may be on the behavioral contexts associated with compensating for memory losses in daily functioning (written cues, visual cues, daily structure, reality orientation through using the person's name, etc.) (Spector et al., 2000; Woods, 2004; Woods et al., 1998) and the issues or events that cue emotional outbursts, depression or anxiety, or other problems (Ayalon et al., 2006; Livingston et al., 2005; Spira & Edelstein, 2006). As can be seen in Figure 10.2, when Mrs. Petrillo's intake coordinator applied these concepts, she developed the following Step 3 inference: As dementia-related declines progress, Mrs. Petrillo reduces her awareness of antecedents and consequences of her behaviors.

Second, Cognitive Cognitive Stimulation was applied primarily to clinically thinking through Mrs. Petrillo's needs regarding her cognitive losses. As a conceptual approach, Cognitive Stimulation Therapy focuses closely on describing and understanding what memory losses and other cognitive declines are occurring, in what domains, and in what order and what rates—and in turn, what may be altered to mitigate, minimize, or slow these declines (Anonymous, 2004; Anonymous, 2007). As also can be seen in the figure, when Mrs. Petrillo's intake coordinator additionally applied these concepts, she developed a further Step 3 inference, as follows: As dementia-related declines progress, Mrs. Petrillo experiences various types of cognitive losses, at different rates of decline.

Step 4: Narrowed Inferences. At Step 4, the clinician's selected theory continues to be used to address still-deeper issues when they exist (Schwitzer, 2006, 2007). At this step, "still-deeper, more encompassing, or more central, causal themes" are formed (Neukrug & Schwitzer, 2006, p. 207). Mrs. Petrillo's counselor continued to use a psychotherapeutic integration of two approaches.

First, continuing to apply Behavior Therapy concepts at Step 4, the intake coordinator presented a single, deepest theoretical inference that she believed to be most fundamental for Mrs. Petrillo from a behavioral perspective: Mrs. Petrillo's problematic behaviors may be responsive to behavioral intervention such as greater daily structure, reinforcing reality orientation, and other behavioral strategies to compensate for early memory loss. Second, continuing to apply Cognitive Stimulation, the coordinator presented a single, deepest theoretical inference that she believed to be most fundamental for Mrs. Petrillo regarding cognitive functioning: Mrs. Petrillo's cognitive losses may be responsive to enhanced stimulation such as joining in activities with others, focused intellectual practice and exercises, and enhancing early

Figure 10.2   Mrs. Sophia Petrillo's Inverted Pyramid Case Conceptualization: Psychotherapeutic Integration of Behavior Therapy and Cognitive Stimulation Therapy

1. IDENTIFY AND LIST CLIENT CONCERNS

Medical history of stroke
Widowed from first husband
Separated from second husband
Living in family arrangement with
    daughter and housemates
History of active, independent living
Irrational behavior
Wintertime nighttime gardening in
    nightgown

Reduced ability to plan menus
Reduced ability to follow a recipe
Reduced ability to organize shopping & outings
Periodic loss of memory of daughter's name
Periodic loss of memory of housemates' names
Calling for deceased husband
Increased sarcasm beyond baseline
Gradual onset of symptoms and disturbances

2. ORGANIZE CONCERNS INTO LOGICAL THEMATIC GROUPINGS

1. Cognitive difficulties: gradual memory loss, gradual confusion, reduced planning and organizing functions
2. Behavioral and affective difficulties: erratic behaviors and decisions, less able to follow plans, increased sarcastic responses

3. THEORETICAL INFERENCES: ATTACH THEMATIC GROUPINGS TO INFERRED AREAS OF DIFFICULTY

Psychotherapeutic Integration

Behavioral Therapy

As dementia-related declines progress, Mrs. Petrillo reduces awareness of antecedents and consequences of her behaviors

Cognitive Stimulation Therapy
As dementia-related declines progress, Mrs. Petrillo experiences various types of cognitive losses, at different rates of decline

4. NARROWED INFERENCES: SUICIDALITY AND DEEPER DIFFICULTIES

Psychotherapeutic Integration

Behavior Therapy

Mrs. Petrillo's problematic behaviors may be responsive to enhanced behavioral intervention such as greater daily structure, practice, and exercises, and enhancing early reminiscences strategies to compensate for early memory loss

Cognitive Stimulation Therapy

Mrs. Petrillo's cognitive losses may be responsive to stimulation such as joining in activities with others, focused intellectual practice and exercises, and enhancing early reminiscences

reminiscences. These two narrowed inferences, together, form the basis for understanding Mrs. Petrillo's current counseling situation.

When all four steps are completed, the client information in Step 1 leads to logical-intuitive groupings on the basis of common denominators in Step 2, the groupings then are explained using theory at Step 3, and then, finally, at Step 4, further deeper explanations are made. From start to finish, the thoughts, feelings, behaviors, and physiological features in the topmost portions are connected on down the pyramid into deepest dynamics.

TREATMENT PLANNING

At this point, Mrs. Petrillo's clinician at the Greater Miami Counseling Center has collected all available information about the problems that have been of concern to her and her daughter. Based upon this information, the counselor developed a five-axis *DSM-IV-TR* diagnosis and then, using the "inverted pyramid" (Neukrug & Schwitzer, 2006; Schwitzer, 1996, 1997), formulated a working clinical *explanation* of Mrs. Petrillo's difficulties and their etiology that we called the *case conceptualization*. This, in turn, guides us to the next critical step in our clinical work, called the *treatment plan*, the primary purpose of which is to map out a logical and goal-oriented strategy for making positive changes in the client's life. In essence, the treatment plan is a road map "for reducing or eliminating disruptive symptoms that are impeding the client's ability to reach positive mental health outcomes" (Neukrug & Schwitzer, 2006, p. 225). As such, it is the cornerstone of our work with not only Mrs. Petrillo, but with all clients who present with disturbing and disruptive symptoms and/or personality patterns (Jongsma & Peterson, 2006; Jongsma et al., 2003a, 2003b; Seligman, 1993, 1998, 2004).

A comprehensive treatment plan must integrate all of the information from the biopsychosocial interview, diagnosis, and case conceptualization into a coherent plan of action. This *plan* comprises four main components, which include (1) a behavioral definition of the problem(s), (2) the selection of achievable goals, (3) the determination of treatment modes, and (4) the documentation of how change will be measured. The *behavioral definition of the problem(s)* consolidates the results of the case conceptualization into a concise hierarchical list of problems and concerns that will be the focus of treatment. The *selection of achievable goals* refers to assessing and prioritizing the client's concerns into a *hierarchy of urgency that* also takes into account the client's motivation for change, level of dysfunction, and real-world influences on his or her problems. The *determination of treatment modes* refers to selection of the specific interventions, which are matched to the uniqueness of the client and to his or her goals and clearly tied to a particular theoretical orientation (Neukrug & Schwitzer, 2006). Finally, the clinician must establish how change will be measured, based upon a number of factors including client records and self-report of change, in-session observations by the clinician, clinician ratings, results of standardized evaluations such as the Beck Anxiety Inventory (Beck & Steer, 1990) or a family functioning questionnaire, pre-post treatment comparisons, and reports by other treating professionals.

The four-step method discussed above can be seen in Figure 6.1 (p. 109) and is outlined below for the case of Mrs. Petrillo, followed by her specific treatment plan.

Step 1: Behavioral Definition of Problems. The first step in treatment planning is to carefully review the case conceptualization, paying particular attention to the results of Step 2 (Thematic Groupings), Step 3 (Theoretical Inferences), and Step 4 (Narrowed Inferences). The identified clinical themes reflect the core areas of concern and distress for the client, while the theoretical and narrowed inferences offer clinical speculation as to their origins. In the case of Mrs. Petrillo, there are two primary areas of concern. The first, "cognitive difficulties," refers to her reduced ability to plan menus, follow a recipe, and organize shopping and outings; her periodic loss of memory of her daughter's name, those of her housemates, and calling for her deceased husband. The second, "behavioral and affective difficulties," refers to her irrational and erratic behavior and decisions, that is, wintertime gardening in her nightgown and increased sarcasm beyond baseline. These symptoms and stresses are consistent with the diagnosis of Dementia of the Alzheimer's Type, With Behavioral Disturbance, With Late Onset (Anonymous, 2004, 2006, 2007; APA, 2000a; Lykestos et al., 2006).

Step 2: Identify and Articulate Goals for Change. The second step is the selection of achievable goals, which is based upon a number of factors, including the most pressing or urgent behavioral, emotional, and interpersonal concerns and symptoms as identified by the client and clinician, the willingness and ability of the client to work on those particular goals, and the realistic (real-world) achievability of those goals (Neukrug & Schwitzer, 2006). At this stage of treatment planning, it is important to recognize that not all of the client's problems can be addressed at once, so we focus initially on those that cause the greatest distress and impairment. New goals can be created as old ones are achieved. In the case of Mrs. Petrillo, the goals are divided into two prominent areas. The first, "cognitive difficulties," requires that we help Mrs. Petrillo to develop an understanding and acceptance of her cognitive impairment, to verbalize thoughts and feelings about these impairments, to develop alternative coping strategies to compensate for her developing cognitive limitations, and to provide psychoeducation and support for her immediate family members. The second, "behavioral and affective difficulties," requires that we help Mrs. Petrillo understand the behavioral and affective symptoms that accompany Alzheimer's disease and develop coping strategies to recognize and minimize their impact on her life.

Step 3: Describe Therapeutic Intervention. This is perhaps the most critical step in the treatment planning process because the clinician must now integrate information from a number of sources, including the case conceptualization, the delineation of the client's problems and goals, and the treatment literature, paying particular attention to *empirically supported treatment* (EST) and *evidence-based practice* (EBP). In essence, the clinician must align his or her treatment approach with scientific evidence from the fields of counseling and psychotherapy. Wampold (2001) identifies two types of evidence-based counseling research: studies that demonstrate "absolute efficacy," that is, the fact that counseling and psychotherapy work, and those that demonstrate "relative efficacy," that is, the fact that certain theoretical/technical approaches work best for certain clients with particular problems (Psychoanalysis, Gestalt Therapy, Cognitive Behavior Therapy, Brief Solution-Focused Therapy, Cognitive Therapy, Dialectical Behavior Therapy, Person-Centered Therapy, Expressive/Creative Therapies, Interpersonal Therapy, and Feminist Therapy); and when delivered through specific treatment modalities (individual, group, and family counseling). In the case of Mrs. Petrillo, we have decided to use a two-pronged integrated approach to therapy, including Behavior Therapy and Cognitive Stimulation Therapy. Behavior Therapy (Lazarus, 2005, 2008; Nye, 1992; Wolpe, 1990) is a highly empirical approach to therapy that "is based on the precepts of classical conditioning, social learning or modeling and operant conditioning" (Neukrug, 2011, p. 255). Drawing heavily from learning theory, it posits in a highly deterministic fashion that all behavior, whether adaptive or maladaptive, is learned either through direct experience or by observing the experiences of other people. These behaviors are learned, maintained, and eliminated through the processes and schedules of reinforcement, punishment, shaping, chaining, and extinction (Neukrug, 2011). As noted above, the role of the therapist is to focus closely on describing and understanding what behaviors (including affective responses) are occurring, when and how they are occurring, what the antecedents and consequences (i.e., what leads to the behaviors and what results from the behaviors) of the behaviors are—and in turn, what may be altered or changed in the behavioral chain to improve these responses; in other words, the model focuses conceptually on the specific factors influencing and resulting from current behaviors, and methods of modifying these factors.

These procedures have been effectively applied in the cases of people struggling with the symptoms of Alzheimer's disease and related neurocognitive impairments (Anonymous, 2007; Ayalon et al., 2006; Livingston et al., 2005; Spector et al., 2000; Spira & Edelstein, 2006). Specific techniques for Mrs. Petrillo include functional analysis of self-care skills, charting/ monitoring of successful implementation of self-care with verbal reinforcement, shaping of appropriate problem-solving skills using cue cards and hand-drawn pictures, client self-monitoring of stress level and anger/sarcasm, caregiver education in behavioral management, including shaping, reinforcement, and extinction, as well as support group for client and family regarding dementia.

Cognitive Stimulation Therapy (Anonymous, 2004, 2007; Livingston et al., 1996) is predicated upon the notion that the cognitive impairments accompanying Alzheimer's disease, including memory, reasoning, planning, and problem-solving are a function of neurobiological deterioration. Cognitive stimulation in the form of cognitive exercises (memory games, puzzles, arts-and-crafts), reminiscence (pictures, songs, cherished objects), and creative-expressive and recreational activities (art, music, play) can and have been proven effective in enhancing neurocognitive functioning (Livingston et al., 1996; Woods, 2004; Woods et al., 1998), which in turn maintains and accentuates daily living skills including self-care, communication, and organization. Specific techniques

for Mrs. Petrillo that are drawn from this approaches include reminiscence/life review exercises comprised of music, pictures, and video, and outings to friends and relatives, creative/ expressive exercises, including art, music, and physical activity, Snoezelen (controlled multisensory) (Anonymous, 2005; Livingston et al., 2005) activities, including visual, auditory, kinesthetic, olfactory, and somatosensory stimulation, relaxation, including progressive muscle work, and deep breathing.

Step 4: Provide Outcome Measures of Change. This last step in treatment planning requires that we specify how change will be measured and indicate the extent to which progress has been made toward realizing these goals (Neukrug & Schwitzer, 2006). The counselor has considerable flexibility in this phase and may choose from a number of objective domains (psychological tests and measures of self-esteem, depression, psychosis, interpersonal relationship, anxiety, etc.), quasi-objective measures (the *DSM-IV-TR's* Axis V GAF scale; pre-post clinician, client, and psychiatric ratings), and subjective ratings (client self-report, clinician's in-session observations). In Mrs. Petrillo's case, we have implemented a number of these, including ongoing measures on the Cohen-Mansfield Agitation Inventory (Cohen-Mansfield, 1991), client and family stated awareness of the symptoms of Alzheimer's disease, client and family report of attendance in psychoeducational support group, client and family report of attendance in Cognitive Stimulation Therapy, and clinician observation of client's communication, self-care, emotional regulation, and behavior control.

The completed treatment plan is now developed through which the counselor, Mrs. Petrillo, and her family will begin their shared work of adjusting to the cognitive, emotional, behavioral, and interpersonal challenges of Alzheimer's disease. The treatment plan appears below and is summarized in Table 10.2.

TREATMENT PLAN

Client: Mrs. Sophia Petrillo

Service Provider: Greater Miami Counseling Center

BEHAVIORAL DEFINITION OF PROBLEMS:

1. Cognitive difficulties—Reduced ability to plan menus, follow a recipe, and organize shopping and outings; periodic loss of memory of daughter's name, those of housemates, and calling for deceased husband

2. Behavioral and affective difficulties—Irrational and erratic behavior and decisions, that is, wintertime gardening in her nightgown and increased sarcasm beyond baseline

GOALS FOR CHANGE:

1. Cognitive difficulties

   • Develop an understanding and acceptance of her cognitive impairment
   • Develop alternative coping strategies to compensate for developing cognitive limitations
   • Verbalize thoughts and feelings about these impairments
   • Provide psychoeducation and support for immediate family members

2. Behavioral and affective difficulties

   • Understand the behavioral and affective symptoms that accompany Alzheimer's disease
   • Develop coping strategies to recognize and minimize their impact
   • Provide psychoeducation and support for immediate family members

THERAPEUTIC INTERVENTIONS:

An ongoing course of individual and family Behavior and Cognitive Stimulation Therapy supplemented with group psychoeducation and skill building

1. Cognitive difficulties

   • Functional analysis of self-care skills
   • Charting/monitoring of successful implementation of self-care with verbal reinforcement
   • Shaping of appropriate problem-solving skills using cue cards and hand-drawn pictures
   • Caregiver education in behavioral management, including shaping, reinforcement, and extinction
   • Support group for client and family regarding dementia
   • Long-term family planning for alternative living arrangements as the level of impairment progresses

2. Behavioral and affective difficulties

   • Reminiscence/life review exercises comprised of music, pictures, video, and outings to friends and relatives
   • Client self-monitoring of stress level and anger/sarcasm
   • Caregiver education in behavioral management, including shaping, reinforcement, and extinction

(Continued)

(Continued)

- Creative/expressive exercises including art, music, and physical activity
- Snoezelen (controlled multisensory) activities including visual, auditory, kinesthetic, olfactory, and somatosensory stimulation
- Relaxation, including progressive muscle work and deep breathing

OUTCOME MEASURES OF CHANGE:

The development of client and family awareness of the symptoms and course of Alzheimer's disease, maintenance of optimal cognitive and behavioral functioning, and long-term care planning as measured by:

- Ongoing measures on the Cohen-Mansfield Agitation Inventory
- Client- and family-stated awareness of the symptoms of Alzheimer's disease
- Client and family report of attendance in psychoeducational support group
- Client and family report of attendance in Cognitive Stimulation Therapy
- Clinician observation of client's communication, self-care, emotional regulation, and behavior control
- Diminished frequency of episodes of erratic behavior
- Family report and clinician observation of reduced client sarcasm
- Family report (through charting and clinician observation) of effective use of behavioral strategies for client's improved coping skills
- Family report of long-term care planning

Table 10.2 Sophia Petrillo's Treatment Plan Summary: Psychotherapeutic Integration of Behavior Therapy and Cognitive Stimulation Therapy

Goals for Change	Therapeutic Interventions	Outcome Measures of Change
Cognitive difficulties	Cognitive difficulties	The development of client and family awareness of the symptoms and course of Alzheimer's disease, maintenance of optimal cognitive and behavioral functioning, and long-term care planning as measured by:
Develop an understanding and acceptance of her cognitive impairment	Functional analysis of self-care skills	
	Charting/monitoring of successful implementation of self-care with verbal reinforcement	
Develop alternative coping strategies to compensate for developing cognitive limitations	Shaping of appropriate problem-solving skills using cue cards and hand-drawn pictures	Ongoing measures on the Cohen-Mansfield Agitation Inventory
Verbalize thoughts and feelings about these impairments	Caregiver education in behavioral management including shaping, reinforcement, and extinction	Client- and family-stated awareness of the symptoms of Alzheimer's disease
	Support group for client and family regarding dementia	
Provide psychoeducation and support for immediate family members	Long-term family planning for alternative living arrangements as the level of impairment progresses	Client and family report of attendance in psychoeducational support group

Goals for Change	Therapeutic Interventions	Outcome Measures of Change
Behavioral and affective difficulties Understand the behavioral and affective symptoms that accompany Alzheimer's disease Develop coping strategies to recognize and minimize their impact Provide psychoeducation and support for immediate family members	Behavioral and affective difficulties Reminiscence/life review exercises comprised of music, pictures, video, and outings to friends and relatives Client self-monitoring of stress level and anger/sarcasm Caregiver education in behavioral management, including shaping, reinforcement, and extinction Creative/expressive exercises, including art, music, and physical activity Snoezelen (controlled multisensory) activities, including visual, auditory, kinesthetic, olfactory, and somatosensory stimulation Relaxation, including progressive muscle work and deep breathing	Client and family report of attendance in Cognitive Stimulation Therapy Clinician observation of client's communication, self-care, emotional regulation, and behavior control Diminished frequency of episodes of erratic behavior Family report and clinician observation of reduced client sarcasm Family report through charting and clinician observation of effective use of behavioral strategies for client's improved coping skills Family report of long-term care planning

CASE 10.3 *GEORGE LOPEZ SHOW'S* GEORGE LOPEZ

INTRODUCING THE CHARACTER

George Lopez is the main character in the *George Lopez Show,* a sitcom that aired on ABC television between 2002 and 2007 and that is now in syndication. It is a "slice of life" show featuring a predominantly Mexican and Mexican American cast. The program features George Lopez, who manages an airplane parts factory; his wife, Angie, who works in the home; their children, Max and Carmen; Mr. Lopez's mother, Benita (Benny); and Angie's father, Victor (Vic) Palermo. The show is family-oriented in nature. It centers on the daily struggles of the Lopez family and the dysfunctional circumstances that bring them together—and the resulting squabbles and frictions within and across the generations, which are oftentimes humorous, but occasionally serious. The central comedic tension is between

Mr. Lopez and his proud and judgmental father-in-law, Vic, who, is a retired physician. Dr. Palermo had always hoped that his daughter would achieve better marital and life status than she did, and thus, George Lopez is forever trying to live up to his father-in-law's expectations of him. Similarly, Angie's mother-in-law, Benny, is forever criticizing her daughter-in-law's cooking, housekeeping skills, and ability to be a good-enough wife to her son. The children, Max and Carmen, struggle with day-to-day adolescent dilemmas and typically provide Mr. Lopez the opportunity to prove his worth, both as a parent, person (and comedian). The following Basic Case Summary and Diagnostic Impressions present our portrayal of the *George Lopez Show's* main character at a recent counseling session as a result of increasing clinically significant distresses related to his complex family life.

Meet the Client

You can assess the client in action by viewing clips of George Lopez's sitcom character video material at the following websites:

- http://www.youtube.com/watch?v=g30LQBLIbZ8 George drives the Batmobile
- http://www.youtube.com/watch?v=NjMom_EaQJ0 Trick or treat me right
- http://www.youtube.com/watch?v=Nkf48tD3teM George and father-in-law, Vic

BASIC CASE SUMMARY

Identifying Information. George Lopez is a 48-year-old Mexican American male who resides in a socioeconomically middle-class household comprising his wife, two children, mother, and father-in-law. Mr. Lopez identifies himself as Roman Catholic. He manages the warehouse at the Power Brothers Aviation Company, where he has progressively advanced through the ranks over his 25-year employment with them. He presented as notably conscious of his appearance, including his average height and weight, recently graying hair, and what he described as "my Mexican features."

Presenting Concern. Mr. Lopez was urged to attend counseling by his wife, Angie, who has become increasingly concerned with the frequency of her husband's headaches and episodes of fatigue, anxiety, and moments of low mood that have bothered her husband since recent changes at work. These changes include corporate cutbacks that have resulted in ongoing furloughs. As a result, Mr. Lopez now has a 1-day furlough without pay per week, along with 1 paid day of working at home instead of at his office. Further, because the manager's position may be permanently cut in the near future, Mr. Lopez feels there is great pressure to compete to "be in the inner circle." As a result, he recently has been encouraged to play golf, play tennis, meet for martinis, and join the Kiwanis Club with his upper-management bosses. He describes this as "like crossing the border again into a whole new world. How does a guy like me hang out with guys like that?"

During the intake, Angie noted that her husband, who typically does not talk about his feelings, has become increasingly irritable, distractible, inattentive at home, and withdrawn from the family, particularly on weekends when he prefers to retreat to the den to watch sports and drink beer with his friends from work. When queried, Mr. Lopez admitted that "I have a lot of responsibilities and a family to support . . . so I like blowing off steam and I get a little cranky once in a while. And okay, sometimes my mood isn't so happy."

Background, Family Information, and Relevant History. George Lopez was born in Tijuana, Mexico, the youngest of three sons to his father, Hernando, who abandoned the family soon after his birth, and mother, Benita (Benny), who worked a number of odd jobs in order to keep her family together. By the time George was 7 years old, his mother began drinking heavily and experienced bouts of depression.

Mr. Lopez attended the Rodrigo Escobar Elementary School in Tijuana where he reports that he was often chastised by his teachers for inattentiveness, failure to focus on his studies, and his seemingly insatiable need to be the center of attention. Nevertheless, Mr. Lopez's memory is that among his endearing childhood qualities were his charm, eloquence, and ability to, as he recalled, "play to my audience." During his middle school years at Tijuana Middle School, Mr. Lopez displayed a propensity for comedy and took an active role in the widely popular school talent shows. It was around that time that he began doing stand-up comedy routines on the streets of Tijuana, which, to his surprise, provided a relatively stable income for his family. By the time Mr. Lopez was of high school age, he had become disinterested in school and recalled that "I was making more money performing on the street than my teacher who was busting her ass in the classroom." However, with the encouragement of his mother, who by that time had been hospitalized several times for the effects of alcoholism, Mr. Lopez persevered in completing his studies.

After graduating from high school, Mr. Lopez crossed the border into the United States and began doing stand-up comedy in local bars, in street festivals, and at local colleges. To his surprise, he became very popular. When Mr. Lopez met Angie, he was 21 and looking forward to a career in comedy; however, they soon had their first child, Max, and his wife convinced him that the family needed him to get a steady job. As a result, he began working in the maintenance department at the Power Brothers Aviation Company, where he quickly earned the respect of his employers and the friendship of his coworkers, who found him funny and loyal. Over the next several years, Mr. Lopez worked diligently at the aviation company while doing occasional evening and weekend stand-up. He advanced to the position of plant manager.

Around that time, Mr. Lopez and his wife were expecting their second child. Mr. Lopez recalls that this was a cause of great stress for him because "I could barely support us with one child . . . how was I going to take care of two children?" Additionally, soon after the birth of the Lopez's second child, Mrs. Lopez's father and his own mother came to live with the family to help out with the child-rearing. However, (a) the friction between him and his father-in-law, who never thought him a good enough husband, and (b) his own mother's constant criticism of his wife have made the household a highly stressful environment. For some time, Mr. Lopez has been occasionally drinking and staying out late after work and has been increasingly irritable when home. He reports having told his wife in the past year that he wanted to quit his job in order to pursue a full-time career as a comedian "because at least there I was having fun." At the same time, until his recent job changes, Mr. Lopez appears to have been managing his multiple but normally expected occupational stresses, culturally appropriate household stresses, and other pressures relatively successfully.

Problem and Counseling History. Mr. Lopez volunteered that he agreed with his wife that he has been having difficulties adjusting to the results of his job cutbacks and furlough, including (a) being at home 2 extra days per week; (b) attempting to work in his home and family environment one of those days per week; and (c) managing financially with 1 day's furlough. He agreed that his mood has been notably low at time, "really nervous" at other times, and increasingly irritable and "moody." In addition, he volunteered that he was experiencing problems with his entry into upper-management culture, which he described as "white country club culture, you know?" As described, he sees this as a new and challenging social, economic, and cultural transition on which his job future might depend.

At the same time, during the intake interview, Mr. Lopez appeared ambivalent about the need for counseling and made it quite clear that he was not the problem and that "I just need a little chance to blow off steam." He was sarcastic throughout the session, making jokes about his family and his circumstances asserting that "this therapy would make a funny routine for my stand-up." He avoided talking in any greater depth about his past or his recent bouts of irritability and often made unpleasant remarks about his father-in-law who "I can't seem to please no matter what I do, especially now that I'm furloughed." He was, nevertheless, oriented in all spheres, articulate albeit glib, and noted that "if I could only get over this bump, I would be as healthy as a bull." Toward the end of the session, Mr. Lopez suggested that his father-in-law and mother should probably get married and move into their own home "and leave us the hell alone."

Goals for Counseling and Course of Therapy to Date. Mr. Lopez said he would come to therapy if "it would make Angie happy," but that he was just "an average guy doing what an average guy does to provide for his family and then blow off steam after an average day." He added that all of his friends at the factory act like he does; they all had the same ups and downs as he is having, but he is just having a more difficult time "getting through it"; and that he loves his family and would "do whatever it takes." At the conclusion of the session, Mr. Lopez did agree to return for short-term counseling with the goal of reducing problematic mood, anxiety, and behavioral symptoms. When asked if he believed it would be beneficial for his entire family to come to counseling, Mr. Lopez said, "Sure we're all crazy, so we might as well all have fun together in here." The plan is for ongoing brief individual counseling to assist the client to return to previous level of functioning.

Diagnostic Impressions

Axis I. 309.28 Adjustment Disorder, Acute, With Mixed Anxiety and Depressed Mood

V62.4 Acculturation Problem

Axis II. V71.09 No Diagnosis on Axis II

Axis III. None

Axis IV. Occupational problem—Job change, job reduction, threat of job loss

Problem with primary support group—Family discord

Axis V. GAF = 70 (Current)

GAF = 80 (Highest level past year)

DISCUSSION OF DIAGNOSTIC IMPRESSION

George Lopez came to counseling at the urging of his wife, who was worried about changes she had noticed in her husband following negative events at his workplace, including a furlough that resulted in reduced pay and more time spent in his household. The changes she noticed included headaches, fatigue, and anxiety. George also had become more irritable, distracted, and inattentive at home, and admitted to feeling depressed at times. In the interview, George described feeling "a little cranky," "really irritable," and "moody," and occasionally drinking with male friends to avoid his household stresses and "blow off steam." In addition, George noted that he was pursuing the specific challenge of making the transition into socioeconomically upper-class Anglo upper-management culture at work in order to better secure his future with the company.

The *DSM-IV-TR* Adjustment Disorders all are clinically significant psychological responses to an identifiable life stressor. To meet the criteria for an Adjustment Disorder, the psychological responses must cause marked distress or clinically significant impairment in functioning, must go beyond normally expected and culturally appropriate reactions, and must not be due to another *DSM-IV-TR* disorder or a medical problem. Adjustment Disorders can occur with depressed mood, anxiety, disturbance in conduct or behavior, or be manifest in a combination of these.

George presented primarily with symptoms and signs of mild depression and moderate anxiety, apparently in direct response to a life event, namely, workplace cutbacks and an at-home furlough. His concerns arose within 3 months of the onset of the workplace stressor. In the absence of any evidence of substance abuse, and without any evidence that his symptoms meet the criteria for another diagnosable Axis I mood or anxiety disorder, the diagnosis is Adjustment Disorder. Because his concerns have lasted fewer than 3 months, the specifier, Acute, is used, and because he reported a combination of depression and anxiety symptoms, the disorder is specified: With Mixed Anxiety and Depressed Mood.

Differential diagnosis requires effectively understanding the client's concerns. Accurately identifying and describing the counseling presentations of Latino/Latina clients may require the counselor's special attention (Bernal & Saez-Santiago, 2006). Depending on certain demographic factors, somatic symptoms (like headaches and fatigue) sometimes are experienced and reported more readily than mood or cognitive symptoms of distress (Guarnaccia, DeLaCancela, & Carrillo, 1989). George Lopez reported headaches and fatigue among his symptoms.

Specific differential considerations when determining an Adjustment Disorder include other relevant Axis I diagnoses. However, George's experiences did not meet the criteria for any diagnosable Mood Disorder or Anxiety Disorder. Adjustment Disorder requires that the client's concerns develop within 3 months of the life event's onset; George presented increasing symptoms shortly after onset of his recent life stressors. Another consideration is whether the client's reactions are normally expected, culturally appropriate reactions that do not produce excessive distress or cause excessive impairment. However, George's concerns were reported to cause clinically significant distress, and some impairment in social functioning at home and the workplace. A separate differential consideration might be whether George's alcohol use warrants a diagnosis of Alcohol Abuse; however, at this moment, his pattern of use seems best described as social or recreational use of alcohol that is not clinically significant.

Further, along with all the various diagnosable disorders, a multiaxial diagnosis also lists Other Conditions That May Be a Focus of Clinical Attention. The client concerns contained in this section (appearing at the end of the *DSM-IV-TR,* following all of the diagnosable disorders)

are not diagnosable mental disorders according to the *DSM* classification system; instead, they sometimes are client problems that are a focus of counseling but not a part of the individual's diagnosable mental disorder. George Lopez's challenges with acculturation into the social hierarchy at work fall within this category.

To round out the diagnosis, George's important family and social stressors are emphasized on Axis IV, and on Axis V his functioning is represented by GAF scores indicating that although at present he is experiencing some mildly serious reactions with some difficulties at work and home, within the recent past he has demonstrated good functioning with only transient, expected difficulties with everyday problems. The information on these axes is consistent with the Axis I diagnosis portrayed by George Lopez in this case.

CASE CONCEPTUALIZATION

When George Lopez visited the Power Brothers Aviation Company's employee assistance program, the counselor's first task was to collect detailed clinical information about the situation leading to George's appointment. The counselor first used this information to develop diagnostic impressions. His concerns were described by Adjustment Disorder and problems of job change, family discord, and acculturation. Next, the counselor developed a case conceptualization. Whereas the purpose of diagnostic impressions is to *describe* the client's concerns, the goal of case conceptualization is to better *understand* and clinically *explain* the person's experiences (Neukrug & Schwitzer, 2006). It helps the counselor understand the conditions leading up to George's Adjustment Disorder and the conditions keeping it going. In turn, case conceptualization sets the stage for treatment planning. Treatment planning then provides a road map that plots out how the counselor and client expect to move from presenting concerns to positive outcomes (Seligman, 1993, p. 157)—helping George reduce his distress and more functionally and successfully deal with his current changes at home and at work.

When forming a case conceptualization, the clinician applies a purist counseling theory, an integration of two or more theories, an eclectic mix of theories, or a solution-focused combination of tactics to his or her understanding of the client. In this case, George's counselor based his conceptualization on a purist theory, Reality Therapy (or Choice Theory). George's counselor applied this model because it is the method of choice at the employee assistance program whenever it appears the client might benefit from an approach that focuses on ways the person is reacting dysfunctionally to unsatisfying relationships and related circumstances (Glasser, 1998, 2001, 2003). The employee assistance program also prefers an approach that emphasizes ways that employees can make better, less painful, and less frustrating choices during times of life challenges (Glasser, 1998, 2001, 2003). The approach also is directive and active and therefore amenable to shorter-term counseling such as for problems of adjustment (Wubbolding et al., 2004; Wubbolding & Colleagues, 1998). Although a potential shortcoming of the model is that clients from ethnic minority backgrounds may confront environments offering them fewer choices due to discrimination or oppression, the counselor believed that the model still would be a good fit helping George focus on the many choices he does have (Wubbolding & Brickell, 1998).

The counselor used the Inverted Pyramid Method of case conceptualization because this method is especially designed to help clinicians more easily form their conceptual pictures of their clients' needs (Neukrug & Schwitzer, 2006; Schwitzer, 1996, 1997). The method has four steps: Problem Identification, Thematic Groupings, Theoretical Inferences, and Narrowed Inferences. The counselor's clinical thinking can be seen in Figure 10.3.

Step 1: Problem Identification. The first step is Problem Identification. Aspects of the presenting problem (thoughts, feelings, behaviors, physiological features), additional areas of concern

besides the presenting concern, family and developmental history, in-session observations, clinical inquiries (medical problems, medications, past counseling, substance use, suicidality), and psychological assessments (problem checklists, personality inventories, mental status exam, specific clinical measures) all may contribute information at Step 1. The counselor "casts a wide net" in order to build Step 1 as exhaustively as possible (Neukrug & Schwitzer, 2006, p. 202). As can be seen in the figure, the counselor identified George Lopez's current primary problems at work (job change, financial loss, need to acculturate to upper management, etc.), primary problems at home (family discord, conflicts with wife, argumentative parents, etc.), physical and mood symptoms of anxiety and depression, use of alcohol, as well as history that was important to George. He attempted to go beyond just listing the primary anxiety and mood problems George presents to cover all of his current challenges and relevant background.

Step 2: Thematic Groupings. The second step is Thematic Groupings. The clinician organizes all of the exhaustive client information found in Step 1 into just a few intuitive-logical clinical groups, categories, or themes on the basis of sensible common denominators (Neukrug & Schwitzer, 2006). Four different ways of forming the Step 2 theme groups can be used: Descriptive-Diagnosis Approach, Clinical Targets Approach, Areas of Dysfunction Approach, and Intrapsychic Approach. As can be seen in Figure 10.3, George's counselor selected the Clinical Targets Approach. This approach sorts together all of the Step 1 information "according to the basic division of behavior, thoughts, feelings, and physiology" (Neukrug & Schwitzer, 2006, p. 205).

The counselor grouped together George's (a) anxiety, depressed mood, and anger into the theme, "distressing feelings"; (b) headache, poor sleep, and fatigue into the theme, "disruptive physiological symptoms"; (c) thoughts, worries, and ruminations about his job situation, finances, family pressures, other current challenges, and loss of his dream life into the theme, "distressing thoughts"; and (d) withdrawing and arguing at home, argumentativeness with family, avoidance of taking on upper-management challenges at work, escape drinking, and other actions into the theme, "dysfunctional behaviors."

So far, at Steps 1 and 2, the counselor has used his clinical assessment skills and his clinical judgment to begin meaningfully understanding George's situation. Now, at Steps 3 and 4, he applies the theoretical approach he has selected. He begins making theoretical inferences to explain the roots underlying George's responses to his situation as they are seen in Steps 1 and 2.

Step 3: Theoretical Inferences. At Step 3, concepts from the counselor's selected theory, Reality Therapy (Choice Theory), are applied to explain the dynamics causing and maintaining George Lopez's problematic thoughts, feelings, behaviors, and physiological responses. The counselor tentatively matches the theme groups in Step 2 with this theoretical approach. In other words, the symptom constellations in Step 2, which were distilled from the symptoms in Step 1, now are combined using theory to show what is believed to be the psychological etiology of George's current needs (Neukrug & Schwitzer, 2006; Schwitzer, 2006, 2007).

According to Reality Therapy (Choice Theory), individuals are born with drives for survival, achievement, love and belonging, independence, and enjoyment, where the need for social relationships is primary. According to the theory, individuals attempt to achieve these through their thoughts, feelings, physiological responses, and actions. Further, individuals have control—or choices—over their thoughts and actions, and less directly, their feelings and physiology. Counseling problems arise when individuals adopt total behavioral approaches that are based in the belief in External Control, which is blaming and critical and indicates the person has not learned how to make choices that best respond to his or her needs and situation.

Instead, approaching situations and events from the basis of Internal Control is adaptive, reduces symptomatic problems, and indicates the person understands he or she has responsibility for, and control of, his or her responses to needs and situations (Glasser, 1998, 2001, 2003).

As can be seen in Figure 10.3, when the counselor applied these Reality Therapy concepts, he explained at Step 3 that the various issues noted in Step 1 (anxiety and low mood, physical symptoms, withdrawal, family conflicts, job troubles), which can be understood in Step 2 to be themes of distressing feelings, disruptive physiological symptoms, distressing thoughts, and dysfunctional behaviors, are caused by George: (a) choosing anxietying behaviors, (b) choosing depressing behaviors, (c) choosing angering behaviors, (d) choosing headaching and fatiguing behaviors, and (e) choosing avoiding and escaping behaviors. These are found on Figure 10.3.

Step 4: Narrowed Inferences. At Step 4, the clinician's selected theory continues to be used to address still-deeper issues when they exist (Schwitzer, 2006, 2007). At this step, "still-deeper, more encompassing, or more central, causal themes" are formed (Neukrug & Schwitzer, 2006, p. 207). Continuing to apply Reality Therapy concepts at Step 4, George Lopez's counselor presented a single, deepest, most-fundamental source of his reasons for referral: "Choosing external-control language in an attempt to deal with unsatisfying family and work relationships." When all four steps are completed, the client information in Step 1 leads to logical-intuitive groupings on the basis of common denominators in Step 2, the groupings then are explained using theory at Step 3, and then, finally, at Step 4, further deeper explanations are made. From start to finish, the thoughts, feelings, behaviors, and physiological features in the topmost portions are connected on down the pyramid into deepest dynamics.

The completed pyramid now is used to plan treatment, where the counselor will challenge George to examine and evaluate his behavioral choices.

Figure 10.3   Sitcom George Lopez's Inverted Pyramid Case Conceptualization Summary: Reality Therapy

1. IDENTIFY AND LIST CLIENT CONCERNS

Anxious feelings	Conflicts with wife
Low mood	Arguments with mother and father-in-law
Anger at home	Conflicts with children
Irritable at home	Job furlough & financial loss
Headaches	Job change to weekly at-home work
Sleep difficulties	Job pressure to acculturate to upper
Beer drinking to socialize and escape	management through socializing, golf,
Distracted at home	and so on
Withdrawn at home	History of low-income background
Inattentive to family	History of giving up comic dream due to
	wife's pregnancy and family financial
	pressure

2. ORGANIZE CONCERNS INTO LOGICAL THEMATIC GROUPINGS

1. Distressing feelings of anxiety, depression, and anger
2. Disruptive physiological symptoms of headache, poor sleep, fatigue
3. Distressing thoughts about job pressures, upper management pressure, family pressures, and loss of dreams for a happy life
4. Dysfunctional behaviors, including withdrawing, arguing and maintaining family conflicts, escape drinking, and avoiding new job demands

3. THEORETICAL INFERENCES: ATTACH THEMATIC GROUPINGS TO INFERRED AREAS OF DIFFICULTY

Choosing paining behaviors

Choosing anxietying behaviors
Choosing depressing behaviors
Choosing angering behaviors
Choosing headaching and
fatiguing behaviors
Choosing avoiding and
escaping behaviors

4. NARROWED INFERENCES: SUICIDALITY AND DEEPER DIFFICULTIES

Choosing external
control language

Choosing external control
language in an attempt
to deal with unsatisfying
family and work
relationships

Treatment Planning

At this point, George's clinician at the Downtown Counseling Center has collected all available information about the problems that have been of concern to him. Based upon this information, the counselor developed a five-axis *DSM-IV-TR* diagnosis and then, using the "inverted pyramid" (Neukrug & Schwitzer, 2006; Schwitzer, 1996, 1997), formulated a working clinical *explanation* of George's difficulties and their etiology that we called the *case conceptualization*. This, in turn, guides us to the next critical step in our clinical work, called the *treatment plan,* the primary purpose of which is to map out a logical and goal-oriented strategy for making positive changes in the client's life. In essence, the treatment plan is a road map *"for reducing or eliminating disruptive symptoms that are impeding the client's ability to reach positive mental health outcomes"* (Neukrug & Schwitzer, 2006, p. 225). As such, it is the cornerstone of our work with not only George, but with all clients who present with disruptive concerns (Jongsma & Peterson, 2006; Jongsma et al., 2003a, 2003b; Seligman, 1993, 1998, 2004).

A comprehensive treatment plan must integrate all of the information from the biopsychosocial interview, diagnosis, and case conceptualization into a coherent plan of action. This *plan* comprises four main components , which include (1) behavioral definition of the problem(s), (2) the selection of achievable goals, (3) the determination of treatment modes, and (4) the documentation of how change will be measured. The *behavioral definition of the problem(s)* consolidates the results of the case conceptualization into a concise hierarchical list of problems and concerns that will be the focus of treatment. The *selection of achievable goals* refers to assessing and prioritizing the client's concerns into a *hierarchy of urgency* that also takes into account the client's motivation for change, level of dysfunction, and real-world influences on his or her problems. The *determination of treatment modes* refers to selection of the specific interventions, which are matched to

the uniqueness of the client and to his or her goals and clearly tied to a particular theoretical orientation (Neukrug & Schwitzer, 2006). Finally, the clinician must establish how change will be measured, based upon a number of factors including client records and self-report of change, in-session observations by the clinician, clinician ratings, results of standardized evaluations such as the Beck Depression Inventory-2 (Beck et al., 1996), or a family functioning questionnaire, pre-post treatment comparisons, and reports by other treating professionals.

The four-step method discussed above can be seen in Figure 6.1 (p. 109) and is outlined below for the case of George, followed by his specific treatment plan.

Step 1: Behavioral Definition of Problems. The first step in treatment planning is to carefully review the case conceptualization, paying particular attention to the results of Step 2 (Thematic Groupings), Step 3 (Theoretical Inferences), and Step 4 (Narrowed Inferences). The identified clinical themes reflect the core areas of concern and distress for the client, while the theoretical and narrowed inferences offer clinical speculation as to their origins. In the case of George, there are four primary areas of concern. The first, "distressing feelings of anxiety, depression, and anger," have compromised his happiness and overall adjustment at work and at home. The second, "disruptive physiological symptoms," refers to headaches, poor sleep, and fatigue. The third, "distressing thoughts about job, upper-management and family pressures, and loss of dreams for a happy life," refers to being distracted and withdrawn at home, inattentive to family, and experiencing conflicts with his wife, children, and in-laws. The fourth, "dysfunctional behaviors," refers to distraction, withdrawal, and inattention at home, maintaining family conflicts, escape drinking, and avoidance of new job demands. These symptoms and stresses are consistent with the diagnosis of Adjustment Disorder, Acute With Mixed Anxiety and Depressed Mood and Acculturation Problems (APA, 2000a; Berry,

2003; Casey, Dorwick, & Wilkinson, 2001; Flores, Ojeda, Yu-Ping, Gee, & Lee, 2006; Strain et al., 1998).

Step 2: Identify and Articulate Goals for Change. The second step is the selection of achievable goals, which is based upon a number of factors, including the most pressing or urgent behavioral, emotional, and interpersonal concerns and symptoms as identified by the client and clinician, the willingness and ability of the client to work on those particular goals, and the realistic (real-world) achievability of those goals (Neukrug & Schwitzer, 2006). At this stage of treatment planning, it is important to recognize that not all of the client's problems can be addressed at once, so we focus initially on those that cause the greatest distress and impairment. New goals can be created as old ones are achieved. In the case of George, the goals are divided into four prominent clusters. The first, "distressing feelings of anxiety, depression, and anger," requires that we help George to understand his feelings of anxiety, depression, and anger, the way they impact his daily functioning, and their triggers. Next we would help him to gain control over, take responsibility for, and reduce the intensity and destructiveness of those feelings. The second, "disruptive physiological symptoms of headache, poor sleep, and fatigue," requires that we assist George to restore a restful sleeping pattern, feel refreshed and energetic during his waking hours, to eliminate his headaches by recognizing their onset and modulating his response through various exercises, and to improve his overall physical functioning. The third, "distressing thoughts about job, upper-management and family pressures, and loss of dreams for a happy life," requires that we help George to understand the origin of his pressures in earlier experiences over living in poverty, identify feelings of resentment, and recognize the fulfilling aspects of his life while building new fantasies. The last, "dysfunctional behaviors," requires that we assist George to regulate his anger and to develop more adaptive responses to stress.

Step 3: Describe Therapeutic Intervention. This is perhaps the most critical step in the treatment planning process because the clinician must now integrate information from a number of sources, including the case conceptualization, the delineation of the client's problems and goals, and the treatment literature, paying particular attention to *empirically supported treatment* (EST) and *evidence-based practice* (EBP). In essence, the clinician must align his or her treatment approach with scientific evidence from the fields of counseling and psychotherapy. Wampold (2001) identifies two types of evidence-based counseling research: studies that demonstrate "absolute efficacy," that is, the fact that counseling and psychotherapy work, and those that demonstrate "relative efficacy," that is, the fact that certain theoretical/technical approaches work best for certain clients with particular problems (Psychoanalysis, Gestalt Therapy, Cognitive Behavior Therapy, Brief Solution-Focused Therapy, Cognitive Therapy, Dialectical Behavior Therapy, Person-Centered Therapy, Expressive/Creative Therapies, Interpersonal Therapy, and Feminist Therapy); and when delivered through specific treatment modalities (individual, group, and family counseling). In the case of George, we have decided to use Reality Therapy (Glasser, 1998, 2001, 2003) due to its emphasis on client recognition of the role of choices in the client's life, how those choices affect the client's happiness (and unhappiness), and how he or she can make healthier and life-affirming choices. The WDEP system (Wubbolding, 2007; Wubbolding & Brickell, 1998; Wubbolding et al., 2004; Wubbolding & Colleagues, 1998) provides the structure for intervention by helping clients to identify their wants (W) and their direction (D), to evaluate the efficacy of their current direction and its outcome (E), and to plan accordingly (P). Given George's general life competencies and past successful adjustment both at home and at work, Reality Therapy's emphasis on strengthening the client's internal locus of control as well fostering insight and change through the therapeutic relationship will assist George to reclaim responsibility in and for his life, as well as to effectively problem-solve. This particular form of counseling/psychotherapy has proven effective in treating a wide range of problems, including anxiety, depression, anger management, and relationship issues (Radtke, Sapp, & Farrell, 1997; Wubbolding, 2000; Wubbolding & Brickell, 1998). Specific techniques for George will include taking responsibility for thoughts, feelings, and behaviors; using physiological and emotional monitoring; recognizing the historical basis for and addressing irrational pressures; practicing statements of responsibility and choice; and developing effective self-regulation and communication skills.

Step 4: Provide Outcome Measures of Change. This last step in treatment planning requires that we specify how change will be measured and indicate the extent to which progress has been made toward realizing these goals (Neukrug & Schwitzer, 2006). The counselor has considerable flexibility in this phase, and may choose from a number of objective domains (psychological tests

and measures of self-esteem, depression, psychosis, interpersonal relationship, anxiety, etc.), quasi-objective measures (the *DSM-IV-TR's* Axis V GAF scale; pre-post clinician, client, and psychiatric ratings), and subjective ratings (client self-report, clinician's in-session observations). In George's case, we have implemented a number of these, including improved pre-post measures on the Beck Depression Inventory (Beck et al., 1996), Beck Anxiety Inventory (Beck & Steer, 1990), and Clinical Anger Scale (Snell et al., 1995); spouse and client report of improvement in overall life, family and work satisfaction, and spouse report of her husband's improvement in mood, activity level, and outlook; and the development of adaptive responses to stress.

The completed treatment plan is now developed through which George will be able to use the techniques of Reality Therapy to reduce his stressful feelings and eliminate his disruptive physiological, emotional, cognitive, and behavioral symptoms. George Lopez's treatment plan is as follows and is summarized in Table 10.3.

TREATMENT PLAN

Client: George Lopez

Service Provider: Downtown Counseling Center

BEHAVIORAL DEFINITION OF PROBLEMS:

1. Distressing feelings of anxiety, depression, and anger

2. Disruptive physiological symptoms of headache, poor sleep, fatigue

3. Distressing thoughts about job pressures, upper-management pressures, family pressures, and loss of dreams for a happy life—Distracted and withdrawn at home, inattentive to family, conflict with his wife, children, and in-laws

4. Dysfunctional behaviors including withdrawing, arguing, and maintaining family conflicts, escape drinking, and avoiding new job demands

(Continued)

(Continued)

GOALS FOR CHANGE:

1. Distressing feelings of anxiety, depression, and anger

   - Understand his feelings of anxiety, depression, and anger and the way they impact his daily functioning
   - Understand the emotional, behavioral, and physiological triggers for these distressing feelings
   - Gain control over, take responsibility for, and reduce the intensity and destructiveness of these feelings
   - Develop self-regulation and self-control strategies for coping with these feelings
   - Learn strategies for long-term coping with these feelings

2. Disruptive physiological symptoms of headache, poor sleep, fatigue

   - Restore a restful sleeping pattern
   - Feel refreshed and energetic during his waking hours
   - Eliminate his headaches by recognizing their onset and modulating his response through various exercises
   - Improve his overall physical functioning through proactive stress management and self-care

3. Distressing thoughts about job pressures, upper-management pressures, family pressures, and loss of dreams for a happy life

   - Understand the nature and origin of these thoughts about pressure in his early formative life and family experiences
   - Identify feelings of resentment for having to sacrifice his life's dream to support a family
   - Recognize the ways that his current family and vocational experiences are fulfilling and develop new fantasies

4. Dysfunctional behaviors including withdrawing, arguing, and maintaining family conflicts, escape drinking, and avoiding new job demands

   - Recognize the cognitive, behavioral, and physiological triggers to his anger
   - Develop more adaptive responses to stress (without reliance upon alcohol, argumentativeness, and withdrawal)

THERAPEUTIC INTERVENTIONS:

A short- to moderate-term course of individual Reality Therapy–centered counseling (2–3 months) that relies on a plan that is simple, attainable, measureable, immediate, controlled, consistent, and committed

1. Distressing feelings of anxiety, depression, and anger

   - Discover how he is choosing to act with anxiety, depression, and anger
   - Identify cognitive, emotional, behavioral, and interpersonal triggers for these feelings

- Identify obstacles to healthy and fulfilling expression of stressful feelings
- Use a feeling-word checklist to identify these feelings
- Accept responsibility for these feelings rather than seeing them as uncontrollable and external

2. Disruptive physiological symptoms of headache, poor sleep, fatigue

- Use physiological monitoring to monitor physical states
- Practice, plan to implement, and provide feedback on the use of relaxation strategies, including deep breathing, progressive muscle relaxation, and guided imagery
- Use of exercise and nutritional planning to optimize healthy functioning

3. Distressing thoughts about job pressures, upper-management pressures, family pressures, and loss of dreams for a happy life

- Recognize the relationship between early poverty and the pressures in his daily life
- Identify basic needs for love, belongingness, power, and freedom and the reality-based obstacles that stand in the way
- Discuss irrational basis for these perceived pressures
- Practice self-reflection and garner feedback for these from valued others (spouse and best friend)
- Use paradoxical intention and reframing to reduce these perceived pressures

4. Dysfunctional behaviors, including withdrawing, arguing, and maintaining family conflicts, escape drinking, and avoiding new job demands

- Recognize the way that he is surrendering choice through these dysfunctional behaviors
- Formulate a workable plan for elimination of these behaviors by focusing on choice and responsibility
- Practice and role-play effective communication with family members

OUTCOME MEASURES OF CHANGE:

The identification of his basic needs, ability to make healthy and responsible choices, development of healthy and fulfilling attitudes toward self, work, and family, accompanied by reduction and eventual elimination of stressful feelings, reactions, and behaviors as measured by:

- Stabilization of clinician's rating of client's GAF to the normal range (>85)
- Client report of improved overall life satisfaction, including attitude toward work
- Improved pre-post scores on the Clinical Anger Scale
- Improved pre-post scores on Beck Depression Inventory II
- Improved pre-post scores on the Beck Anxiety Inventory
- Client and spouse's report of improved overall mood, attitude, and behavior at home, including reduced conflicts
- Client's report of ways in which he has taken responsibility and made responsible choices for internal stress and outward distress

Table 10.3 Sitcom George Lopez's Treatment Plan Summary: Reality Therapy

Goals for Change	Therapeutic Interventions	Outcome Measures of Change
Distressing feelings of anxiety, depression, and anger	Distressing feelings of anxiety, depression, and anger	The identification of his basic needs, ability to make healthy and responsible choices, development of healthy and fulfilling attitudes toward self, work, and family, accompanied by reduction and eventual elimination of stressful feelings, reactions, and behaviors as measured by:
Understand his feelings of anxiety, depression, and anger and the way they impact his daily functioning	Discover how he is choosing to act with anxiety, depression, and anger	
Understand the emotional, behavioral, and physiological triggers to these distressing feelings	Identify cognitive, emotional, behavioral, and interpersonal triggers for these feelings	
	Identify obstacles to healthy and fulfilling expression of stressful feelings	
Gain control over, take responsibility for, and reduce the intensity and destructiveness of these feelings	Use a feeling-word checklist to identify these feelings	Stabilization of clinician's rating of client's GAF to the normal range (>85)
	Accept responsibility for these feelings rather than seeing them as uncontrollable and external	Client report of improved overall life-satisfaction, including attitude toward work
Develop self-regulation and self-control strategies for coping with these feelings	Disruptive physiological symptoms of headache, poor sleep, fatigue	Improved pre-post scores on the Clinical Anger Scale
Learn strategies for long-term coping with these feelings	Use physiological monitoring to monitor physical states	Improved pre-post scores on Beck Depression Inventory II
Disruptive physiological symptoms of headache, poor sleep, fatigue	Practice, plan to implement, and provide feedback on the use of relaxation strategies, including deep breathing, progressive muscle relaxation, and guided imagery	Improved pre-post scores on the Beck Anxiety Inventory
Restore a restful sleeping pattern	Use of exercise and nutritional planning to optimize healthy functioning	Client and spouse's report of improved overall mood, attitude, and behavior at home, including reduced conflicts
Feel refreshed and energetic during his waking hours	Distressing thoughts about job pressures, upper-management pressures, family pressures, and loss of dreams for a happy life	Client's report of ways in which he has taken responsibility and made responsible choices for internal stress and outward distress
Eliminate his headaches by recognizing their onset and modulating his response through various exercises	Recognize the relationship between early poverty and the pressures in his daily life	
Improve his overall physical functioning through proactive stress management and self-care	Identify basic needs for love, belongingness, power, and freedom and the reality-based obstacles that stand in the way	
Distressing thoughts about job pressures, upper-management pressures, family pressures, and loss of dreams for a happy life	Discuss irrational basis for these perceived pressures	
	Practice self-reflection and garner feedback for these from valued others (spouse and best friend)	

Goals for Change	Therapeutic Interventions	Outcome Measures of Change
Understand the nature and origin of these thoughts about pressure in his early formative life and family experiences	Use paradoxical intention and reframing to reduce these perceived pressures	
Identify feelings of resentment for having to sacrifice his life's dream to support a family	<u>Dysfunctional behaviors, including withdrawing, arguing, and maintaining family conflicts, escape drinking, and avoiding new job demands</u>	
Recognize the ways that his current family and vocational experiences are fulfilling and develop new fantasies	Recognize the way that he is surrendering choice through these dysfunctional behaviors	
<u>Dysfunctional behaviors, including withdrawing, arguing, and maintaining family conflicts, escape drinking, and avoiding new job demands</u>	Formulate a workable plan for elimination of these behaviors by focusing on choice and responsibility	
Recognize the cognitive, behavioral, and physiological triggers to his anger	Practice and role-play effective communication with family members	
Develop more adaptive responses to stress (without reliance upon alcohol, argumentativeness, and withdrawal)		

CASE 10.4 *STAR TREK: THE NEXT GENERATION'S* DATA

INTRODUCING THE CHARACTER

Lieutenant Commander Data is the android character on the television series, *Star Trek: The Next Generation,* which aired on CBS for 178 episodes between 1987 and 1994. The television series also was made into several full-length motion pictures, including *Star Trek: Generations* (Carson, 1994) produced by Paramount Pictures. *Star Trek* was originally created by visionary Gene Roddenberry and ran for 78 episodes on television in the early 1960s. Although the original show (*Star Trek: TOS*–The Original Series) was short-lived, its legacy has endured to include numerous successful spinoff television series,

movies, television cartoons, and books. In the original series, Leonard Nimoy played the half-human, half-Vulcan Mr. Spock who was forever at odds due to his hybrid origins. In that tradition, in *The Next Generation* series, Lieutenant Commander Data functioned as a powerful vehicle for the discourse surrounding what it takes to be truly human. Lieutenant Commander Data is continually presented with challenges that lead him and his crewmates to question the meaning of "being real." In the following basic case summary and diagnostic impressions, we picture Data's depressed mood, the effects of a medical procedure on his memory, and his pressing concerns about identity and faith.

Meet the Client

You can assess the client in action by viewing clips of Lieutenant Commander Data's video material at the following websites:

- http://www.youtube.com/watch?v= DLIU5tC3LAs Data feels laughter
- http://www.youtube.com/watch?v= XeyplUvxztE A tribute to Data
- http://www.youtube.com/watch?v= GYp2dx652ho Is Data human?

BASIC CASE SUMMARY

Identifying Information. Data is an android who identifies himself as biracial with both machine and human ethnicities. He is the science officer aboard the U.S.S. *Enterprise* space vessel with the rank of lieutenant commander. He and his ship have been assigned to a mission exploring deep space for the past 5 years. Data's appearance features pale skin, golden eyes, and ship officer's uniform.

Presenting Concern. Data was referred to the ship's counselor, Deanna Troi, on the recommendation of Captain Jean-Luc Picard, who reported that "Data has been acting very sluggish lately and I've grown concerned about his ability to function effectively at his post." The Captain reported that for about the past 2 or 3 weeks, Data appears to "feel empty" much of time; no longer seems very interested in intellectual jousting or visiting the holodeck for virtual recreation in his off hours; seems to move slowly about his everyday tasks; and has mentioned several times that he has mused about "just shutting off." In addition, the captain noted that Data has had large gaps in memory ever since a neural-network procedure was performed on him in the year 2324.

Background, Family Information, and Relevant History. Lieutenant Commander Data's origins were quite different from those of his crewmates

as he was created rather than born. In telling his story, Data spoke with affection of Dr. Noonien Soong, a brilliant cybernetic evolutionist with a specialty in the creation of sentient androids. Data was created in the year 2314 A.D. on the planet Omicron Theta by Dr. Soong, who had been performing cutting-edge experiments with the "positronic neural-network"—which was a near perfect duplicate of the human brain and nervous system. Dr. Soong's achievement, the creation of Data along with his brother Lore, brought Dr. Soong much adulation but also raised concerns that, according to the Star Fleet panel of ethics, "He was trifling in the shadow of God."

According to available health and mental health records, because Data was created, rather than born, he did not have a childhood in the conventional sense of the word. According to available files, during that early period, his favorite story, one read to him by Dr. Soong's wife Dr. Juliana Tanna, was "Pinocchio." Data was particularly enamored with the story of "Pinocchio" because like the mythical wooden puppet, he too wanted to be real. Data recalled believing that "As long as I could store the entire compendium of human knowledge and observe humans in all facets of their existence, I too could become real." In the year 2336, Data was deactivated by Dr. Soong because he had broken into the laboratory to steal an "emotion chip," a complex, highly unstable microchip capable of the processing of complex human emotions. Disappointed in his "son," Dr. Soong stripped clean Data's neural network so that he would forget his act of defiance and shipped him anew to Star Fleet Academy to be reprogrammed as a science officer. Data appears to have lost all previously remembered knowledge regarding his earlier existence, previously learned information about the pursuit of the human experience, and learned material about his identity formation.

At Star Fleet, Data rose quickly through the ranks by virtue of his vast intellect, ability to translate any language, his fearlessness, and great strength. He won the admiration and respect of his fellow cadets and became fast friends with

Geordi La Forge who would later be assigned with him to his first commission aboard the U.S.S. *Enterprise*, Star Fleet's flagship. Data enjoyed the camaraderie aboard the *Enterprise*, embraced each opportunity to visit new planets and new people in hopes that he could somehow learn what it meant to be truly alive. Although all traces of the earlier theft and reprogramming were taken from Data's memory, he had "neural flashbacks" and dislocated fragments of memories of the story of Pinocchio. During such moments, Lieutenant Commander Data sought out the company of his friend, Geordi, and the two would have long conversations about the differences between man and machine. He often asked his friend if he thought that "I would ever be real?"

On the 15th anniversary of Data's successful reprogramming, Captain Picard received an order from Star Fleet to return his science officer for reprogramming and redeployment on a deep space science lab. In a bold act of defiance, Captain Picard argued that Data was not real and, instead a machine, the property of the U.S.S. *Enterprise*. This came as a surprise to Data who always considered the Captain to be his friend; however, Data had failed to realize that the Captain's efforts to dehumanize him were really designed to keep him aboard the *Enterprise*. In a court trial aboard the ship's holodeck, a virtual platform, Data's Star Fleet attorney argued that by virtue of having earned the Star Fleet Command Decoration for Gallantry, a Medal of Honor with Clusters, the Legend of Honor, and the Star of Cross, as well as by virtue of befriending the crew of the *Enterprise*, he was as much human as anyone else. Data lost the battle, but won the war, and was declared human by the virtual tribunal and given his choice of where to serve. He chose to remain aboard the *Enterprise* as a member of its crew. Although Data initially thought that this was the best decision, he was not convinced by the tribunal's ruling that he was indeed human and began to experience difficulty carrying out his daily functions without feeling what crewmate Geordi La Forge later noted to be "sadness." Unfamiliar with this strange emotional

experience, Data welcomed the visit with Counselor Troi.

Problem and Counseling History to Date. Data punctually presented himself to Counselor Troi. On arrival at the interview, Data did appear to be moving and thinking sluggishly, and agreed that lately he has been ruminating about shutting off, but has resisted his temptation to act on these self-harming ideations. He expressed concern that "I've felt similarly slow before, but never like this, and it has been going on for almost 3 human weeks now." He expressed concern that his diminished ability to concentrate, think, and act decisively might harm his effectiveness in his assigned post. Further, because his energy levels seemed low, he was worried that Geordi and other crewmates would abandon him since he "just cannot drag myself to the holodeck or the recreation chamber to relax with them." Data said that if he knew was the experience of human crying was like, he might engage in it forthwith. On the topic of memory, Data candidly admitted that the neural procedure performed on him left him with the inability to recall previously available information. He believed this was "greatly interfering with my self advancement and very worrisome." He added that he also was using excessive neural energy trying to "solve some important questions about who I am and what I believe about God and the universe." He expressed a desire to talk about these two issues in counseling, but said "I don't know if I have the energy or inner resources."

Goals for Counseling and Course of Therapy to Date. After consulting with Captain Picard, Counselor Troi determined that Lieutenant Commander Data was not malfunctioning in any mechanical way, but was simply "acting outside of the parameters of his programming." Upon further consultation with the ship's memory banks and a virtual conversation with Dr. Soong, it was decided that rather than once again neutralizing and reprogramming Data, that an attempt would be made to provide him with a course of traditional counseling, as would be done with any other (human) member of the crew. The primary goal is to resolve mood-related symptoms in order to assist Data in returning to his previous level of effective functioning.

Secondary goals are to assist Data to better adapt to his loss of memory and, ideally, resolve his identity- and faith-based questions.

Diagnostic Impressions

Axis I.   296.22, Major Depressive Disorder, Single Episode, Moderate

294.0 Amnestic Disorder Due to Neural Network Trauma, Chronic

313.82 Identity Problem

V62.89 Religious or Spiritual Problem

Axis II.   V71.09 No Diagnosis on Axis II

Axis III.   Neural Network Trauma

Axis IV.   Other psychosocial and environmental problems—Discord with scientist-creator, threat of neutralization and reprogramming

Axis V.   GAF = 60 (at intake)

GAF = 81 (highest on record)

DISCUSSION OF DIAGNOSTIC IMPRESSIONS

Lieutenant Commander Data was referred to the ship's counselor by his captain, who was worried about several domains of Data's functioning. The captain was concerned that Data was experiencing difficulties found in each of these areas: mood; amnesia; and problems with identity and spirituality.

Each section of the *DSM-IV-TR* classification system contains a group of diagnoses that share qualitatively similar symptoms or features. For instance, the Mood Disorders section contains all of the disorders associated with a disturbance in mood (including depressive disorders and bipolar disorders); the Delirium, Dementia, Amnestic Disorders, and Other Cognitive Disorders section contains a variety of mental disorders all featuring significant deficits in cognitive functioning; and the Other Conditions That May Be a Focus of Clinical Attention all are nondiagnosable client problems that are a focus of counseling but

not a part of the individual's diagnosable mental disorder. The ship's counselor explored concerns in each of these areas.

First, the counselor explored Data's depressive symptoms. Data reported diminished interest in his usual activities and loss of pleasure from formerly enjoyable recreational and other interests. He described feeling "empty" and having thoughts about "shutting off." In the interview he appeared fatigued and sluggish, and admitted having difficulty concentrating and thinking effectively. He has experienced these symptoms for more than 2 weeks, and they are interfering with his ability to function at his post and elsewhere. Data's presentation meets the criteria of a Major Depressive Episode. Mood Episodes are the building blocks for making a mood disorder diagnosis.

Lieutenant Commander Data has experienced no Manic or Hypomanic Episodes; and therefore, the diagnosis is Major Depressive Disorder. The current episode is the first that he has experienced. In turn, the course is specified as Single

Episode. Finally, his current episode is described: He experiences meet the criteria for a Major Depressive Episode. He is experiencing distress along with more than minor impairment in occupational functioning.

Conversely, his symptoms are not substantially beyond those needed for the diagnosis and are not causing severe problems with work or social functioning. Therefore, the severity specifier, Moderate, is the best fit.

One differential consideration might be Adjustment Disorder With Depressed Mood. Adjustment Disorders With Depressed Mood are negative affective reactions to life stressors in the absence of another diagnosable Axis I disorder. In this case, Data's symptoms conform to the specific criteria for a Major Depressive Episode, which go beyond the general criteria set for Adjustment Disorder.

Next, the counselor explored Data's memory loss. He described memory impairment whereby he was unable to recall information that he previously knew and could recall (including previously remembered knowledge about his earlier existence, the pursuit of the human experience, and his identity formation). This memory impairment was the direct result of a medical procedure causing trauma to his neural network (a human client might have experienced head trauma with associated brain damage). Data reports clinically significant distress associated with his loss of memory. This kind of amnesia indicates a diagnosis of Amnestic Disorder Due to a General Medical Condition. The specific medical condition is listed so that the specific diagnosis is Amnestic Disorder to Due Neural Network Trauma. His memory loss has lasted more than 1 month, so the specifier Chronic, is used.

There are various differential diagnoses when considering a disorder centering on amnesia. Delirium and dementia due to various medical etiologies, substance use, or other causes may involve memory impairment combined with impaired consciousness (delirium) or multiple cognitive deficits (dementia). Likewise, disruptions in thinking can occur with a Major Depressive Disorder. However, Data's symptoms are

characterized only by memory loss without any other cognitive disturbances or deficits, and a specific medical etiology has been identified.

Finally, the counselor explored the questions about identity and spiritual dilemmas over which Data was concerned. These client concerns were not diagnosable mental disorders according to the *DSM* classification system; instead, they are client problems or issues that are a focus of treatment. We decided to list Identity Problem, and Religious or Spiritual Problem. Spiritual and religious identity questions can overlap with other aspects mental health (Elkins, 1995), and may warrant evaluation during clinical assessment with some clients (Griffith & Griggs, 2001). Although Data's identity and spiritual concerns were associated with his diagnosable depressive mood and amnesia, we believed they were of enough clinical importance, and might warrant sufficient clinical attention during counseling, to merit inclusion on Axis I.

To complete the diagnosis, Data's Neural Network Trauma *(sic)* is listed on Axis III, his relevant psychosocial stressors are emphasized on Axis IV, and on Axis V his functioning is represented by GAF scores indicating that within the recent past he was demonstrating good functioning and the absence of concerns beyond everyday problems, and that at present he is experiencing moderately serious symptoms affecting occupational and other functioning that led to his referral. The information on these axes is consistent with the Axis I diagnoses describing Lieutenant Commander Data's reasons for referral.

CASE CONCEPTUALIZATION

When Lieutenant Commander Data reported to the ship's counselor, she conducted a detailed intake interview, collecting as much information as possible about the symptoms and situations leading to Data's arrival at counseling. Based on the intake, the ship's counselor developed diagnostic impressions, describing Data's presenting concerns a single episode of Major Depressive Disorder, Amnestic Disorder, and identity and spiritual problems. Next, a case conceptualization was developed. Whereas the purpose of diagnostic impressions is to *describe* the client's concerns, the goal of case conceptualization is to better *understand* and clinically *explain* the person's experiences (Neukrug & Schwitzer, 2006). It helps the counselor understand the etiology leading to Data's depressive and amnestic disorders and other counseling interests, and the factors maintaining these concerns. In turn, case conceptualization sets the stage for treatment planning. Treatment planning then provides a road map that plots out how the counselor and client expect to move from presenting concerns to positive outcomes (Seligman, 1993, p. 157)—helping Lieutenant Commander Data improve his low mood and related symptoms, resolve his questions of identity and spirituality, and better manage the effects of the amnesia he developed as result of a medical procedure.

When forming a case conceptualization, the clinician applies a purist counseling theory, an integration of two or more theories, an eclectic mix of theories, or a solution-focused combination of tactics to his or her understanding of the client. In this case, the ship's counselor based her conceptualization on psychotherapeutic integration of two theories (Corey, 2009). Psychotherapists very commonly integrate more than one theoretical approach in order to form a conceptualization and treatment plan that will be as efficient and effective as possible for meeting the client's needs (Dattilo & Norcross, 2006; Norcross & Beutler, 2008). In other words, counselors using the psychotherapeutic integration method attempt to flexibly tailor their clinical efforts to "the unique needs and contexts of the individual client" (Norcross & Beutler, 2008, p. 485). Like other counselors using integration, Data's counselor chose this method because she had not found one individual theory that was comprehensive enough, by itself, to address all of the "complexities," "range of client types," and "specific problems" seen among her everyday caseload (Corey, 2009, p. 450).

Specifically, the ship's counselor selected an integration of (a) Cognitive Behavior Therapy and (b) Existential Counseling. She selected this approach based on Lieutenant Commander Data's presentation of depressive mood concerns along with unresolved issues pertaining to identity and spirituality, and her knowledge of current outcome research with clients experiencing these types of concerns (Critchfield & Smith-Benjamin, 2006; Fotchmann & Gelenberg, 2005; Hollon, Thase, & Markowitz, 2002; Russell, 2007; Livesley, 2007; Westen & Morrison, 2001). According to the research, Cognitive Behavior Therapy is one treatment approach indicated when assisting clients with depressive disorders (Fotchmann & Gelenberg, 2005; Hollon et al., 2002; Westen & Morrison, 2001), whereas an integrated approach emphasizing existential counseling is one treatment of choice for addressing questions of identity, search for meaning, and anxieties about the conditions of living and death (Russell, 2007; Van Deurzen, 1991; Yalom, 1980, 2003). Data's counselor is comfortable theoretically integrating these approaches.

The counselor used the Inverted Pyramid Method of case conceptualization because this method is especially designed to help clinicians more easily form their conceptual pictures of their clients' needs (Neukrug & Schwitzer, 2006; Schwitzer, 1996, 1997). The method has four steps: Problem Identification, Thematic Groupings, Theoretical Inferences, and Narrowed Inferences. The counselor's clinical thinking can be seen in Figure 10.4.

Step 1: Problem Identification. The first step is Problem Identification. Aspects of the presenting problem (thoughts, feelings, behaviors, physiological features), additional areas of concern besides the presenting concern, family and developmental history, in-session observations, clinical inquiries (medical problems, medications, past counseling, substance use, suicidality), and psychological assessments (problem checklists, personality inventories, mental status exam, specific clinical measures) all may contribute information at Step 1. The counselor "casts a wide net" in order to build step 1 as exhaustively as possible (Neukrug & Schwitzer,

2006, p. 202). As can be seen in Figure 10.4, the ship's counselor identified Lieutenant Commander Data's primary concerns (major depression and related behavioral and cognitive symptoms); secondary concerns (pertaining to memory losses due to a medical procedure); and additional counseling issues (identity and spiritual questions). She attempted to go beyond just the depressive observations that led to his referral, in order to be descriptive as she could.

Step 2: Thematic Groupings. The second step is Thematic Groupings. The clinician organizes all of the exhaustive client information found in Step 1 into just a few intuitive-logical clinical groups, categories, or themes, on the basis of sensible common denominators (Neukrug & Schwitzer, 2006). Four different ways of forming the Step 2 theme groups can be used: Descriptive-Diagnosis Approach, Clinical Targets Approach, Areas of Dysfunction Approach, and Intrapsychic Approach. As can be seen in Figure 10.4, Lieutenant Commander Data's counselor selected the Descriptive-Diagnosis Approach. This approach sorts together all of the various Step 1 information about the client's adjustment, development, distress, or dysfunction "to show larger clinical problems as reflected through a diagnosis" (Neukrug & Schwitzer, 2006, p. 205).

The ship's counselor grouped together all of Data's various affective, cognitive, behavioral, and physiological symptoms of a single mood disorder into the overarching descriptive-diagnostic theme, Major Depressive Disorder. Similarly, she grouped Data's memory symptoms into a single theme pertaining to Amnestic Disorder Due to a General Medical Condition. Finally, she grouped together Data's persistent issues of self into the theme, Counseling Questions of Identity and Spirituality. The counselor's conceptual work at Step 2 gave her a way to think about Lieutenant Commander Data's functioning and concerns more insightfully.

Step 3: Theoretical Inferences. At Step 3, concepts from the counselor's theoretical integration of two approaches—Cognitive Behavior Therapy and Existential Counseling—are applied to explain the experiences causing, and the mechanisms maintaining, Lieutenant Commander Data's problematic thoughts, feelings, and behaviors. The counselor tentatively matches the theme groups in Step 2 with this theoretical approach. In other words, the symptom constellations in Step 2, which were distilled from the symptoms in Step 1, now are combined using theory to show what are believed to be the underlying causes or psychological etiology of Data's current needs (Neukrug & Schwitzer, 2006; Schwitzer, 2006, 2007).

First, Cognitive Behavior Therapy was applied primarily to Data's depressive needs. According to Cognitive Behavior Therapy (Beck, 1995, 2005; Ellis, 1994; Ellis & MacLaren, 2005), irrational thinking, faulty beliefs, or other forms of cognitive errors lead individuals to engage in problematic behaviors and to experience negative moods and attitudes. As can be seen in Figure 10.4, when the counselor applied these Cognitive Behavior Therapy concepts, she explained at Step 3 that the various depressive symptoms noted in Step 1 (feeling empty, poor thinking and actions, etc.), which can be understood in Step 2 to be a theme of a major depressive disorder, are rooted in or caused by: (a) the irrational belief that "Without my memory, I can't advance toward being human, and therefore I am worthless" and (b) catastrophizing in the form of the belief that "If I can't remember and become human, there is no reason to live and function."

Second, Existential Counseling was applied primarily to Data's counseling questions of self, identity, spirituality, and meaning. According to the theory, Existential Counseling is appropriate for clients addressing problems about living, dealing with feelings of alienation, and experiencing developmental crisis pertaining to death and meaning (Van Deurzen, 2002). The approach assists such clients to confront their questions of self; widen their perspectives of themselves, the universe, and their roles; and clarify what provides their current and future life with meaning

(Van Deurzen, 2002). Existential counselors conceptualize client needs from the viewpoint of increasing clients' self-determination (Van Deurzen, 2002; Vontress, Johnson, & Epp, 1999). As also can be seen in the figure, when the ship's counselor applied these existential counseling concepts, she additionally explained at Step 3 that the various Step 1 issues (doubts and questions about "who I am," etc.), which can be understood in Step 2 to be a theme of counseling questions of identity and spirituality, are rooted in or caused by Data's fears and anxieties about conditions of life and death, place in the universe, and God's perceptions of him.

Step 4: Narrowed Inferences. At Step 4, the clinician's selected theory continues to be used to address still-deeper issues when they exist (Schwitzer, 2006, 2007). At this step, "still-deeper, more encompassing, or more central, causal themes" are formed (Neukrug & Schwitzer, 2006, p. 207). Lieutenant Commander Data's counselor continued to use a psychotherapeutic integration of two approaches.

First, continuing to apply Cognitive Behavior Therapy concepts at Step 4, Data's counselor presented a single, deepest, most-fundamental faulty belief that she believed to be most explanatory and causal regarding Data's primary reasons for referral: the deepest irrational self-statement that "if I can't be human I don't deserve to, or want to, exist." Second, continuing to apply Existential Counseling, the ship's counselor presented a single, most deeply rooted explanation, as follows. Data believes his fears and anxieties about self and the universe are intolerable and he has no power to solve them. This deepest theme is consistent with Existential Counseling, which aims to assist clients to become more present in their self-exploration, support clients in confronting their existential anxieties, and facilitate clients' redefining of self (Bugental, 1990). These two narrowed inferences, together, form the basis for understanding the etiology and maintenance of Lieutenant Commander Data's difficulties.

When all four steps are completed, the client information in Step 1 leads to logical-intuitive groupings on the basis of common denominators in Step 2, the groupings then are explained using theory at Step 3, and then, finally, at Step 4, further deeper explanations are made. From start to finish, the thoughts, feelings, behaviors, and physiological features in the topmost portions are connected on down the pyramid into deepest dynamics.

TREATMENT PLANNING

At this point, Data's clinician at the U.S.S. *Enterprise's* Counseling Bay has collected all available information about the problems that have been of concern to him and his captain. Based upon this information, the counselor developed a five-axis *DSM-IV-TR* diagnosis and then, using the "inverted pyramid" (Neukrug & Schwitzer, 2006; Schwitzer, 1996, 1997), formulated a working clinical *explanation* of Data's difficulties and their etiology that we called the *case conceptualization*. This, in turn, guides us to the next critical step in our clinical work, called the *treatment plan,* the primary purpose of which is to map out a logical and goal-oriented strategy for making positive changes in the client's life. In essence, the treatment plan is a road map *"for reducing or eliminating disruptive symptoms that are impeding the client's ability to reach positive mental health outcomes"* (Neukrug & Schwitzer, 2006, p. 225). As such, it is the cornerstone of our work with not only Data, but with all clients who present with disturbing and disruptive symptoms and/or personality patterns (Jongsma & Peterson, 2006; Jongsma et al., 2003a, 2003b; Seligman, 1993, 1998, 2004).

A comprehensive treatment plan must integrate all of the information from the biopsychosocial interview, diagnosis, and case conceptualization into a coherent plan of action. This *plan* comprises four main components, which include

Figure 10.4 Lieutenant Commander Data's Inverted Pyramid Case Conceptualization: Psychotherapeutic Integration of Cognitive Behavior Therapy and Existential Counseling

1. IDENTIFY AND LIST CLIENT CONCERNS

Feeling "empty"
Loss of interest in daily activities
Poor concentration
Poor ability to think clearly
Poor ability to act decisively
Thoughts of "shutting off"
Fatigue & sluggishness interfering
 with daily duties
Desire to engage in human crying
History of Neural Network Trauma

Doubts and questions about "who I am"
Unsure how to move forward with "self-
 advancement"
Questions of self as machine versus individual
Unable to recall previously known information
 about human experience
Unable to recall previously known information
 about own identity formation
Unable to recall other, earlier learned
 information

2. ORGANIZE CONCERNS INTO LOGICAL THEMATIC GROUPINGS

1. Major Depressive Disorder
2. Amnestic Disorder due to a General Medical Condition
3. Counseling questions of identity and spirituality

3. THEORETICAL INFERENCES: ATTACH THEMATIC GROUPINGS TO INFERRED AREAS OF DIFFICULTY

Psychotherapeutic integration

Cognitive Behavior Therapy
Irrational belief: "Without my memory, I can't advance toward being human, and therefore I am worthless"

Catastrophizing: "If I can't remember and become human, there is no reason to live and function"

Existential Counseling
Fears and anxieties about conditions of life and death, place in the universe, and God's perception of him

4. NARROWED INFERENCES: SUICIDALITY AND DEEPER DIFFICULTIES

Psychotherapeutic Integration

Cognitive Behavior Therapy

Deepest faulty belief: "If I can't be human I don't deserve to, or want to, exist"

Existential Counseling

Believes his fears and anxieties about self and the universe are intolerable and he has no power to solve them

(1) A behavioral definition of the problem(s), (2) the selection of achievable goals, (3) the determination of treatment modes, and (4) the documentation of how change will be measured. The *behavioral definition of the problem(s)* consolidates the results of the case conceptualization into a concise hierarchical list of problems and concerns that will be the focus of treatment. The *selection of achievable goals* refers to assessing and prioritizing the client's concerns into a *hierarchy of urgency* that also takes into account the client's motivation for change, level of dysfunction, and real-world influences on his or her problems. The *determination of treatment modes* refers to selection of the specific interventions, which are matched to the uniqueness of the client and to his or her goals and clearly tied to a particular theoretical orientation (Neukrug & Schwitzer, 2006). Finally, the clinician must establish how change will be measured, based upon a number of factors including client records and self-report of change, in-session observations by the clinician, clinician ratings, results of standardized evaluations such as the Beck Anxiety Inventory (Beck & Steer, 1990) or a family functioning questionnaire, pre-post treatment comparisons, and reports by other treating professionals.

The four-step method discussed above can be seen in Figure 6.1 (p. 109) and is outlined below for the case of Data, followed by his specific treatment plan.

Step 1: Behavioral Definition of Problems. The first step in treatment planning is to carefully review the case conceptualization, paying particular attention to the results of Step 2 (Thematic Groupings), Step 3 (Theoretical Inferences), and Step 4 (Narrowed Inferences). The identified clinical themes reflect the core areas of concern and distress for the client, while the theoretical and narrowed inferences offer clinical speculation as to their origins. In the case of Data, there are three primary areas of concern. The first, "major depressive disorder," refers to his feelings of emptiness, fatigue, and sluggishness; loss of interest in daily activities; poor concentration; inability to think clearly and act decisively; and

desire to engage in human crying. The second, "amnestic disorder due to a general medical condition," refers to his inability to recall previously known information about human experience, his own identity formation, and earlier learned information. The third, "counseling questions of identity and spirituality," refers to his doubts and questions about who he is, what he believes about God and the universe, and about himself as machine as opposed to being real. These symptoms and stresses are consistent with the diagnosis of Major Depressive Disorder, Single Episode, Moderate; Amnestic Disorder Due to Neural Network Trauma, Chronic; Identity Problem; and Religious or Spiritual Problem (Andrews, Slade, Sunderland, & Anderson, 2007; APA, 2000a, 2000b; Erikson, 1950; Hollon et al., 2002; Livesley, 2007; Tsai, 2008; Yudofsky & Hales, 2007).

Step 2: Identify and Articulate Goals for Change. The second step is the selection of achievable goals, which is based upon a number of factors, including the most pressing or urgent behavioral, emotional, and interpersonal concerns and symptoms as identified by the client and clinician, the willingness and ability of the client to work on those particular goals, and the realistic (real-world) achievability of those goals (Neukrug & Schwitzer, 2006). At this stage of treatment planning, it is important to recognize that not all of the client's problems can be addressed at once, so we focus initially on those that cause the greatest distress and impairment. New goals can be created as old ones are achieved. In the case of Data, the goals are divided into three prominent areas. The first, "major depressive disorder," requires that we help Data to understand the basis for his depression, identify its triggers, replace negative with positive self-talk, use behavioral strategies to overcome depression, learn and implement problem-solving strategies to avoid depressive outcome, learn and implement relapse prevention strategies, and to develop a positive, life-affirming activities and a supportive social network. The second, "Amnestic Disorder Due to a General Medical Condition," requires that we help Data to complete neuropsychiatric and neuropsychological evaluations, to understand the dysfunctional neural network basis of his memory problems, to develop alternate cognitive strategies to compensate for his memory impairment, to explore feelings related to his impairment, to identify and refute irrational thinking that contributes to his guilt and shame over cognitive inefficiency. The third, "counseling questions about identity and spirituality," requires that we help Data to clarify his spiritual concepts by describing elements of his spiritual quest, to explore his concept of and relationship with a higher power, and to resolve issues that prevent faith or belief from developing and growing; and with regard to identity, to explore and resolve anxieties that flow from realization of aloneness, meaninglessness, and inevitable nonbeing, to identify maladaptive coping mechanisms such as losing control, avoiding autonomy and playing the victim, to take responsibility for his life so that he may live authentically, and to develop a will to meaning.

Step 3: Describe Therapeutic Intervention. This is perhaps the most critical step in the treatment planning process because the clinician must now integrate information from a number of sources, including the case conceptualization, the delineation of the client's problems and goals, and the treatment literature, paying particular attention to *empirically supported treatment* (EST) and *evidence-based practice* (EBP). In essence, the clinician must align his or her treatment approach with scientific evidence from the fields of counseling and psychotherapy. Wampold (2001) identifies two types of evidence-based counseling research: studies that demonstrate "absolute efficacy," that is, the fact that counseling and psychotherapy work, and those that demonstrate "relative efficacy," that is, the fact that certain theoretical/technical approaches work best for certain clients with particular problems (Psychoanalysis, Gestalt Therapy, Cognitive Behavior Therapy, Brief Solution-Focused Therapy, Cognitive Therapy, Dialectical Behavior Therapy, Person-Centered Therapy, Expressive/Creative Therapies,

Interpersonal Therapy, and Feminist Therapy); and when delivered through specific treatment modalities (individual, group, and family counseling). In the case of Data, we have decided to use a two-pronged integrated approach to therapy. This is comprised first of Cognitive Behavior Therapy (CBT) (Beck, 1995, 2005; Ellis, 1994; Ellis & MacLaren, 2005), which has been found to be highly effective in counseling and psychotherapy with adults who experience the symptoms of Major Depressive Disorder (Fochtmann & Gelenberg, 2005; Hollon et al., 2002; Westen & Morrison, 2001). CBT relies on a variety of cognitive techniques (reframing, challenging irrational thoughts, and cognitive restructuring) and behavioral techniques (reinforcement for and shaping of adaptive behavior, extinction of maladaptive behaviors, systematic desensitization, exposure with response. Specific techniques for Data include helping him to express painful feelings and irrational thoughts regarding cognitive deficiencies related to his medical condition as well as to what it means to be truly human, to identify triggers for depressive thoughts, feelings, and behaviors, to replace negative with positive self-talk, to use behavioral strategies to overcome depression including reinforcement for achievements and completed tasks, bibliotherapy and psychopharmacology, and to assist him in developing and engaging in a regular schedule of vocational, relational, and avocational activities.

Existential Therapy (Bugental, 1990; Van Deurzen, 1991, 2002; Yalom, 1980, 2003) is predicated on the belief that "people are born into a world which likely has no inherent meaning or purpose" (Neukrug, 2011, p. 151) and that they struggle to find meaning by overcoming internal and external obstacles to feelings of authenticity or being fully alive. While we attempt to defend against inevitable feelings of loneliness, meaninglessness, and despair with maladaptive responses such as neurotic guilt and anxiety, it is tireless self-exploration and the relationship with a highly empathetic, existentially knowledgeable and directive therapist that can help clients move to a position of choice and the "will to meaning" (Frankl, 1968). It is only from this most advanced evolved place that clients can construct and live a lifestyle free of internal impediments to happiness and fulfillment. Existential Therapy has been found to be effective for clients struggling with depression and medical issues as well as with deep and painful questions about religion, identity, and meaning (Goldenberg, Kosloff, & Greenberg, 2006; Keshen, 2006). Specific techniques for Data that are drawn from this approach include educating him in the philosophy of existentialism and Existential Therapy; using listening, empathy, and dialectical inquiry to explore his existential issues and defenses; using acceptance, confrontation, encouragement, and paradoxical intention to provoke deeper examination; and both dereflecting and refocusing him on possibilities rather than limitations.

Step 4: Provide Outcome Measures of Change. This last step in treatment planning requires that we specify how change will be measured and indicate the extent to which progress has been made toward realizing these goals (Neukrug &

Schwitzer, 2006). The counselor has considerable flexibility in this phase, and may choose from a number of objective domains (psychological tests and measures of self-esteem, depression, psychosis, interpersonal relationship, anxiety, etc.), quasi-objective measures (the *DSM-IV-TR's* Axis V GAF scale; pre-post clinician, client, and psychiatric ratings); and subjective ratings (client self-report, clinician's in-session observations). In Data's case, we have implemented a number of these, including pre-post measures on the Beck Depression Inventory, post measures of GAF functioning in the normal range (>85), clinician-observed and client-reported use of positive self-talk, client-reported increased self-reliance and reduced dependency, resolution of grief, and compliance with psychopharmacological treatment

The completed treatment plan is now developed through which the counselor and Data will begin their shared work of reducing his depression and dependency and building a healthy self-image and relationship style. Lieutenant Commander Data's treatment plan appears below, and a summary can be found in Table 10.4.

TREATMENT PLAN

Client: Lieutenant Commander Data

Service Provider: U.S.S. *Enterprise* NCC-1701-D Counseling Bay

BEHAVIORAL DEFINITION OF PROBLEMS:

1. Major depressive disorder—Feelings of emptiness, fatigue and sluggishness, loss of interest in daily activities, poor concentration, inability to think clearly and act decisively, and desire to engage in human crying.

2. Amnestic Disorder Due to a General Medical Condition. Inability to recall previously known information about human experience, his own identity formation, and earlier learned information

3. Counseling questions of identity and spirituality—Doubts and questions about who he is, what he believes about God and the universe and about himself as machine as opposed to being real

GOALS FOR CHANGE:

1. Major Depressive Disorder

   - Express painful feelings related to early life experiences that reinforce and maintain depression
   - Identify triggers for depressive thoughts, feelings, and behaviors
   - Replace negative with positive self-talk
   - Use behavioral strategies to overcome depression
   - Bibliotherapy for depression
   - Psychopharmacology for depression
   - Develop and engage in regular schedule of fulfilling vocational, interpersonal, and avocational activities

2. Amnestic Disorder Due to a General Medical Condition

   - Complete neuropsychiatric and neuropsychological evaluations
   - Understand the dysfunctional neural network basis of his memory problems
   - Develop alternate cognitive strategies to compensate for his memory impairment
   - Explore feelings related to his impairment
   - Identify and refute irrational thinking that contributes to his guilt and shame over cognitive inefficiency
   - Explore thoughts and feelings about possible neurosurgery

3. Counseling questions of identity and spirituality

   - Clarify his spiritual concepts by describing elements of his spiritual quest
   - Explore his concept of and relationship with a higher power
   - Resolve issues that prevent faith or belief from developing and growing
   - Explore and resolve anxieties that flow from realization of aloneness, meaninglessness, and inevitable nonbeing
   - Identify maladaptive coping mechanisms such as losing control, avoiding autonomy, and playing the victim
   - Acknowledge responsibility for his life and pursue authenticity
   - Develop a will to meaning

(Continued)

(Continued)

THERAPEUTIC INTERVENTIONS:

A short- to moderate-term course of individual cognitive behavioral and existential counseling, supplemented with group support (6–9 months)

1. Major Depressive Disorder

   • Express painful feelings and irrational thoughts regarding cognitive deficiencies related to his medical condition as well as to what it means to be truly human
   • Identify triggers for depressive thoughts, feelings, and behaviors
   • Replace negative with positive self-talk
   • Use behavioral strategies to overcome depression, including reinforcement for achievements and completed tasks and mentoring new Star Fleet cadets
   • Developing and engaging in a regular schedule of vocational, relational, and avocational activities
   • Bibliotherapy and psychopharmacology

2. Amnestic Disorder Due to a General Medical Condition

   • Group support for cognitive impairment
   • Individual and group neurocognitive re-education

3. Counseling questions of identity and spirituality

   • Education in the philosophy of existentialism and Existential Therapy
   • Using listening, empathy, and dialectical inquiry to explore his existential issues and defenses
   • Using acceptance, confrontation, encouragement, and paradoxical intention to provoke deeper examination
   • Reflecting and refocusing on possibilities rather than limitations

OUTCOME MEASURES OF CHANGE:

The elimination of depressive thoughts and feelings related to the medical problem, development of an existential awareness of self and will to meaning, clarification of spirituality and identity issues as measured by:

   • Pre-post measures on the Beck Depression Inventory
   • Post measures of GAF function in the normal range (>85)
   • Client self-reported increased in acceptance of medical condition and development of compensatory skill set
   • Client-reported understanding and application of principles of Existential Therapy
   • Clinician-observed and client-reported spiritual awareness and acceptance
   • Client-reported overall life and self-satisfaction
   • Optimal job performance

Table 10.4   Lieutenant Commander Data Treatment Plan Summary: Psychotherapeutic Integration of Cognitive Behavior Therapy and Existential Counseling

Goals for Change	Therapeutic Interventions	Outcome Measures of Change
Major Depressive Disorder Express painful feelings related to early life experiences that reinforce and maintain depression Identify triggers for depressive thoughts, feelings, and behaviors Replace negative with positive self-talk Use behavioral strategies to overcome depression Bibliotherapy for depression Psychopharmacology for depression Develop and engage in regular schedule of fulfilling vocational, interpersonal, and avocational activities *Amnestic Disorder Due to a General Medical Condition* Complete neuropsychiatric and neuropsychological evaluations Understand the dysfunctional neural network basis of his memory problems Develop alternate cognitive strategies to compensate for his memory impairment Explore feelings related to his impairment Identify and refute irrational thinking that contributes to his guilt and shame over cognitive inefficiency	Major Depressive Disorder Express painful feelings and irrational thoughts regarding cognitive deficiencies related to his medical condition as well as to what it means to be truly human Identify triggers for depressive thoughts, feelings, and behaviors Replace negative with positive self-talk Use behavioral strategies to overcome depression, including reinforcement for achievements and completed tasks and mentoring new Star Fleet cadets Developing and engaging in a regular schedule of vocational, relational, and avocational activities Bibliotherapy and psychopharmacology *Amnestic Disorder Due to a General Medical Condition* Group support for cognitive impairment Individual and group neurocognitive reeducation *Counseling questions of identity and spirituality* Education in the philosophy of existentialism and Existential Therapy Using listening, empathy, and dialectical inquiry to explore his existential issues and defenses Using acceptance, confrontation, encouragement, and paradoxical intention to provoke deeper examination Reflecting and refocusing on possibilities rather than limitations	The elimination of depressive thoughts and feelings related to the medical problem, development of an existential awareness of self and will to meaning, clarification of spirituality and identity issues as measured by: Pre-post measures on the Beck Depression Inventory Post measures of GAF function in the normal range (>85) Client self-reported increase in acceptance of medical condition and development of compensatory skill set Client-reported understanding and application of principles of Existential Therapy Clinician-observed and client-reported spiritual awareness and acceptance Client-reported overall life and self-satisfaction Optimal job performance

(Continued)

Table 10.4 (Continued)

Goals for Change	Therapeutic Interventions	Outcome Measures of Change
Explore thoughts and feelings about possible neurosurgery		
Counseling questions of identity and spirituality		
Clarify his spiritual concepts by describing elements of his spiritual quest		
Explore his concept of and relationship with a higher power		
Resolve issues that prevent faith or belief from developing and growing		
Explore and resolve anxieties that flow from realization of aloneness, meaninglessness, and inevitable nonbeing		
Identify maladaptive coping mechanisms such as losing control, avoiding autonomy, and playing the victim		
Acknowledge responsibility for his life and pursue authenticity		
Develop a will to meaning		

CASE 10.5   *WILL AND GRACE'S* JACK McFARLAND

INTRODUCTION OF THE CHARACTER

Jack McFarland is one member of a four-character ensemble cast of the NBC sitcom *Will and Grace,* which aired on NBC between 1998 and 2006. Jack McFarland, a flamboyant, hyperactive gay man who was obviously comfortable with his sexual identity, formed the hub of the show's cast. Jack also was known by a handful of nicknames, including Jackie, Poodle, Just Jack, and Jack McFairy Land. Although Jack's portrayal conforms to several perennial "campy" stereotypes pertaining to gay male identity, *Will and Grace* is notable as the first prime-time American television series to come out of the closet and present homosexuality in a matter-of-fact and, most often, highly comedic and endearing fashion.

Beyond Jack, the cast comprised Will Truman, an attorney who also is gay and was recently outed by Jack; Will's best friend and roommate, Grace Adler; and the group's wealthy, overly entitled, and deeply superficial designer friend, Karen Walker. The show attempted to comfortably, and often quite provocatively, deal with the vicissitudes of gay life—but also turned its searingly intelligent light on such issues as relationships, mortality, social justice, gender, racial politics, and of course, homophobia. Chronically unemployed and unattached, Jack was forever trying to find himself, as well as someone else with whom to share his life and many talents. In the following basic case summary and diagnostic impressions, we fine-tune Jack's dynamics and life concerns in order to portray the (a) depressed mood symptoms, (b) difficulties with maintaining focus and managing activity level, and (c) clinically significant personality features he might experience.

Meet the Client

You can assess the client in action by viewing clips of Jack McFarland's video material at the following websites:

- http://www.youtube.com/watch?v= mARNVXhVy3U Nurse Jack
- http://www.youtube.com/watch?v= U0jV5XU-jrI Jack, the tap-dancing fool
- http://www.youtube.com/watch?v= ESsovl8ow00 Will asks Jack for advice
- http://www.youtube.com/watch?v= 5IiTyiWZggM Will meets Jack

---

Basic Case Summary

Identifying Information. Jack McFarland is a 34-year-old white male who identifies himself as having a gay sexual identity. He resides in a rented apartment in a cooperative on the Upper East Side of New York City. Mr. McFarland has worked in the theater, retail sector, and health

sciences, and describes himself as currently being "between careers." He is single and describes himself as being "between boyfriends." His primary support group includes his closest friends, Will, Grace, and Karen, whom believes "know me better than anybody . . . and still like me!"

Regarding the therapeutic alliance, prior to scheduling an appointment at the Upper East Side Counseling Center, Mr. McFarland made several phone calls to the intake coordinator requesting a therapist who "really gets gay guys." Once assured that the counseling staff was competent in their skills and attitudes pertaining to minority sexual orientation clients, Mr. McFarland quickly scheduled and eagerly arrived for his first appointment.

Presenting Concern. Mr. McFarland communicated a mixed message about his presenting concerns. In written intake materials, he indicated that he wanted to address relationship concerns; he provided an unsolicited list of his "most admirable qualities," and replied on his screening form that "I just can't find the right guy for me." However, during the interview itself, it became clearer that he had set the appointment because he was becoming increasing concerned about the reemergence of depressed mood, fatigue, self-doubting thoughts, and other apparent depressive signs that he has experienced "on and off" throughout his adult life. In addition, in the meeting, he raised concern about his difficulty "paying attention and staying on task when I want to" and "just staying in my seat, or staying in one place, long enough." He said this second set of concerns was irritating to his friends at times and he is concerned that these symptoms might be contributing to his obstacles finding a lasting career and a lasting intimate relationship.

Background, Family Information, and Relevant History. Mr. McFarland was born in Westchester County, New York, an only child to parents who separated several months before his birth. His mother, Judith, worked as a cocktail waitress and exotic dancer who struggled to make ends meet, and who told her son while he was growing up that "Your father didn't have what it takes to hang in there." When Mr. McFarland was 6 years of age, Judith remarried to Daniel. Mr. McFarland described his stepfather as "gentle" and "just great" and said he has developed a very close bond with him.

Mr. McFarland attended Westchester Elementary and Middle Schools, where he very early on developed an interest and apparent natural affinity for the theater, and was often chosen for the lead role in school plays, particularly musicals. Looking back, Mr. McFarland said he "enjoyed dressing up and pretending I was different people . . . and the applause wasn't too bad either." Mr. McFarland recalls that by his early adolescence he had become comfortable with his own awareness of his gay sexual identity. Regarding his parents at that time, he believed his stepfather was aware of Jack's homosexuality; however, "My mom must have had gay blinders on." Throughout high school, Mr. McFarland continued to enjoy theatric endeavors and performed in a local community theater. He recalled dating a number of older men who "seemed to really get me." Those relationships were typically short-lived. Next Mr. McFarland attended Westchester Community College, which he hoped would garner him attention through which he could build his acting portfolio. It was during his college years that Mr. McFarland met Will Truman who would later become his best friend.

Although successful in theater and other extracurricular activities throughout elementary, middle and high school, and community college, Mr. McFarland also recalls difficulties "sticking with one thing." He remembers that despite adequate ability, he did poorly in math classes and high school physics due to abundant careless mistakes. He recalled "being in trouble" often for "not being in my seat" when required in class, not paying attention when given a task or assignment in school, or a chore at home (such as taking out the trash or washing the car). Further, he recalls often being unprepared for class due to losing his books, assignments, and pens; and in theatre productions forgetting or losing his

scripts and, sometimes, costumes and props. Likewise, he recalls that "for as long as I can remember in school" he had to use extreme concentration to "make it in my seat through the whole school day." He often was made to stay after school for being fidgety and distracting to those around him. Both in school and at home or in his neighborhood, he recalls being known at times as "motor mouth."

At age 19, a significant event for Mr. McFarland was his decision to make a donation at the local sperm bank for profit because "I was between jobs and didn't have a dime. . . ." This was significant primarily because later in life he encountered a son who resulted from his donation.

During his 20s, Mr. McFarland continued his seemingly random dating and became increasingly cynical about relationships. When he was 26, Mr. McFarland began a search for his father, only to find out that he had died several years before.

After promising yet unfulfilling jobs as a backup dancer, most noticeably to Jennifer Lopez, Mr. McFarland decided that perhaps his talents could be best used in fashion retail. While working at Macy's one Christmas, he reconnected with his college friend, Will Truman, who by that time had come out of the closet "just as I predicted." Upon Will's invitation, Mr. McFarland moved into his friend's apartment and soon married Rosario, Will's housekeeper, so that "the poor darling could finally get her green card." When Will's best friend, Grace, lost her own job, she moved in with the two men and Mr. McFarland decided to move out. However, he continued to spend nearly all of his time with Will and Grace, and out of desperation, opened a one-table café in their hallway called Jacques' Place. During a one-man show, Mr. McFarland met Karen, Will and Grace's socialite friend who "was a gal I could really relate to." "She got me entirely." Mr. McFarland reflected on his sporadic job history and series of impulsive career choices, as well as his short-lived impulsive lifestyle and social changes; he noted that "I seemed to have the same troubles 'staying in my seat' in jobs and friendships and romantic relationships that I did in school." He noted his various colleagues, friends, and intimate partners "really found my bouncing around hard to take sometimes."

Among his professional and social relationships, he characterized his friendship with Karen as a highlight, noting that she was particularly supportive when Mr. McFarland's son, Elliot, came to visit. Awkward at first, Mr. McFarland became comfortable in the role of "sorta kinda dad" to Elliot, and for the first time in his life "felt really important." Elliot's stay in New York was short-lived, and soon after his departure, Mr. McFarland said he "fell into a depression" because aside from his close relationship with Will, Grace, and Karen, he "felt all alone again . . . and this was no act." On further inquiry by the therapist, Mr. McFarland identified other "periods of depression," which he thought might have begun around the time of his entry into community college and seemed to "come and go" over his adult years.

Problem and Counseling History. Mr. McFarland reports having spent several unproductive years in psychotherapy earlier in life on the recommendation of his mother when "she finally realized I was queer . . . duh!!!" Mr. McFarland did not find counseling necessary or helpful at that time, but recalled enjoying the process of talking to someone who listened attentively to him.

Over the last several years, Mr. McFarland had been able to rely on his friends for emotional support and understanding when relationships failed; however, he was beginning to think that "maybe I need a real shrink." Further, although Mr. McFarland says he often feels "really down" when intimate relationships come to an end, on further inquiry he was able to recall at least four different occasions in which his mood became recognizably depressed; he lost interest in his usual social gatherings, theater outings, and movie-going; lost his appetite; fell asleep successfully but had difficulty staying asleep throughout the night; and, disturbingly to him, experienced self-doubts and the sense that he might be worthless in many important ways. He could not recall exactly, but thought these periods lasted somewhere between a few days and 6 weeks. He reports that he would "lay around" for several

days or weeks, and then rally his resources to begin aerobics classes at the gym, jog in the park, and return to seeing friends until his good mood gradually returned. He reported once feeling so down that he underwent a physical, but that his primary-care physician found no neurological or biochemical concerns. Jack admitted drinking alcohol socially and trying cocaine in his early 20s, but denies these are problematic patterns for him.

In recounting the story, Mr. McFarland spoke at an almost feverish pace, barely taking a breath between sentences, as if driven by a motor. When he finally did take a breath, Mr. McFarland settled back into the couch, sighed deeply, and began weeping. His otherwise upbeat and frenetic demeanor gave way to far more somber tones as he questioned out loud "why can everybody else find a guy and I can't . . . I mean, Christ, everyone goes home with someone every night, but not me." Mr. McFarland said he had only recently begun to question his worth both as a person and a relationship partner, and was beginning to believe that "maybe there is something wrong with me . . . I mean, if my father left me, why would any other guy want to stay?" Typically relying upon his charm, quick-talking humor, and ability to "keep them laughing" to attract and maintain work situations, friendships, and intimate relationships, Mr. McFarland now appeared disillusioned with himself and lamented that "I think I'm going to be alone forever."

Overall, two main themes emerged via the client's written materials and intake interview. The first theme comprises a long-standing history of inattention and hyperactivity first apparent in childhood and present throughout adolescence, young adulthood, and adulthood, which appears to have probably interfered with his ability to engage successfully and productively in school, work, and social endeavors. The second theme comprises what appear to be recurrent episodes of Major Depressive Disorder, which the client has tolerated for time periods and then self-alleviated with aerobic exercise and social support-seeking.

Goals for Counseling and Course of Therapy to Date. As of this writing, Mr. McFarland has attended one extensive evaluation session as authorized by his insurance carrier. He has identified a problem history that appears salient to his current presenting mood and hyperactivity-inattention concerns. He has identified important family-of-origin issues that he believes are important in understanding his pattern of relationship failures, career instability, and presenting symptoms; and responded that he is committed to "using all the therapy they'll give me, man, because my ship is sinking fast."

Diagnostic Impressions

Axis I.   296.31 Major Depressive Disorder, Recurrent (With Interepisode Recovery), Current Episode Mild

   314.01 Attention-Deficit/Hyperactivity Disorder, Combined Type, in Partial Remission

Axis II.   Histrionic Personality Disorder Features

Axis III.   None

Axis IV.   Occupational problems—Unemployment

   Problems related to the social environment—Living without intimate relationship

Axis V.   GAF = 60 (current)

   GAF = 75 (highest level past year)

DISCUSSION OF DIAGNOSTIC IMPRESSIONS

Jack McFarland set up a counseling appointment at the Upper East Side Counseling Center on his own volition and was worried about several domains of his everyday adjustment. He had been experiencing clinically significant concerns in two areas: mood, and attention and activity.

Each section of the *DSM-IV-TR* classification system contains a group of diagnoses that share qualitatively similar symptoms or features. For instance, the Mood Disorders section contains all of the disorders associated with a disturbance in mood (including depressive disorders and bipolar disorders); and the Disorders Usually First Diagnosed in Infancy, Childhood, or Adolescence section contains disorders that all share the feature of first occurring early in the life cycle, but many of which, like Attention-Deficit/Hyperactivity Disorder (ADHD), may continue into adulthood.

Jack McFarland's first concern pertained to his mood. In the interview, he reported experiencing depressed mood, along with fatigue, feelings of low self-worth, sleep difficulty, and diminished interest in usually enjoyable activities and interests. Further, he reported that he has experienced multiple life periods in which these problems have reappeared. In turn, his mood problems are characterized by recurrent episodes of depression and related symptoms. In the absence of any evidence of abuse of a substance (such as alcohol) or effects of medical problem (like hypothyroidism), his current low mood and diminished social interests, physiological symptoms (pertaining to sleep and fatigue), and cognitive symptoms (pertaining to self-reproach) meet the criteria for a Major Depressive Episode. Mood Episodes are used as building blocks for making a mood disorder diagnosis.

Mr. McFarland has experienced no Manic or Hypomanic Episodes; therefore, the diagnosis is Major Depressive Disorder. He has experienced a series of depressive episodes, but in between the episodes he reports full relief from his symptoms, the course is specified as: Recurrent (With Full Interepisode Recovery). With regard to his current episode, he experiences the minimum criteria for a Major Depressive Episode and reports only minor impairment in usual social and other activities. This makes the severity specifier, Mild, is the best fit.

One differential diagnosis regarding mood that might be considered is Dysthymic Disorder, since he has experienced depressive symptoms variously for many years. Dysthymic Disorder describes a long-term experience of mild but ever-present depression. However, this diagnosis requires at least 2 years of symptoms prior to the person's first Major Depressive Episode, which Jack does not report, and requires the continuous presence of symptoms, which is not the case with Jack.

Jack McFarland's second concern pertained to his ability to attend to the world around him and manage his activity level. In the interview, Jack complained about his inability to pay close attention when needed, and to stay on task when required. He reported difficulty organizing tasks, and remembered making careless mistakes in school. Further, Jack complained about an inability to "stay in one place" for a long enough span of time. He remembered being in disciplinary trouble in school for fidgeting, distracting others, and being a "motor mouth." Likewise, he exhibited a frenetic demeanor in the counseling session. His problematic behaviors occur in multiple settings, including but not limited to work, and they are causing impairment in his social functioning.

This combination of symptoms is characteristic of Attention-Deficit/Hyperactivity Disorder. This diagnosis is suggested when either abundant inattention symptoms are present, abundant hyperactive symptoms are present, or when both sets are present. Mr. McFarland is experiencing both sets of maladaptive behaviors about equally, indicating a subtype of Combined Type. Because he is an adult who, at present, has symptoms that seem to no longer exhaustively meet the full diagnostic criteria, the specifier, In Partial Remission, is noted.

Diagnoses including other anxiety disorders, Bipolar Disorder, substance-related disorders, and personality disorders all are differential considerations. However, Mr. McFarland's presentation and history conform with the features of Attention-Deficit/Hyperactivity Disorder, In Partial Remission.

In addition to Jack McFarland's primary presenting problems, on Axis II problematic personality features and defenses can be listed even when they do not reflect a diagnosable Personality Disorder, if these personality characteristics are important to understanding the client's functioning and are maladaptive for the person. Based on the personality features portrayed in this case, we provided the notation, Histrionic Personality Disorder Features, to describe Jack's pattern of "excessive emotionality and attention seeking," which have some maladaptive qualities associated with his intimate relationships and other interpersonal contexts (APA, 2000, p. 685).

To wrap up the diagnosis, Mr. McFarland's important social pressures are emphasized on Axis IV, and on Axis V his functioning is represented by GAF scores ranging from a recent period of good functioning with only normally expected, transient, everyday reactions and concerns, to the current period of moderate symptoms causing moderate difficulties in social and other areas, which led to his counseling appointment. The information on these axes is consistent with the information on Axes I and II.

CASE CONCEPTUALIZATION

When Jack McFarland set up an appointment at the Upper East Side Counseling Center, he was scheduled for an initial intake appointment, the purpose of which was to engage Jack in counseling and obtain as much assessment information as possible about the symptoms and situations leading to his decision to seek counseling. Included among the intake materials were a thorough history, client report, counselor observations, and written evaluation findings. Based on the intake, Jack McFarland's counselor developed diagnostic impressions, describing his presenting concerns by Major Depressive Disorder, ADHD in partial remission, as well as histrionic personality features and psychosocial environmental problems with employment and intimate relationships. A case conceptualization next was developed. Whereas the purpose of diagnostic impressions is to *describe* the client's concerns, the goal of case conceptualization is to better *understand* and clinically *explain* the person's experiences (Neukrug & Schwitzer, 2006). It helps the counselor understand the etiology leading to Jack's depressive disorder, hyperactivity and attention symptoms, and personality features, and the factors maintaining these concerns. In turn, case conceptualization sets the stage for treatment planning. Treatment planning then provides a road map that plots out how the counselor and client expect to move from presenting concerns to positive outcomes (Seligman, 1993, p. 157)—helping Jack McFarland improve his low mood and related symptoms, and reducing the problematic aspects of psychological dependence.

When forming a case conceptualization, the clinician applies a purist counseling theory, an integration of two or more theories, an eclectic mix of theories, or a solution-focused combination of tactics, to his or her understanding of the client. In this case, Mr. McFarland's counselor based his conceptualization on psychotherapeutic integration of two theories (Corey, 2009). Psychotherapists very commonly integrate more than one theoretical approach in order to form a conceptualization and treatment plan that will be as efficient and effective as possible for meeting the client's needs (Dattilo & Norcross, 2006; Norcross & Beutler, 2008). In other words, counselors using the psychotherapeutic integration method attempt to flexibly tailor their clinical efforts to "the unique needs and contexts of the individual client" (Norcross & Beutler, 2008, p. 485). Like other counselors using integration, Mr. McFarland's clinician chose this method because he had not found one individual theory that was comprehensive enough, by itself, to

address all of the "complexities," "range of client types," and "specific problems" seen among his everyday caseload (Corey, 2009, p. 450).

Specifically, Jack McFarland's counselor selected an integration of (a) Cognitive Behavior Therapy and (b) Brief Psychodynamic Therapy. The counselor selected this approach based on the combination of mood, behavioral, intrapersonal, and interpersonal issues the client presented, and his own knowledge of the current outcome research and clinical literature pertaining to best practices with clients experiencing these sorts of concerns (Critchfield & Smith-Benjamin, 2006; Fotchmann & Gelenberg, 2005; Henggeler, Schoenwald, Borduin, Rowland, & Cunningham, 1998; Hollon, Thase, & Markowitz, 2002; Livesley, 2007; McWilliams, 1994, 1999; Westen & Morrison, 2001). According to the research, Cognitive Behavior Therapy is one treatment approach indicated when assisting clients with depressive disorders (Fotchmann & Gelenberg, 2005; Hollon et al., 2002; Westen & Morrison, 2001), whereas an integrated approach emphasizing Interpersonal Psychotherapy is indicated for treatment personality dynamics such as Mr. McFarland's (Critchfield & Smith-Benjamin, 2006; Livesley, 2007). This type of integration of psychodynamic and cognitive behavioral approaches is the primary model employed at the Upper East Side Counseling Center.

The counselor used the Inverted Pyramid Method of case conceptualization because this method is especially designed to help clinicians more easily form their conceptual pictures of their clients' needs (Neukrug & Schwitzer, 2006; Schwitzer, 1996, 1997). The method has four steps: Problem Identification, Thematic Groupings, Theoretical Inferences, and Narrowed Inferences. The counselor's clinical thinking can be seen in Figure 10.5.

Step 1: Problem Identification. The first step is Problem Identification. Aspects of the presenting problem (thoughts, feelings, behaviors, physiological features), additional areas of concern besides the presenting concern, family and developmental history, in-session observations, clinical inquiries (medical problems, medications, past counseling, substance use, suicidality), and psychological assessments (problem checklists, personality inventories, mental status exam, specific clinical measures) all may contribute information at Step 1. The counselor "casts a wide net" in order to build Step 1 as exhaustively as possible (Neukrug & Schwitzer, 2006; p. 202). As can be seen in Figure 10.5, the counselor at Upper East Side Counseling Center identified Jack McFarland's primary concerns for coming in (his symptoms of depression, regretful self-reproach about job and relationship instability), other apparently important dynamics (his inattentive, hyperactive, excessively emotional, and attention-seeking behaviors), his developmental history (parental, family, and earlier experiences), and current situations (job, relationship, and friendship factors). The psychotherapist attempted to go beyond just the concerns that led Jack to seek an appointment in order to be as descriptive as he could.

Step 2: Thematic Groupings. The second step is Thematic Groupings. The clinician organizes all of the exhaustive client information found in Step 1 into just a few intuitive-logical clinical groups, categories, or themes, on the basis of sensible common denominators (Neukrug & Schwitzer, 2006). Four different ways of forming the Step 2 theme groups can be used: Descriptive-Diagnosis Approach, Clinical Targets Approach, Areas of Dysfunction Approach, and Intrapsychic Approach. As can be seen in the figure, Jack's counselor selected the Intrapsychic Approach. This approach sorts together all of the Step 1 information about the "client's adjustment, development, distress, or dysfunction" in order "to show clinical patterns in the ways life events are associated with the person's personal experience and identity" (Neukrug & Schwitzer, 2006, p. 205).

Interestingly, the counselor grouped together all of the factors in Step 1 into just two themes capturing the two intrapsychic patterns he believes Jack McFarland has been dealing with throughout his adolescence, young adulthood,

and adulthood. Specifically, he grouped: all of the Step 1 data pertaining to depressed mood, low self-worth, and regrets into the theme, "recurrent low mood and other symptoms of depression, along with low-self-worth and regret about parental, past, and current relationships and job history"; and all of the Step 1 data pertaining to hyperactivity, inattention, emotionality, and attention-seeking into the theme, "long-standing hyperactivity, inattention, excessive emotionality and attention-seeking, all of which deflect intimate relationships and defeat job success." In this case example, the counselor used the Intrapsychic Approach to group much diverse information together to show how external life experiences have been associated with Mr. McFarland's experience of self.

So far, at Steps 1 and 2, the counselor has used his intake skills and clinical judgment to begin meaningfully understanding Jack McFarland's situation. Now, at Steps 3 and 4, he applies an integration of the two theoretical approaches he has selected. He begins making theoretical inferences to interpret and explain the processes underlying the client's problematic dynamics as they are seen in Steps 1 and 2.

Step 3: Theoretical Inferences. At Step 3, concepts from the counselor's theoretical integration of two approaches—Cognitive Behavior Therapy and Brief Psychodynamic Therapy—are applied to explain the experiences causing, and the mechanisms maintaining, Jack McFarland's problematic thoughts, feelings, and behaviors. The counselor tentatively matches the theme groups in Step 2 with this theoretical approach. In other words, the symptom constellations in Step 2, which were distilled from the symptoms in Step 1, now are combined using theory to show what are believed to be the underlying causes or psychological etiology of Jack McFarland's current needs (Neukrug & Schwitzer, 2006; Schwitzer, 2006, 2007).

First, Cognitive Behavior Therapy was applied primarily to Mr. McFarland's depressive needs and his faulty cognitive and behavioral efforts to regulate these. According to Cognitive Behavior Therapy (Beck, 1995, 2005; Ellis, 1994; Ellis & MacLaren, 2005), irrational thinking, faulty beliefs, or other forms of cognitive errors lead individuals to engage in problematic behaviors and to experience negative moods and attitudes. As can be seen in Figure 10.5, when the counselor applied these Cognitive Behavior Therapy concepts, he explained at Step 3 that the various issues noted in Step 1 (depressed mood, etc.), which can be understood in Step 2 to be a theme of recurrent low mood, low self-worth, and regret, are maintained by two irrational self-statements: (a) "My father left me and my mother does not want to really know me; this tells me anyone who really knows me will not love me or approve of me and will leave me"; and (b) "Rejection is too painful and therefore I must not become too attached to anyone or any situation."

Second, Brief Psychodynamic Therapy was applied primarily to Mr. McFarland's hyperactive and attention-seeking needs, and to amplify what already was inferred about his thinking and behaviors from the cognitive approach. Psychodynamic Therapy infers that adult psychological concerns are influenced by parental and family relationships and other early formational experiences—and infers that irrational forces, unconscious motives, and attempts to defend against early psychodevelopmental hurts and injuries lead to the problematic moods, thoughts, and behaviors confronting adult clients (Auld & Hyman, 1991; Leiper & Maltby, 2004; McWilliams, 1994, 1999; Patton & Meara, 1992). In turn, from the perspective of Psychodynamic Therapy, generally speaking, the individual's problematic symptoms often are rudimentary attempts to cover over, defend against, or compensate for inner conflicts (Auld & Hyman, 1991; Leiper & Maltby, 2004; McWilliams, 1994, 1999; Patton & Meara, 1992). As also can be seen in the figure, Jack McFarland's counselor interpreted his problematic intrapersonal and interpersonal behaviors to be psychodynamic defenses (deflection, projection, denial, sublimation, reaction formation) helping Jack defend against fears of abandonment.

Step 4: Narrowed Inferences. At Step 4, the clinician's selected theory continues to be used to address still-deeper issues when they exist (Schwitzer, 2006, 2007). At this step, "still-deeper, more encompassing, or more central, causal themes" are formed (Neukrug & Schwitzer, 2006, p. 207). Jack McFarland's counselor continued to use a psychotherapeutic integration of two approaches.

First, continuing to apply Cognitive Behavior Therapy concepts at Step 4, Jack's counselor presented a single, deepest, most-fundamental core faulty belief that he believed to be most explanatory and causal regarding his primary reasons for referral: the deepest irrational self-statement that "others certainly will reject me if they get to know me and therefore I must avoid, at all costs, allowing anyone to become too close to me." Second, continuing to apply Brief Psychodynamic Therapy, the counselor presented a single, most deeply rooted intrapsychic conflict. This is an especially important step in contemporary—brief—psychodynamic approaches. Whereas traditional, time-unlimited psychodynamic therapy may identify and address a wide range of conflicts, brief psychodynamic therapists "usually rely on identifying an explicit focus, such as a core conflict or relational theme" and then actively work to challenge defenses related to the core conflict that has been identified (Leiper & Maltby, 2004, p. 144; Messer & Warren, 1995). In Mr. McFarland's case, at Step 4, the counselor distilled his core conflict to be: Fear of abandonment and the disintegration of self that would result from abandonment. These two narrowed inferences, together, form the basis for understanding the etiology and maintenance of Mr. McFarland's difficulties.

When all four steps are completed, the client information in Step 1 leads to logical-intuitive groupings on the basis of common denominators in Step 2, the groupings then are explained using theory at Step 3, and then, finally, at Step 4, further deeper explanations are made. From start to finish, the thoughts, feelings, behaviors, and physiological features in the topmost portions are connected on down the pyramid into deepest dynamics.

Figure 10.5   Jack McFarland's Inverted Pyramid Case Conceptualization Summary: Psychotherapeutic Integration of Brief Psychodynamic Psychotherapy and Cognitive Behavior Therapy

1. IDENTIFY AND LIST CLIENT CONCERNS

Early history of father abandonment
History of mother's "blinders" to gay identity
History of dating older men "who get me"
Child, adolescent, and adult inability to pay attention
Child, adolescent, and adult inability to stay on task
"Motor mouth"
Inability to remain interested in one job for extended time
Inability to stay invested in one relationship for extended time

Job instability
Relationship instability
Excessive emotionality
Excessive attention-seeking
Interferes with interpersonal relationships
Recurrent periods of low mood
Fatigue
Low self-worth
Self-reproach
Sleep difficulties
Diminished interest in activities

2. ORGANIZE CONCERNS INTO LOGICAL THEMATIC GROUPINGS

1. Recurrent low mood and other symptoms of depression along with low self-worth and regret about parental, past, and current relationship and job history
2. Long-standing hyperactivity, inattention, excessive emotionality, and attention-seeking, all of which deflect intimate relationships and defeat job success

3. THEORETICAL INFERENCES: ATTACH THEMATIC GROUPINGS TO INFERRED AREAS OF DIFFICULTY

Psychotherapeutic Integration

Cognitive Behavior Therapy

Irrational self-statement:

1. My father left me and my mother does not want to really know me; this tells me anyone who really knows me will not love me or approve of me and will leave me
2. Rejection is too painful, and therefore I must not become too attached to anyone or any situation

Brief Psychodynamic Psychotherapy
Jack uses a group of psychodynamic defenses—deflection, projection, denial, sublimation, reaction formation—to defend against fears of abandonment

4. NARROWED INFERENCES: SUICIDALITY AND DEEPER DIFFICULTIES

Psychotherapeutic Integration

Cognitive Behavior Therapy

Core faulty belief: Others certainly will reject me if they get to know me, and therefore I must avoid, at all costs, allowing anyone to become too close to me

Brief Psychodynamic Therapy

Fear of abandonment and the disintegration of self that would result from abandonment

TREATMENT PLANNING

At this point, Mr. McFarland's clinician at the Upper East Side Counseling Center has collected all available information about the problems that have been of concern to him. Based upon this information, the counselor developed a five-axis *DSM-IV-TR* diagnosis and then, using the "inverted pyramid" (Neukrug & Schwitzer, 2006; Schwitzer, 1996, 1997), formulated a working clinical *explanation* of Jack's difficulties and their etiology that we called the *case conceptualization*. This, in turn, guides us to the next critical step in our clinical work, called the *treatment plan,* the primary purpose of which is to map out a logical and goal-oriented strategy for making positive changes in the client's life. In essence, the treatment plan is a road map *"for reducing or eliminating disruptive symptoms that are impeding the client's ability to reach positive mental health outcomes"* (Neukrug & Schwitzer, 2006, p. 225). As such, it is the cornerstone of our work with not only Jack, but with all clients who present with counterproductive and disruptive symptoms and/or personality patterns (Jongsma & Peterson, 2006; Jongsma, Peterson, & McInnis, 2003a, 2003b; Seligman, 1993, 1998, 2004).

A comprehensive treatment plan must integrate all of the information from the biopsychosocial interview, diagnosis, and case conceptualization into a coherent plan of action. This *plan* comprises four main components, which include (1) a behavioral definition of the problem(s), (2) the selection of achievable goals, (3) the determination of treatment modes, and (4) the documentation of how change will be measured. The *behavioral definition of the problem(s)* consolidates the results of the case conceptualization into a concise hierarchical list of problems and concerns that will be the focus of treatment. The *selection of achievable goals* refers to assessing and prioritizing the client's concerns into a *hierarchy of urgency* that also takes into account the client's motivation for change, level of dysfunction, and real-world influences on his or her problems. The *determination of treatment modes* refers to selection of the specific

interventions, which are matched to the uniqueness of the client and to the client's goals and clearly tied to a particular theoretical orientation (Neukrug & Schwitzer, 2006). Finally, the clinician must establish how change will be measured, based upon a number of factors including client records and self-report of change, in-session observations by the clinician, clinician ratings, results of standardized evaluations such as the Beck Anxiety Inventory (Beck & Steer, 1990) or a family functioning questionnaire, pre-post treatment comparisons, and reports by other treating professionals.

The four-step method discussed above can be seen in Figure 6.1 (p. 109) and is outlined below for the case of Jack, followed by his specific treatment plan.

Step 1: Behavioral Definition of Problems. The first step in treatment planning is to carefully review the case conceptualization, paying particular attention to the results of Step 2 (Thematic Groupings), Step 3 (Theoretical Inferences), and Step 4 (Narrowed Inferences). The identified clinical themes reflect the core areas of concern and distress for the client, while the theoretical and narrowed inferences offer clinical speculation as to their origins. In the case of Mr. McFarland, there are two primary areas of concern. The first, "recurrent low mood and other symptoms of depression along with low self-worth and regret about parental, past and current relationship and job history," refers to recurrent periods of low mood, fatigue, low self-worth, self-reproach, sleep difficulties, job and relationship instability, and diminished interest in activities. The second, "long-standing hyperactivity, inattention, excessive emotionality and attention seeking," refers to inability to stay invested in one relationship for an extended period of period of time, inability to stay interested in one job for extended time, excessive emotionality and attention seeking, child, adolescent, and adult inability to pay attention and stay on task. These symptoms and stresses are consistent with the diagnosis of Major Depressive Disorder, Recurrent (With Interepisode Recovery), Current

Episode, Mild; and ADHD, Combined Type, in Partial Remission (APA, 2000a; Barkley, 2006; Conners, 2008; Depression Guideline Panel, 1993; Dobson, 1993; Hollon, Thase, & Markowitz, 2002; Tippins & Reiff, 2004).

Step 2: Identify and Articulate Goals for Change. The second step is the selection of achievable goals, which is based upon a number of factors, including the most pressing or urgent behavioral, emotional, and interpersonal concerns and symptoms as identified by the client and clinician, the willingness and ability of the client to work on those particular goals, and the realistic (real-world) achievability of those goals (Neukrug & Schwitzer, 2006). At this stage of treatment planning, it is important to recognize that not all of the client's problems can be addressed at once, so we focus initially on those that cause the greatest distress and impairment. New goals can be created as old ones are achieved. In the case of Mr. McFarland, the goals are divided into two prominent areas. The first, "recurrent low mood and other symptoms of depression along with low self-worth and regret about parental, past and current relationship and job history," requires that we help Mr. McFarland to understand the relationship between early father abandonment and his life-long depression, understand the relationship between his mother's denial of his homosexuality and his historic relationship instability, recognize and resolve the irrational thoughts regarding his self-worth and worth to others, alleviate his depressive symptoms by exploring his unconscious defense mechanisms, identify career directions, and improve the overall quality of his life, including sleep, appetite, activity level, and self-care. The second, "long-standing hyperactivity, inattention, excessive emotionality and attention seeking," requires that we help Mr. McFarland to understand the signs and symptoms of ADHD throughout the life span and accept it as a chromic adjustment issue, recognize the particular impact of ADHD on relationship, parental, vocational, and avocational stability, reduce impulsive actions while increasing concentration and focus on low-interest

activities, minimize interference of ADHD symptoms on his daily life, sustain attention and concentration for consistently longer periods of time, gain awareness of and control excessive emotionality stemming from early parental conflicts and maladaptive defense mechanisms.

Step 3: Describe Therapeutic Intervention. This is perhaps the most critical step in the treatment planning process because the clinician must now integrate information from a number of sources, including the case conceptualization, the delineation of the client's problems and goals, and the treatment literature, paying particular attention to *empirically supported treatment* (EST) and *evidence-based practice* (EBP). In essence, the clinician must align his or her treatment approach with scientific evidence from the fields of counseling and psychotherapy. Wampold (2001) identifies two types of evidence-based counseling research: studies that demonstrate "absolute efficacy," that is, the fact that counseling and psychotherapy work, and those that demonstrate "relative efficacy," that is, the fact that certain theoretical/technical approaches work best for certain clients with particular problems (Psychoanalysis, Gestalt Therapy, Cognitive Behavior Therapy, Brief Solution-Focused Therapy, Cognitive Therapy, Dialectical Behavior Therapy, Person-Centered Therapy, Expressive/Creative Therapies, Interpersonal Therapy, and Feminist Therapy); and when delivered through specific treatment modalities (individual, group, and family counseling).

In the case of Mr. McFarland, we have decided to use a two-pronged or integrated approach to therapy composed of Cognitive Behavior Therapy and Brief Psychodynamic Therapy. Cognitive Behavior Therapy (Beck, 1995, 2005; Ellis, 1994; Ellis & MacLaren, 2005), has been found to be highly effective in counseling and psychotherapy with adults (and adolescents) who experience the symptoms of Depression (Fochtman & Gelenberg, 2005; Hollon et al., 2002; Westen & Morrison, 2001). The approach relies on a variety of cognitive techniques (reframing, challenging irrational thoughts, and cognitive restructuring) and behavioral techniques (reinforcement for and shaping of adaptive behavior, extinction of maladaptive behaviors, systematic desensitization, and exposure with response prevention) (Ball et al., 2006; Frank et al., 2005; Milkowitz, 2008). Techniques drawn from this approach will include identifying and challenging irrational depressogenic thoughts related to low self-worth, developing a schedule for self-care and health maintenance, as well as shaping and reinforcing affirmative self-statements and beliefs. They will also include exploring the role of unresolved feelings of abandonment and rejection; using dream analysis, free association, and exploration of transference to understand and modify defense mechanisms contributing to depression and attention-seeking; encouraging the client to share feelings of sadness and rejection paired with positive support and relaxation; scheduling an intake with a career counselor; referral to psychiatrist for possible psychopharmacotherapy; training in the use of relaxation including breathing; biofeedback; muscle relaxation, and guided imagery; identification of a "coach" from among close friends to provide feedback for focused and unfocused behavior; and bibliotherapy for ADHD awareness. We will also use Brief Psychodynamic Psychotherapy, a variant of classical Freudian Psychoanalysis, which posits that interpersonal and intrapersonal conflicts stem from early family-of-origin relationships, and the way that they become represented or internalized in the form of maladaptive (and adaptive) defensive mechanisms and styles, unhealthy (and healthy) relationship preferences, and self-image (Auld & Hyman, 1991; Davanloo, 2005; Leiper & Maltby, 2004; McWilliams, 1994, 1999; Patton & Meara, 1992). The techniques that flow from this theoretical position are more directly, and at times confrontationally, applied and in a shorter time frame (Corey, 2009), and borrow from cognitive therapy (Seligman & Reichenberg, 2007). They include the more traditional components of analysis such as interpretation of dreams, defenses, and transference; and may also include supportive yet confrontational techniques such as "head-on collision" to disrupt and modify defenses and "pressuring" the client to address deeper and maladaptive

emotional and behavioral issues. Techniques drawn from this approach will also include "pressuring" to explore his defense-based ways of relating to others; monitoring his dreams, fantasies, and relationship with the counselor in order to relate past and current relational styles; teaching problem-solving skills for impulse control; and analyzing the transference relationship.

Step 4: Provide Outcome Measures of Change. This last step in treatment planning requires that we specify how change will be measured and indicate the extent to which progress has been made toward realizing these goals (Neukrug & Schwitzer, 2006). The counselor has considerable flexibility in this phase and may choose from a number of objective domains (psychological tests and measures of self-esteem, depression, psychosis, interpersonal relationship, anxiety, etc.), quasi-objective measures (the *DSM-IV-TR's* Axis V GAF scale; pre-post clinician, client, and psychiatric ratings), and subjective ratings (client self-report, clinician's in-session observations). In Mr. McFarland's case, we have implemented a number of these, including pre-post measure on the Beck Depression Inventory-II (Beck, Steer, & Brown, 1996), pre-post measures on the Beck Depression Inventory and Conners 3 (Conners, 2008), post-only measures of GAF functioning in the mild range (>70), client self-reported awareness and clinician observation of understanding of defenses, client self-reported awareness of and ability to regulate mood and behavior, clinician-observed improvement in impulse, behavior, and emotional control, client self-report of productive career training and vocational planning, client-reported stable relationship, and compliance with psychopharmacotherapy for depression and ADHD.

The completed treatment plan is now developed through which the counselor and Mr. McFarland will begin their shared work of ameliorating his depression, improving the quality of his relationships, and assisting him in the management of his ADHD. The treatment plan is described below and summarized in Table 10.5.

TREATMENT PLAN

Client: Jack McFarland

Service Provider: Upper East Side Counseling Center

BEHAVIORAL DEFINITION OF PROBLEMS:

1. Recurrent low mood and other symptoms of depression along with low self-worth and regret about parental, past and current relationship and job history—Recurrent periods of low mood, fatigue, low self-worth, self-reproach, sleep difficulties, job and relationship instability, and diminished interest in activities

2. Long-standing hyperactivity, inattention, excessive emotionality and attention seeking— Inability to stay invested in one relationship for an extended period of period of time, inability to stay interested in one job for extended time, excessive emotionality and attention seeking; child, adolescent, and adult inability to pay attention and stay on task

GOALS FOR CHANGE:

1. Recurrent low mood and other symptoms of depression along with low self-worth and regret about parental, past and current relationship and job history

2. Understand the relationship between early father abandonment and his lifelong depression

3. Explore the relationship between his mother's denial of his homosexuality and his historic relationship instability

4. Recognize and resolve the irrational thoughts regarding his self-worth and worth to others

5. Alleviate his depressive symptoms by exploring his unconscious defense mechanisms

6. Identify career directions

7. Improve the overall quality of his life including sleep, appetite, activity level, and self-care

8. Long-standing hyperactivity, inattention, excessive emotionality and attention seeking

9. Understand the signs and symptoms of ADHD throughout the lifespan and accept it as a chromic adjustment issue

10. Recognize the particular impact of ADHD on relationship, parental, vocational, and avocational stability

11. Reduce impulsive actions while increasing concentration and focus on low-interest activities

12. Minimize interference of ADHD symptoms in his daily life

13. Sustain attention and concentration for consistently longer periods of time

14. Gain awareness of and control excessive emotionality stemming from early parental conflicts and maladaptive defense mechanisms

(Continued)

(Continued)

THERAPEUTIC INTERVENTIONS:

A short- to moderate-term course (6–9 months) of integrated Cognitive Behavior and Brief Psychodynamic Psychotherapy supplemented with career planning and relaxation training

1. Recurrent low mood and other symptoms of depression along with low self-worth and regret about parental, past and current relationship and job history

   - Identify and challenge irrational depressogenic thoughts related to low self-worth
   - Shape and reinforce affirmative self-statements and beliefs
   - Explore the role of unresolved feelings of abandonment and rejection
   - Use dream analysis, free association, and interpretation of transference to understand and modify defense mechanisms contributing to depression and attention-seeking
   - Developing a schedule for self-care and health maintenance
   - Encouragement to share feelings of sadness and rejection paired with positive support and relaxation
   - Schedule intake with a career counselor
   - Referral to psychiatrist for possible psychopharmacotherapy

2. Long-standing hyperactivity, inattention, excessive emotionality and attention-seeking

   - "Pressuring" to explore his defense-based ways of relating to others
   - Monitor dreams, fantasies, and relationship with the counselor in order to relate past and current relational styles
   - Teach problem-solving skills for impulse control and attention-focusing based on self-reinforcement
   - Train in the use of relaxation, including breathing, biofeedback, muscle relaxation, and guided imagery
   - Identify a "coach" from among close friends to provide feedback for focused and unfocused behavior
   - Bibliotherapy for ADHD awareness
   - Attend adult ADHD support group
   - Psychiatric consultation for possible psychopharmacotherapy

OUTCOME MEASURES OF CHANGE:

A reduction in the adverse impact of symptoms of ADHD, elimination of depression, greater capacity for self-regulation, and vocational/interpersonal stability as measured by:

- Pre-post measures on the Beck Depression Inventory
- Pre-post measures on the Conners 3
- Post-only measures of GAF functioning in the mild range (>70)
- Client self-reported awareness and clinician observation of understanding of defenses
- Client self-reported awareness of and ability to regulate mood and behavior
- Clinician-observed improvement in impulse, behavior, and emotional control
- Client self-report of productive career training and vocational planning
- Client-reported stable relationship
- Compliance with psychopharmacotherapy for depression and ADHD

Table 10.5   Jack McFarland's Treatment Plan Summary: Psychotherapeutic Integration of Brief Psychodynamic Psychotherapy and Cognitive Behavior Therapy

Goals for Change	Therapeutic Interventions	Outcome Measures of Change
Recurrent low mood and other symptoms of depression along with low self-worth and regret about parental, past and current relationship and job history	Recurrent low mood and other symptoms of depression along with low self-worth and regret about parental, past and current relationship and job history	A reduction in the adverse impact of symptoms of ADHD, elimination of depression, greater capacity for self-regulation and vocational/interpersonal stability as measured by:
Understand the relationship between early father abandonment and his life-long depression	Identify and challenge irrational depressogenic thoughts related to low self-worth	Pre-post measures on the Beck Depression Inventory
Explore the relationship between his mother's denial of his homosexuality and his historic relationship instability	Shape and reinforce affirmative self-statements and beliefs	Pre-post measures on the Conners 3
	Explore the role of unresolved feelings of abandonment and rejection	Post-only measures of GAF functioning in the mild range (>70)
Recognize and resolve the irrational thoughts regarding his self-worth and worth to others	Use dream analysis, free association, and interpretation of transference to understand and modify defense mechanism contributing to depression and attention-seeking	Client self-reported awareness and clinician observation of understanding of defenses
Alleviate his depressive symptoms by exploring his unconscious defense mechanisms	Developing a schedule for self-care and health maintenance	Client self-reported awareness of and ability to regulate mood and behavior
Identify career directions	Encouragement to share feelings of sadness and rejection paired with positive support and relaxation	Clinician-observed improvement in impulse, behavior, and emotional control
Improve the overall quality of his life, including sleep, appetite, activity level, and self-care	Schedule intake with a career counselor	Client self-report of productive career training and vocational planning
	Referral to psychiatrist for possible psychopharmacotherapy	
Long-standing hyperactivity, inattention, excessive emotionality, and attention-seeking	Long-standing hyperactivity, inattention, excessive emotionality, and attention-seeking	Client-reported stable relationship
Understand the signs and symptoms of ADHD throughout the life span and accept it as a chromic adjustment issue	"Pressuring" to explore his defense-based ways of relating to others	Compliance with psychopharmacotherapy for depression and ADHD
	Monitor dreams, fantasies, and relationship with the counselor in order to relate past and current relational styles	
Recognize the particular impact of ADHD on relationship, parental, vocational, and avocational stability	Teach problem-solving skills for impulse control and attention-focusing based on self-reinforcement	
	Train in the use of relaxation, including breathing, biofeedback, muscle relaxation, and guided imagery	

(Continued)

Table 10.5 (Continued)

Goals for Change	Therapeutic Interventions	Outcome Measures of Change
Reduce impulsive actions while increasing concentration and focus on low-interest activities Minimize interference of ADHD symptoms in his daily life Sustain attention and concentration for consistently longer periods of time Gain awareness of and control excessive emotionality stemming from early parental conflicts and maladaptive defense mechanisms	Identify a "coach" from among close friends to provide feedback for focused and unfocused behavior Bibliotherapy for ADHD awareness Attend adult ADHD support group Psychiatric consultation for possible psychopharmacotherapy	

FOLLOW-UP: DIAGNOSIS, CASE CONCEPTUALIZATION, AND TREATMENT PLANNING THEMES—CHAPTER SUMMARY

This chapter presented a demanding clinical caseload comprising five adult clients: Jack Bauer, Sophia Petrillo, George Lopez, Lieutenant Commander Data, and Jack McFarland. Mrs. Petrillo is an older adult. Interestingly, this caseload had a gender balance of one female client and four males. Among the caseload's diversity were four American clients: Of these, Jack Bauer, Mrs. Sophia Petrillo, and Jack McFarland are white and have European cultural heritages; and George Lopez is Mexican American. Rounding out the group is Lieutenant Commander Data, who we characterized as bi-racial with both human and machine ethnicities. Upper, upper-middle, and middle socioeconomic statuses were represented by this group of clients. All of these clients, with the exception of Jack McFarland, identified themselves as heterosexual.

Among this chapter's clients, Jack McFarland sought counseling services on his own accord at

the Upper East Side Counseling Center, and both George Lopez and Mrs. Petrillo sought outpatient counseling at the urging of family members. On the other hand, Jack Bauer and Lieutenant Commander Data both were mandated to visit counseling by their superiors.

Among the concerns presented by our clients in the chapter's caseload, Jack Bauer sought assistance for concerns characterized diagnostically as Posttraumatic Stress Disorder, along with Bereavement and antisocial personality features; Lieutenant Commander Data presented a single episode of moderate Major Depression, along with Amnestic Disorder Due to the general medical condition, "Neural Network Trauma" (sic) and spiritual questions; Mrs. Petrillo was observed experiencing symptoms of the Alzheimer's type of dementia; sitcom character George Lopez was dealing with an Adjustment Disorder with anxiety and depressed mood, and Acculturation Problems; whereas Jack McFarland had concerns described diagnostically as recurrent episodes of mild Major Depression, as well as ADHD, which as in partial remission in adulthood, and Histrionic Personality features. Taken together, the caseload comprised a mix of concerns connected to adjustments and life events, mood and anxiety, and psychological problems due to medical conditions.

Looking at the counseling theories represented, their counselors formed case conceptualizations and then treatment plans based on Cognitive Behavior Therapy, Reality Therapy, and three psychotherapeutic integrations: Behavior Therapy with Cognitive Stimulation Therapy, Cognitive Behavior Therapy with Existential Counseling, and Cognitive Behavior Therapy with Brief Psychodynamic Psychotherapy.

In their treatment plans, these clients' counselors expressed hopes that their clients would achieve such as outcomes as: resolving post-traumatic stress symptoms and antisocial thoughts and actions (Jack Bauer), resolving symptoms associated with depression and clarifying identity and spiritual questions (Data), establishing family support and long-term care to maintain optimal cognitive and behavioral functioning (Mrs. Petrillo), developing abilities to address basic needs, make healthy choices, and have fulfilling attitudes about self and family and work (George Lopez), and reduce the adverse impacts of ADHD and depression and increase self-management (Jack McFarland).

STUDY QUESTIONS AND LEARNING ACTIVITIES

Based on your understanding of this chapter's cases, consider and respond to these Study Questions and Learning Activities:

1. This caseload is a demanding one.

   a. If you were assigned this group of clients, what would be your initial reactions to their individual characteristics and differences? Their reasons for referral?

   b. What would you identify as your greatest strengths for assisting these five clients? Your areas of greatest need for growth?

2. In their Basic Case Summaries, this chapter's counselors focused on their clients' earlier developmental and family experiences, presenting concerns, assessment of current distress, and areas and life roles in which they were experiencing difficulties, client strengths, and hopes for change. There was an emphasis on Jack Bauer's developmental and family history plus his recent and current stresses, traumas, and losses; psychological and biological (biomechanical) origins of Data's mood and identity problems; patterns, severity, and consequences of Mrs. Petrillo's onset of dementia symptoms; George Lopez's early as well as young adult and adult development, and cultural transitions, as factors in his current concerns; and similarly, Jack McFarland's early family and developmental as well as young adult and adult developmental experiences.

   a. Keeping in mind that the initial counseling meeting, screening session, or intake interview usually requires the counselor to balance rapport and trust-building, on one hand, and assessment and information-gathering, on the other hand, what would you identify as your greatest strengths when engaging these five clients in the counseling process, and gathering the clinical information needed to conceptualize and plan for their counseling process? Your areas of greatest need for growth?

   b. Looking at the five Basic Case Summaries, how does this type of clinical writing differ from your everyday thinking and conversation about people? What are your levels of comfort, skill, and experience, with this type of professional writing? What steps can you take to further develop or improve these skills?

   c. What suggestions would you have for one or more of the counselors in this chapter regarding missing, overlooked, or underemphasized—or overemphasized—information gathered and reported in the Basic Case Summaries? What would you like to have known more about? What methods could be used—clinical interview questions, observations, psychological measures, or other means—to find the additional information you would seek?

3. This chapter illustrated *DSM-IV-TR* diagnoses found in the following sections: Disorders Usually First Diagnosed in Infancy, Childhood, or Adolescence (even when the client is an adult, ADHD is found in this section); Delirium, Dementia, and Amnestic and Other Cognitive Disorders; Mood Disorders; Anxiety Disorders; Adjustment Disorders; and Personality Disorders—plus Other Conditions That May Be a Focus of Clinical Attention.

   a. How familiar are you with these sections of the *DSM-IV-TR?* What is your comfort level using the *DSM-IV-TR* to explore these sets of concerns? Which of these groups of disorders are likely to be most important to you in the practicum, internship, residency, or professional practice settings in which you hope to work?

   b. What are your attitudes, reactions, or thoughts concerning diagnosis of childhood disorders? Concerning the diagnosis of behavioral consequences of problematic substance use? Concerning diagnosing life-long patterns characterized as personality disorders? How can you further explore or develop your professional attitudes about diagnosis of these types of concerns?

   c. What will be your next steps in gaining greater comfort and skills at diagnosis of the attention-deficit and disruptive behavior disorders of childhood? Dementia? Amnestic Disorders? Mood, Anxiety, and Adjustment Disorders? Personality disorders?

   d. What are your attitudes, reactions, or thoughts concerning use of Axis IV to record psychosocial and environmental stressors (such as Jack Bauer's loss of his wife and discord with his daughter) and Axis III to record general medical problems (such as Mrs. Petrillo's stroke)? What will be your next steps in gaining greater comfort and skills with these axes?

   e. Among this group of clients, Axis V Global Assessment of Functioning (GAF) scores ranged from 60 (Jack Bauer, Data, and Jack McFarland all were estimated with moderate symptoms) to 70 (George's mild symptoms with some dysfunction at work and other roles). What are your attitudes, reactions, or thoughts concerning use of Axis V GAF scores to estimate the client's overall level of functioning? Do you agree with the counselors' estimates found in this chapter? What will be your next steps in gaining greater comfort and skills estimating Axis V GAF scores?

4. This chapter's cases included two examples of case conceptualization and treatment planning using purist counselor theories and three examples of psychotherapeutic integration.

   a. What is your level of familiarity with the various adult counseling theories illustrated in this chapter: Cognitive Behavior Therapy and Behavior Therapy? Existential Counseling, and Psychodynamic Psychotherapy? Cognitive Stimulation Therapy? What do you believe are their relative strengths and weaknesses? For which individuals do they seem to be a good match? For what types of client concerns do they seem to be potentially effective? What do the evidence and discussions found in the current literature say about this?

   b. Which of these theories seem to be a good fit with your own attitudes and skills? Which interest you the most?

   c. To learn more, review the resources and references cited in the chapter, interview a practicing counselor who uses these theories in his or her everyday work, seek clinical supervision from a supervisor experienced with the approach, enroll in a special topics class, or look for continuing education workshops and conference presentations covering these approaches.

   d. What are your thoughts, reactions, and comfort level integrating multiple psycho-therapeutic approaches to address the needs of your clients? Which theories are you most likely, or least likely, to consider integrating into your approach? How will you decide when, with whom, and in what ways, to integrate multiple approaches? To consider and learn more about integrating approaches such as Cognitive Behavior Therapy with Existential Counseling or with Brief Psychodynamic Psychotherapy, or Behavior and Cognitive Stimulation Therapies, interview a practicing counselor who uses an integration of these theories in his or her everyday work, seek clinical supervision from a supervisor experienced with psychotherapeutic integration of these theories, or seek other professional consultations and learning opportunities.

5. The case conceptualizations found in this chapter began with casting a wide net for client concerns and dynamics, next forming intuitive-logical groupings to begin better understanding the clients' presentations, and then applying counseling theories to make clinical inferences about the clients' situations.

   a. How does this type of professional clinical thinking differ from your everyday thinking, conversation, and analysis about people? What are your levels of comfort, skill, and experience at this type of clinical thinking? What steps can you take to further develop or improve your conceptualizing skills?

   b. What are your thoughts, reactions, and critique of the ways these counselors grouped together: Jack Bauer's PTSD, Bereavement, and antisocial features—or Data's Major Depressive Disorder, Amnestic Disorder, and other counseling questions? Mrs. Petrillo's Cognitive Difficulties versus her Behavioral and Affective Difficulties? For George Lopez, distressing feelings, disruptive physiological symptoms, distressing thoughts, and dysfunctional behaviors? For Jack McFarland, two interesting groupings of recurrent mood and self-worth problems, distinguished from long-standing hyperactivity and other intrapersonal and interpersonal concerns? Do you agree with each of these thematic groupings? How might you have organized these differently, more usefully, or more effectively?

   c. What are your thoughts and reactions pertaining to the ways the counselors applied the various theoretical approaches in order to explain, make inferences about, and prepare for treatment planning with these clients? What were your reactions to the counselors' presentations of Jack Bauer's faulty beliefs and faulty core belief (Cognitive Behavior Therapy)? Lieutenant Commander Data's irrational and faulty beliefs and catastrophizing (Cognitive Behavior Therapy) and fears and anxieties and life conditions and the self (Existential Counseling)? Mrs. Petrillo's reduced awareness of behavioral antecedents and consequences (Behavioral Therapy) and various cognitive declines (Cognitive Stimulation)? George Lopez's choosing paining behaviors and external-control language (Reality Therapy)? Jack McFarland's irrational self-statements and core faulty beliefs (Cognitive Behavior Therapy) and use of defenses against fear of abandonment and disintegration of self (Psychodynamic Therapy)? Do you agree with the ways the counselor used the various theories with these clients? How might you have applied the theories differently, more usefully, or more effectively?

6. A fully developed treatment plan was presented for each of the individuals comprising this chapter's caseload. The treatment plans provide goals for change, interventions, and outcome measures.

   a. How does this type of clinical writing, thinking, and preparation for the professional counseling process differ from your everyday approach to engaging in helpful relationships with people? What are your levels of comfort, skill, and experience with this type of professional writing, thinking, and preparation? What steps can you take to further develop or improve your treatment planning skills for the types of practicum, internship, residency, or work settings that are of most interest to you?

   b. This chapter's treatment plans first list goals for change for each "client" character, next apply the selected counseling theory to clearly state the interventions and approaches to be used, and finally identify ways to measure the expected changes. What are your thoughts, reactions, and critique of the ways this chapter's counselors prepared Jack Bauer's, Data's, Mrs. Petrillo's, George Lopez's, and Jack McFarland's treatment plans? What interests you most about these plans? What raises questions for you?

   c. What are your thoughts and reactions pertaining to: cognitive behavioral techniques (Jack Bauer), use of behavioral and stimulation therapies (Mrs. Petrillo), reality therapy methods (George Lopez), cognitive behavioral techniques and existential approaches

(Data), and cognitive behavioral techniques and psychodynamic approaches (Jack McFarland) outlined as interventions? With which are you most familiar? Least familiar? Unfamiliar? Which will you select to learn more about through further reading, clinical supervision, or other professional development? Alternatively, which do not seem to be close fits with your own preferred approach?

d. These clients' counselors used counselor observation, client report, change scores on psychological measures and the GAF, behavioral reports, and other means to measure outcomes. As you review the outcome measures found on Jack Bauer's, Mrs. Petrillo's, George Lopez's, Data's, and Jack McFarland's treatment plans, consider these questions: Do the measures seem realistic and accomplishable? Are they concrete and specific enough to indicate change? Are they sensitive to the needs of the client? Which of these measures will become a regular part of your own repertoire, which might you decline to use, and what additional measures might you add to your own list? What new skills and competencies might you need to develop in order to effectively report on your own clients' outcomes?

7. Now, working independently, with a partner, or in a small group, select your own "client" from among the pop culture world of Adults in Television Sitcoms and Comedies. Develop your own narrative about the client's arrival at counseling. Then, prepare a fully completed Basic Case Summary, Diagnostic Impressions, Case Conceptualization, and Treatment Plan!

11

CHARACTERS IN MUSIC, MUSICALS, AND ADVERTISING

The Cases of Fred the Baker, Maria, Billie Jean, Eleanor Rigby, and the Geico Caveman

PREVIEW: POPULAR CULTURE THEMES

In this section, you will meet a group of characters who have been drawn from popular songs, Broadway musicals, and television advertising. Although we are attracted to music for different reasons, including the melody, the lyrics, or the rhythm, music videos provide us with an opportunity to engage with a particular song at a much deeper level. Similarly, musicals, by virtue of their multisensory appeal, are capable of drawing us in to a particular place, period in time, or life of a character. Television commercials are self-contained stories that often center on the life of a unique and entertaining individual.

Before exploring the lives of each of the characters, it is important to consider the role of popular song, music, and advertising in shaping our perception of people. Advertising, for example, far from a humanitarian force, is designed primarily to sell us a product, idea, or lifestyle. The implicit and explicit messages in television (and print) ads appeal to sensation-seeking needs of the audience (Leone & D'Arienzo, 2000), and capitalize upon our preconceived and often stereotypical perceptions of masculinity and femininity (Lamb & Brown, 2007; Lamb, Brown, & Tappan, 2009; Packwood-Freeman & Merskin, 2006) as well as mental health and mental illness (Rubin, 2006a). Music has historically been a powerful cultural force (Brooks, McCarthy, Ondaatje, & Zakaras, 2004; Vuust & Frith, 2008) and, in our society, a mirror into personal experience, particularly of adolescents (Gardstrom, 1999). With regard to musicals, it has been suggested that in addition to its entertainment value, the genre has offered powerful social, gender, and political commentary (Coleman & Sebesta, 2008; Jones, 2003). However, concern has come from many corners regarding the potentially destructive influence of certain musical genres, including heavy metal and rap (Lacourse, Claes, & Villenueve, 1999; Selfhout, Delsing, ter Bogt, & Meeus, 2008).

With regard to the specific characters in this section, Fred Wozniak is known to us as the dutiful and diligent Dunkin' Donuts baker who rises each morning before dawn with his singular task of making the donuts—in rain, shine, or snow. A symbol of steadfast dedication to customer satisfaction, Fred's motto of "time to make the donuts" has become an anthem to the American worker and part of our lexicon. In our presentation, Fred struggles with an Adjustment Disorder. Maria is the innocent and romantic female lead character in Leonard Bernstein's masterful and timeless musical tale about warring New York street gangs. Her songs of hope, love, and sadness have been sung for generations. In our presentation, Maria struggles with Acute Stress Disorder (ASD) and Bereavement. When the late Michael Jackson wrote the song "Billie Jean" for his record-breaking album *Thriller,* and then created a musical video around it to showcase his magical dancing, few could have anticipated its historic appeal. However, the back story of its main character, a pregnant teenage girl, has become anthemic. In our presentation, Billie Jean struggles with Delusional Disorder and Post-traumatic Stress Disorder (PTSD). Similarly, the Beatles' John Lennon and Paul McCartney could not have anticipated the widespread popularity and appeal of the tragic protagonist of their song "Eleanor Rigby," the lonely and lamenting church keep. In our presentation, Eleanor struggles with Mood Disorder Due to Hypothyroidism and Mild Mental Retardation. And finally, there is the caveman, whom we have named Neander Thal, the brunt of jokes in the highly popular and ubiquitous Geico Insurance commercials. While buying insurance is, as the commercial proclaims, "So easy a caveman can do it," this character struggles in many significant ways. In our presentation, the Caveman struggles with Adjustment Disorder and Acculturation Problem.

On the surface, this improbable group of characters may share very little in common as they differ in age, nationality, race, gender, and species and have been drawn from distant corners of the entertainment world. However, at their core, these are very real people with touching and very real stories, from Maria's shattered optimism to Eleanor's intractable sadness and loneliness to the frustration, resentment, and anger of the Geico Caveman, who suffers the very real stings of racial discrimination. In contrast to the dramatic tale of Billie Jean, Fred the Baker may seem rather mundane; however, he too must address significant life issues as he transitions from one phase of his life to the next. Taken together, Fred the Baker, Maria, Billie Jean, Eleanor Rigby, and the Geico Caveman will challenge your clinical decision-making.

APPROACHES TO LEARNING

As you learn about this group of characters, pay attention to:

- The different symptom patterns in adjustment disorders and other, more severe and long-standing disorders.
- The manner in which popular culture and, in particular, music and stage shows depict more severe psychological disturbance such as psychosis.
- How major life transitions such as retirement, the loss of a spouse, or having a child affect men and women differently.
- The way that different demographic groups experience acculturation and disenfranchisement, and how that might result in counseling needs.
- How you as a counselor might orient yourself differently to a client with ASD as opposed to PTSD.

CASE 11.1   DUNKIN' DONUTS' FRED THE BAKER

INTRODUCING THE CHARACTER

Fred is the well-known and much beloved Dunkin' Donuts baker featured in the company's print and television advertisements from 1982 to 1997. He was played by long-time character actor Michael Vale, who died at age 83 in December 2005. Dunkin' Donuts is an international retail chain that makes and sells its own coffee and donuts, and has been doing so since 1950. The "It's worth the trip" advertising campaign featuring Fred the Baker first aired in 1982 and was wildly successful. The campaign, was replaced by the equally successful "America Runs on Dunkin" campaign, which has only recently been supplanted with the "You Can Do It" slogan. Fred was the behind-the-scenes owner of a Dunkin' Donuts bakery who, like his counterparts in the U.S. Postal Service, would rise early in the morning and trudge to work through all kinds of weather because, in his words, "It's time to make the donuts." This trademark slogan became iconic in popular culture, representing the loyalty, perseverance, and passion of the American worker. Interestingly, Dunkin' Donuts customers were actually surveyed in anticipation of Fred's impending retirement, and after receiving their "permission," he was honored in Boston with a parade followed by Free Donut Day on September 22, 1997. The following basic case summary and diagnostic impressions describe the clinically significant distress we believe Fred may have confronted during the life-cycle transition of retirement.

Meet the Client

You can assess the client in action by viewing clips of Fred the Baker's video material at the following websites:

- http://www.youtube.com/watch?v=83mJ QXiG8Bw A Dunkin' Donuts Christmas
- http://www.youtube.com/watch?v= gwfrBbNo5Jg Time to make the donuts
- http://www.youtube.com/watch?v=5_ mfiw_lD9s&p=028D0C49D86F0BAB&p laynext=1&index=48 Fun in the kitchen with Fred

BASIC CASE SUMMARY

Identifying Information. Fred "the Baker" Wozniak is a 72-year-old retired white man of Polish heritage who lives in Boston, Massachusetts. Until recently, he was a career baker. He worked as the sole proprietor of one of

the busiest Dunkin' Donuts stores in Massachusetts for 15 years, prior to which he was a company baker at the main plant in Amherst, Massachusetts. Mr. Wozniak lives at home with his wife, Tatiana, to whom he has been married for 46 years.

Presenting Concern. Mr. Wozniak was referred through the Dunkin' Donuts employee assistance program (EAP) to the Greater Boston Community Mental Health Center, with a presenting concern of depression. According to his wife, since his retirement, Mr. Wozniak has been "sleeping all day, lying around on the couch, and refusing to even go out." Mr. Wozniak had also shown little interest in visiting long-time friends or family members who live close by. Mrs. Wozniak also noted that during her husband's sleep "he thrashes about, sleep walks, and is always mumbling 'Time to make the donuts.'"

Background, Family Information, and Relevant History. Fred Wozniak was born in Worcester, Massachusetts, the first of six children to Stefan and Yadwiga Wozniak, first-generation immigrants from Gdansk, Poland. He characterized his parents as "pursuing the American dream" and said that his parents took great pride in being Americans and honored their countries, both old and new, by having a large family. Fred, their first-born, remembers being "lavished with attention and love," and said he felt encouraged to "make my parents proud." His birth was soon followed in rapid succession by that of five other children, and because his parents had to work long hours in order to support their family, he was typically left in charge. This did not seem to faze Mr. Wozniak while growing up, and he readily embraced the role of big brother and assistant to his parents.

Mr. Wozniak made no plans to go to college and instead put his full energies into his studying and specializing in the high school culinary arts vocational track, from which he graduated with honors. Soon after graduating from high school, Mr. Wozniak enlisted in the military and spent several years overseas as the company cook, where he gained recognition and a reputation for responsibility, diligence, and willingness to feed his fellow man "no matter where we were in battle." After being honorably discharged from the military, Mr. Wozniak returned to Worcester and soon after married his teenage sweetheart, Tatiana. Enthusiastically looking forward to parenthood, the couple had triplets, followed by twins. Although overjoyed to have "a family as large as the one I grew up in," he recalled "not being quite ready to raise that many children." He immediately took a job at the local Dunkin' Donuts factory, working the early morning shift so that "I could be home with my family when the kids got home from school." Mr. Wozniak was a model employee who took great pride in his product and soon rose to the position of plant manager. Over the next several years, he and his wife raised their children to be close with family, work hard, and "give back to others."

When Mr. Wozniak was in his mid-50s, both of his parents died tragically in a subway accident. Although shocked and deeply saddened by this loss, Mr. Wozniak recalled thinking to himself, "I never realized how quickly things changed, and I started to worry that I really needed to make sure that my family was well taken care of, just in case something happened to me."

At age 60, Mr. Wozniak and his wife decided that they would take their life's savings and purchase a Dunkin' Donuts franchise. By that time, Mr. Wozniak's celebrity in the Worcester/Boston area, as well as his skill and dedication, resulted in one of the highest earning franchises in the entire Dunkin' Donuts chain. He continued to work long hours in order to ensure the success of his shop and received additional monies by playing the role of Fred the Baker on television commercials. However, the long hours standing on his feet, reaching into and out of an oven, and waking up early in the morning as well as his fondness for glazed crullers resulted in Type II diabetes and severe arthritis in his ankles. After working continuously for more than 55 years, Mr. Wozniak sold his beloved donut shop, and along with his wife, decided to "spend the rest of my life with my family," which by that time had grown to include 13 grandchildren and four great grandchildren. It was with great excitement and anticipation that everyone, according to his wife,

"looked forward to Poppa's retirement." They were quite surprised when soon after he left formal employment that Mr. Wozniak seemed to lose his interest in living.

Problem and Counseling History. Mr. and Mrs. Wozniak both attended his initial session at the Dunkin' Donuts Employee Assistance Program (DDEAP). The Wozniaks arrived 15 minutes late for the intake session and were clearly distressed. According to Mrs. Wozniak, "You'd think after 50 years working in the city, he'd know how to find his way around." Mr. Wozniak shot back, "Just point to the donut store and I know where to go . . . I never realized the city was so big." Mr. Wozniak presented as a tall, heavy-set man who sat rather uncomfortably in his chair, looking around the room, and in particular at the clinician's diplomas, in which regard he commented, "I never thought I'd end up in a therapist's office . . . a man lives his life, does his job, and this is where it all ends up?!" Mr. Wozniak indicated that he had never had a need for counseling and that "My job has been therapy enough for me, but I have to admit, I am feeling a little lost these days." Mr. Wozniak went on to describe the difficulty he has had adjusting to life without work and described periods of restlessness, irritability, and "this weird feeling like I've lost a big part of myself." He described difficulty falling asleep at night and "not eating much . . . not even my precious vanilla glazed crullers." Mr. Wozniak, a proud man, asserted that "I think once I find a new routine, something to feel good about, I'll be a lot better." Mr. Wozniak denies any suicidal ideation. His recent annual physical exam ruled out any effects of his diabetes or chronic arthritis, or medications treating these conditions, on his mood or behavior

Goals for Counseling and Course of Therapy to Date. Mr. Wozniak reluctantly agreed to return to the counseling center "to make my wife happy." He did express an interest in joining a local branch of Retired Bakers Anonymous (RBA) so that he could assist others who were having similar difficulties adjusting to retirement. Goals are to assist the client in returning to his previously adaptive levels of mood and functioning and to promote an effective retirement transition.

Diagnostic Impressions

Axis I.   309.0 Adjustment Disorder, Acute, With Depressed Mood

Axis II.   V71.09 No Diagnosis on Axis II

Axis III.   Type II Diabetes

Arthritis, Rheumatoid

Axis IV.   Problems related to the social environment—Adjustment to retirement, life-cycle transition

Axis V.   GAF = 60 (at intake)

GAF = 85 (highest level obtained from client's company medical records)

DISCUSSION OF DIAGNOSTIC IMPRESSIONS

Fred Wozniak was referred to the Greater Boston Community Mental Health Center through his EAP because of changes in his mood and behavior following his recent retirement. These changes included depressed mood, sleeping throughout the day, and lack of energy and ambition. He described feeling restless and irritable. He also reported some difficulties with sleep and appetite since retiring.

The *Diagnostic and Statistical Manual of Mental Disorders, Fourth Edition, Text Revision (DSM-IV-TR)* Adjustment Disorders all are clinically significant psychological responses to an identifiable life stressor. To meet the criteria for an Adjustment Disorder, the psychological responses must cause marked distress or clinically significant impairment in functioning, must go beyond normally expected and culturally appropriate reactions, and must not be due to another *DSM-IV-TR* disorder or a medical problem. Adjustment Disorders can occur with depressed mood, anxiety, disturbance in conduct or behavior, or have a combination of these.

In this case, Fred the Baker presented clinically significant responses to the life cycle transition of retirement, including mildly depressed mood and other signs of mild depression. His changes in mood and behavior arose within 3 months of the

onset of the stressor. In the absence of any evidence of substance abuse, and without any evidence that his symptoms meet the criteria for another diagnosable Axis I mood or anxiety disorder, the diagnosis is Adjustment Disorder. Because his concerns have lasted fewer than 3 months, the specifier Acute is used, and because he reported primarily depressive symptoms, the disorder is specified With Depressed Mood.

Distinguishing among physical, cognitive, affective, and behavioral factors influencing changes in older adult clients' functioning requires the counselor's special attention (Schlossberg, 1995). In this case, one consideration is whether Mr. Wozniak's depressive symptoms are a direct consequence of one of his general medical conditions, diabetes or arthritis. However, these were ruled out during his recent physical exam.

Besides general medical conditions, specific differential considerations when determining an Adjustment Disorder include other relevant Axis I diagnoses. However, Mr. Wozniak's experiences did not meet the criteria for any diagnosable Mood Disorder or Anxiety Disorder. Adjustment Disorder requires that the client's concerns develop within 3 months of the life event's onset; Mr. Wozniak presented increasing symptoms shortly after onset of his recent life stressors. Another consideration is whether the client's reactions are normally expected, culturally appropriate reactions that do not produce excessive distress or cause excessive impairment. However, his concerns were reported to cause clinically significant distress and some impairment in social functioning.

To finish the diagnosis, Mr. Wozniak's medical conditions are listed on Axis III, his relevant life stressor is emphasized on Axis IV, and on Axis V his functioning is represented by Global Assessment of Functioning (GAF) scores indicating that although at present he is experiencing moderate difficulties with functioning, earlier in the year he has demonstrated good functioning and the absence of concerns beyond everyday problems. The information on these axes is consistent with the Axis I diagnosis indicated.

CASE CONCEPTUALIZATION

During Fred the Baker's initial Dunkin' Donuts EAP appointment, his counselor at the Greater Boston Community Mental Health Center conducted a thorough intake and collected detailed information. The counselor first used this information to develop diagnostic impressions. Mr. Wozniak's EAP concerns were described as Adjustment Disorder associated with the stressor of retirement. Next, the counselor developed a case conceptualization. Whereas the purpose of diagnostic impressions is to *describe* the client's concerns, the goal of case conceptualization is to better *understand* and clinically *explain* the person's experiences (Neukrug & Schwitzer, 2006). It helps the counselor understand the sources of his difficulties and the factors maintaining them. In turn, case conceptualization sets the stage for treatment planning. Treatment planning then provides a road map that plots out how the counselor and client expect to move from presenting concerns to positive outcomes (Seligman, 1993, p. 157)—helping Fred better adjust to retirement.

When forming a case conceptualization, the clinician applies a purist counseling theory, an integration of two or more theories, an eclectic mix of theories, or a solution-focused combination of tactics, to his or her understanding of the client. In this case, Mr. Wozniak's counselor based his conceptualization on a purist theory, Person-Centered Therapy. The counselor selected this approach because it is the primary counseling method used at the Greater Boston Community Mental Health Center when the clinician believes the client has the capabilities to use the therapeutic experience to gain self-understanding, improve self-direction, make his or her own constructive changes, and act effectively and productively, and when facilitating the client's own self-directed adjustment seems to be a desired outcome (Rogers, 1986)—as in the case of Mr. Wozniak, who has a lifelong history of successful adjustment.

The counselor used the Inverted Pyramid Method of case conceptualization because this method is especially designed to help clinicians more easily form their conceptual pictures of their clients' needs (Neukrug & Schwitzer, 2006; Schwitzer, 1996, 1997). The method has four steps: Problem Identification, Thematic Groupings, Theoretical Inferences, and Narrowed Inferences. The counselor's clinical thinking can be seen in Figure 11.1.

Step 1: Problem Identification. The first step is Problem Identification. Aspects of the presenting problem (thoughts, feelings, behaviors, physiological features), additional areas of concern besides the presenting concern, family and developmental history, in-session observations, clinical inquiries (medical problems, medications, past counseling, substance use, suicidality), and psychological assessments (problem checklists, personality inventories, mental status exam, specific clinical measures) all may contribute information at Step 1. The counselor "casts a wide net" in order to build Step 1 as exhaustively as possible (Neukrug & Schwitzer, 2006, p. 202). As can be seen in Figure 11.1, the counselor identified at Step 1 all of Fred's main reasons for his current visit (low mood and other depressive symptoms following retirement); information about his adjustment before the current transition (past feelings of pride, success, etc.); and physical ailments. The counselor went beyond just listing "retirement" as the main reason for referral and was as complete as he could be about the present and relevant past.

Step 2: Thematic Groupings. The second step is Thematic Groupings. The clinician organizes all of the exhaustive client information found in Step 1 into just a few intuitive-logical clinical groups, categories, or themes on the basis of sensible common denominators (Neukrug & Schwitzer, 2006). Four different ways of forming the Step 2 theme groups can be used: Descriptive-Diagnosis Approach, Clinical Targets Approach, Areas of Dysfunction Approach, and Intrapsychic Approach. As can be seen in the figure, Mr. Wozniak's counselor selected the Clinical Targets Approach. This approach sorts together all of the Step 1 information into "the basic division of behavior, thoughts, feelings, and physiology" (Neukrug & Schwitzer, 2006, p. 205).

The counselor formed the following groupings: (a) Past versus present thoughts (combining past satisfaction in giving back, current lack of identified interests); (b) Past versus present behaviors (work as a war cook, franchise ownership, early morning baker, lying around house, restless behavior, low motivation to act); (c) Past versus present mood (pride, depressed mood, irritability); and (d) Past versus present physiology (development of diabetes and arthritis; sleep difficulties, fatigue, and low energy). His conceptual work at Step 2 gave the counselor a way to begin organizing Fred the Baker's areas of functioning more clearly.

So far, at Steps 1 and 2, the counselor has used his clinical assessment skills and his clinical judgment to begin meaningfully understanding Mr. Wozniak's needs. Now, at Steps 3 and 4, he applies the theoretical approach he has selected. He begins making theoretical inferences to understand the processes underlying the client's concerns as they are seen in Steps 1 and 2.

Step 3: Theoretical Inferences. At Step 3, concepts from the counselor's selected therapy, Person-Centered Therapy, are applied to explain the factors maintaining Mr. Wozniak's present adjustment difficulties. The counselor tentatively matches the theme groups in Step 2 with this theoretical approach. In other words, the symptom constellations in Step 2, which were distilled from the symptoms in Step 1, now are combined using theory to show what are believed to be the underlying causes or psychological etiology of Mr. Wozniak's current needs (Neukrug & Schwitzer, 2006; Schwitzer, 2006, 2007).

According to Person-Centered Therapy, individuals are capable of self-understanding and self-direction. Further, under the correct conditions, individuals progressively experience greater self-realization, fulfillment, autonomy, self-determination, and self-perfection as their lives progress, in a process referred to as the actualizing tendency (Broadley, 1999). The needed conditions are empathy, accurate understanding, and positive regard from the important others in our lives (Bohart & Greenberg, 1997; Rogers, 1961, 1977)—along with other situations that create for us a growth-producing climate. In other words, when their interpersonal climate is growth-producing, individuals move forward toward their own self-fulfillment across the life span (Thorne, 2002). Conversely, according to the theory, lack of empathy, accurate understanding, and positive regard from the important others in our lives—and the absence of roles and situations that are growth-producing—can disrupt or derail forward actualizing movement and result in maladjustment (Broadley, 1999; Rogers, 1961, 1977, 1986).

As can be seen in Figure 11.1, when the counselor applied these Person-Centered Therapy concepts, he explained at Step 3 that the various issues noted in Step 1 (the various recent and current symptoms of depression, etc.), which can be understood to be themes of past versus present thoughts, behaviors, mood, and physiology at Step 2, together comprise a situation in which Fred is experiencing "loss of primary sources of self-worth and self-actualization." According to Person-Centered Therapy inferences, lacking these sources of worth and actualization (i.e., losing important relationships with customers, staff, and business associates that provided empathy and positive regard; losing productive satisfactions and giving back and successes of being an American small businessman and cook) has led to Mr. Wozniak's changes in mood, thinking, actions, and physical well-being. The theme appears on Figure 11.1.

Step 4: Narrowed Inferences. At Step 4, the clinician's selected theory continues to be used to address still-deeper issues when they exist (Schwitzer, 2006, 2007). At this step, "still-deeper, more encompassing, or more central, causal themes" are formed (Neukrug & Schwitzer, 2006, p. 207). Continuing to apply Person-Centered Therapy concepts at Step 4, Mr. Wozniak's counselor presented the deeper implication of his loss of sources of self-worth from his work life, specifically, "Questioning the enduring value of his life." The counselor borrows from Erikson's psychosocial stage model of development (Crain, 1992; Erikson, 1950; Miller, 1993) to infer that Mr. Wozniak is grappling with the question of whether, on one hand, his life will have been of enduring value, he will leave a positive mark on the world through his years of work life and family life, and he will have been an example for others to follow (known as generativity), or, on the other hand, his life has been narrow, and therefore produces letdown and feelings of psychological impoverishment (known as stagnation). According to the theory, solving this question is needed for Mr. Wozniak to return to his progress toward self-actualization. These developmental concepts are compatible and can be helpful when applying the Person-Centered Theory to a client's life transitions (Rogers, 1986).

When all four steps are completed, the client information in Step 1 leads to logical-intuitive groupings on the basis of common denominators in Step 2, the groupings then are explained using theory at Step 3, and then, finally, at Step 4, further deeper explanations are made. From start to finish, the thoughts, feelings, behaviors, and physiological features in the topmost portions are connected on down the pyramid into deepest dynamics.

The completed pyramid now is used to plan treatment, in which the counselor will engage Mr. Wozniak with congruence, unconditional positive regard, and accurate empathy to promote his transition from past to present sources of self-worth and self-actualization, and resolve his questions of generativity versus stagnation at retirement.

TREATMENT PLANNING

At this point, Mr. Wozniak's clinician at DDEAP has collected all available information about the problems that have been of concern to him and his wife. Based upon this information, the counselor developed a five-axis *DSM-IV-TR* diagnosis and then, using the "inverted pyramid" (Neukrug & Schwitzer, 2006; Schwitzer, 1996, 1997), formulated a working clinical *explanation* of Mr. Wozniak's difficulties and their etiology that we called the *case conceptualization.* This, in turn, guides us to the next critical step in our clinical work, called the *treatment plan,* the primary purpose of which is to map out a logical and goal-oriented strategy for making positive changes in the client's life. In essence, the treatment plan is a road map *"for reducing or eliminating disruptive symptoms that are impeding the client's ability to reach positive mental health outcomes"* (Neukrug & Schwitzer, 2006, p. 225). As such, it is the cornerstone of our work with not only Mr. Wozniak, but with all clients who present with disruptive symptoms (Jongsma, Peterson, & McInnis, 2003a, 2003b; Jongsma & Peterson, 2006; Seligman, 1993, 1998, 2004).

A comprehensive treatment plan must integrate all of the information from the biopsychosocial interview, diagnosis, and case conceptualization into a coherent plan of action. This *plan* comprises four main components, which include (1) A behavioral definition of the problem(s), (2) the selection of achievable goals, (3) the determination of treatment modes, and (4) the documentation of how change will be measured. The *behavioral*

Figure 11.1   Fred the Baker's Inverted Pyramid Case Conceptualization Summary: Person-Centered Counseling

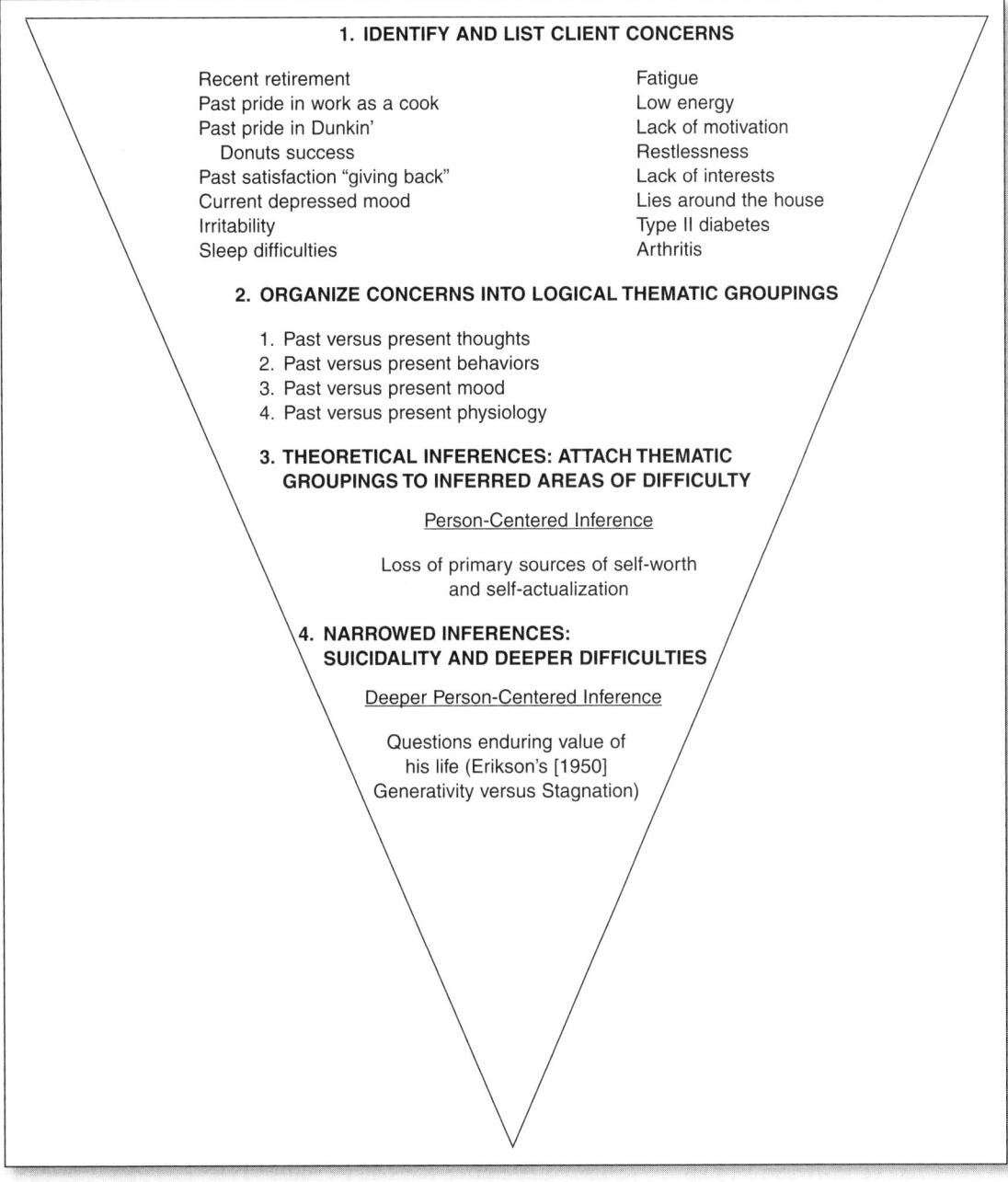

1. IDENTIFY AND LIST CLIENT CONCERNS

Recent retirement
Past pride in work as a cook
Past pride in Dunkin'
   Donuts success
Past satisfaction "giving back"
Current depressed mood
Irritability
Sleep difficulties

Fatigue
Low energy
Lack of motivation
Restlessness
Lack of interests
Lies around the house
Type II diabetes
Arthritis

2. ORGANIZE CONCERNS INTO LOGICAL THEMATIC GROUPINGS

1. Past versus present thoughts
2. Past versus present behaviors
3. Past versus present mood
4. Past versus present physiology

**3. THEORETICAL INFERENCES: ATTACH THEMATIC
GROUPINGS TO INFERRED AREAS OF DIFFICULTY**

Person-Centered Inference

Loss of primary sources of self-worth
and self-actualization

**4. NARROWED INFERENCES:
SUICIDALITY AND DEEPER DIFFICULTIES**

Deeper Person-Centered Inference

Questions enduring value of
his life (Erikson's [1950]
Generativity versus Stagnation)

definition of the problem(s) consolidates the results of the case conceptualization into a concise hierarchical list of problems and concerns that will be the focus of treatment. The *selection of achievable goals* refers to assessing and prioritizing the client's concerns into a *hierarchy of urgency* that also takes into account the client's motivation for change, level of dysfunction, and real-world influences on his or her problems. The *determination of treatment modes* refers to selection of the specific interventions, which are matched to the uniqueness of the client and to his or her goals and clearly tied to a particular theoretical orientation (Neukrug & Schwitzer, 2006). Finally, the clinician must establish how change will be measured, based upon a number of factors, including client records and self-report of change, in-session observations by the clinician, clinician ratings, results of standardized evaluations such as the Beck Depression Inventory (Beck, 1996) or a family functioning questionnaire, pre-post treatment comparisons, and reports by other treating professionals.

The four-step method discussed above can be seen in Figure 6.1 (p. 109) and is outlined below for the case of Mr. Wozniak, followed by his specific treatment plan.

Step 1: Behavioral Definition of Problems. The first step in treatment planning is to carefully review the case conceptualization, paying particular attention to the results of Step 2 (Thematic Groupings), Step 3 (Theoretical Inferences), and Step 4 (Narrowed Inferences). The identified clinical themes reflect the core areas of concern and distress for the client, while the theoretical and narrowed inferences offer clinical speculation as to their origins. In the case of Mr. Wozniak, there are four primary areas of concern. The first, "past versus present thoughts," refers to the difference between his historic pride in his work as a cook and success in the business world with his current negative and pessimistic thinking and outlook. The second, "past versus current behaviors," refers to

his sleep difficulties, fatigue and low energy, lack of interest, and lying around the house. The third, "past versus present mood," refers to the difference between his historic optimism, good mood, and even temperament with his current depressed mood and pessimism. The fourth, "past versus current physiology," refers to the difference between his historic high energy level and calm demeanor with his current irritability and restlessness. These symptoms and stresses are consistent with the diagnosis of Adjustment Disorder, Acute With Depressed Mood, and medical conditions on Axis III (Diabetes and Rheumatoid Arthritis) (APA, 2000a; Casey, Dorwick, & Wilkinson, 2001; Strain et al., 1998).

Step 2: Identify and Articulate Goals for Change. The second step is the selection of achievable goals, which is based upon a number of factors, including the most pressing or urgent behavioral, emotional, and interpersonal concerns and symptoms as identified by the client and clinician, the willingness and ability of the client to work on those particular goals, and the realistic (real-world) achievability of those goals (Neukrug & Schwitzer, 2006). At this stage of treatment planning, it is important to recognize that not all of the client's problems can be addressed at once, so we focus initially on those that cause the greatest distress and impairment. New goals can be created as old ones are achieved. In the case of Mr. Wozniak, the goals are divided into four prominent clusters. The first, "past versus present thoughts," requires that we help Mr. Wozniak to explore his health and mortality issues and address his self-defeating thoughts. The second, "past versus current behaviors," requires that we assist Mr. Wozniak to improve the quality of his daily activities and motivation to engage in them. The third, "past versus current mood," requires that we explore the basis for Mr. Wozniak's depressed mood and help him to improve it. The last, "past versus current physiology," requires that we assist Mr. Wozniak in improving his overall health and health care behaviors.

Step 3: Describe Therapeutic Interventions. This is perhaps the most critical step in the treatment planning process because the clinician must now integrate information from a number of sources, including the case conceptualization, the delineation of the client's problems and goals, and the treatment literature, paying particular attention to *empirically supported treatment* (EST) and *evidence-based practice* (EBP). In essence, the clinician must align his or her treatment approach with scientific evidence from the fields of counseling and psychotherapy. Wampold (2001) identifies two types of evidence-based counseling research: studies that demonstrate "absolute efficacy," that is, the fact that counseling and psychotherapy work, and those that demonstrate "relative efficacy," that is, the fact that certain theoretical/ technical approaches work best for certain clients with particular problems (Psychoanalysis, Gestalt Therapy, Cognitive Behavior Therapy, Brief Solution-Focused Therapy, Cognitive Therapy, Dialectical Behavior Therapy, Person-Centered Therapy, Expressive/Creative Therapies, Interpersonal Therapy, and Feminist Therapy); and when delivered through specific treatment modalities (individual, group, and family counseling). In the case of Mr. Wozniak, we have decided to use Person-Centered Counseling (Bohart & Greenberg, 1997; Broadley, 1999; Carkhuff, 2000; Raskin & Rogers, 2000; Rogers, 1961, 1977) due to its humanistic emphasis on each person's inherent capacity for self-determination, growth, and actualization. Given Mr. Wozniak's past successes and achievements as well as previous positive self-regard, the therapeutic conditions of unconditional positive regard, genuineness, empathy, and congruence would help him to understand the unforeseen emotional, behavioral, and cognitive stresses of retirement and the importance of maintaining his health. Additionally, the nondirective nature of client-centered counseling would facilitate Mr. Wozniak's adjustment to his entirely different life after work, and plan for as well as enjoy the fruits of his "golden years." The highly supportive nature of this type of counseling with the elderly, particularly those who are coping with retirement (Lowis, Edwards, & Burton, 2009) and medical conditions (Chewning & Sleath, 1996; Eales, Keating, & Damsma, 2001), in conjunction with psychoeducation (Haight & Gibson, 2005) and creative activities (Butler, 2001; Duffey, 2005) has been found to be effective with adults at this stage of life who are coping with issues similar to Mr. Wozniak's. Specific techniques will include life review, retirement planning, health care maintenance, and diabetes group support.

Step 4: Provide Outcome Measures of Change. This last step in treatment planning requires that we specify how change will be measured and indicate the extent to which progress has been made toward realizing these goals (Neukrug & Schwitzer, 2006). The counselor has considerable flexibility in this phase, and may choose from a number of objective domains (psychological tests and measures of self-esteem, depression, psychosis, interpersonal relationship, anxiety, etc.), quasi-objective measures (the *DSM-IV-TR's* Axis V GAF scale; pre-post clinician, client, and psychiatric ratings), and subjective ratings (client self-report, clinician's in-session observations). In Mr. Wozniak's case, we have implemented a number of these, including pre-post measures on the Retirement Satisfaction Inventory (Floyd et al., 1992) and Beck Depression Inventory-II (Beck, Steer, & Brown, 1996), client report of improvement in overall life satisfaction and spouse's report of her husband's improvement in mood, activity level, and outlook

The completed treatment plan is now developed through which the counselor and Mr. Wozniak will be able to use emotional, behavioral, and cognitive awareness and skills to address mortality issues and enjoy, along with his wife, the retirement years. Fred the Baker's treatment plan follows and is summarized in Table 11.1.

TREATMENT PLAN

Client: Fred Wozniak

Service Provider: Greater Boston Community Mental Health Center

BEHAVIORAL DEFINITION OF PROBLEMS:

1. Past versus present thoughts—The difference between his historic pride in his work as a cook and success in the business world with his current negative and pessimistic thinking and outlook

2. Past versus present behaviors—The difference between his past enthusiasm, initiative, restful sleep, and focused/productive behavior with his current sleep difficulties, fatigue, and low energy, lack of interests, lying around the house

3. Past versus current mood—The difference between his historic optimism, good mood, and even temperament with his current depressed mood and pessimism

4. Past versus present physiology—Difference between his historic high energy level and calm demeanor with his current irritability and restlessness

GOALS FOR CHANGE:

1. Past versus present thoughts

   • Gradual reduction and elimination of self-defeating thoughts
   • Exploration of thoughts regarding retirement
   • Understanding and expression of mortality concerns

2. Past versus current behaviors

   • Improve the quality of sleep and activities of daily living (ADLs)
   • Develop fulfilling post-retirement activity plan, including leisure and family-related activities

3. Past versus current mood

   • Exploration of relationship between retirement and current mood
   • Improvement in mood
   • Insight into and elimination of depression

4. Past versus current physiology

   • Improved physical self-care, including nutrition and exercise
   • Strengthen compliance with medical treatment

THERAPEUTIC INTERVENTIONS:

A short-term course of individual client-centered counseling (2–3 months) supplemented with psychoeducational group support.

1. Past versus current thoughts

   - Engage in life review with focus on accomplishments
   - Attend retirement-based psychoeducational support group
   - Identify and refute irrational thoughts about productivity and self-worth
   - Identify fear-based thoughts related to diabetes and aging

2. Past versus current behaviors

   - Volunteer in the Dunkin' Donuts Entrepreneurial Mentoring Program
   - Structured plan to travel and visit with children and grandchildren

3. Past versus current mood

   - Express feelings of disappointment and loss related to retirement
   - Verbalize understanding of the relationship between depressed mood and thoughts and feelings regarding retirement and mortality

4. Past versus current physiology

   - Consultation with a nutritionist with specific experience in diabetes management
   - Membership in local retiree's exercise group
   - Practice relaxation techniques, including guided imagery and focused breathing
   - Enlist assistance and support of spouse around medical concerns and care
   - Attendance in diabetes support group supplemented with bibilotherapy on diabetes

OUTCOME MEASURES OF CHANGE:

The development of congruence between his ideal and actual self, improved self-esteem, greater capacity for understanding and expression of feelings, healthy attitudes toward retirement, improved mood and energy level, productive and enjoyable use of leisure time, and good health as measured by:

- Stabilization of clinician's rating of client's GAF to the mild range (>70)
- Pre-post improvement of scores on Retirement Satisfaction Inventory
- Client report of improved overall life satisfaction
- Improved pre-post scores on Beck Depression Inventory II
- Client self-reported compliance with medical and health-related/exercise activities
- Spouse's report of improved overall mood, outlook, and activity level

Table 11.1   Fred the Baker's Treatment Plan Summary: Person-Centered Therapy

Goals for Change	Therapeutic Interventions	Outcome Measures of Change
Past versus present thoughts	Past versus current thoughts	The development of congruence between his ideal and actual self, improved self-esteem, greater capacity for understanding and expression of feelings, healthy attitudes toward retirement, improved mood and energy level, productive and enjoyable use of leisure time, and good health as measured by:
Gradual reduction and elimination of self-defeating thoughts	Engage in life review with focus on accomplishments	
	Attend retirement-based psychoeducational support group	
Exploration of thoughts regarding retirement	Identify and refute irrational thoughts about productivity and self-worth	
Understanding and expression of mortality concerns	Identify fear-based thoughts related to diabetes and aging	Stabilization of clinician's rating of client's GAF to the mild range (>70)
Past versus current behaviors		
Improve the quality of sleep and activities of daily living (ADLs)	Past versus current behaviors	Pre-post improvement of scores on Retirement Satisfaction Inventory
	Volunteer in the Dunkin' Donuts Entrepreneurial Mentoring Program	
Develop fulfilling post-retirement activity plan including leisure and family-related activities	Structured plan to travel and visit with children and grandchildren	Client report of improved overall life-satisfaction
	Past versus current mood	Improved pre-post scores on Beck Depression Inventory II
Past versus current mood		
Exploration of relationship between retirement and current mood	Express feelings of disappointment and loss related to retirement	Client self-reported compliance with medical and health-related/exercise activities
Improvement in mood	Verbalize understanding of the relationship between depressed mood and thoughts and feelings regarding retirement and mortality	Spouse's report of improved overall mood, outlook, and activity level
Insight into and elimination of depression		
Past versus current physiology	Past versus current physiology	
Improved physical self-care including nutrition and exercise	Consultation with a nutritionist with specific experience in diabetes management	
	Membership in local retiree's exercise group	
Strengthen compliance with medical treatment	Practice relaxation techniques, including guided imagery and focused breathing	
	Enlist assistance and support of spouse around medical concerns and care	
	Attendance in diabetes support group supplemented with bibilotherapy on diabetes	

CASE 11.2 *WEST SIDE STORY'S* MARIA

INTRODUCING THE CHARACTER

Maria is the female lead in the 1957 Broadway musical *West Side Story,* which was written by Arthur Laurents, with music composed by Leonard Bernstein and lyrics by Stephen Sondheim. Four years later, it was made into an Oscar-award-winning film of the same title starring Natalie Wood. The story follows two rival New York City street gangs and is loosely based upon William Shakespeare's *Romeo and Juliet.* In a somewhat classical character portrayal, in both the play and the movie Maria is presented as a stunning young woman with a gentle demeanor and elements of old-world charm.

At the beginning of the story, the audience is introduced to the Sharks and the Jets, two warring gangs in New York City. As the "rumble" musically unfolds, the audience soon understands that the thuggery and bravado that is wielded along with knives and chains is a metaphor for the deep racial and cultural tensions that divide the Puerto Rican Sharks and the Caucasian Jets. Maria, sister of Bernardo, who is the leader of the Sharks, falls in love with Tony, who is a member of the rival gang. The poignancy of the love story is counterposed against the brutal racial violence between the two factions. Ultimately, the violence first takes the life of Bernardo and then that of Tony, leaving Maria behind to mourn the senseless losses of both her brother and her lover. The following basic case summary and diagnostic impressions present our portrayal of Maria's distressing and dysfunctional reactions to witnessing the story's violent traumatic events and her normally expected grief reactions.

Meet the Client

You can assess the client in action by viewing clips of Maria's video material at the following websites:

- http://www.youtube.com/watch?v=4 oxfOncYiag *A Boy Like That*
- http://www.youtube.com/watch?v=5_ QffCZs-bg *Tonight*
- http://www.youtube.com/watch?v= Ye7PlyIcCro *I Feel Pretty*

BASIC CASE SUMMARY

Identifying Information. Maria is an 18-year-old Puerto Rican high school student who lives in a two-bedroom apartment in the Bowery section of New York City with her cousin and friend, Anita. Maria is a recent transfer student from San Juan High School in Puerto Rico. She reported that she was several weeks pregnant.

Presenting Concern. Maria was escorted to the Bowery Community Services Center by Anita, who has become increasingly concerned by her friend's behavior, saying that Maria has been having "*ataques de nervios*" (attacks of the nerves). She noted that Maria has not eaten for the last several days, has refused to leave the apartment in order to attend classes, has been "talking crazy like she wants to die," and has not been taking care of herself. Anita dates these changes to the death of Maria's boyfriend Tony during a gang fight the previous week.

Anita also said that ever since witnessing the murder from a close-by window, Maria has avoided going anywhere near the Bowery streets where the violence took place. Anita also reported that although previously her friend has "always been a calm girl," ever since the stabbings Maria has become a *"persona nerviosa"* (a nervous person). Anita said that Maria does not sleep very much, but that when she does, she hears her calling out in their apartment during nightmares. Also according to Anita, during the day Maria seems to be in a daze, is not able to focus on school or even simple activities like watching television. Correspondingly, in the interview, Maria did not appear to be completely present in the room, and said she has been feeling "like I am watching myself walk through the world."

Background, Family Information, and Relevant History. Maria was born in Cidra, a small municipality of Puerto Rico, the oldest of three female children to parents who lived in poverty. Maria's father, Raul Escobar, whom Anita and Maria both described as a calm yet very rigid and traditional man, worked alongside his wife, Costanza, in a local garment factory. Wanting more for their daughter, Raul Escobar and Costanza encouraged Maria to do well in school and made plans for her to marry Chino Rodriguez, who had earlier relocated to New York City. Their apparent hope was that she could live with her brother Bernardo while she got to know Chino. The parents did not know that both Chino and Bernardo had become members of a New York street gang.

Described by Anita as "a dreamer who loved romance novels and soap operas," Maria wanted more out of life and wanted to marry someone of her own choice rather than a man chosen for her by her parents. As a result, Maria boarded a bus the day after she finished her sophomore year in high school and traveled to New York to live with her friend Anita, a dressmaker. There, she enrolled in Fiorello LaGuardia High School and became active in the school's musical department. While staging a production of *Romeo and Juliet,* she met Tony, to whom she was immediately attracted. Anita vehemently protested the relationship because Tony was Anglo and belonged to a rival gang, the Jets.

Following Maria's junior year in high school, her parents, with whom she had remained in contact, urged her to return to Puerto Rico so that she could begin plans to marry the man they had selected for her. Mr. and Mrs. Escobar were not aware that by that time Maria was already in love with Tony and deeply embroiled in the social politics of the neighborhood gangs. Her friend, Anita, also urged her to return home so that she could be safe from the "poison of the street gangs." As it was described in the interview, in spite of the desires of both her cousin and her parents, Maria chose to remain in New York and planned to leave high school to get a job in a local garment factory so that she and Tony could have their own life. At the time that she was brought to the counseling center by Anita, Tony had recently been killed in a violent gang battle that Maria had witnessed.

Problem and Counseling History. Maria was accompanied by her friend Anita to the first counseling session and seemed almost inert. Slumping in her chair and staring at the floor, Maria offered very little of the above information, interjecting at times "I just want to die," and "life has no meaning without Tony." She answered questions in a monosyllabic fashion, offering little spontaneous information, and crying almost continually throughout the interview. She made minimal eye contact, moved and talked very slowly, and was unkempt and poorly groomed. At one point, when Anita was providing details surrounding Tony's death, Maria erupted into a rage that she directed toward Anita who firmly yet lovingly comforted and quieted her. Maria commented that she came to New York to have a better life and had now discovered "the true meaning of anger and hatred." Maria asserted that she did not want to be in counseling and that perhaps she should return to her family in Puerto Rico to "do my parents bidding and lead the life they wanted me to."

Goals for Counseling and Course of Therapy to Date. Shortly after Tony's death, she was referred to the school clinic where the psychiatrist recommended medication "for what I think he called depression"; however Maria was worried about the effect of any drug on her pregnancy. The clinic psychiatrist had been concerned about Maria's complaints that she was not sleeping, was having nightmares about and flashbacks to Tony's murder, and was reluctant to walk past the schoolyard where the slaying occurred.

This evaluation session suggests that Maria may be experiencing symptoms of Acute Stress Disorder (ASD) with possible graduation in time to PTSD. Although Maria refused a request that she return to the clinic psychiatrist for follow-up, she agreed at the urging of her cousin to remain in New York for at least the next school year. She also agreed to return for regular ongoing counseling sessions at the Bowery Community Services Center for "*consejo*" (advice or counsel). Immediate goals are to develop and implement an individual counseling treatment plan addressing acute stress symptoms. Eventual goals are to resolve grief and loss issues via individual counseling and/or participation in a support group.

Diagnostic Impressions

Axis I.   308.3 Acute Stress Disorder

V62.82 Bereavement

Axis II.   V71.09 No Diagnosis on Axis II

Axis III. Pregnancy, Early Stages

Axis IV.   Problem related to social environment—Death of intimate partner

Other psychosocial and environmental problems—Exposure to gang violence, exposure to hostile racial climate

Axis V.   GAF = 50 (current)

GAF = 95 (highest level past year)

DISCUSSION OF
DIAGNOSTIC IMPRESSIONS

Maria was brought to the Bowery Community Services Center because her cousin was concerned about her "being in a daze," not sleeping or at other times having nightmares, and having difficulties concentrating on school or focusing on television shows. In the interview, Maria appeared not quite emotionally present and said she feels as though she is "watching herself." As the case discussed, she recently witnessed her boyfriend's murder during gang violence.

The predominant feature shared by all of the diagnosable disorders found in the Anxiety Disorders section of the *DSM-IV-TR* is the presence of panic, increased arousal, excessive worry, or other signs of anxiety that cause distress or impairment. Among these are Acute Stress Disorder and PTSD, both of which, by definition, occur only in the aftermath of, or as a result of, a traumatic life event.

This case described Maria's clinically significant negative reactions to her exposure to a traumatic experience in which she witnessed the actual death of someone close to her. She also witnessed serious injury to others during the gang fight. She reacted with intense fear and horror at her boyfriend's death. These characteristics meet the *DSM-IV-TR* definition of a traumatic event. Following the event, Maria has been experiencing dissociative symptoms, including: reduced awareness of her surroundings (she feels "in a daze"), derealization (she has the sensation of watching herself), and feelings of numbed detachment. She has been reexperiencing the event during nightmares. She has also been avoiding conversation when it centers on the event. She has signs of anxiety, including sleep disruption. According to the case timeline, it has been several days since the traumatic event. These factors indicate a diagnosis of Acute Stress Disorder.

Differential diagnosis requires effectively understanding the client's concerns. Accurately identifying and describing the counseling presentations of Latino/Latina clients may require the counselor's special attention (Bernal & Saez-Santiago, 2006). In this case, Maria's cousin described her dissociative and other symptoms in the cultural context of becoming a *persona nerviosa* who was experiencing *ataques de nervios*. Accurate assessment and diagnosis may require clinicians to recognize and understand such cultural contexts and meanings in their work with some of their Hispanic clients (Mendez-Villarrubia & LaBruzza, 1994).

Specific differential diagnoses might include PTSD and Adjustment Disorder. However, PTSD requires more than 1 month of symptoms, whereas ASD is the diagnosis of choice when symptoms occur within 1 month of a severe stressor and have not lasted beyond 4 weeks (should her symptoms persist, the diagnosis may later change to PTSD). Whereas Adjustment Disorders are negative reactions to any sort of life stressors, in this case, Maria has experienced exposure to an extreme stressor meeting the diagnostic definition of trauma, and her reactions conform to the specific constellation of symptoms characteristic of ASD and PTSD, which go beyond the general criteria set for Adjustment Disorder.

Further, along with all the various diagnosable disorders, a multiaxial diagnosis also lists Other Conditions That May Be a Focus of Clinical Attention. The client concerns contained in this section (appearing at the end of the *DSM-IV-TR,* following all of the diagnosable disorders) are not diagnosable mental disorders according to the *DSM* classification system; instead, they sometimes are client problems that are a focus of counseling but not a part of the individual's diagnosable mental disorder. Maria's grief reactions, or Bereavement, are in this category.

To round out the diagnosis, Maria's pregnancy is listed on Axis III because the baby is a painful reminder of her dead boyfriend, her critical psychosocial stressors are emphasized on Axis IV, and on Axis V her functioning is represented by GAF scores indicating that although at present she is experiencing serious difficulties that are impairing her functioning, before the trauma she had been demonstrating superior functioning. The information on these axes is consistent with the Axis I diagnosis indicated.

CASE CONCEPTUALIZATION

The counselor to whom Maria was assigned at the Bowery Community Services Center closely listened to Maria and collected information. Her counselor first used this information to develop diagnostic impressions. Her concerns were described by ASD and Bereavement. Next, her counselor developed a case conceptualization. Whereas the purpose of diagnostic impressions is to *describe* the client's concerns, the goal of case conceptualization is to better *understand* and clinically *explain* the person's experiences (Neukrug & Schwitzer, 2006). It helps the counselor understand the etiology leading to Maria's acute stress reactions and the factors maintaining them. In turn, case conceptualization sets the stage for treatment planning. Treatment planning then provides a road map that plots out how the counselor and client expect to move from presenting concerns to positive outcomes (Seligman, 1993, p. 157)—ideally, assisting Maria to manage or eliminate the problematic trauma reactions and related concerns that led her cousin to bring her to the center.

When forming a case conceptualization, the clinician applies a purist counseling theory, an integration of two or more theories, an eclectic mix of theories, or a solution-focused combination of tactics, to his or her understanding of the client. In this case, Maria's counselor based her conceptualization on a purist theory, Cognitive Behavior Therapy. She selected this approach based on her knowledge of current outcome research with clients experiencing ASD, PTSD, and similar reactions (Bradley, Greene, Russ, Dutra, & Westen, 2005; Foa & Keane, 2000). Cognitive Behavior Therapy also an approach of choice at the Bowery Community Services Center.

The counselor used the Inverted Pyramid Method of case conceptualization because this method is especially designed to help clinicians more easily form their conceptual pictures of their clients' needs (Neukrug & Schwitzer, 2006; Schwitzer, 1996, 1997). The method has four steps: Problem Identification, Thematic Groupings, Theoretical Inferences, and Narrowed Inferences. The counselor's clinical thinking can be seen in Figure 11.2.

Step 1: Problem Identification. The first step is Problem Identification. Aspects of the presenting problem (thoughts, feelings, behaviors, physiological features), additional areas of concern besides the presenting concern, family and developmental history, in-session observations, clinical inquiries (medical problems, medications, past counseling, substance use, suicidality), and psychological assessments (problem checklists, personality inventories, mental status exam, specific clinical measures) all may contribute information at Step 1. The counselor "casts a wide net" in order to build Step 1 as exhaustively as possible (Neukrug & Schwitzer, 2006, p. 202). As can be seen in Figure 11.2, the counselor collected information about the violent traumatic loss Maria witnessed, her symptoms of depersonalization and derealization (being in a daze, etc.), her physical and other related concerns (poor sleep, poor concentration, etc.), avoidance; about her low mood and other signs of grief and loss; and about the other stressors in her life (acculturation, pregnancy, separation

from parents, etc.). Her counselor tried to go beyond the presenting acute stress to be sure she collected information about grief and Maria's co-occurring life stresses.

Step 2: Thematic Groupings. The second step is Thematic Groupings. The clinician organizes all of the exhaustive client information found in Step 1 into just a few intuitive-logical clinical groups, categories, or themes, on the basis of sensible common denominators (Neukrug & Schwitzer, 2006). Four different ways of forming the Step 2 theme groups can be used: Descriptive-Diagnosis Approach, Clinical Targets Approach, Areas of Dysfunction Approach, and Intrapsychic Approach. As can be seen in the figure, Maria's counselor selected the Areas of Dysfunction Approach. This approach sorts together all of the Step 1 information into "areas of dysfunction according to important life situations, life themes, or life roles and skills" (Neukrug & Schwitzer, 2006, p. 205).

The counselor grouped together (a) witnessing the gang violence and her subsequent acute stress reactions into the theme, "post-trauma symptoms and stresses"; (b) her low mood and other signs of bereavement into the theme, "grief and loss"; and (c) her teenage pregnancy, separation from parents, and cultural changes into the theme, "multiple additional life-circumstance stresses." The counselor's conceptual work at Step 2 gave her a way to begin understanding and explaining Maria's areas of functioning and areas of concern more clearly and meaningfully.

So far, at Steps 1 and 2, the counselor has used her clinical assessment skills and her clinical judgment to begin meaningfully understanding Maria's needs. Now, at Steps 3 and 4, she applies the theoretical approach she has selected. She begins making theoretical inferences to interpret and explain the processes or roots underlying Maria's concerns as they are seen in Steps 1 and 2.

Step 3: Theoretical Inferences. At Step 3, concepts from the counselor's selected theory, Cognitive Behavior Therapy, are applied to explain the experiences and the mechanisms that are maintaining Maria's problematic thoughts, feelings, and behaviors. The counselor tentatively matches the theme groups in Step 2 with this theoretical approach. In other words, the symptom constellations in Step 2, which were distilled from the symptoms in Step 1, now are combined using theory to show what is believed to be the psychological etiology of Maria's current needs (Neukrug & Schwitzer, 2006; Schwitzer, 2006, 2007).

According to Cognitive Behavior Therapy (Beck, 1995, 2005; Ellis, 1994; Ellis & MacLaren, 2005), irrational thinking, faulty beliefs, or other forms of cognitive errors lead individuals to engage in problematic behaviors and to experience negative moods and attitudes. As can be seen in Figure 11.2, when the counselor applied these Cognitive Behavior Therapy concepts, she explained at Step 3 that the various issues noted in Step 1 (witnessing trauma, avoiding and re-experiencing, anxiety, grief feelings, dealing with change and pregnancy), which can be understood to be themes of (a) posttrauma symptoms and stresses, (b) grief and loss, and (c) additional life-circumstance stresses (Step 2), are rooted in or caused by a collection of faulty beliefs that witnessing her boyfriend's violent death is so awful she cannot recover, survive her grief, find any point to succeeding in life, or find any reason for wanting her baby. These faulty beliefs are fully spelled out in Figure 11.2.

Step 4. Narrowed Inferences. At Step 4, the clinician's selected theory continues to be used to address still-deeper issues when they exist (Schwitzer, 2006, 2007). At this step, "still-deeper, more encompassing, or more central, causal themes" are formed (Neukrug & Schwitzer, 2006, p. 207). Continuing to apply Cognitive Behavior Therapy concepts at Step 4, Maria's counselor presented a single, deepest, most-fundamental cognitive error that she believed to be most explanatory and causal regarding Maria's current psychotherapeutic needs: the deepest faulty core belief that "What I

have seen is too horrific, and what I have lost is too great, for me to ever survive, and so I am helpless to be anything besides a *persona nerviosa* and suffer *ataques de nervios* from which I cannot recover" (see Figure 11.2). When all four steps are completed, the client information in Step 1 leads to logical-intuitive groupings on the basis of common denominators in Step 2, the groupings then are explained using theory at Step 3, and then, finally, at Step 4, further deeper explanations are made. From start to finish, the thoughts, feelings, behaviors, and physiological features in the topmost portions are connected on down the pyramid into deepest dynamics.

The completed pyramid now is used to plan treatment, where Maria's counselor will assist Maria to examine her cognitive distortions.

TREATMENT PLANNING

At this point, Maria's clinician at the Bowery Community Services Center has collected all available information about the problems that have been of concern to Maria and the clinician who performed her assessment. Based upon this information, the counselor developed a five-axis *DSM-IV-TR* diagnosis and then, using the "inverted pyramid" (Neukrug & Schwitzer, 2006; Schwitzer, 1996, 1997), formulated a working clinical *explanation* of Maria's difficulties and their etiology that we called the *case conceptualization.* This, in turn, guides us to the next critical step in our clinical work, called the *treatment plan,* the primary purpose of which is to map out a logical and goal-oriented strategy for making positive changes in the client's life. In essence, the treatment plan is a road map "for reducing or eliminating disruptive symptoms that are impeding the client's ability to reach positive mental health outcomes" (Neukrug & Schwitzer, 2006, p. 225). As such, it is the cornerstone of our work with not only Maria, but with all clients who present with disturbing and disruptive symptoms and/or personality patterns (Jongsma, Peterson, & McInnis, 2003a, 2003b; Jongsma & Peterson, 2006; Seligman, 1993, 1998, 2004).

Figure 11.2   Maria's Inverted Pyramid Case Conceptualization Summary: Cognitive Behavior
Therapy

1. IDENTIFY AND LIST CLIENT CONCERNS

Witnessed violent death of boyfriend

Witnessed gang war violence

Sleep difficulties

Fatigue

Poor appetite

Unkempt appearance

Poor concentration

Feeling as though "watching herself"

Feeling "in a daze"

Avoiding conversation about stabbing

Low mood

Crying in session

Sluggish in session

Feelings of grief and loss

Cultural differences

Separation from parents

Geographic relocation

Teenage pregnancy

2. ORGANIZE CONCERNS INTO LOGICAL THEMATIC GROUPINGS

1. Posttrauma symptoms and stresses
2. Grief and loss
3. Multiple additional life-circumstance stresses

**3. THEORETICAL INFERENCES: ATTACH THEMATIC
GROUPINGS TO INFERRED AREAS OF DIFFICULTY**

<u>Cognitive Distortions</u>

1. Seeing my boyfriend and his gang killed was so awful
   I will never be able to recover and return to
   an everyday life ever again
2. I cannot go on without my boyfriend
   and I will never survive my grief
3. Without my boyfriend there is no point
   to remaining here, attending high school,
   or succeeding in America
4. Without my boyfriend, there is no reason to want
   to bring my baby into this terrible world and this bad place

**4. NARROWED INFERENCES:
SUICIDALITY AND DEEPER DIFFICULTIES**

<u>Deeper Cognitive Distortion</u>

What I have seen is too horrific, and what I have
lost is too great, for me to ever survive, and so
I am helpless to be anything besides a
persona nerviosa and suffer *ataques
de nervios* from which I cannot recover

A comprehensive treatment plan must integrate all of the information from the biopsychosocial interview, diagnosis, and case conceptualization into a coherent plan of action. This plan comprises four main components, which include (1) a behavioral definition of the problem(s), (2) the selection of achievable goals, (3) the determination of treatment modes, and (4) the documentation of how change will be measured. The *behavioral definition of the problem(s)* consolidates the results of the case conceptualization into a concise hierarchical list of problems and concerns that will be the focus of treatment. The *selection of achievable goals* refers to assessing and prioritizing the client's concerns into a *hierarchy of urgency* that also takes into account the client's motivation for change, level of dysfunction, and real-world influences on his or her problems. The *determination of treatment modes* refers to selection of the specific interventions, which are matched to the uniqueness of the client and to his or her goals and clearly tied to a particular theoretical orientation (Neukrug & Schwitzer, 2006). Finally, the clinician must establish how change will be measured, based upon a number of factors, including client records and self-report of change, in-session observations by the clinician, clinician ratings, results of standardized evaluations such as the Beck Depression Inventory (Beck & Steer, 1990) or a family functioning questionnaire, pre-post treatment comparisons, and reports by other treating professionals.

The four-step method discussed above can be seen in Figure 6.1 (p. 109) and is outlined below for the case of Maria Escobar, followed by her specific treatment plan.

Step 1: Behavioral Definition of Problems. The first step in treatment planning is to carefully review the case conceptualization, paying particular attention to the results of Step 2 (Thematic Groupings), Step 3 (Theoretical Inferences), and Step 4 (Narrowed Inferences). The identified clinical themes reflect the core

areas of concern and distress for the client, while the theoretical and narrowed inferences offer clinical speculation as to their origins. In the case of Maria, there are three primary areas of concern. The first, "posttrauma symptoms and stresses," refers to her feeling as though watching herself, feeling in a daze, and avoidance of conversations about the stabbing. The second, "grief and loss," refers to her low mood, feelings of loss, sleep difficulties, fatigue, poor appetite, unkempt appearance, and poor concentration. The third, "multiple additional life-circumstance stressors," refers to her pregnancy, separation from parents, geographic relocation, and cultural differences that isolate her. These symptoms and stresses are consistent with the diagnosis of ASD and Bereavement (APA, 2000a; Bradley et al., 2005; Bryant et al., 2008; Neeyer, 2000; Servaty-Seib, 2004).

Step 2: Identify and Articulate Goals for Change. The second step is the selection of achievable goals, which is based upon a number of factors, including the most pressing or urgent behavioral, emotional, and interpersonal concerns and symptoms as identified by the client and clinician, the willingness and ability of the client to work on those particular goals, and the realistic (real-world) achievability of those goals (Neukrug & Schwitzer, 2006). At this stage of treatment planning, it is important to recognize that not all of the client's problems can be addressed at once, so we focus initially on those that cause the greatest distress and impairment. New goals can be created as old ones are achieved. In the case of Maria, the goals are divided into three prominent areas. The first, "posttrauma symptoms and stresses," requires that we help Maria to relieve the symptoms of acute posttraumatic stress and verbalize an understanding of how the symptoms of ASD develop. The second, "grief and loss," requires that we help Maria to appropriately grieve her loss and improve her overall daily functioning. The third, "multiple additional life-circumstance stressors," requires that we help Maria to develop post–high school/postpregnancy plans and determine the role she would like her parents to play in her life.

Step 3: Describe Therapeutic Interventions. This is perhaps the most critical step in the treatment planning process because the clinician must now integrate information from a number of sources, including the case conceptualization, the delineation of the client's problems and goals, and the treatment literature, paying particular attention to *empirically supported treatment* (EST) and *evidence-based practice* (EBP). In essence, the clinician must align his or her treatment approach with scientific evidence from the fields of counseling and psychotherapy. Wampold (2001) identifies two types of evidence-based counseling research: studies that demonstrate "absolute efficacy," that is, the fact that counseling and psychotherapy work, and those that demonstrate "relative efficacy," that is, the fact that certain theoretical/technical approaches work best for certain clients with particular problems (Psychoanalysis, Gestalt Therapy, Cognitive Behavior Therapy, Brief Solution-Focused Therapy, Cognitive Therapy, Dialectical Behavior Therapy, Person-Centered Therapy, Expressive/Creative Therapies, Interpersonal Therapy, and Feminist Therapy); and when delivered through specific treatment modalities (individual, group, and family counseling). In the case of Maria, we have decided to use Cognitive Behavior Therapy (Beck, 1995, 2005; Ellis, 1994; Ellis & MacLaren, 2005), which has been found to be highly effective in counseling and psychotherapy with adults (and adolescents) who experience the symptoms of ASD (Bradley et al., 2005; Bryant et al., 2008). The approach relies on a variety of cognitive techniques (reframing, challenging irrational thoughts, and cognitive restructuring) and behavioral techniques (reinforcement for and shaping of adaptive behavior, extinction of maladaptive behaviors, systematic desensitization, and

exposure with response prevention) (Ball et al., 2006; Frank et al., 2005; Milkowitz, 2008). Maria's bereavement issues will be addressed through a combination of individual and group techniques that have been found similarly useful (Fiorini & Mullen, 2006; Kaczmarek & Backlund, 1991; Neimeyer, 2000; Servaty-Seib, 2004). Specific techniques for Maria will include cognitive and behavioral trauma work, individual and group bereavement counseling, and postpregnancy family and vocational planning.

Step 4: Provide Outcome Measures of Change. This last step in treatment planning requires that we specify how change will be measured and indicate the extent to which progress has been made toward realizing these goals (Neukrug & Schwitzer, 2006). The counselor has considerable flexibility in this phase, and may choose from a number of objective domains (psychological tests and measures of self-esteem, depression, psychosis, interpersonal relationship, anxiety, etc.), quasi-objective measures (the *DSM-IV-TR's* Axis V GAF scale; pre-post clinician, client, and psychiatric ratings), and subjective ratings (client self-report, clinician's in-session observations). In Maria's case, we have implemented a number of these, including pre-post measure on the Beck Depression Inventory-II and Grief Evaluation Measure, post measures of GAF functioning in the mild range (>70), client and her cousin's report of improved daily functioning and clinician observation of ability to discuss and cope with her loss.

The completed treatment plan is now developed through which the counselor and Maria will work through the traumatic loss of her boyfriend Tony, develop and implement plans for her pregnancy, and make decisions about whether to remain in New York to pursue vocational training or return to Puerto Rico to live with her parents. The treatment plan appears below and is summarized in Table 11.2.

TREATMENT PLAN

Client: Maria Escobar

Service Provider: Bowery Community Services Center

BEHAVIORAL DEFINITION OF PROBLEMS:

1. Posttrauma symptoms and stresses—Feeling as though watching herself, feeling in a daze, and avoidance of conversations about the stabbing

2. Grief and loss—Low mood, feelings of loss, sleep difficulties, fatigue, poor appetite, unkempt appearance, and poor concentration

3. Multiple additional life-circumstance stress—Pregnancy, separation from parents, geographic relocation, and cultural differences that separate her

GOALS FOR CHANGE:

1. Posttrauma symptoms and stresses
   - Relieve the symptoms of acute posttrauma stress
   - Verbalize an understanding of how the symptoms of ASD develop

2. Grief and loss
   - Appropriately grieve the loss of her boyfriend
   - Improvement in overall daily functioning and mood

3. Multiple additional life-circumstance stresses
   - Develop post–high school/postpregnancy vocational plan
   - Determine the role her parents will play in her life

THERAPEUTIC INTERVENTIONS:

A moderate-term course of individual cognitive-behavior and bereavement counseling (6–9 months)

1. Posttrauma symptoms and stresses
   - Participate in imaginal and in vivo exposure with response prevention to elements of traumatic event
   - Practice thought-stopping for unwanted and intrusive recollections
   - Modify irrational thoughts about the trauma and her perceived role
   - Learn skills of eye movement desensitization and reprocessing (EMDR) to reduce emotional and physiological reactivity to trauma recollections
   - Participation in trauma-focused group therapy
   - Discuss and implement relapse strategies for ASD symptoms

2. Grief and loss

   • Verbalize circumstances of loss and identify related feelings and thoughts
   • Explore feelings of anger, sadness, and guilt related to loss
   • Identify positive characteristics of lost loved one
   • Identify and understand the stages of grief
   • Develop and engage in healthy mourning ritual

3. Multiple additional life-circumstance stresses

   • Schedule appointments at local health care center for duration of pregnancy
   • Pregnancy counseling and decision-making regarding post-pregnancy planning, including the possibility of adoption
   • Reestablish connection with parents in Puerto Rico
   • Join local chapter of Puerto Rican/American cultural association

OUTCOME MEASURES OF CHANGE:

Alleviation of symptoms of Acute Stress Disorder related to her recent loss, return to daily functionality and decision-making about her future as measured by:

   • Pre-post measures on the Beck Depression Inventory
   • Pre-post measures of improvement on the Grief Evaluation Measure
   • Post measures of GAF functioning in the mild range (>70)
   • Client and cousin reports of improved daily functioning, including and self-care
   • Clinician observation of ability to discuss the recent loss
   • Report by health center social worker of clear and constructive post-pregnancy planning

Table 11.2   Maria's Treatment Plan Summary: Cognitive Behavior Therapy

Goals for Change	Therapeutic Interventions	Outcome Measures of Change
Posttrauma symptoms and stresses	Posttrauma symptoms and stresses	Alleviation of symptoms of Acute Stress Disorder related to her recent loss, return to daily functionality and decision-making about her future as measured by:
Relieve the symptoms of acute posttrauma stress	Participate in imaginal and in vivo exposure with response prevention to elements of traumatic event	
Verbalize an understanding of how the symptoms of ASD develop	Practice thought-stopping for unwanted and intrusive recollections	Pre-post measures on the Beck Depression Inventory
Grief and loss	Modify irrational thoughts about the trauma and her perceived role	Pre-post measures of improvement on the Grief Evaluation Measure
Appropriately grieve the loss of her boyfriend	Learn skills of EMDR to reduce emotional and physiological reactivity to trauma recollections	Post measures of GAF functioning in the mild range (>70)
Improvement in overall daily functioning and mood	Participation in trauma-focused group therapy	

(Continued)

Table 11.2 (Continued)

Goals for Change	Therapeutic Interventions	Outcome Measures of Change
Multiple additional life-circumstance stresses Develop post–high school/ post-pregnancy vocational plan Determine the role her parents will play in her life	Discuss and implement relapse strategies for ASD symptoms Grief and loss Verbalize circumstances of loss and identify related feelings and thoughts Explore feelings of anger, sadness, and guilt related to loss Identify positive characteristics of lost loved one Identify and understand the stages of grief Develop and engage in healthy mourning ritual Multiple additional life-circumstance stresses Schedule appointments at local health care center for duration of pregnancy Pregnancy counseling and decision-making regarding post-pregnancy planning, including the possibility of adoption Reestablish connection with parents in Puerto Rico Join local chapter of Puerto Rican/ American cultural association	Client and cousin reports of improved daily functioning, including and self-care Clinician observation of ability to discuss the recent loss Report by health center social worker of clear and constructive postpregnancy planning

CASE 11.3   THE *THRILLER* ALBUM'S BILLIE JEAN

INTRODUCING THE CHARACTER

Billie Jean is the title character in the song of the same name by pop artist Michael Jackson, who first released the song on his 1982 album, *Thriller.* The work's producer was the legendary Quincy Jones. The song is a passionate assertion that its performer is not the father of Billie Jean's infant child. In the song, Billie Jean is introduced as "a beauty queen from movie scene" who tells the singer that the child to whom she recently gave birth belongs to him. The singer protests that "Billie Jean is not my lover, she's just a girl who claims that I am the one, but the kid is not my son." The young woman continues to taunt, harass, and stalk the singer, claiming that the child is indeed his. Although a magnificently choreographed and performed song that soon rose to the top of the pop charts, it was as much an anthem against casual and irresponsible sex as it was a tribute to Michael's Jackson's many varied talents. Debate continues about the Billie Jean song's historical origins: some critics claim the musical work tells a purely fictional story, while Michael Jackson's family and others argue that Billie Jean was an amalgam of the groupies who idolized and followed the Jackson 5 when Michael was a mere child.

We believe Michael Jackson's song describes a nonbizarre, romantic delusion. In the basic case summary and diagnostic impressions below, we expand on Billie Jean's probable delusional disorder and also present what we portray as her negative reactions to a recent sexual trauma.

Meet the Client

You can assess the client in action by viewing the Billie Jean song lyrics at the following website:

- http://www.lyricsfreak.com/m/michael+jackson/billie+jean_20092703.html

You can also view the song being performed at the following websites:

- http://www.youtube.com/watch?v=Zi_XLOBDo_Y Billie Jean by Michael Jackson
- http://www.youtube.com/watch?v=Y8KjO1BsGb0 Michael Jackson performing Billie Jean

BASIC CASE SUMMARY

Identifying Information. Billie Jean Beachman is a socioeconomically middle class, 15-year-old African American girl who resides in Los Angeles, California, and is a student at Quincy Jones High School. She was referred to counseling by Ms. Michelle Grimes, her case worker from the L.A. Department of Families and

Children. Billie Jean's fashionable attire and stylish appearance, featuring a sequined "Michael Jackson" style single glove, was noted to be significant.

Presenting Concern. Ms. Grimes reports that Billie Jean was assigned to her caseload shortly after the birth of the teen's first child several months ago. Ms. Grimes referred Billie Jean for evaluation and treatment due to her concerns that her mental health status might limit her ability to adequately care for her newborn baby. Prior to referral, Billie Jean had been participating in an ongoing support group for teen mothers at the Motown Family Guidance Center. According to Ms. Grimes, Billie Jean's recent apparent "obsession" with a local pop singer, Michael Jackson, raised concerns in the group. She reported that Billie Jean has been using almost all of her group time to talk about her "secret" that Michael Jackson is her baby's father. Further, Billie Jean's pregnancy and subsequent son were the result of a sexual assault.

Billie Jean appears to be exhibiting problematic symptoms suggesting re-experience of trauma, including writing about sexual assault themes in her high school English classes, enacting a rape scene in her drama club, and making up a song about forcible sex that she sang for her support group members. However, when queried by her group leader and later by Ms. Grimes about what was clearly known to be a rape, Billie Jean indicated that "I don't have anything to tell you," "Nope, there's nothing that happened to me except loving a rock star," "I don't remember anything like that; I just like writing stories and songs that way." She also easily reacts in her support group, in classrooms, and in private meetings with irritable outbursts and angry retorts when challenged about her baby's origins. Further, teachers report she seems "on edge" and distracted much of the time, which might be explainable by being a new teen mother. Ms. Grimes expressed specific concerns that Billie Jean does not seem to have the energy or desire to attend to her baby as needed, and reacts angrily with yelling when the baby cries excessively.

Background, Family Information, and Relevant History. Billie Jean was born in Los Angeles, California, the second of three children to Monica and Bernardino Beachman. Her early upbringing, educational experiences, and developmental advances appear to have been normally expected and uneventful. However, beginning in middle school, due to work schedules, Billie Jean was more often left in the care of an elderly neighbor who, while providing support and encouragement, appears to have provided inadequate supervision. According to previous reports, Billie Jean, in order to be accepted and included among her older sister's teenage cohort, began to develop a precocious interest in sexual experimentation and alcohol and marijuana use. Correspondingly, she often was the target of sexually aggressive middle and high school boys, who easily manipulated her with gifts of favorite music CDs, trips to pop rock concerts, and access to alcohol or marijuana. She continued to express a strong interest in her older sister's teenage cohort, was an avid collector of pop music and rock and roll and movie posters, especially those with strong teen themes, and apparently became problematically obsessive about the retro music and videos of the Jackson 5, and current music and videos of Michael Jackson.

Problem and Counseling History. Referral information indicates that about 11 months ago, after clandestinely leaving the home of her neighbor-caretaker late at night to look around the neighborhood for activity, she was surprised by an attack of three 19-year-old men who were her sister's acquaintances. Reportedly she was held down and sexually assaulted by at least two of the assailants. As a result, she spent the next 3 days in Los Angeles Community Hospital. At the end of that period, it was discovered that she was pregnant.

After giving birth, Billie Jean and her infant continued living with her parents and sisters. Her parents appear to be supportive; her sister denies having any knowledge of the sexual assault event or the perpetrators. Billie Jean named her son

Michael Jr. after the pop star, Michael Jackson. Billie Jean was encouraged to return to school while her son remained in her mother's care; however, this proved too stressful for the new mother. Billie Jean began skipping school and coming home to be with her child and said to her mother one day, "I think this is really Michael Jackson's baby." Billie Jean began spending her monthly financial allotment on Michael Jackson albums and videos, writing love letters to him, and telling everyone she knew that Michael was her child's father. At one point, she left the house in the middle of the night with the infant in order to travel to Chicago where Michael Jackson was performing. She was detained by the police at the L.A. bus station and returned home to her mother. She insisted that "if Michael could only see his baby he'd know that it was his and our lives together would be perfect."

Further, Mrs. Beachman noted that her daughter's behavior changed drastically several months after the assault, as she would stare off into space, complain that she felt strange all over her body, was nervous and frightened all the time, and had difficulty sleeping. At this point, the family sought assistance from the Department of Families and Children, resulting in Billie Jean's work with Ms. Grimes and participation in the Motown Family Guidance Center support group for teen mothers. At the time of this intake, Ms. Grimes believes Billie Jean requires more intensive mental health care beyond the provision of routine social services and the support group. Billie Jean's parents have assumed primary caretaking for the infant at present.

Goals for Counseling and Course of Therapy to Date. Billie Jean Beachman arrived punctually for her intake appointment accompanied by her mother, Monica Beachman, and her Department of Families and Children social worker, Ms. Grimes. Billie Jean loosely held her infant son and seemed not to notice his irritability, hunger, and discomfort. At times, Billie Jean's mother took the child from her arms and said impatiently, "No, Billie Jean, do it this way." During these interchanges, Billie Jean stared past her mother with disinterest and abruptly asked seemingly irrelevant questions such as "How far is it to Chicago from here?" "I think my baby could have a career in music like his father." Billie Jean was oriented to person but it is unclear whether she was oriented to time or place because she seemed dazed when responding. She had difficulty reciting serial 7s, but she did know the name of the president of the United States. She could perform simple computations, but was unable to provide appropriate responses to analogies such as "in what way are a wheel and a ball alike." When directly asked questions about her child, Billie Jean smiled and said, "He was a special gift to me," and had no clear awareness of the violent circumstances surrounding the baby's conception.

Taken together, Billie Jean appears to be experiencing symptoms of PTSD, including re-experiencing in the form of reenactment via her writing and creative expression; avoidance in the form of inability to recall or remember, and cognitive and affective detachment; and increased arousal in the form of angry irritability and poor concentration. She also appears to be experiencing a nonbizarre delusion of the erotomanic type centering on her unfounded belief about the father of her infant. The plan is for intensive ongoing psychotherapy with goals of addressing increasing Billie Jean's functioning in the post-trauma context. See treatment plan for specific goals for change.

Diagnostic Impressions

Axis I. 297.1 Delusional Disorder, Erotomanic Type

309.81 Posttraumatic Stress Disorder, Acute, With Delayed Onset

Axis II. V71.09 No Diagnosis on Axis II

Axis III. Recent childbirth

Axis IV. Other psychosocial and environmental problem—Exposure to sexual assault

Axis V. GAF = 40 (current)

GAF = 60 (highest level past year)

DISCUSSION OF DIAGNOSTIC IMPRESSIONS

Billie Jean was referred to counseling by her case worker, who was worried about two domains of Billie Jean's functioning. She believed Billie Jean might be experiencing delusions as well as the aftereffects of a trauma.

Each section of the *DSM-IV-TR* classification system contains a group of diagnoses that share qualitatively similar symptoms or features. For instance, the predominant feature shared by all of disorders in the Schizophrenic and Other Psychotic Disorders section is the presence of

psychotic symptoms: delusions, prominent hallucinations, disorganized speech, disorganized behavior, or catatonic behavior. Likewise, the predominant feature shared by all of the diagnosable disorders found in the Anxiety Disorders section of the *DSM-IV-TR* is the presence of increased arousal, excessive worry, or other signs of anxiety that cause distress or impairment, including panic. Among these are ASD and PTSD, both of which, by definition, occur only in the aftermath of, or as a result of, a traumatic life event. Before moving on to a discussion of differential diagnoses for Billie Jean, it is important to note that African Americans are disproportionately diagnosed with serious mental health problems compared with European Americans, and that counselors should be familiar with the potential for racial bias in diagnosis (Schwartz & Feisthamel, 2009).

The counselor first looked at concerns about Billie Jean and delusions. Despite actual evidence to the contrary, Billie Jean maintains the firm belief that singer Michael Jackson is the father of her baby. She claims this belief when talking to other people, writes letter to Jackson, and insists that he should see the baby. She has held this belief for several months. This delusion involves the real-life situation of having loved and being loved at a distance, appeared in Billie Jean in the absence of any hallucinations or other signs of the onset of Schizophrenia, and in the absence of any other overtly odd or bizarre behavior. Assuming there is no evidence that Billie Jean's delusional ideation is the consequence of a general medical condition or the result of substance use, a Delusional Disorder is suggested.

Differential diagnoses that already have been ruled out include Schizophrenia, Psychotic Disorder Due to a Medical Condition, and Substance-Induced Psychotic Disorder. This is of note partly because there is evidence that in the past, mental health professionals have sometimes tended to overdiagnosis the presentation of psychotic symptoms among their African American clients (Strakowski, McElroy, Keck, & West, 1996). Another differential consideration is a mood disorder with psychotic features—for example, Major Depressive Disorder, Single Episode, Severe With Mood Congruent Psychotic Features, With Postpartum Onset. However, Billie Jean's mood and behavior do not meet the criteria for a Major Depressive Episode. Similarly, PTSD, in and of itself, results in distressing changes in thoughts and perceptions. However, here again, Billie Jean's delusional belief is not accounted for by the characteristic criteria for PTSD. Dissociative Disorders also might be considered; however, the characteristic features of the relevant dissociative diagnoses are the inability to recall important personal information (Dissociative Amnesia) or the presence of two or more distinct

personalities (Dissociative Identity Disorder), neither of which is a good match with Billie Jean's presentation.

The counselor next looked at concerns about Billie Jean's posttraumatic symptoms. This case described what we portrayed as Billie Jean's clinically significant negative reactions to her exposure to the traumatic experience of being sexually assaulted by three men in her neighborhood. She experienced an event characterized by threat to her physical integrity (she was held against her will and raped) and was subjected to threat of injury and serious physical damage. Her reactions are assumed to have included intense fear and helplessness. These characteristics meet the *DSM-IV-TR* definition of a traumatic event. (As a side note, in younger children, trauma can result from "any event or series of events that overwhelms, overstimulates, or creates extreme fear in the child, causing permanent or temporary interruption of normal developmental processes or tasks" (Munson, 2001, p. 184).

Since the assault, Billie Jean has been reexperiencing the event by writing school papers with rape themes, portraying rape scenes in her drama club, and singing a song about forcible sex. At the same time, she has been avoiding recalling the event by denying it took place when the topic arises in conversation, reporting an inability to recall that the assault occurred, and developing feelings of detachment. She has signs of anxiety, including nervousness, generalized fearfulness, trouble sleeping, and irritable outbursts. According to the case timeline, Billie Jean's symptoms have been present for several months. These factors suggest a diagnosis of PTSD. Because symptoms have persisted more than 3 months, the specifier, Chronic, is listed.

Differential diagnoses might include ASD and Adjustment Disorder. However, ASD allows for a maximum duration of symptoms of 1 month, whereas PTSD fits when symptoms have lasted beyond 4 weeks. Whereas Adjustment Disorders are negative reactions to any sort of life stressors, in this case, Billie Jean has experienced exposure to an extreme stressor meeting the diagnostic definition of trauma, and her reactions conform to the specific constellation symptoms characteristic of PTSD and ASD, which go beyond the general criteria set for Adjustment Disorder.

To finish the diagnosis, Billie Jean's pregnancy is listed on Axis III, her critical stressor is emphasized on Axis IV, and on Axis V her functioning is represented by GAF scores ranging from the presence of moderate symptoms within the past year, to the current major impairments she is experiencing that led to her referral. The information on these axes is consistent with the Axis I diagnoses describing Billie Jean's experiences and presentation.

CASE CONCEPTUALIZATION

When Billie Jean Beachman arrived for her first counseling appointment, her screening counselor collected as much information as possible about the symptoms and situations leading to her referral by her case worker. Included among the intake materials were a thorough history; client report; the reports of Billie Jean's case worker, the Quincy Jones High School counselor, and mother; counselor observations; and mental status and written psychological data. Based on the intake, Billie Jean's counselor developed diagnostic impressions, describing her presenting concerns as Delusional Disorder, plus PTSD. A case conceptualization next was developed.

At the Los Angeles counseling center to which Billie Jean was referred, Brief Solution-Focused Counseling is used. The Center employs a brief solution-focused model because it is believed to be an efficient and effective method of providing services, and outcome studies suggest the approach can be successful with a range of presenting problems (De Jong & Berg, 2002; MacDonald, 1994). Whereas the purpose of diagnostic impressions is to *describe* the client's concerns, the goal of case conceptualization as it is applied to Brief Solution-Focused Counseling is to better *understand* and clinically *organize* the person's experiences (Neukrug & Schwitzer, 2006). It helps the counselor determine the

circumstances leading to Billie Jean's PTSD, and the factors maintaining her presenting concerns. In turn, case conceptualization sets the stage for treatment planning. Treatment planning then provides a road map that plots out how the counselor and client expect to move from presenting concerns to positive outcomes (Seligman, 1993, p. 157)—helping Billie Jean return to her previous level of functioning.

Generally speaking, when forming a theoretically based case conceptualization, the clinician applies a purist counseling theory, an integration of two or more theories, an eclectic mix of theories that focuses extensively on diagnosis, history, and etiology; by comparison, when forming a solution-focused case conceptualization, the counselor applies an eclectic combination of solution-focused, or solution-creating, tactics to his or her immediate understanding of the client and engages quickly in identifying and reaching goals (Berg, 1994; DeShazer & Dolan, 2007; Gingerich & Eisengart, 2000).

Billie Jean's counselor used the Inverted Pyramid Method of case conceptualization because this method is especially designed to help clinicians more easily form their conceptual pictures of their clients' needs (Neukrug & Schwitzer, 2006; Schwitzer, 1996, 1997). Generally speaking, when the method is used with a theory-based conceptual model, there are four steps: Problem Identification, Thematic Grouping, Theoretical Inferences, and Narrowed Inferences. However, when the Brief Solution-Focused Counseling model is applied, only the first two steps are needed: Problem Identification and Thematic Grouping. From a solution-focused perspective, it is these two steps that focus attention on what clients want and need and what concerns will be explored and resolved (Bertolino & O'Hanlon, 2002). Brief Solution-Focused counselors make carefully thought-out professional clinical decisions at Steps 1 and 2 of the pyramid; they are sure to have a rational framework for their decisions, rather than applying techniques and approaches at random (Lazarus, Beutler, & Norcross, 1992; Norcross & Beutler, 2008). Billie Jean's counselor's solution-focused clinical thinking can be seen in Figure 11.3.

Step 1: Problem Identification. The first step is Problem Identification. Aspects of the presenting problem (thoughts, feelings, behaviors, physiological features), additional areas of concern besides the presenting concern, family and developmental history, in-session observations, clinical inquiries (medical problems, medications, past counseling, substance use, suicidality), and psychological assessments (problem checklists, personality inventories, mental status exam, specific clinical measures) all may contribute information at Step 1. The counselor "casts a wide net" in order to build Step 1 as exhaustively as possible (Neukrug & Schwitzer, 2006, p. 202). As can be seen in Figure 11.3, the counselor identified Billie Jean's recent sexual trauma (gang rape, held against will, etc.), her various posttraumatic presenting symptoms (denial and inability to recall assault, writing about and acting out forced sex, anxiety and sleep problems, etc.), facts and events pertaining to her pregnancy and childbirth, her various thoughts and actions associated with her romantic delusion (belief Michael Jackson is child's father, obsession with "being in love with rock star," running away to Chicago, etc.), and mental status factors. The counselor attempted to go beyond just the most pressing presenting symptoms in order to be descriptive as she could.

Step 2: Thematic Groupings. The second step is Thematic Groupings. The clinician organizes all of the exhaustive client information found in Step 1 into just a few intuitive-logical clinical groups, categories, or themes, on the basis of sensible common denominators (Neukrug & Schwitzer, 2006). Four different ways of forming the Step 2 theme groups can be used: Descriptive-Diagnosis Approach, Clinical Targets Approach, Areas of Dysfunction Approach, and Intrapsychic Approach. As can be seen in the figure, Billie Jean's counselor selected the Clinical Targets Approach. This approach sorts together all of the Step 1 information "according to the basic division of behavior, thoughts, feelings, and physiology" (Neukrug & Schwitzer, p. 205).

The counselor grouped together: (a) all of Billie Jean's problematic posttraumatic cognitive, affective, and physiological concerns connected to dissociation, memory loss, anger, nervousness, and so on, plus all of Billie Jean's problematic posttraumatic behavioral concerns connected to reenacting the trauma, and so on; and (b) all of Billie Jean's problematic romantic delusional cognitive and behavioral symptoms connected to her untrue belief that Michael Jackson is her child's father. The counselor selected the Clinical Targets Approach to organize Billie Jean's concerns from a Solution-Focused Counseling perspective on the rational basis that she planned to emphasize cognitive interventions that she believed would lead to good solutions with adolescents such as Billie Jean (Vernon, 2009).

With this two-step conceptualization completed, the client information in Step 1 leads to logical-intuitive groupings on the basis of common denominators in Step 2, and the counselor is ready to engage the client in planning and implementing Brief Solution-Focused Counseling.

TREATMENT PLANNING

At this point, Billie Jean's clinician at the L.A. Department of Children and Families has collected all available information about the problems that have been of concern to Billie Jean and the professionals who performed her assessment. Based upon this information, the counselor developed a five-axis *DSM-IV-TR* diagnosis and then, using the "inverted pyramid" (Neukrug & Schwitzer, 2006; Schwitzer, 1996, 1997), formulated a working clinical *explanation* of Billie Jean's difficulties and their etiology that we called the *case conceptualization.* This, in turn, guides us to the next critical step in our clinical work, called the *treatment plan,* the primary purpose of which is to map out a logical and goal-oriented strategy for making positive changes in the client's life. In essence, the

Figure 11.3 Billie Jean's Inverted Pyramid Case Conceptualization Summary: Brief Solution-Focused Counseling Emphasizing Cognitive Interventions With Adolescents

1. IDENTIFY AND LIST CLIENT CONCERNS

Recent sexual assault by 3
    neighborhood men
Held against her will, raped
Intense fear and helplessness
Pregnancy and birth resulting
    from gang rape
Portraying rape scenes in theater
    class
Writing about rape in school papers
Singing a song about forced sex
Denies assault occurred
Inability to recall assault
Feelings of detachment
Seems dazed

Nervousness & anxiety
Sleep troubles
Angry outbursts
Delusional belief about Michael Jackson
Talks in group counseling about Michael
    Jackson
Sees self as "loving a rock star"
Attempted to visit Michael Jackson
    in Chicago
Attends to baby's needs but is
    distracted by delusion

2. ORGANIZE CONCERNS INTO LOGICAL THEMATIC GROUPINGS

1. Problematic posttraumatic cognitive, affective, and
   physiological symptoms (dissociation, dazed, memory loss,
   angry outbursts, nervousness, and anxiety, sleep trouble)
   plus problematic posttraumatic behavioral symptoms
   (portraying, writing about, singing about forced sex;
   denying event)
2. Problematic romantic delusional cognitive and behavioral
   symptoms (delusional belief that Michael Jackson is child's
   father; talks openly about "secret" of Michael Jackson
   fatherhood; describes self "in love with rock star";
   attempted to travel to Chicago; distracted from
   effective mothering by delusion)

**3. THEORETICAL INFERENCES: ATTACH THEMATIC
GROUPINGS TO INFERRED AREAS OF DIFFICULTY**

**4. NARROWED INFERENCES: SUICIDALITY
AND DEEPER DIFFICULTIES**

treatment plan is a road map "for reducing or eliminating disruptive symptoms that are impeding the client's ability to reach positive mental health outcomes" (Neukrug & Schwitzer, 2006, p. 225). As such, it is the cornerstone of our work with not only Billie Jean, but with all clients who present with disturbing and disruptive symptoms and/or personality patterns (Jongsma et al., 2003a, 2003b; Jongsma & Peterson, 2006; Seligman, 1993, 1998, 2004).

A comprehensive treatment plan must integrate all of the information from the biopsychosocial interview, diagnosis, and case conceptualization into a coherent plan of action. This plan comprises four main components, which include (1) a behavioral definition of the problem(s), (2) the selection of achievable goals, (3) the determination of treatment modes, and (4) the documentation of how change will be measured. The *behavioral definition of the problem(s)* consolidates the results of the case conceptualization into a concise hierarchical list of problems and concerns that will be the focus of treatment. The *selection of achievable goals* refers to assessing and prioritizing the client's concerns into a *hierarchy of urgency* that also takes into account the client's motivation for change, level of dysfunction and real-world influences on his or her problems. The *determination of treatment modes* refers to selection of the specific interventions, which are matched to the uniqueness of the client and to his or her goals and clearly tied to a particular theoretical orientation (Neukrug & Schwitzer, 2006). Finally, the clinician must establish how change will be measured, based upon a number of factors, including client records and self-report of change, in-session observations by the clinician, clinician ratings, results of standardized evaluations such as the Beck Depression Inventory (Beck & Steer, 1990) or a family functioning questionnaire, pre-post treatment comparisons, and reports by other treating professionals.

The four-step method discussed above can be seen in Figure 6.1 (p. 109) and is outlined below for the case of Billie Jean Beachman, followed by her specific treatment plan.

Step 1: Behavioral Definition of Problems. The first step in solution-focused treatment planning is to carefully review the case conceptualization, paying particular attention to the results of Step 2 (Thematic Groupings). The identified clinical themes reflect the core areas of concern and distress for the client. In the case of Billie Jean, there are two primary areas of concern. The first, "problematic posttraumatic cognitive, affective, physiological and behavioral symptoms," refers to her nervousness, anxiety, and intense fear and helplessness, sleep troubles, angry outbursts, denial of and inability to recall the assault, feelings of detachment; writing about rape in school papers, singing a song about forced sex, and portraying rape scenes in theater class. The second, "problematic romantic delusional cognitive and behavioral symptoms," refers to her delusional belief that Michael Jackson is her child's father, obsessive thinking about Michael Jackson, perception of herself as loving a rock star, attempting to visit Michael Jackson in Chicago, and distraction from child care by the delusion. These symptoms and stresses are consistent with the diagnosis of Delusional Disorder, Erotomanic Type; PTSD, Acute With Delayed Onset (APA, 2000a; Brunello et al., 2001; Kessler et al., 2001; Bradley et al., 2005; Bryant et al., 2008; Munro, 1999).

Step 2: Identify and Articulate Goals for Change. The second step is the selection of achievable goals, which is based upon a number of factors, including the most pressing or urgent behavioral, emotional, and interpersonal concerns and symptoms as identified by the client and clinician, the willingness and ability of the client to work on those particular goals, and the realistic (real-world) achievability of those goals (Neukrug & Schwitzer, 2006). At this stage of treatment planning, it is important to recognize that not all of the client's problems can be addressed at once, so we focus initially on those that cause the greatest distress and impairment. New goals can be created as old ones are achieved. In the case of Billie Jean, the goals are divided into two prominent areas. The first, "problematic post-traumatic cognitive, affective, physiological and behavioral symptoms," requires that we help Billie Jean to verbalize an understanding of how the symptoms of PTSD develop, to reduce the negative impact that the traumatic event had on her life, to develop and implement effective coping skills, and to recall the traumatic event without becoming overwhelmed with stressful feelings or dissociating. The second, "problematic romantic delusional cognitive and behavioral symptoms," requires that we help Billie Jean to control or eliminate active psychotic symptoms and to focus her thoughts on reality so she may effectively take care of her child and herself.

Step 3: Describe Therapeutic Interventions. This is perhaps the most critical step in the treatment planning process because the clinician must now integrate information from a number of sources, including the case conceptualization, the delineation of the client's problems and goals, and the treatment literature, paying particular attention to *empirically supported treatment* (EST) and *evidence-based practice* (EBP). In essence, the clinician must align his or her treatment approach with scientific evidence from the fields of counseling and psychotherapy. Wampold (2001) identifies two types of evidence-based counseling research: studies that demonstrate "absolute efficacy," that is, the fact that counseling and psychotherapy work, and those that demonstrate "relative efficacy," that is, the fact that certain theoretical/technical approaches work best for certain clients with particular problems (Psychoanalysis, Gestalt Therapy, Cognitive Behavior Therapy, Brief Solution-Focused Therapy, Cognitive Therapy, Dialectical Behavior Therapy, Person-Centered Therapy, Expressive/Creative Therapies, Interpersonal Therapy, and Feminist Therapy); and when delivered through specific treatment modalities (individual, group, and family counseling).

In the case of Billie Jean, we have decided to use Brief Solution-Focused Therapy (De Jong &

Berg, 2002; De Shazer & Dolan, 2007; Gingerich & Eisengart, 2000; Gutterman, 2006) emphasizing cognitive interventions with adolescents (Corcoran & Stephenson, 2000; Thompson & Henderson, 2011; Hopson & Kim, 2005; Lines, 2002; Vernon, 2009). This counseling approach is "pragmatic, anti-deterministic and future oriented [and as such] offers optimism, and hope about the ability of the client to change" (Neukrug, 2011, p. 426). It de-emphasizes psychopathology and the past, and instead focuses on the client's strengths, resources, and skills in order to generate solutions to the problems and concerns. Forward looking and quickly moving, Solution-Focused Therapy's basic assumptions include: change is constant and inevitable, clients have the inherent skills and abilities to change, small steps lead to big changes, exceptions to problems do occur and can be used for change, and the future is both created and negotiable, as well as simple axioms such as "if it ain't broke, don't fix it," "if it works, do more of it," and "if it's not working, do something different" (Neukrug, 2011).

We view Brief Solution-Focused Therapy as being particularly useful in Billie Jean's case due to its emphasis on change, the future, and tapping into the client's resources and skills. Additionally, solution-focused treatment is fast-moving, makes use of creative techniques (art, play, and narrative) with children and adolescents, and relies on challenging, strength-based questioning that can be highly engaging with adolescents. Billie Jean would be referred to a day-treatment program where she can receive individual, family, group, and psychoeducational support. Specific techniques for her posttraumatic symptoms include education and orientation to brief-solution focused treatment, goal setting with regard to Posttraumatic Stress Disorder symptoms, "scaling" of her posttraumatic symptoms to provide context and perspective as well as a starting point for change and then ongoing scaling to gauge improvement, use of the miracle question to help her begin to cognitively process the possibility of change, externalizing the symptoms by using solution talk and creating hypothetical solutions, identifying and complimenting Billie Jean on past and current use of skills to solve problems, amplification of previously successful strategies for self-care, using preferred-goal, evaluative, coping, exception-seeking and solution-focused questions and psychiatric referral for possible psychopharmacotherapy. Specific techniques for her delusional symptoms include assessing the pervasiveness of Billie Jean's thought disorder, explaining the nature of thought disorder, and using the above solution-focused methods to help restructure her beliefs about the relationship with Michael Jackson, her parental role, and the relationship with her parents.

Step 4: Provide Outcome Measures of Change. This last step in treatment planning requires that we specify how change will be measured and indicate the extent to which progress has been made toward realizing these goals (Neukrug & Schwitzer, 2006). The counselor has considerable flexibility in this phase and may choose from a number of objective domains (psychological tests and

measures of self-esteem, depression, psychosis, interpersonal relationship, anxiety, etc.), quasi-objective measures (the *DSM-IV-TR's* Axis V GAF scale; pre-post clinician, client, and psychiatric ratings), and subjective ratings (client self-report, clinician's in-session observations). In Billie Jean's case, we have implemented a number of these, including pre-post measures on the Clinician-administered PTSD Scale for Children and Adolescents (Newman et al., 2006) and Parenting Stress Index-II (PSI-II) (Abidin, 1997), post-only measures of GAF functioning in the mild to moderate range (60–70), clinician-observed and client/parent report of reduction in affective, cognitive, physiological, and behavioral symptoms of PTSD, and caseworker report of improved parenting skills.

The completed treatment plan is now developed through which the counselor, Billie Jean, and her family will work through the traumatic experience, alleviate her psychotic symptoms, and restore her to a level of adaptive functioning. Billie Jean's treatment plan is as follows and is summarized in Table 11.3.

TREATMENT PLAN

Client: Billie Jean Beachman

Service Provider: L.A. Department of Families and Children

BEHAVIORAL DEFINITION OF PROBLEMS:

1. Problematic posttraumatic cognitive, affective, physiological, and behavioral symptoms—Nervousness, anxiety, and intense fear and helplessness, sleep troubles, angry outbursts, denial of and inability to recall the assault, feelings of detachment; writing about rape in school papers, singing a song about forced sex, and portraying rape scenes in theater class

2. Problematic romantic delusional cognitive and behavioral symptoms—Delusional belief that Michael Jackson is child's father, obsessive thinking about Michael Jackson, perception of self as "loving a rock star," attempting to visit Michael Jackson in Chicago, and distraction from child care by the delusion

GOALS FOR CHANGE:

1. Problematic posttraumatic cognitive, affective, physiological, and behavioral symptoms
   • Verbalize an understanding of how the symptoms of PTSD develop
   • Reduce the negative impact of traumatic event

- Develop and implement effective coping skills
- Recall the traumatic event without becoming overwhelmed with stressful feelings or dissociating

2. Problematic romantic delusional cognitive and behavioral symptoms
   - Control or eliminate active psychotic symptoms
   - Focus thoughts on reality for purposes of effective self- and child care
   - Support of reality-based peer relationships

THERAPEUTIC INTERVENTIONS:

A moderate-term course of individual, family, and group Solution-Focused Therapy (6–9 months)

1. Problematic posttraumatic cognitive, affective, physiological, and behavioral symptoms
   - Education and orientation to brief solution-focused treatment
   - Goal setting with regard to Posttraumatic Stress Disorder symptoms
   - "Scaling" of posttraumatic symptoms to provide context and perspective as well as a starting point for change
   - Ongoing scaling to gauge improvement
   - Use of the miracle question to help her begin to cognitively process the possibility of change
   - Externalizing the symptoms by using solution talk and creating hypothetical solutions
   - Identifying and complimenting past and current use of skills to solve problems
   - Amplification of previously successful strategies for self-care
   - Using preferred-goal, evaluative, coping, exception-seeking, and solution-focused questions
   - Psychiatric referral for possible psychopharmacotherapy

2. Problematic romantic delusional cognitive and behavioral symptoms
   - Assessing the pervasiveness of thought disorder
   - Explaining the nature of thought disorder
   - Using the above solution-focused methods to help restructure beliefs about the relationship with Michael Jackson, parental role, and the relationship with parents
   - Psychiatric referral for possible psychopharmacotherapy

OUTCOME MEASURES OF CHANGE:

Alleviation of symptoms of posttraumatic stress and delusional disorders. Return to adaptive level of functioning, resumption of positive child care as measured by:

- Pre-post measures on the Clinician-administered PTSD Scale for Children and Adolescents (CAPS-CA)
- Pre-post measures on the Parent Stress Index-II (PSI-II)
- Post-only measure of GAF functioning in the mild to moderate range (60–70)
- Clinician-observed reduction in affective, cognitive, physiological, and behavioral symptoms of PTSD
- Client and parent reports of reduction in affective, cognitive, physiological, and behavioral symptoms of PTSD
- Caseworker report of improved parenting skills of client

Table 11.3   Billie Jean's Treatment Plan Summary: Brief Solution-Focused Counseling Emphasizing Cognitive Interventions With Adolescents

Goals for Change	Therapeutic Interventions	Outcome Measures of Change
Problematic posttraumatic cognitive, affective, physiological and behavioral symptoms	Problematic posttraumatic cognitive, affective, physiological, and behavioral symptoms	Alleviation of symptoms of posttraumatic stress and delusional disorders
Verbalize an understanding of how the symptoms of PTSD develop	Education and orientation to brief-solution focused treatment	Return to adaptive level of functioning, resumption of positive child care as measured by:
Reduce the negative impact of traumatic event	Goal setting with regard to posttraumatic stress disorder symptoms	Pre-post measures on the Clinician-administered PTSD Scale for Children and Adolescents (CAPS-CA)
Develop and implement effective coping skills	"Scaling" of posttraumatic symptoms to provide context and perspective as well as a starting point for change	
Recall the traumatic event without becoming overwhelmed with stressful feelings or dissociating	Ongoing scaling to gauge improvement	Pre-post measures on the Parent Stress Index-II (PSI-II)
	Use of the miracle question to help her begin to cognitively process the possibility of change	Post-only measure of GAF functioning in the mild to moderate range (60–70)
Problematic romantic delusional cognitive and behavioral symptoms	Externalizing the symptoms by using solution talk and creating hypothetical solutions	Clinician-observed reduction in affective, cognitive, physiological, and behavioral symptoms of PTSD
Control or eliminate active psychotic symptoms	Identifying and complimenting past and current use of skills to solve problems	
Focus thoughts on reality for purposes of effective self- and child care	Amplification of previously successful strategies for self-care	Client and parent reports of reduction in affective, cognitive, physiological, and behavioral symptoms of posttraumatic stress disorder
Support of reality-based peer relationships	Using preferred-goal, evaluative, coping, exception-seeking and Solution-Focused questions	Caseworker report of improved parenting skills of client
	Psychiatric referral for possible psychopharmacotherapy	
	Problematic romantic delusional cognitive and behavioral symptoms	
	Assessing the pervasiveness of thought disorder	
	Explaining the nature of thought disorder	
	Using the above solution-focused methods to help restructure beliefs about the relationship with Michael Jackson, parental role, and the relationship with parents	
	Psychiatric referral for possible psychopharmacotherapy	

CASE 11.4   THE *REVOLVER* ALBUM'S ELEANOR RIGBY

INTRODUCING THE CHARACTER

Eleanor Rigby is the namesake of John Lennon's and Paul McCartney's 1966 Beatles song that appeared on the album *Revolver.* In the song, Eleanor Rigby is the female protagonist in the gripping and poignant story of a melancholy and lonely woman who is associated with her local parish church and its rector, Father McKenzie.

When we meet Eleanor Rigby, she is picking up the rice in the church where a wedding has been, living in a dream, waiting at the window and "wearing the face that she keeps in a jar by the door." The song is both a personal lament and one of solidarity with all the lonely people. "The song ends with Eleanor dying in the church while tending to her duties, being buried along with her name" and Father McKenzie "wiping the dirt from his hands as he walks from the grave."

The song marked a transition for the Beatles from playful performers of widely popular love songs to more serious studio musicians who could write as effortlessly and powerfully of death and loneliness as they could joyful pop. Picking up where the Beatles left off, in the following basic case summary and diagnostic impressions, we further develop Eleanor's scenario in order to illustrate a mood disorder due to a medical condition and the diagnosis of Mental Retardation.

Meet the Client

You can assess the client in action by viewing the Eleanor Rigby song lyrics at the following website:

- http://www.lyricsfreak.com/b/beatles/eleanor+rigby_10026674.html

You can also view the song being performed at the following websites:

- http://www.youtube.com/watch?v=lFeMhdXIqWc
- http://www.youtube.com/watch?v=Ht-qVldmP00

BASIC CASE SUMMARY

Identifying Information. Eleanor Rigby is a 62-year-old British woman who resides alone in a private apartment on the campus of St. Peter's Parish Church in Woolton, Liverpool. She has been a widow for about 40 years. She volunteered that she is of the Anglican faith and is devout. She is employed as a church assistant to Father Nigel McKenzie of St. Peter's Parish Church. She arrived, 30 minutes early for the interview, by public transportation. Although she appeared dressed appropriately for the interview, her hair required some attention and her dress did not appear recently cleaned. Although engaged, she appeared tired.

Presenting Information. Ms. Rigby was referred to the Liverpool City Services Clinic by Father Nigel McKenzie, who was concerned about her ongoing depressed mood, pessimistic and doubtful thinking and rumination, occasional teariness, and slowness performing her daily tasks. He reported that although she has seemed "about this depressed" for many years, he made the referral because he has found faith-based counseling to be ineffective, and he is concerned about her future situation as she ages and retires, or as he eventually moves on to a new parish assignment.

Along with her mood symptoms, Father McKenzie shared some available records indicating that earlier in life, while in the school system, Eleanor had been identified as a student with a measured IQ of about 70.

Background, Family Information, and Relevant History. Eleanor Rigby was born in Liverpool, England, the only child to John and Frances Rigby. Mr. Rigby worked as a craft mason, and was a devout Anglican man who was a part-time vicar and made substantial time and service contributions to St. Peter's Parish Church. Mrs. Rigby worked part-time in the parish kindergarten.

Ms. Rigby remembers her childhood and school years through her late teens as happy ones. She recalls enjoying attending the church kindergarten and parish events "because my parents were always right around the corner." She denied any memories of low mood, poor sleep or appetite, periods of teariness or pessimism outside what would be normally expected across the childhood life cycle.

She does recall having difficulties academically and eventually falling behind her peers "and I hated to lose my girlfriends when they moved on without me." Correspondingly, according to older records, sometime before age 10 Ms. Rigby was identified by her teachers as a student with difficulty grasping concepts expected for her grade. Ms. Rigby underwent individual testing for intellectual functioning at this time and once again a few years later. Results suggested a subaverage intellectual functioning with IQ equaling about 70. Ms. Rigby's memory and records indicate that she was generally successfully adjusted to daily activities and tasks but less capable in academic classrooms. With assistance from the parish, her parents were able to enroll her in the Lady Beatrice Campbell Dame School, where she received specialized academic experiences.

Socially, Ms. Rigby functioned moderately well. At about age 20, she married a man about the same age as her, whom she described as "my love from way back then." Her husband was a junior assistant craft mason and one of her father's colleagues; Eleanor and her husband met at a church function. By Eleanor's recall, "that was my favorite time of life." Sadly, however, her husband died of an illness about 2 years later. Father McKenzie reported that at that time an arrangement was made for Ms. Rigby to be employed by the parish and has received a salary and room and board ever since. Overall, Ms. Rigby has been able to function in her role as church assistant with close attention, structure, feedback, and support from Father McKenzie. Likewise, with close support and structure, she has been able to manage daily living tasks such as self-care, basic cooking and eating, cleaning and dressing, and so on. However, it is Father McKenzie's opinion that without close supervision she would be less able or unable to maintain her current self-care level. She is able to use public transportation with supervision (Father McKenzie boarded her on the bus to this counseling appointment, and a staff member will board her for her return home), but rarely socializes, interacts with the community, or uses services outside the church grounds.

Problem and Counseling History. Ms. Rigby appears to have been experiencing a mood disorder for about the past 15 years. Father McKenzie recalled that Ms. Rigby's mood seemed to decline during her "mid 40s." He said at that time, she became more visibly "depressed," was teary on occasion, and seemed irritable at times. She also was more pessimistic. Ms. Rigby herself remembers "just having trouble sleeping" and said that she began feeling "really tired all the time." She said she also began gaining weight, and on inquiry from the counselor, mentioned that her menstrual periods became more irregular as well. Outside of the earlier loss of her husband, neither Father McKenzie nor the client could identify any situational change or other significant event that might have accounted for her chance in mood and related symptoms.

Her symptoms have been unresponsive to faith-based counseling. She was referred to a family medical clinic for a full physical exam conjointly with this psychological intake. Results of her medical exam indicate a clinically significant finding of low thyroid function (clinically significant thyroid stimulating hormone [TSH] levels) consistent with her mood and related symptoms.

Goals for Counseling and Course of Therapy to Date. Ms. Rigby has been seen for one intake interview and one medical physical exam to date. She appeared somewhat strained by the need to attend meetings and appointments off the church campus but is agreeable to further services. Father McKenzie has agreed to supervise her attendance and participation. At this early stage, the primary goals are to continue supportive and life-skills counseling and follow through with appropriate medical intervention for a probable mood disorder due to hypothyroidism.

Diagnostic Impressions

Axis I.   293.83 Mood Disorder Due to Hypothyroidism, With Depressive Symptoms

Axis II.   317 Mental Retardation, Mild

Axis III.   Hypothyroidism

Axis IV.   Problems related to the social environment—Living alone, social disconnection

Other psychosocial and environmental problems—Daily functioning when adequate support and supervision are unavailable

Axis V.   GAF = 61 (current)

GAF = 70 (highest level recent years)

DISCUSSION OF
DIAGNOSTIC IMPRESSIONS

Eleanor Rigby was referred to the Liverpool City Services Clinic by Father McKenzie because she was experiencing what he recognized as symptoms of a depressive disorder. He had noticed her ongoing depressed mood and tearfulness; pessimistic, doubting, ruminating thinking; and fatigue. Eleanor also reported difficulties sleeping, feeling fatigued, and gaining weight. In addition to the primary reason for referral, records indicated that on the basis of testing while a student, Ms. Rigby was reported to have a measured IQ of about 70.

Each section of the *DSM-IV-TR* classification system contains a group of diagnoses that share qualitatively similar symptoms or features. For example, all of the diagnoses contained in the section, Mental Disorders Due to a General Medical Condition, are characterized by psychological and behavioral symptoms that are directly due to the physiological effects of medical problems. These include dementias, amnestic disorders, psychotic disorders, mood disorders, anxiety disorders, sexual dysfunctions, and sleep disorders that are the result of a medical condition. Likewise, the Disorders Usually First Diagnosed in Infancy, Childhood, or Adolescence section contains disorders that all share the feature of

first occurring early in the life cycle; these include some concerns, like Mental Retardation, that may continue into adulthood.

Eleanor's presenting concerns related to a depressed mood. Her low mood, tearfulness, physical symptoms, and changes in thought all are characteristic of a Major Depressive Episode. Onset was thought to be during her early 40s. Outside of the early loss of her husband, no significant psychosocial stressors were associated with her depression. She did report the physical symptom of irregular menstrual periods, and her counselor referred her for a general physical exam along with the counseling intake. Lab test results from the physical exam revealed low thyroid function (clinically significant TSH levels) consistent with her mood and related symptoms. In such cases the diagnosis is a Mental Disorder Due to a General Medical Condition, more specifically: Mood Disorder Due to Hypothyroidism, With Depressive Symptoms.

Differential diagnoses might include Major Depressive Disorder, Dysthymic Disorder, or Adjustment Disorder With Depressed Mood. However, because the counselor expertly referred Ms. Rigby for a physical exam, evidence was found indicating that her low mood and related symptoms were, instead, the direct consequence of a medical problem.

Eleanor's intellectual functioning, although not the principal diagnosis or the primary reason for referral, should also be noted since it might be clinically significant in relation to her functioning. A multiaxial diagnosis presents all the various diagnosable disorders and other conditions that might be a focus of clinical attention on Axis I—except for the Personality Disorders and Mental Retardation, which are reported on Axis II. In other words, Axis II answers the questions: "Is there evidence of mental retardation?" and "Does the client evidence any long-term pattern of maladaptive character traits that cause significant impairment or distress" (LaBruzza & Mendez-Villarrubia, 1994, p. 86). The listing of mental retardation and personality disorders on a separate axes is done simply to ensure that these situations are not overlooked while the clinician is attending to Axis I disorders, which usually are more pronounced (APA, 2000a).

The diagnosis of Mental Retardation requires significantly below-average intellectual functioning as demonstrated by a score of 70 or lower on an individually administered, standardized IQ test. There also must be some impairment in everyday functioning, in areas such as self-care, home living, self-direction, academic or work skills, leisure, or health and safety. When a person's IQ scores falls between 71–84, the category, Borderline Intellectual Functioning, is listed on Axis II. Borderline Intellectual Functioning is found in the section Other Conditions That May Be a Focus of Clinical Attention. (As an aside, other *DSM-IV-TR* diagnoses requiring formal standardized psychological testing plus impairment in functioning are the Axis I Learning Disorders: Reading Disorder, Mathematics Disorder, Disorder of Written Expression, and Learning Disorders Not Otherwise Specified.) Eleanor Rigby was tested at about an IQ of 70, and has been living successfully and relatively independently with the support and assistance provided by Father McKenzie. Her IQ score falls between 50–70, and therefore the degree of mental retardation is listed as Mild.

To round out the diagnosis, the medical condition associated with the diagnosis listed on Axis I must be listed on Axis III, Eleanor Rigby's

social stressors are emphasized on Axis IV, and on Axis V her functioning is represented by GAF scores ranging from the presence of only mild symptoms within the past year, to the current, mildly serious symptoms affecting mood and other functioning, which led to her referral. The information on all five axes is consistent.

CASE CONCEPTUALIZATION

Upon arrival at the Liverpool City Services Clinic, Eleanor Rigby's intake counselor collected as much information as possible about the symptoms and situations leading to her referral. Included among the intake materials were a thorough history, client report, the reports of Father McKenzie, counselor observations, available records pertaining to intellectual and psychological assessments, and important data from her medical exam. Based on the intake, Eleanor Rigby's counselor developed diagnostic impressions, describing her presenting concerns as a Depressive Mood Disorder due to a General Medical Condition, namely, Hypothyroidism, and also noted mild mental retardation. Next, a case conceptualization was developed.

At the Liverpool City Services Clinic, Brief Solution-Focused Counseling is used. The clinic employs a brief solution-focused model because it is believed to be an efficient and effective method of providing services, and outcome studies suggest the approach can be successful with a range of presenting problems (De Jong & Berg, 2002; MacDonald, 1994). Whereas the purpose of diagnostic impressions is to *describe* the client's concerns, the goal of case conceptualization as it is applied to Brief Solution-Focused Counseling is to better *understand* and clinically *organize* the person's experiences (Neukrug & Schwitzer, 2006). It helps the counselor determine the factors pertaining to Eleanor Rigby's depressive disorder and hypothyroidism. In turn, case conceptualization sets the stage for treatment planning. Treatment planning then provides a road map that plots out how the counselor and client expect to move from presenting concerns to positive outcomes (Seligman, 1993, p. 157)—helping

Eleanor Rigby elevate her mood and achieve an improved level of functioning.

Generally speaking, when forming a theoretically based case conceptualization, the clinician applies a purist counseling theory, an integration of two or more theories, an eclectic mix of theories that focuses extensively on diagnosis, history, and etiology; by comparison, when forming a solution-focused case conceptualization, the counselor applies an eclectic combination of solution-focused, or solution-creating, tactics to his or her immediate understanding of the client and engages quickly in identifying and reaching goals (Berg, 1994; De Shazer & Dolan, 2007; Gingerich & Eisengart, 2000).

Eleanor's counselor used the Inverted Pyramid Method of case conceptualization because this method is especially designed to help clinicians more easily form their conceptual pictures of their clients' needs (Neukrug & Schwitzer, 2006; Schwitzer, 1996, 1997). Generally speaking, when the method is used with a theory-based conceptual model, there are four steps: Problem Identification, Thematic Groupings, Theoretical Inferences, and Narrowed Inferences. However, when the Brief solution-focused Counseling model is applied, only the first two steps are needed: Problem Identification and Thematic Grouping. From a solution-focused perspective, it is these two steps that focus attention on what clients want and need and what concerns will be explored and resolved (Bertolino & O'Hanlon, 2002). Brief Solution-Focused counselors make carefully thought-out professional clinical decisions at Steps 1 and 2 of the pyramid; they are sure to have a rational framework for their decisions, rather than applying techniques and approaches at random (Lazarus et al., 1992; Norcross & Beutler, 2008). Eleanor's counselor's solution-focused clinical thinking can be seen in Figure 11.4.

Step 1: Problem Identification. The first step is Problem Identification. Aspects of the presenting problem (thoughts, feelings, behaviors, physiological features), additional areas of concern besides the presenting concern, family and developmental history, in-session observations, clinical inquiries (medical problems, medications, past counseling, substance use, suicidality), and psychological assessments (problem checklists, personality inventories, mental status exam, specific clinical measures) all may contribute information at Step 1. The counselor "casts a wide net" in order to build Step 1 as exhaustively as possible (Neukrug & Schwitzer, 2006, p. 202). As can be seen in Figure 11.4, the counselor listed all of the information she had about Eleanor's symptoms of depression (low mood, teariness, fatigue, etc.), all of the clinical information from Eleanor's medical exam pertaining to her thyroid (hypothyroidism, disrupted menstrual cycle, etc.), all of the testing data and psychosocial information pertaining to Eleanor's mental retardation, and notes about Eleanor's life history (loss of husband, previous counseling). She attempted to be as thorough as she could in order to fully describe Eleanor Rigby's needs.

Step 2: Thematic Groupings. The second step is Thematic Groupings. The clinician organizes all of the exhaustive client information found in Step 1 into just a few intuitive-logical clinical groups, categories, or themes, on the basis of sensible common denominators (Neukrug & Schwitzer, 2006). Four different ways of forming the Step 2 theme groups can be used: Descriptive-Diagnosis Approach, Clinical Targets Approach, Areas of Dysfunction Approach, and Intrapsychic Approach. As can be seen in the figure, Eleanor's counselor selected the Descriptive-Diagnosis Approach. This approach sorts together all of the various Step 1 information about the client's adjustment, development, distress, or dysfunction "to show larger clinical problems as reflected through a diagnosis" (Neukrug & Schwitzer, 2006, p. 205).

The counselor made just two straightforward, clear groupings: (a) mild depressive mood disorder due to hypothyroidism and (b) mild mental retardation with relatively good ability for daily functioning. Although quite straightforward, the counselor's conceptual work at Step 2 using the Descriptive-Diagnosis Approach gave her a clear way to organize the aims of the Brief Solution-Focused Counseling in which she and Eleanor would engage.

Figure 11.4   Eleanor Rigby's Inverted Pyramid Case Conceptualization Summary: Brief Solution-Focused Counseling

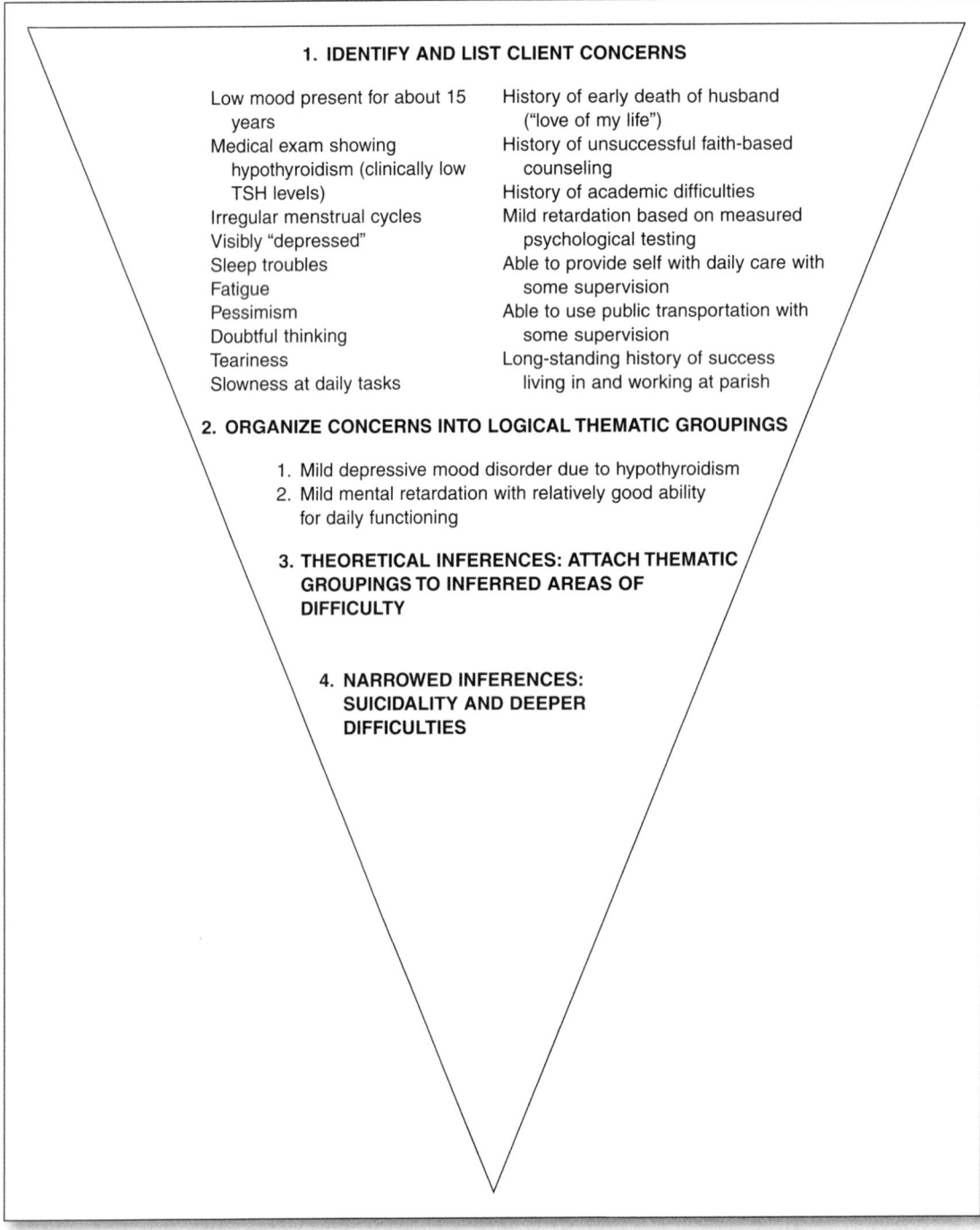

1. IDENTIFY AND LIST CLIENT CONCERNS

Low mood present for about 15 years

Medical exam showing hypothyroidism (clinically low TSH levels)

Irregular menstrual cycles

Visibly "depressed"

Sleep troubles

Fatigue

Pessimism

Doubtful thinking

Teariness

Slowness at daily tasks

History of early death of husband ("love of my life")

History of unsuccessful faith-based counseling

History of academic difficulties

Mild retardation based on measured psychological testing

Able to provide self with daily care with some supervision

Able to use public transportation with some supervision

Long-standing history of success living in and working at parish

2. ORGANIZE CONCERNS INTO LOGICAL THEMATIC GROUPINGS

1. Mild depressive mood disorder due to hypothyroidism
2. Mild mental retardation with relatively good ability for daily functioning

3. THEORETICAL INFERENCES: ATTACH THEMATIC GROUPINGS TO INFERRED AREAS OF DIFFICULTY

4. NARROWED INFERENCES: SUICIDALITY AND DEEPER DIFFICULTIES

TREATMENT PLANNING

At this point, Eleanor's clinician at the Liverpool City Services Clinic has collected all available information about the problems that have been of concern. Based upon this information, the counselor developed a five-axis *DSM-IV-TR* diagnosis and then, using the "inverted pyramid" (Neukrug & Schwitzer, 2006; Schwitzer, 1996, 1997), formulated a working clinical *explanation* of Eleanor Rigby's difficulties and their etiology that we called the *case conceptualization*. This, in turn, guides us to the next critical step in our clinical work, called the *treatment plan,* the primary purpose of which is to map out a logical and goal-oriented strategy for making positive changes in the client's life. In essence, the treatment plan is a road map "for reducing or eliminating disruptive symptoms that are impeding the client's ability to reach positive mental health outcomes" (Neukrug & Schwitzer, 2006, p. 225). As such, it is the cornerstone of our work with not only Eleanor Rigby, but with all clients who present with disturbing symptoms and/or problematic patterns (Jongsma et al., 2003a, 2003b; Jongsma & Peterson, 2006; Seligman, 1993, 1998, 2004).

A comprehensive treatment plan must integrate all of the information from the biopsychosocial interview, diagnosis, and case conceptualization into a coherent plan of action. This plan comprises four main components, which include (1) a behavioral definition of the problem(s), (2) the selection of achievable goals, (3) the determination of treatment modes, and (4) the documentation of how change will be measured. The *behavioral definition of the problem(s)* consolidates the results of the case conceptualization into a concise hierarchical list of problems and concerns that will be the focus of treatment. The *selection of achievable goals* refers to assessing and prioritizing the client's concerns into a *hierarchy of urgency* that also takes into account the client's motivation for change, level of dysfunction, and real-world influences on his or her problems. The *determination of treatment modes* refers to selection of the specific interventions, which are matched to the uniqueness of the client and to his or her goals and clearly tied to a particular theoretical orientation (Neukrug & Schwitzer, 2006). Finally, the clinician must establish how change will be measured, based upon a number of factors, including client records and self-report of change, in-session observations by the clinician, clinician ratings, results of standardized evaluations such as the Beck Anxiety Inventory (Beck & Steer, 1990) or a family functioning questionnaire, pre-post treatment comparisons, and reports by other treating professionals.

The four-step method discussed above can be seen in Figure 6.1 (p. 109) and is outlined below for the case of Eleanor Rigby, followed by her specific treatment plan.

Step 1: Behavioral Definition of Problems. The first step in solution-focused treatment planning is to carefully review the case conceptualization, paying particular attention to the results of Step 2 (Thematic Groupings). The identified clinical themes reflect the core areas of concern and distress for the client. In the case of Eleanor, there are two primary areas of concern. The first, "mild depressive mood disorder due to hypothyroidism," refers to her sleep troubles, fatigue, pessimism, doubtful thinking, teariness, and slowness on daily tasks related to previously diagnosed hypothyroidism. The second, "mild mental retardation," refers to her history of academic difficulties, her need for some supervision in order to provide self- and daily care, attend to workplace needs, and use public transportation; and general overall successful living in and working at the parish. These symptoms and stresses are consistent with the diagnosis of Mood Disorder Due to Hypothyroidism, With Depressive Symptoms; Mental Retardation, Mild (APA, 2000a; Grabe et al., 2005; King, Hodapp, & Dykens, 2005; Saravanan, Visser, & Dayan, 2006).

Step 2: Identify and Articulate Goals for Change.
The second step is the selection of achievable
goals, which is based upon a number of factors,
including the most pressing or urgent behavioral,
emotional, and interpersonal concerns and symptoms as identified by the client and clinician, the
willingness and ability of the client to work on
those particular goals, and the realistic (real-
world) achievability of those goals (Neukrug &
Schwitzer, 2006). At this stage of treatment planning, it is important to recognize that not all of
the client's problems can be addressed at once,
so we focus initially on those that cause the
greatest distress and impairment. New goals can
be created as old ones are achieved. In the case
of Eleanor Rigby, the goals are divided into two
prominent areas. The first, "mild depressive
symptoms due to hypothyroidism," requires that
we assist her to learn about the relationship
between her medical condition and her depressed
mood, to schedule regular visits to the city health
clinic in order to maintain her TSH levels, and to
learn about the importance of proper nutrition and
physical health care. The second, "mild mental
retardation," requires that we help Eleanor to optimize her overall level of adaptive functioning.

Step 3: Describe Therapeutic Interventions. This is
perhaps the most critical step in the treatment planning process because the clinician must now integrate information from a number of sources,
including the case conceptualization, the delineation of the client's problems and goals, and the
treatment literature, paying particular attention
to *empirically supported treatment* (EST) and
evidence-based practice (EBP). In essence, the
clinician must align his or her treatment approach
with scientific evidence from the fields of counseling and psychotherapy. Wampold (2001) identifies
two types of evidence-based counseling research:
studies that demonstrate "absolute efficacy," that is,
the fact that counseling and psychotherapy work,
and those that demonstrate "relative efficacy,"
that is, the fact that certain theoretical/technical
approaches work best for certain clients with
particular problems (Psychoanalysis, Gestalt
Therapy, Cognitive Behavior Therapy, Brief

Solution-Focused Therapy, Cognitive Therapy,
Dialectical Behavior Therapy, Person-Centered
Therapy, Expressive/Creative Therapies,
Interpersonal Therapy, and Feminist Therapy); and
when delivered through specific treatment modali-
ties (individual, group, and family counseling).

In the case of Eleanor Rigby, we have decided
to use Brief Solution-Focused Therapy (De Jong
& Berg, 2002; De Shazer & Dolan, 2007;
Gingerich & Eisengart, 2000; Gutterman, 2006).
This counseling approach is "pragmatic, anti-
deterministic and future oriented [and as such]
offers optimism, and hope about the ability of the
client to change" (Neukrug, 2011, p. 426). It de-
emphasizes psychopathology and the past, and
instead focuses on the client's strengths,
resources, and skills in order to generate solutions to the problems and concerns. Forward
looking and quickly moving, Solution-Focused
Therapy's basic assumptions include that change
is constant and inevitable, clients have the inherent skills and abilities to change, small steps lead
to big changes, exceptions to problems do occur
and can be used for change, and the future is both
created and negotiable; as well as simple axioms
such as "if it ain't broke, don't fix it," "if it
works, do more of it," and "if it's not working,
do something different" (Neukrug, 2011).

We view Brief Solution-Focused Therapy as
being particularly useful in Eleanor's case due to
its emphasis on change, the future, and tapping
into the client resources and skills. In spite of her
medical and developmental challenges, she does
indeed work, take care of herself, and relate with
others. Rather than delve into her personality
structure, it is most pragmatic to strengthen her
overall coping skills so that she may best function in her day-to-day life. This approach, which,
in addition, focuses on empowerment, hope, and
the strengthening of support networks, has been
found to be particularly useful in case management with clients coping with persistent challenges (Greene et al., 2006). Specific techniques
for Eleanor Rigby include asking a simplified
version of the "miracle question" to assess goals
for change, using preferred-goal, evaluative,
coping, exception-seeking and solution-focused

questions, "scaling" both her depression and desired mood to provide context and perspective as well as a starting point for change, identifying and complimenting Eleanor on her use of skills, amplification of previously successful strategies for self-care, reframing her mood problems as the result of a medical condition that she can address as she has other basic self-care issues, and referral to both a medical support group and endocrinologist for management of her thyroid condition.

Step 4: Provide Outcome Measures of Change. This last step in treatment planning requires that we specify how change will be measured and indicate the extent to which progress has been made toward realizing these goals (Neukrug & Schwitzer, 2006). The counselor has considerable flexibility in this phase and may choose from a number of objective domains (psychological tests and measures of self-esteem, depression, psychosis, interpersonal relationship, anxiety, etc.), quasi-objective measures (the

DSM-IV-TR's Axis V GAF scale; pre-post clinician, client, and psychiatric ratings), and subjective ratings (client self-report, clinician's in-session observations). In Eleanor's case, we have implemented a number of these, including pre-post measures on the Beck Depression Inventory-II (Beck et al., 1996), post-only improvement on the Adaptive Behavior Assessment System-II (Harrison & Oakland, 2000), post-only measures of GAF functioning in the mild range (>70), client self-reported awareness of and ability to address medical challenge, Father McKenzie's report of improved overall self-care and improved mood, and clinician-observed improvement in mood and physical well-being.

The completed treatment plan is now developed through which the counselor and Eleanor will begin their shared work of enhancing her overall coping and adaptive skills, including her physical and mental health. Eleanor Rigby's treatment plan appears below, and a summary can be found in Table 11.4.

TREATMENT PLAN

Client: Eleanor Rigby

Service Provider: Liverpool City Services Clinic

BEHAVIORAL DEFINITION OF PROBLEMS:

1. Mild Depressive Mood Due to Hypothyroidism—Sleep troubles, fatigue, pessimism, doubtful thinking, teariness, and slowness on daily tasks

2. Mild Mental Retardation—History of academic difficulties; need for some supervision in order to provide self- and daily care, attend to workplace needs, and use public transportation; general overall successful living in and working at the parish

GOALS FOR CHANGE:

1. Mild Depressive Mood Due to Hypothyroidism

   • Learn about the relationship between the medical condition and depression

(Continued)

(Continued)

- Develop a routine schedule of medical health care to maintain TSH levels
- Develop knowledge of and ability to apply nutritional and physical health care skills

2. Mild Mental Retardation

- Optimize overall level of adaptive functioning

THERAPEUTIC INTERVENTIONS:

A moderate- to long-term course (9–12 months) of Brief Solution-Focused Therapy supplemented with group support

1. Mild Depressive Mood Due to Hypothyroidism

- Asking a simplified version of the "miracle question" to assess goals for change
- Using preferred-goal, evaluative, coping, exception-seeking, and solution-focused questions
- Reframing mood problems as the result of a medical condition that can be addressed
- "Scaling" her depression and desired mood to provide context and perspective as well as a starting point for change
- Amplification of previously successful strategies for self-care
- Referral to developmentally appropriate medical support group
- Referral to endocrinologist for management of thyroid condition

2. Mild Mental Retardation

- Using preferred-goal, evaluative, coping, exception-seeking, and solution-focused questions to enhance coping skills
- Amplification of previously successful strategies for adaptive functioning
- Identifying and complimenting on use of skills
- Referral to a social and daily-living skills support group

OUTCOME MEASURES OF CHANGE:

The reinforcement and strengthening of already-present coping skills and alleviation of depression through appropriate medical care as measured by:

- Pre-post measures on the Beck Depression Inventory
- Post-only improvement on the Adaptive Behavior Assessment System-II
- Post-only measures of GAF functioning in the mild range (>70)
- Client self-reported awareness of and ability to address medical challenge
- Father McKenzie's report of improved overall self-care and improved mood
- Clinician-observed improvement in mood and physical well-being

Table 11.4   Eleanor Rigby's Treatment Plan Summary: Brief Solution-Focused Counseling

Goals for Change	Therapeutic Interventions	Outcome Measures of Change
<u>Mild depressive mood due to hypothyroidism</u> Learn about the relationship between the medical condition, and depression Develop a routine schedule of medical healthcare to maintain TSH levels Develop knowledge of and ability to apply nutritional and physical health care skills <u>Mild mental retardation</u> Optimize overall level of adaptive functioning	<u>Mild depressive mood due to hypothyroidism</u> Asking a simplified version of the "miracle question" to assess goals for change, Using preferred-goal, evaluative, coping, exception-seeking, and solution-focused questions Reframing mood problems as the result of a medical condition that can be addressed "Scaling" her depression to provide context and perspective as well as a starting point for change Amplification of previously successful strategies for self-care Referral to developmentally appropriate medical support group Referral to endocrinologist for management of thyroid condition. <u>Mild mental retardation</u> Using preferred-goal, evaluative, coping, exception-seeking and Solution-Focused questions to enhance coping skills Amplification of previously successful strategies for adaptive functioning Identifying and complimenting on use of skills Referral to a social and daily-living skills support group	The reinforcement and strengthening of already-present coping skills and alleviation of depression through appropriate medical care as measured by: Pre-post measures on the Beck Depression Inventory Post-only improvement on the Adaptive Behavior Assessment System-II Post-only measures of GAF functioning in the mild range (>70) Client self-reported awareness of and ability to address medical challenge Father McKenzie's report of improved overall self-care and improved mood Clinician-observed improvement in mood and physical well-being

CASE 11.5   GEICO INSURANCE COMPANY'S CAVEMAN

INTRODUCING THE CHARACTER

The "Caveman" is the trademarked character in an ongoing Geico Insurance advertising campaign created in 2004 by Joe Lawson of the Martin Agency. In its national effort to convince would-be customers that purchasing insurance through its online portal was incredibly simple, Geico introduced the slogan, "So easy a caveman can do it." The figurehead of this campaign was, naturally, a Neanderthal-like character who simply wanted to pursue life, liberty, and happiness in the same way that others around him did. The increasingly complex commercials evolved to include a group of cavemen in "normal, everyday activities," including bowling, walking through an airport, and hanging out at a bar. In each of these television commercials, the cavemen, who thought that they were living an otherwise normal and uneventful life, continually confront advertisements for Geico Insurance with the slogan reminding them that they are less than human. Although the ads were widely popular, the producers' attempts to spin these commercials into a television series were met with less than far-reaching enthusiasm. Clever and satirical, these television commercials highlight the issue of racial politics. The following basic case summary and diagnostic impressions describe Caveman's adjustment and acculturation concerns, characterized by emotional and behavioral symptoms that cause him distress.

Meet the Client

You can assess the client in action by viewing clips of Caveman's video material at the following websites:

- http://www.youtube.com/watch?v=m9 Dognr3BII Cavemen chat
- http://www.youtube.com/watch?v=3Mg_JIceCvk Caveman and friends bowling

- http://www.youtube.com/watch?v=sPP fYKbO-1M Caveman plays tennis with Billie Jean King
- http://www.youtube.com/watch?v= iomlEcaeZgQ Therapy for the Caveman
- http://www.youtube.com/watch?v= 3F3qzfTCDG4 The Caveman protests

---

BASIC CASE SUMMARY

Identifying Information. Neander Thal is a 31-year old man of Cavemanian origins. Mr. Thal has been residing in an apartment in Cincinnati, Ohio, for the past 6 months. He was relocated from his home in the country of Cavemanland by his company in order to serve as senior manager of the company's U.S. branch headquarters located in Cincinnati. He resides with two Cavemanian coworkers who relocated with him. Mr. Thal was motivated and engaged in the interview. He appeared appropriate for a professional interview and, notably, was dressed in hair style and dress of his native Cavemanland.

Presenting Concern. Mr. Thal was self-referred to the Lawson Martin Clinical Practice. In his written intake materials, he endorsed symptoms, including sleep disturbance, worry, anxiety, social isolation, and pessimism. His written narrative description of his concern highlighted a theme of "feeling like I don't fit in" and "starting to doubt myself." He identified his problems as beginning about 3 weeks after arrival at his U.S. work assignment. In the interview, Mr. Thal reported that "I never thought I'd need counseling" and "I hope you don't think I'm wasting your time" but said "I'm getting really worried about myself."

Background, Family Information, and Relevant History. Mr. Thal was born in the Neander Valley of Cavemanland and was the middle of three boys. Both parents worked in the computer industry. Mr. Thal reported that his childhood and teen years were relatively uneventful. He remembers generally enjoying his parent and family relationships; however, he recalls substantial competition among the brothers, notably on the soccer field, bowling league, and in academics at school. He recalls they also competed for friendships and membership in the most prestigious social cliques and for dating opportunities with girls and later young women.

According to the client's report, all three brothers attended schools at about the same time, and for much of their college years, they all attended the Caveman Institute of Technology. Mr. Thal majored in international business. He recalls his first geographic move was right after university graduation, when he began his first job with his current company in a new city outside of the Neander Valley, about 6 hours from "home." He remembers feeling "a little down" and "lonely" for a few weeks, but said that he was able to begin making new social acquaintances and friends among his new coworkers, by visiting open-mic nights at a coffee shop, and by joining a bowling league.

He reports that after about 5 years and two promotions, he became regional supervisor for Neander Valley operations. At this time, he relocated to his home city; reestablished long-standing friendships; and began a committed intimate relationship with a "high school sweetheart" with whom he shared an executive apartment. He reports that at times he did feel self-doubts about his ability to succeed at work and "worried that one day they'd find out I wasn't really that good." He also reported being "plagued" by fears that one day some "better looking guy with a

better car" would "steal my girlfriend." In fact, he reported that his moments of apparently unfounded jealousy increased over time, and did lead to the relationship's ending when his then-girlfriend "just got too tired of all my worries about losing her, I guess." His corporate success continued up until his very recent relocation to Cincinnati.

Problem and Counseling History. Mr. Thal has been seen for one evaluation meeting as per his health maintenance organization (HMO). He reports that at present he spends "almost all of my waking moments" worrying about "what the people around me think of me." He ruminates about his perception that "no matter where I go in town, people snicker and laugh and point at me." Although he is able to fall asleep at night, he is having difficulty staying asleep and "wakes up about every hour." He reports being fatigued and in the interview looked tired. He describes "started to feel nervous all of the time" and as a result of his worries about being ridiculed, sometimes goes without lunch during the day to avoid going into the streets and to a sandwich shop; and has avoided joining a bowling league here. He grew irritable when describing feeling "like I'll never fit in. People here won't even give me a chance just because I look different. Darn it, they don't even know me!" He also said he "could cut my hair like them, or shave my beard like them, or dress like them, but is that what I have to do to get along?" He appears aware of steps to take make the social transition in a new city and location but feels unable to take these steps.

Goals for Counseling and Course of Therapy to Date. Recommendation is for time-limited psychotherapy to address the problematic thoughts and perceptions interfering with the client's successful life-situation adjustment.

Diagnostic Impressions

Axis I.   309.9 Adjustment Disorder, Acute, With Anxiety

V62.89 Acculturation Problem

Axis II.   V71.09 No Diagnosis on Axis II

Axis III. None

Axis IV.   Problems related to social environment—Geographic relocation, problems with acculturation

Axis V.   GAF = 70 (current)

GAF = 88 (highest level past year)

DISCUSSION OF
DIAGNOSTIC IMPRESSIONS

Neander Thal came into the Lawson Martin Clinical Practice presenting difficulties associated with his geographic relocation to Cincinnati from his home country. He indicated that he was feeling symptoms of anxiety and worry, was having trouble sleeping through the night, felt socially isolated, and was pessimistic. He reported very good adjustment prior to his relocation and, in fact, recalled an earlier occasion during which he made a geographic change inside his home country without undue symptoms of distress.

The *DSM-IV-TR* Adjustment Disorders all are clinically significant psychological responses to an identifiable life stressor. To meet the criteria for an Adjustment Disorder, the psychological responses must cause marked distress or clinically significant impairment in functioning, must go beyond normally expected and culturally appropriate reactions, and must not be due to another *DSM-IV-TR* disorder or a medical problem. Adjustment Disorders can occur with depressed mood, anxiety, disturbance in conduct or behavior, or have a combination of these.

Mr. Thal presented symptoms focused primarily around the experience of mild anxiety. He reported ruminating about others' judgments about him, constant worry, and nervousness. He was avoiding normal social situations such as restaurants, and failed to take steps to address his social isolation such as joining a bowling league. He exhibited physical symptoms of anxiety such as sleep disruption and fatigue. His concerns emerged within 3 months of the onset of his relocation. In the absence of any evidence of substance abuse, and without any evidence that his symptoms meet the criteria for another diagnosable Axis I mood or anxiety disorder, the diagnosis is Adjustment Disorder. Because his concerns have lasted fewer than 3 months, the specifier Acute is used, and because he reported primarily anxiety symptoms, the disorder is specified With Anxiety.

Specific differential considerations when determining an Adjustment Disorder include other relevant Axis I diagnoses. However, Mr. Thal's experiences did not meet the criteria for any diagnosable Anxiety Disorder. Adjustment Disorder requires that the client's concerns develop within 3 months of the life event's onset; Mr. Thal presented increasing symptoms shortly after the stresses of his relocation and social and cultural transition. Another consideration is whether the client's reactions are normally expected, culturally appropriate reactions that do not produce excessive distress or cause excessive impairment. However, Neander Thal's concerns were reported to cause clinically significant distress and some impairment in social functioning and in the workplace.

Further, along with all the various diagnosable disorders, a multiaxial diagnosis also lists Other Conditions That May Be a Focus of Clinical Attention. The client concerns contained in this section (appearing at the end of the *DSM-IV-TR,* following all of the diagnosable disorders) are not diagnosable mental disorders according to the *DSM* classification system; instead, they sometimes are client problems that are a focus of counseling but not a part of the individual's diagnosable mental disorder. Mr. Thal's challenges with acculturation are in this category. Acculturation encompasses concerns about attitudinal and behavioral differences or internal changes encountered when moving between two cultures (Arthur, 2004; Pederson, 1991); when these concerns result in physiological, psychological, or social stresses, they may be a clinically important focus of counseling (Poyrazli, Kavanaugh, Baker, & Al-Timimi, 2004).

To complete the diagnosis, Mr. Thal's important social stressors are emphasized on Axis IV, and on Axis V his functioning is represented by GAF scores indicating that although at present he is experiencing some mildly serious symptoms and some mild difficulties in social and work and home functioning, within the recent past he has demonstrated good functioning with only normally expected difficulties with everyday problems. The information on these axes is consistent with the Axis I diagnoses reflecting Neander Thal's adjustment situation.

CASE CONCEPTUALIZATION

During Mr. Thal's intake session at the Lawson Martin Clinical Practice, his counselor collected as much information as possible about his current adjustment difficulties and relevant history. The counselor first used this information to develop diagnostic impressions. Mr. Thal's concerns were described by Adjustment Disorder With Anxiety. Next, the counselor developed a case conceptualization. Whereas the purpose of diagnostic impressions is to *describe* the client's concerns, the goal of case conceptualization is to better *understand* and clinically *explain* the person's experiences (Neukrug & Schwitzer, 2006). It helps the counselor understand the circumstances leading to the Adjustment Disorder and the factors maintaining it. In turn, case conceptualization sets the stage for treatment planning. Treatment planning then provides a road map that plots out how the counselor and client expect to move from presenting concerns to positive outcomes (Seligman, 1993, p. 157)—helping Mr. Thal reduce his anxiety and positively change his reactions and behaviors during his current adjustment to Cincinnati.

When forming a case conceptualization, the clinician applies a purist counseling theory, an integration of two or more theories, an eclectic mix of theories, or a solution-focused combination of tactics to his or her understanding of the client. In this case, Mr. Thal's counselor based his conceptualization on a purist theory, Adlerian Therapy (or Individual Psychology). The counselor selected this approach because it is the counseling method of choice at the Lawson Martin Clinical Practice whenever it appears the client might benefit from a model that has strengths from a multicultural perspective; Adlerian Therapy emphasizes the importance of cultural context and, specifically, individual behavior and adjustment in the context of societal constraints and influences (Carlson & Englar-Carlson, 2008; Nystul, 1999). The clinical practice also prefers Adlerian Therapy when an approach is needed that emphasizes health rather than pathology, and a holistic perspective on life (Nystul, 1999). This approach also is amenable to time-limited counseling, such as for an adjustment disorder (Carlson, Watts, & Maniacci, 2006). The Lawson Martin staff believe the Adlerian approach reflects best practice with clients such as Neander Thal.

The counselor used the Inverted Pyramid Method of case conceptualization because this method is especially designed to help clinicians more easily form their conceptual pictures of their clients' needs (Neukrug & Schwitzer, 2006; Schwitzer, 1996, 1997). The method has four steps: Problem Identification, Thematic Groupings, Theoretical Inferences, and Narrowed Inferences. The counselor's clinical thinking can be seen in Figure 11.5.

Step 1: Problem Identification. The first step is Problem Identification. Aspects of the presenting problem (thoughts, feelings, behaviors, physiological features), additional areas of concern besides the presenting concern, family and developmental history, in-session observations, clinical inquiries (medical problems, medications, past counseling, substance use, suicidality), and psychological assessments (problem checklists, personality inventories, mental status exam, specific clinical measures) all may contribute information at Step 1. The counselor "casts a wide net" in order to build Step 1 as exhaustively as possible (Neukrug & Schwitzer, 2006, p. 202). As can be seen in Figure 11.5, the counselor identified all of Mr. Thal's current presenting problems (worry, avoidance, and anxiety symptoms), plus his past difficulties with workplace self-doubt, and romantic relationship self-doubt and its consequences.

Step 2: Thematic Groupings. The second step is Thematic Groupings. The clinician organizes all of the exhaustive client information found in Step 1 into just a few intuitive-logical clinical groups, categories, or themes, on the basis of sensible common denominators (Neukrug & Schwitzer, 2006). Four different ways of forming the Step 2 theme groups can be used: Descriptive-Diagnosis Approach, Clinical Targets Approach, Areas of Dysfunction Approach, and Intrapsychic Approach. As can be seen in Figure 11.5, Mr. Thal's counselor selected the Intrapsychic Approach. This approach sorts together all of the Step 1 information about the "client's adjustment, development, distress, or dysfunction" in order "to show clinical patterns in the ways life events are associated with the person's personal experience and identity" (Neukrug & Schwitzer, 2006, p. 205).

Interestingly, the counselor grouped together all of the factors in Step 1 into just one theme, capturing the intrapsychic pattern he believes Mr. Thal has been dealing with since early in his work life, in his intimate relationships, as well as during his current acculturation. Specifically, he grouped all of the Step 1 data into the theme: "patterns of anxiety symptoms, avoidance, and worry about not succeeding, not fitting in, not being good enough, and not being desirable enough."

So far, at Steps 1 and 2, the counselor has used his intake evaluation skills and clinical judgment to begin meaningfully understanding Mr. Thal's situation. Now, at Steps 3 and 4, he applies the theoretical approach he has selected. He begins making theoretical inferences to interpret and explain the processes underlying Caveman's problematic dynamics as they are seen in Steps 1 and 2.

Step 3: Theoretical Inferences. At Step 3, constructs from the selected theory, Adlerian Therapy (or Individual Psychology), are applied to explain the roots of Mr. Thal's past and present adjustment difficulties. The counselor tentatively matches the theme group in Step 2 with this theoretical approach. In other words, the symptom constellation formed in Step 2, which distilled together all of the symptoms in Step 1, now are combined using theory to show what are believed to be the underlying causes or psychological etiology of Neander Thal's clinical needs (Neukrug & Schwitzer, 2006; Schwitzer, 2006, 2007).

According to Adlerian Therapy, psychological health is characterized by a drive or striving for goal accomplishment, self-perfection, connection, and cooperation with other people, and meaningfulness in our lives; this allows us to overcome normally expected feelings of doubt or inferiority (Sweeney, 1998). By comparison, psychological difficulties can arise from *feelings of inferiority* that are beyond those normally expected. Specifically, the theory suggests that when an individual develops problematic feelings of inferiority (in Adlerian language, Secondary Feelings of Inferiority), he or she may turn to maladaptive thoughts (in Adlerian language, private logic), interpersonal behaviors (in Adlerian language, problems with social interest and social concern), or other defenses, such as compensations, or striving for superiority. According to Adlerian Therapy, family psychological dynamics, sibling birth order, and social context all influence the development of feelings of inferiority. Mr. Thal's family of brothers would be one focus of the counselor's attention (Carlson et al., 2006; Watts, 2003).

As can be seen in Figure 11.5, when Mr. Thal's counselor applied these Adlerian constructs, he explained at Step 3 that the anxiety and related problems and consequences at Step 1, which formed a pattern of worry about not succeeding and not fitting in and not being desirable enough (Step 2), are understood to be Adlerian problems of (a) feelings of inferiority and (b) low social inference. The feelings of inferiority contribute to avoiding social interactions and not fully meeting social interests, characteristics of low social inference (Adler, 1964; Watts, 2007).

Step 4: Narrowed Inferences. At Step 4, the clinician's selected theory continues to be used to address still-deeper issues when they exist (Schwitzer, 2006, 2007). At this step, "still-deeper, more encompassing, or more central, causal themes" are formed (Neukrug & Schwitzer, 2006, p. 207). Continuing to apply Adlerian concepts at Step 4, Mr. Thal's counselor presented a single, deepest, most-fundamental inference that he believed to be most explanatory of Mr. Thal's difficulties: Inferiority Complex, captured by a fear of being unlovable and of not being good enough (Carlson et al., 2006; Watts, 2003). When all four steps are completed, the client information in Step 1 leads to logical-intuitive groupings on the basis of common denominators in Step 2, the groupings then are explained using theory at Step 3, and then, finally, at Step 4, further deeper explanations are made. From start to finish, the thoughts, feelings, behaviors, and physiological features in the topmost portions

are connected on down the pyramid into deepest dynamics.

The completed pyramid now is used to plan treatment, in which the counselor and Neander Thal will address his inferiority complex.

TREATMENT PLANNING

At this point, Mr. Thal's clinician at the Lawson Martin Clinical Practice has collected all available information about the problems that have been of concern to him. Based upon this information, the counselor developed a five-axis *DSM-IV-TR* diagnosis and then, using the "inverted pyramid" (Neukrug & Schwitzer, 2006; Schwitzer, 1996, 1997), formulated a working clinical *explanation* of Neander Thal's difficulties and their etiology that we called the *case conceptualization*. This, in turn, guides us to the next critical step in our clinical work, called the *treatment plan,* the primary purpose of which is to map out a logical and goal-oriented strategy for making positive changes in the client's life. In essence, the treatment plan is a road map "for reducing or eliminating disruptive symptoms that are impeding the client's ability to reach positive mental health outcomes" (Neukrug & Schwitzer, 2006, p. 225). As such, it is the cornerstone of our work with not only Mr. Thal, but with all clients who present with disturbing or disruptive symptoms and/or personality patterns (Jongsma et al., 2003a, 2003b; Jongsma & Peterson, 2006; Seligman, 1993, 1998, 2004).

A comprehensive treatment plan must integrate all of the information from the biopsychosocial interview, diagnosis, and case conceptualization into a coherent plan of action. This plan comprises four main components, which include (1) a behavioral definition of the problem(s), (2) the selection of achievable goals, (3) the determination of treatment modes, and (4) the documentation of how change will be measured. The *behavioral definition of the problem(s)* consolidates the results of the case conceptualization into a concise

Figure 11.5 Geico Caveman's Inverted Pyramid Case Conceptualization Summary: Adlerian Therapy

1. IDENTIFY AND LIST CLIENT CONCERNS

Current worry
Current anxiety
Currently feels nervous
Feelings of social isolation
Pessimism
Worry about ability to adjust
Rumination about people's reactions
Thoughts about changing appearance
   to fit in
Avoiding lunch to avoid being in public
Avoiding taking action of joining
   bowling league

Plagued by fears of inadequacy in past romantic
   relationship
Jealousy and worry in past romantic
   relationship
Loss of relationship due to own fears and
   behaviors
Recent arrival in United States
New work responsibilities
Past self-doubts of having weakness
   "found out" at work

2. ORGANIZE CONCERNS INTO LOGICAL THEMATIC GROUPINGS

1. Pattern of anxiety symptoms, avoidance, and worry about
   not succeeding, not fitting in, not being good enough,
   desirable enough

3. THEORETICAL INFERENCES: ATTACH THEMATIC GROUPINGS TO INFERRED AREAS OF DIFFICULTY

Adlerian Inferences About Areas of Difficulty

Feelings of inferiority
Low social inference

4. NARROWED INFERENCES: SUICIDALITY AND DEEPER DIFFICULTIES

Narrowed Adlerian Inference

Inferiority Complex (Fear of
being unlovable and of
not being enough)

hierarchical list of problems and concerns that will be the focus of treatment. The *selection of achievable goals* refers to assessing and prioritizing the client's concerns into a *hierarchy of urgency* that also takes into account the client's motivation for change, level of dysfunction, and real-world influences on his or her problems. The *determination of treatment modes* refers to selection of the specific interventions, which are matched to the uniqueness of the client and to his or her goals and clearly tied to a particular theoretical orientation (Neukrug & Schwitzer, 2006). Finally, the clinician must establish how change will be measured, based upon a number of factors, including client records and self-report of change, in-session observations by the clinician, clinician ratings, results of standardized evaluations such as the Beck Depression Inventory-II (Beck, 1996) or a family functioning questionnaire, pre-post treatment comparisons, and reports by other treating professionals.

The four-step method discussed above can be seen in Figure 6.1 (p. 109), and is outlined below for the case of Neander Thal, followed by his specific treatment plan.

Step 1: Behavioral Definition of Problems. The first step in treatment planning is to carefully review the case conceptualization, paying particular attention to the results of Step 2 (Thematic Groupings), Step 3 (Theoretical Inferences), and Step 4 (Narrowed Inferences). The identified clinical themes reflect the core areas of concern and distress for the client, while the theoretical and narrowed inferences offer clinical speculation as to their origins. In the case of Mr. Thal, there is one primary areas of concern, "a pattern of anxiety symptoms and behavior." This area of concern refers to his sleep disturbance, nervousness, feelings of social isolation, concerns over ability to adjust, ruminations about peoples' reactions, thoughts about changing appearance to fit in, avoidance of social activities including lunch and bowling, feelings of inadequacy, jealousy in romantic relationships, and loss of relationships due to fears, self-doubts. These symptoms and stresses are consistent with the diagnosis of Adjustment Disorder, Acute, With Anxiety and Acculturation Problems (APA, 2000a; Berry, 2003; Casey, Dorwick, & Wilkinson, 2001; Flores, Ojeda, Yu-Ping, Gee, & Lee, 2006; Strain et al., 1998).

Step 2: Identify and Articulate Goals for Change. The second step is the selection of achievable goals, which is based upon a number of factors, including the most pressing or urgent behavioral, emotional, and interpersonal concerns and symptoms as identified by the client and clinician, the willingness and ability of the client to work on those particular goals, and the realistic (real-world) achievability of those goals (Neukrug & Schwitzer, 2006). At this stage of treatment planning, it is important to recognize that not all of the client's problems can be addressed at once, so we focus initially on those that cause the greatest distress and impairment. New goals can be created as old ones are achieved. In the case of Neander Thal, the goals center on one prominent cluster: "a pattern of anxiety symptoms." The specific goals for Mr. Thal include developing insight into the historical source of his inferiority feelings, increasing and expanding his social interest, exploring his "style of life" for adaptive and maladaptive elements, decreasing fears and feelings of rejection and self-doubt, developing acceptance of himself and his appearance, understanding and re-organizing his private logic for the purpose of self.

Step 3: Describe Therapeutic Interventions. This is perhaps the most critical step in the treatment planning process because the clinician must now integrate information from a number of sources, including the case conceptualization, the delineation of the client's problems and goals, and the treatment literature, paying particular attention to *empirically supported treatment* (EST) and *evidence-based practice* (EBP). In essence, the clinician must align his or her treatment approach with scientific evidence from the fields of counseling and psychotherapy. Wampold (2001) identifies two types of evidence-based counseling research: studies that demonstrate "absolute efficacy," that is, the fact that counseling and psychotherapy work, and those that demonstrate "relative efficacy," that is, the fact that certain theoretical/technical approaches work best for certain clients with particular problems (Psychoanalysis, Gestalt Therapy, Cognitive Behavior Therapy, Brief Solution-Focused Therapy, Cognitive Therapy, Dialectical Behavior Therapy, Person-Centered Therapy, Expressive/Creative Therapies, Interpersonal Therapy, and Feminist Therapy); and when delivered through specific treatment modalities (individual, group, and family counseling). In the case of Caveman, we have decided to use Adlerian Therapy (Adler, 1964; Dinkmeyer & Sperry, 2000) due to its humanistic and interpersonal emphasis on each person's capacity for power, connection, and self-fulfillment. Given Mr. Thal's complex family history and the detrimental effect it has had on the development of his self-image and interpersonal relationship schema, the supportive yet directive nature of Alderian Therapy will provide the counselor with a useful therapeutic orientation to his problems and effective strategies for change. Use of Adlerian Therapy has proven useful for clients with similar concerns as Caveman (Carlson et al., 2006; Oberst & Stewart, 2003). Specific techniques for Mr. Thal will include examination of his early recollections and family constellation to understand their formative roles, dream analysis to explore and modify his private logic and social schema, role-playing to explore new patterns of behavior, thoughts, and

feelings, "spitting in his soup" to demonstrate faulty private logic, and creating tasks centered on social interactions.

Step 4: Provide Outcome Measures of Change. This last step in treatment planning requires that we specify how change will be measured and indicate the extent to which progress has been made toward realizing these goals (Neukrug & Schwitzer, 2006). The counselor has considerable flexibility in this phase and may choose from a number of objective domains (psychological tests and measures of self-esteem, depression, psychosis, interpersonal relationship, anxiety, etc.), quasi-objective measures (the *DSM-IV-TR's* Axis V GAF scale; pre-post clinician, client, and psychiatric ratings), and subjective ratings (client self-report, clinician's in-session observations). In Caveman's case, we have implemented a number of these, including pre-post comparisons of effective and fulfilling social attitudes and interactions, client self-reported awareness of improved self-regard and style of life, counselor observation of self-affirming private logic, and pre-post improvement on the Beck Anxiety Inventory.

The completed treatment plan is now developed through which the counselor and Mr. Thal will begin their shared work of improving his relationships with others, his self-regard, and overall style of life. The treatment plan is described below and summarized in Table 11.5.

TREATMENT PLAN

Client: Neander Thal

Service Provider: Lawson Martin Clinical Practice

BEHAVIORAL DEFINITION OF PROBLEMS:

1. Pattern of Anxiety Symptoms—Sleep disturbance, nervousness, feelings of social isolation, concerns over ability to adjust, ruminations about peoples' reactions, thoughts about changing

appearance to fit in, avoiding social activities, including lunch and bowling, feelings of inadequacy, jealousy in romantic relationships, loss of relationships due to fears, self-doubts

GOALS FOR CHANGE:

1. Pattern of anxiety symptoms

- Increase insight into the historical source of inferiority feelings
- Increase and expand social interest
- Explore "style of life" for adaptive and maladaptive elements
- Decrease fears and feelings of rejection and self-doubt
- Develop acceptance of himself and his appearance
- Understand and reorganize private logic for the purpose of self-enhancement
- Explore and enhance personal courage to enhance the overall quality of life

THERAPEUTIC INTERVENTIONS:

A short- to moderate-term course of individual Adlerian counseling (3–6 months)

1. Pattern of anxiety symptoms

- Encourage and support client to explore his style of life, feelings of inferiority, private logic, compensatory behavior, and goals for change
- Examine early recollections and family constellation to understand their formative role
- Dream analysis to explore and modify private logic and social schema
- Role-playing to explore new patterns of behavior, thoughts, and feelings
- "Spit in the client's soup" to demonstrate faulty private logic
- Set and accomplish tasks centered on social interactions

OUTCOME MEASURES OF CHANGE:

The development of positive feelings of worth, social interest and involvement, adaptive private logic, and a happiness and self-contented style of life will be measured by:

- Pre-post comparisons of effective and fulfilling social attitudes and interactions
- Client self-reported awareness of improved self-regard and style of life
- Counselor observation of self-affirming private logic
- Pre-post improvement on Beck Anxiety Inventory
- Pre-post measures on the Social Interest Inventory II
- Pre-post improvement of overall functioning as measured by GAF scores in the mild range (>70)
- Increased number of friends, friendly interactions, and accepted social invitations

Table 11.5   Geico Caveman's Treatment Plan Summary: Adlerian Therapy

Goals for Change	Therapeutic Interventions	Outcome Measures of Change
Pattern of anxiety symptoms	Pattern of anxiety symptoms	The development of positive feelings of worth, social interest and involvement, adaptive private logic, and a happiness and self-contented style of life will be measured by:
Increase insight into the historical source of inferiority feelings	Encourage and support client to explore his style of life, feelings of inferiority, private logic, compensatory behavior, and goals for change	
Increase and expand social interest	Examine early recollections and family constellation to understand their formative role	Pre-post comparisons of effective and fulfilling social attitudes and interactions
Explore "style of life" for adaptive and maladaptive elements	Dream analysis to explore and modify private logic and social schema	Client self-reported awareness of improved self-regard and style of life
Decrease fears and feelings of rejection and self-doubt	Role-playing to explore new patterns of behavior, thoughts, and feelings	Counselor observation of self-affirming private logic
Develop acceptance of himself and his appearance	"Spit in the client's soup" to demonstrate faulty private logic	Pre-post improvement on Beck Anxiety Inventory
Understand and reorganize private logic for the purpose of self enhancement	Set and accomplish tasks centered on social interactions	Pre-post measures on the Social Interest Inventory II
Explore and enhance personal courage to enhance the overall quality of life		Pre-post improvement of overall functioning as measured by GAF scores in the mild range (>70)
		Increased number of friends, friendly interactions, and accepted social invitations

FOLLOW-UP: DIAGNOSIS, CASE CONCEPTUALIZATION, AND TREATMENT PLANNING THEMES—CHAPTER SUMMARY

This chapter presented a varied clinical caseload comprising three adult clients, Fred the Baker, Eleanor Rigby, and Caveman, and two adolescents: Maria and Billie Jean. Among the caseload's diversity were Maria, a Puerto Rican teenager living in New York City; Billie Jean, an African American teenager living in Los Angeles; an Anglo-American client, Fred the Baker; and two international clients, Eleanor Rigby, an English woman in Liverpool, and Caveman, who

we presented as being from Cavemanland but currently working in Cincinnati, Ohio. Upper-middle, middle, and working-class socioeconomic statuses were represented by this group of clients. We identified all of these clients as heterosexual.

Among this chapter's clients, Fred the Baker and Caveman sought counseling services on their own accord—Caveman at a private clinical practice and Fred through his EAP. Maria and Eleanor Rigby were urged to visit the Bowery Community Services Center and Liverpool City Services Clinic, respectively, by people in their lives. Finally, Billie Jean was required to attend counseling by her L.A. Department of Families and Children Services caseworker.

Among the concerns presented by the clients making up the chapter's caseload, Fred the Baker sought assistant for concerns characterized diagnostically as Adjustment Disorder With Depressed Mood; Maria presented symptoms of ASD, along with Bereavement; Billie Jean also was dealing with posttrauma reactions, described diagnostically as PTSD, along with Delusional Disorder; Eleanor Rigby's concerns were identified as depressive symptoms of a Mood Disorder Due to a General Medical Condition, namely, Hypothyroidism, as well as a background history of mild Mental Retardation; and finally, like Fred, Caveman presented Adjustment Disorder, in this case with anxiety, and problems associated with acculturation.

Turning to the counseling theories represented, these clients' counselors formed case conceptualizations and then treatment plans based on Person-Centered Counseling, Cognitive Behavior Therapy, Adlerian Therapy, and in two cases, Brief Solution-Focused Counseling.

In their treatment plans, these clients' counselors expressed hopes that their clients would achieve such as outcomes as development of congruence between ideal and actual self and improved self-esteem (Fred the Baker), alleviation of ASD symptoms (Maria) and PTSD and delusional disorder symptoms (Billie Jean), strengthening of already-present coping skills and alleviation of depression (Eleanor Rigby), and development of positive self-worth, social interest, and self-contented lifestyle (Caveman).

STUDY QUESTIONS AND LEARNING ACTIVITIES

Based on your understanding of this chapter's cases, consider and respond to these Study Questions and Learning Activities:

1. This caseload is a varied one.

   a. If you were assigned this group of clients, what would be your initial reactions to their individual characteristics and differences? Working with both adults and adolescents? Their reasons for referral?

   b. What would you identify as your greatest strengths for assisting these five clients? Your areas of greatest need for growth?

2. In their Basic Case Summaries, this chapter's counselors focused on their clients' earlier developmental and family experiences, presenting concerns, assessment of current distress, and areas and life roles in which they were experiencing difficulties, client strengths, and hopes for change. There was an emphasis on: Fred the Baker's developmental and adult life history plus his current transition; the traumatic events leading to, and symptoms and severity of, Maria's onset of acute stress; the extremely traumatic events leading to, and patterns and severity of, Billie Jean's difficulties; Eleanor Rigby's current coping as well as her early and adult development and life history and record of Mental Retardation; and likewise, Caveman's current transition experience but also his developmental and past adult history.

   a. Keeping in mind that the initial counseling meeting, screening session, or intake interview usually requires the counselor to balance rapport and trust-building, on one hand, and assessment and information-gathering, on the other hand, what would you identify as your greatest strengths when engaging these five clients in the counseling process, and gathering the clinical information needed to conceptualize and plan for their counseling process? Your areas of greatest need for growth?

   b. Looking at the five Basic Case Summaries, how does this type of clinical writing differ from your everyday thinking and conversation about people? What are your levels of comfort, skill, and experience with this type of professional writing? What steps can you take to further develop or improve these skills?

   c. What suggestions would you have for one or more of the counselors in this chapter regarding missing, overlooked, or underemphasized—or overemphasized—information gathered and reported in the Basic Case Summaries? What would you like to have known more about? What methods could be used—clinical interview questions, observations, psychological measures, or other means—to find the additional information you would seek?

3. This chapter illustrated *DSM-IV-TR* diagnoses found in the following sections: Disorders Usually First Diagnosed in Infancy, Childhood, or

Adolescence (Mental Retardation is found in this section even when the client is an adult), Mental Disorders due to a General Medical Condition Not Elsewhere Classified, Schizophrenic and Other Psychotic Disorders, Anxiety Disorders, and Adjustment Disorders—plus Other Conditions That May Be a Focus of Clinical Attention.

a. How familiar are you with these sections of the *DSM-IV-TR?* What is your comfort level using the *DSM-IV-TR* to explore these sets of concerns? Which of these groups of disorders are likely to be most important to you in the practicum, internship, residency, or professional practice settings in which you hope to work?

b. What are your attitudes, reactions, or thoughts concerning diagnosis of childhood disorders? Concerning the diagnosis of behavioral consequences of problematic substance use? Concerning diagnosing lifelong patterns characterized as personality disorders? How can you further explore or develop your professional attitudes about diagnosis of these types of concerns?

c. What will be your next steps in gaining greater comfort and skills at diagnosis of mental retardation? Mental disorders that are due to a medical condition? Psychotic Disorders other than Schizophrenia (like Delusional Disorder)? Anxiety and Adjustment Disorders?

d. What are your attitudes, reactions, or thoughts concerning use of Axis IV to record psychosocial and environmental stressors (such as Maria's exposure to gang violence, and to a hostile racial climate) and Axis V to record general medical problems (such as Billie Jean's recent childbirth)? What will be your next steps in gaining greater comfort and skills with these axes?

e. Among this group of clients, Axis V GAF scores ranged from 40 (Billie Jean's impairment in reality testing) to 70 (Caveman's mild symptoms). What are your attitudes, reactions, or thoughts concerning use of Axis V GAF scores to estimate the client's overall level of functioning? Do you agree with the counselors' estimates found in this chapter? What will be your next steps in gaining greater comfort and skills estimating Axis V GAF scores?

4. This chapter's cases included three examples of case conceptualization and treatment planning using purist counselor theories, and two applications of Brief Solution-Focused Counseling.

a. What is your level of familiarity with the various adult counseling theories illustrated in this chapter: Person-Centered Counseling? Cognitive Behavior Therapy? Adlerian Therapy? What do you believe are their relative strengths and weaknesses? For which individuals do they seem to be a good match? For what types of client concerns do they seem to be potentially effective? What do the evidence and discussions found in the current literature say about this?

b. Which of these theories seems to be a good fit with your own attitudes and skills? Which interest you the most?

c. To learn more, review the resources and references cited in the chapter, interview a practicing counselor who uses these theories in his or her everyday work, seek clinical supervision from a supervisor experienced with the approach, enroll in a special topics class, or look for continuing education workshops and conference presentations covering these approaches.

d. What are your thoughts, reactions, and comfort level employing a Brief Solution-Focused approach to address the needs of your clients? What knowledge or skills will you need to be an effective Brief Solution-Focused counselor?

e. How will you decide when, with whom, and in what ways to employ Brief Solution-Focused approaches? To consider and learn more about solution-focused counseling strategies, interview a practicing counselor who uses a solution focus in his or her everyday work, seek clinical supervision from a supervisor experiencing with solution-focused counseling, or seek other professional consultations and learning opportunities.

5. The case conceptualizations found in this chapter began with casting a wide net for client concerns and dynamics, next formed intuitive-logical groupings to begin better understanding the clients' presentations, and then applied counseling theories to make clinical inferences about the clients' situations.

a. How does this type of professional clinical thinking differ from your everyday thinking, conversation, and analysis about people?

What are your levels of comfort, skill, and experience with this type of clinical thinking? What steps can you take to further develop or improve your conceptualizing skills?

b. What are your thoughts, reactions, and critique of the ways these counselors grouped together: Fred's past versus present thoughts, behaviors, mood, and physiology? Maria's posttrauma stresses, grief, and additional stresses? Billie Jean's problematic post-traumatic symptoms, and her problematic romantic delusional symptoms? Eleanor's mild depressive mood due to hypothyroidism, and mild mental retardation with good daily functioning? Caveman's single theme, a pattern of anxiety about not being desirable enough? Do you agree with each of these thematic groupings? How might you have organized these differently, more usefully, or more effectively?

c. What are your thoughts and reactions pertaining to the ways the counselors applied the various theoretical approaches in order to explain, make inferences about, and prepare for treatment planning with these clients? What were your reactions to the counselors' presentations of: Fred the Baker's loss of sources of self-worth and questions about his enduring value (Person-Centered Counseling)? Maria's cognitive distortions (Cognitive Behavior Therapy)? Caveman's inferiority and low social inference (Adlerian Therapy)? Do you agree with the ways the counselor used the various theories with these clients? How might you have applied the theories differently, more usefully, or more effectively?

6. A fully developed treatment plan was presented for each of the individuals comprising this chapter's caseload. The treatment plans provide goals for change, interventions, and outcome measures.

a. How does this type of clinical writing, thinking, and preparation for the professional counseling process differ from your everyday approach to engaging in helpful relationships with people? What are your levels of comfort, skill, and experience with this type of professional writing, thinking, and preparation? What steps can you take to further develop or improve your treatment planning skills for the types of practicum,

internship, residency, or work settings that are of most interest to you?

b. This chapter's treatment plans first list goals for change for each "client" character, next apply the selected counseling theory to clearly state the interventions and approaches to be used, and finally identify ways to measure the expected changes. What are your thoughts, reactions, and critique of the ways this chapter's counselors prepared Fred's, Maria's, Billie Jean's, Eleanor's, and Caveman's treatment plans? What interests you most about these plans? What raises questions for you?

c. What are your thoughts and reactions pertaining to the Person-Centered approaches (Fred), Cognitive Behavioral techniques (Maria), Adlerian methods (Caveman), and Solution-Focused components (Billie Jean and Eleanor) outlined as interventions? With which are you most familiar? Least familiar? Unfamiliar? Which will you select to learn more about through further reading, clinical supervision, or other professional development? Alternatively, which do not seem to be close fits with your own preferred approach?

d. These clients' counselors used counselor observation, client report, change scores on psychological measures and the GAF, behavioral reports, and other means to measure outcomes. As you review the outcome measures found on Fred's, Maria's, Billie Jean's, Eleanor's, and Caveman's treatment plans, consider these questions: Do the measures seem realistic and accomplishable? Are they concrete and specific enough to indicate change? Are they sensitive to the needs of the client? Which of these measures will become a regular part of your own repertoire, which might you decline to use, and what additional measures might you add to your own list? What new skills and competencies might you need to develop in order to effectively report on your own clients' outcomes?

7. Now, working independently, with a partner, or in a small group, select your own "client" from among the pop culture world of Characters in Music, Musicals, and Advertising. Develop your own narrative about the client's arrival at counseling. Then, prepare a fully completed Basic Case Summary, Diagnostic Impressions, Case Conceptualization, and Treatment Plan!

12

CHARACTERS IN LITERATURE AND COMICS

The Cases of Annie Wilkes, Miss Celie, Chief Bromden, Peter Parker, and Christopher Robin

PREVIEW: POPULAR CULTURE THEMES

In this final section, we will bring together a fascinating array of characters that have initially come to us through the written word. Drawn from the imaginations of the some of the most widely read authors of our time, including Stephen King, Alice Walker, Ken Kesey, A. A. Milne, and Stan Lee of Marvel Comics fame, these characters, who differ as widely in their demography as they do in their stories, share in common uniquely interesting lives. Although they also differ in their print mediums of origin—novel, children's story, and comic book—each of the protagonists in these rich tales has a story to tell.

There are numerous popular literary media, modes, and devices for delivering narratives about people's lives, including novels, magazines, comics, newspaper, and advertisement (Danesi, 2008). Whether the stories are framed historically or reflect on contemporary themes, they reflect both personal and cultural meaning. Mythologist

Joseph Campbell recognized the transcultural and panhistoric nature of myths and legends, and wove together an intricate and colorful tapestry of the human experience (Campbell, 1968; Campbell & Moyers, 1991). So powerful are these stories drawn from the world's literature that their themes have been integrated into our popular culture psyche in the form of movies and television shows (Indick, 2004; Murphy, 1996) and the entirety of the superhero genre (Rubin, 2006b).

With regard to the specific characters in this section, Annie Wilkes, star along with her love interest and kidnapping victim Paul Sheldon, is determined to have a hand in rewriting the great American romance story of Misery Chastain. An eerie psychological thriller later made into a movie that garnered an Oscar for its female lead, the story is a dark psychological thriller that remains popular to date. In our presentation, Annie Wilkes struggles with Bipolar Disorder and Antisocial Personality Features. Miss Celie is the unlikely heroine in Alice Walker's Pulitzer prize–winning novel *The Color Purple,* which was adapted by Steven Spielberg into an Academy Award–winning film—a testament to the power of the tale of its victorious protagonist. In our presentation, Miss Celie struggles with Posttraumatic Stress Disorder (PTSD) and Dysthymic Disorder. Chief Bromden is the tall and oppressed character, along with Randle Patrick (R. P.) McMurphy of Ken Kesey's award-winning novel *One Flew Over the Cuckoo's Nest,* which also was made into an award-winning film of the same title. In our presentation, the Chief struggles with Schizophrenia and Alcohol Abuse. Peter Parker, aka, Spider-Man, originally appeared in issue 15 of Marvel Comics' *Amazing Fantasy.* The angst-ridden teen has cast his web across comic book pages for over four decades and more recently came to the silver screen in a series of record-breaking blockbuster movies starring Tobey Maguire and Kirsten Dunst. In our presentation, Peter struggles with Major Depressive Disorder and Personality Changes Due to a Radioactive Spider Bite. And finally, there is forever young Christopher Robin, the main character in A. A. Milne's beloved children's stories about Winnie the Pooh, Tigger, and adventures in the Hundred Acre Wood. The stories have captured the imaginations of children for more than 80 years; have been made into numerous films and books; and their images have been cast onto every conceivable consumer product for children of all ages. In our presentation, Christopher Robin struggles with Asperger's Syndrome.

Taken together, these characters form a powerful ensemble, drawn from different literary eras and genres as well as from different corners of society. They range in age from childhood to middle age and portray the full range of human experience, from the whimsical fantasies of an innocent little boy to the painful psychotic experience of a middle-aged woman. These particular characters fly by virtue of either their imaginations or spider webs, experience the depths of despair and the heights of elation. They experience captivity, either at the hands of society or of their own making, wrestle with demons, both inner and outer, and constantly strive to achieve security, safety, connection, and meaning. Annie Wilkes, Miss Celie, Chief Bromden, Peter Parker, and Christopher Robin will team up to stimulate your imagination and continue to strengthen your diagnostic, case conceptualization, and treatment planning skills.

APPROACHES TO LEARNING

As you learn about this group of characters, pay attention to:

- The way that Disorders First Evidenced in Infancy, Childhood, or Adolescence—particularly Autism Spectrum Disorders—are depicted in popular literature.
- How discussions of real-life psychological problems are represented in comic books and fiction.
- The relationship between chronic and acute psychological problems in the characters in this section and how this coincides with your knowledge of the *Diagnostic and Statistical Manual (DSM).*
- The manner in which the adjustment problems and counseling needs of different racial, ethnic, gender, and age groups are portrayed in popular culture in general and in literature in particular.

CASE 12.1 *MISERY'S* ANNIE WILKES

INTRODUCING THE CHARACTER

Annie Wilkes is the main character in the 1987 Stephen King novel, *Misery,* which in 1990 was made into a motion picture directed by Rob Reiner. Annie Wilkes is a former nurse who was acquitted of charges that she murdered numerous patients, including children, who were under her care. The details of Ms. Wilkes's early life are rather sketchy; however, when the story of *Misery* opens, Ms. Wilkes, while driving to her secluded Colorado home, finds famous romance novelist, Paul

Sheldon, unconscious on the side of the road. Ms. Wilkes takes the battered author back to her home and nurses him to health. Over the course of the story, Sheldon quickly discovers that Ms. Wilkes is obsessed with the main character of his novel, *Misery Chastain.* Believing that it was divine providence that brought Paul Sheldon to her, and that it was her mission to nurse him back to health so that he could complete his novel, Annie Wilkes compels him to rewrite the series when she learns that he has killed off her beloved character. His recuperation soon turns into a horror story, complete with torture at Ms. Wilkes's hands, and his growing realization that this "fan" is psychotic and very likely guilty of the numerous murders with which she was charged. Although Sheldon ultimately liberates himself from his sadistic captor, the psychological and physical scars of his captivity leave the reader and film-goer with images of the haunting scenes that transpired in Annie Wilkes's secluded mountain cabin.

Using *Misery* as our jumping-off point, the following basic case summary and diagnostic impressions describe (a) a long-term pattern characterized by periods of severe, abnormally elevated and expansive mood, co-occurring with (b) another enduring pattern of inner experience and behavior characterized by disregard for and violation of the rights of others, both of which we conceive Annie Wilkes to have been experiencing.

Meet the Client

You can assess the client in action by viewing clips of Annie Wilkes's video material at the following websites:

- http://www.youtube.com/watch?v=i5 OlolbLXvw Annie hurts Paul for lying
- http://www.youtube.com/watch?v=64 RdMFheer4 Annie from all sides

---

BASIC CASE SUMMARY

Identifying Information. Annie Wilkes is a 42-year-old, unmarried, white woman who lives alone in a modest home in the North Mountains

of Colorado and is a retired nurse. She has no living relatives, spends most of her time in isolation, and apparently, with the exception of monthly visits to town for groceries, passes her time alone reading and re-reading the romance novels of Paul Sheldon. She is particularly drawn to his multivolume Misery series and considers herself to be "Sheldon's biggest fan."

Presenting Concern. Ms. Wilkes was referred to the Overlook Psychotherapy Center by her attorney, John Frederick, seeking support for his client's case against the Colorado District Hospital. In his referral, Mr. Frederick indicated that while he was able to win an acquittal for Ms. Wilkes on multiple murder charges, he believed her countersuit against the State of Colorado for wrongful termination could be strengthened with psychiatric support. During the course of preparing for trial, Ms. Wilkes had acknowledged to Mr. Frederick that psychiatric disorders had run in her family and that she had been prone to what she referred to as "my little mood swings."

Background, Family Information, and Relevant History. Annaliese "Annie" Wilkes was born in Bakersfield, California, the only child of Frederick and Amanda Wilkes, junior college teachers who had met while in an alcohol rehabilitation program in San Diego. Mrs. Wilkes's pregnancy was complicated by the stress of frequent fighting with her husband, which occasionally became violent. Bedridden for the last 2 months of her pregnancy, Mrs. Wilkes was severely depressed and delivered Annie 4 weeks early via emergency cesarean section.

In spite of her traumatic beginnings, Ms. Wilkes was an otherwise healthy and vital infant who was described by her mother as being unusually curious and active. She performed well in school and preferred the company of adults to that of children. She often remained after school in order to avoid going home as her parents fought frequently, began drinking again, and were verbally abusive toward her. There are reports that as an elementary school–aged child, she frequently ran away from home for one or two nights at a time.

When Ms. Wilkes was 10, she was removed from her parents' care and placed with a cousin in a neighboring town, where she learned that her mother had long suffered with Bipolar Disorder and Alcohol Abuse. Ms. Wilkes had only sporadic contact with her parents during her adolescence and returned to their care when she was a high school junior as her cousin had passed away. While living with her cousin, she was suspected of hunting down and torturing squirrels and rabbits in the neighboring park, and on at least one occasion, of setting a swing set on fire in the park. However, she appeared to participate successfully at school and earned good enough grades to continue advancing.

Upon returning home, Ms. Wilkes immersed herself in her school work and vowed that she would choose a profession in which she could help others; she chose nursing. Ms. Wilkes had planned to attend nursing school immediately after high school but experienced what in retrospect she called "my first bout." A month after graduating from high school, Ms. Wilkes began acting erratically, going for days at a time without sleeping, filling out numerous applications for nursing jobs, and to nursing schools, as well as visiting hospital emergency rooms so that "I could get a first-hand look at what I would be doing when I became a nurse." With the help of her family physician, Ms. Wilkes was placed on medication that seemed to quiet her and allowed her to attain sufficient stability to enter nursing school. Ms. Wilkes never took the time nor had the interest to cultivate romantic relationships, as "I was dedicated to the mission of helping children."

Ms. Wilkes was the top student throughout nursing school and developed an affinity for children. She often remained in the hospital long after her training in order to provide comfort to the infants in the neonatal intensive care unit. In looking back, Ms. Wilkes recalled thinking, "They were so little and helpless and I knew what that was like, so I gave them my heart." Ms. Wilkes's parents were absent for her nursing school graduation ceremony, and what could have been the happiest day of her life turned out to be one of the saddest, and she recalled vowing "to never be the kind of person that they were."

Ms. Wilkes's nursing career was very rewarding, and she was recognized early on for her unique skills in working with children; however, at age 32 her performance was tarnished when an infant died while under her care, and she was blamed for the death. She was placed on probation, and soon after she had another episode requiring psychiatric hospitalization and suspension of her nursing license. That particular "episode," as she referred to it, was marked by taking on double shifts as well as per diem work, and in her words, "The desire to help as many children as I could." A coworker described her behavior as "incredibly energetic . . . Annie could do the work of five of us, sometimes for a week or more at a time, but when she crashed, it was as if she was a zombie for 2 days." Another coworker said that "when Annie was on top, you could hardly keep up with all her ideas about making the hospital better, and 'fixing' the patients, and improving efficiency. You could hardly keep with her!"

After discharge from the hospital, Ms. Wilkes resigned her job, moved across the state, and registered with a nursing temp company. Over the next 2 years, Ms. Wilkes provided home health care to infants and children, several of whom died of mysterious circumstances that were blamed directly on her. She was prosecuted by the State's Attorney's office but acquitted on all charges. Her nursing license was revoked and she returned to Bakersfield to live in her childhood home, alone, broken, and without direction. She decided to sue both the hospital that discharged her and the State Licensing Board that revoked her license.

Problem and Counseling History. Ms. Wilkes was referred to the Overlook Psychotherapy Center by her attorney, who believed that her chances for a successful lawsuit would depend on her ability to demonstrate that her erratic behavior was related to her traumatic upbringing, that her symptoms were under control, and that she had developed sufficient insight. Ms. Wilkes presented as a very tense and rigid woman who was dressed in very simple clothing and who was meticulously groomed. Oriented in all spheres, Ms. Wilkes spoke in a very measured and articulate fashion about her mental health problems and the circumstances surrounding the revocation of her nurse's license. She did not accept the diagnosis of Bipolar Disorder given to her while hospitalized, insisting instead "that would mean I'm just like my momma, and I'm nothing like her." She did acknowledge, however, that "I do like to take a nip late at night before bedtime; it helps me to fall asleep." When asked about the death of the children who were in her care, Ms. Wilkes broke down and sobbed inconsolably, and once she was able to contain herself, she said almost inaudibly, "Those children had no hope, and I took care of them the best way I could."

Goals for Counseling and Course of Therapy to Date. Staff of the Overlook Psychotherapy Center have declined to participate as consultants to Ms. Wilkes's legal team. Given her reason for referral, psychiatric history, the inconsistencies in her accounts of the deaths, and her erratic behavior, Miss Wilkes was referred to a Denver psychiatric center for a thorough assessment and treatment. On the basis of that referral, a full report of the resulting diagnostic impressions, conceptualization, and treatment plan are attached to this outpatient intake summary.

Diagnostic Impressions

Axis I.   296.44 Bipolar Disorder, Most Recent Episode Manic, Severe With Mood Congruent Psychotic Features, In Partial Remission

Axis II.   301.7 Antisocial Personality Disorder

Axis III.   None

Axis IV.   Problems with primary support group—History of emotional abuse by parents

Occupational problems—Job loss, revocation of professional license

Other psychosocial and environmental problems—Geographic isolation from adequate medical, mental health, and social services

Axis V.   GAF = 40 (at intake)

GAF = 59 (highest level past year)

DISCUSSION OF DIAGNOSTIC IMPRESSIONS

Annie Wilkes arrived at the Overlook Psychotherapy Center, presenting a history of recurring episodes characterized by expansive mood, along with: inflated self-esteem; grandiose beliefs that she could improve hospital efficiency and "help" innumerable pediatric patients; noticeably decreased need for sleep; flights of ideas and racing thoughts; and markedly increased goal-directed activities in her nursing position. During these symptomatic periods, she experienced psychotic features in the form of delusions that murdering young hospital children was a way to "fix" them. In between recurrent episodes, she experienced periods described by others as a "crash" during which she was "zombie"-like; however, no clear episodes of major depression were noted in her history.

The *DSM-IV-TR's* Mood Disorders section includes all of the Axis I diagnosable disorders that feature a disturbance in mood. The Mood Disorders include Depressive Disorders (in which the client experiences unipolar depression), Bipolar Disorders (in which the client experiences manic, hypomanic, or mixed episodes), and mood disorders that are due to substance use or a medical condition.

Annie Wilkes's mood problems were characterized by recurrent episodes of expansive mood and other symptoms characteristic of mania. In the absence of any evidence that her symptoms are the consequences of abuse of a substance (such as alcohol) or effects of a medical problem (like hyperthyroidism), Annie Wilkes's expansive mood, grandiosity, physiological symptoms, cognitive symptoms, and behavioral symptoms meet the criteria for a Manic Episode. Manic Episodes are used as building blocks for making a Mood Disorder diagnosis.

Annie Wilkes apparently has experienced no clear Major Depressive Episodes. However, when a person has experienced at least one Manic Episode, the diagnosis is Bipolar I Disorder, regardless of whether or not he or she also has experienced any Major Depressive Episodes. Annie has experienced a series of Manic Episodes. In these situations, the Most Recent Episode is described. Therefore, the diagnosis is Bipolar I Disorder, Most Recent Episode Manic. During her most recent episode, she experienced substantial symptoms in excess of the minimum needed to make the diagnosis. Further, she had psychotic delusions confusing murder with saving children's lives. Themes of death may be congruent with disturbances in mood, and themes pertaining to being a savior are congruent with mania. Therefore, the severity specifier to be listed is Severe With Mood Congruent Psychotic Features. Presently she appears to have only a few symptoms (she still reports sleep disturbances and appears to have some mild disturbances of thought); therefore, the specifier, In Partial Remission, is used.

Differential diagnoses might include Bipolar II Disorder, in which less severe and shorter lasting hypomanic episodes rather than manic episodes are experienced, and Cyclothymic Disorder, in which hypomanic and mildly depressive episodes both are experienced. However, Annie Wilkes's manic symptoms clearly conform to the criteria for Manic Episodes. Psychotic Disorders such as Schizophrenia and Schizoaffective Disorder share features of delusions and mood disruption with Bipolar I disorder. However, Annie does not exhibit any of the additional characteristics of the schizophrenic disorders such as disorganized speech or behavior or flattened affect.

In addition to Bipolar I Disorder, the diagnosis of a personality disorder was considered. A multiaxial diagnosis presents all the various diagnosable disorders and other conditions that might be a focus of clinical attention on Axis I except for the Personality Disorders and Mental Retardation, which are reported on Axis II. In other words, Axis II answers the questions: "Does the client evidence any long-term pattern of maladaptive character traits that cause significant impairment or distress?" "Does the client [present symptoms and experiences that] meet the criteria for any of the [diagnosable] personality disorders?" as well as whether Mental Retardation is present (LaBruzza & Mendez-Villarrubia, 1994, p. 86).The *DSM-IV-TR's* Personality Disorders section contains 11 disorders characterized by pervasive, inflexible, stable, and enduring maladaptive patterns of personality—marked by inner experiences, interpersonal relationships, and other behaviors that deviate from what is normally expected from the person's cultural context—that have been present since adolescence or early adulthood.

Annie Wilkes's history reflects a pervasive pattern of disregarding and violating the rights of others, including committing clandestine murder and kidnapping. She has recurrently failed to conform to social norms, professional ethics, and laws; disregarded others' safety; and shown lack of remorse and indifference to the pain and suffering she causes. Taken together, this pattern suggests a diagnosis of Antisocial Personality Disorder.

Bipolar I Disorder can be an exceptionally disruptive condition for individuals who experience it, and Manic Episodes can produce extreme changes in personality and severe changes in behavior (Federman & Thomson, 2010). Correspondingly, one differential consideration is whether Annie Wilkes's personality features and behaviors appear only during Manic Episodes; if so, no additional personality disorder diagnosis is needed. However, her failure to conform to social norms and unlawful behaviors (she is suspected of additional murders when not experiencing mania), her reckless disregard for others (background history suggests she is suspected of kidnapping a paperback novelist), as well as her lack of remorse and indifference to having harmed others, are seen even beyond the parameters of her periodic Manic Episodes and therefore present a pervasive and inflexible pattern that warrants additional listing on Axis II.

To wrap up the diagnosis, Annie Wilkes's substantial social stressors are emphasized on Axis IV, and on Axis V her functioning is represented by Global Assessment of Functioning (GAF) scores indicating some impairment in reality testing at present, and, at her highest recent point of functioning, the presence of some moderately serious symptoms. The information on these axes is consistent with the Axis I and Axis II diagnoses reflecting Annie's history and current situation.

CASE CONCEPTUALIZATION

The first task for Annie Wilkes's Overlook Psychotherapy Center clinician was to conduct a detailed assessment of her history and current functioning. The counselor first used this information to develop diagnostic impressions. Annie Wilkes's patterns were described by Bipolar Disorder along with Antisocial Personality Features. Next, the counselor developed a case conceptualization. Whereas the purpose of diagnostic impressions is to *describe* the client's concerns, the goal of case conceptualization is to better *understand* and clinically *explain* the person's experiences (Neukrug & Schwitzer, 2006). It helps the counselor understand the etiology

leading to some of Annie's problematic concerns and the factors maintaining these issues. In turn, case conceptualization sets the stage for treatment planning. Treatment planning then provides a road map that plots out how the counselor and client expect to move from presenting concerns to positive outcomes (Seligman, 1993, p. 157)—helping Annie control or reduce her problematic mood episodes, behavior, and personality dynamics.

When forming a case conceptualization, the clinician applies a purist counseling theory, an integration of two or more theories, an eclectic mix of theories, or a solution-focused combination of tactics to his or her understanding of the client. In this case, Ms. Wilkes's counselor based his conceptualization on a purist theory, Cognitive Behavior Therapy. He selected this approach based on his knowledge of current outcome research with clients experiencing Bipolar Disorder and personality disorders (Critchfield & Smith-Benjamin, 2006; Jones, 2004; Livesley, 2007; Looper & Kirmayer, 2002; Scott & Gutierrez, 2004). Cognitive Behavior Therapy also is consistent with this counselor's professional therapeutic viewpoint and that of his clinical setting, the Overlook Psychotherapy Center.

The counselor used the Inverted Pyramid Method of case conceptualization because this method is especially designed to help clinicians more easily form their conceptual pictures of their clients' needs (Neukrug & Schwitzer, 2006; Schwitzer, 1996, 1997). The method has four steps: Problem Identification, Thematic Groupings, Theoretical Inferences, and Narrowed Inferences. The counselor's clinical thinking can be seen in Figure 12.1.

Step 1: Problem Identification. The first step is Problem Identification. Aspects of the presenting problem (thoughts, feelings, behaviors, physiological features), additional areas of concern besides the presenting concern, family and developmental history, in-session observations, clinical inquiries (medical problems, medications, past counseling, substance use, suicidality), and psychological assessments (problem checklists, personality inventories, mental status exam, specific clinical measures) all may contribute information at Step 1. The counselor "casts a wide net" in order to build Step 1 as exhaustively as possible (Neukrug & Schwitzer, 2006, p. 202). As can be seen in Figure 12.1, Annie's clinician had a wide range of material to capture, including manic episode symptoms of Bipolar Disorder; psychotic symptoms associated with her manic episodes; information about her work history and legal problems; important childhood behaviors; data about her traumatic developmental and family experiences; and notes about her alcohol use. He worked to include as much information as possible about Annie's presenting concern, collateral concerns, and history.

Step 2: Thematic Groupings. The second step is Thematic Groupings. The clinician organizes all of the exhaustive client information found in Step 1 into just a few intuitive-logical clinical groups, categories, or themes, on the basis of sensible common denominators (Neukrug & Schwitzer, 2006). Four different ways of forming the Step 2 theme groups can be used: Descriptive-Diagnosis Approach, Clinical Targets Approach, Areas of Dysfunction Approach, and Intrapsychic Approach. As can be seen in the figure, Annie Wilkes's counselor selected the Areas of Dysfunction Approach. This approach sorts together all of the Step 1 information into "areas of dysfunction according to important life situations, life themes, or life roles and skills" (Neukrug & Schwitzer, 2006, p. 205).

The counselor grouped together (a) all of the effects of Annie's non-psychotic manic episode symptoms and signs of Bipolar Disorder (erratic mood, excessive energy, denial, etc.) into the theme, "dealing with routine effects of Bipolar Disorder"; (b) all of the effects and results of her psychotic symptoms (confusing murder with helping, etc.) into the theme, "dealing with the psychotic effects of Bipolar Disorder"; and (c) all of the effects and outcomes of her interpersonal trauma growing up (childhood conduct, parent history, her antisocial beliefs and actions,

etc.), into the theme, "dealing with the learned experiences of a traumatic household background and foster care." The counselor's conceptual work at Step 2 gave him a way to begin usefully understanding and explaining Annie's areas of functioning and built a bridge to the steps that follow.

So far, at Steps 1 and 2, the counselor has used his clinical assessment skills and his clinical judgment to begin meaningfully understanding Annie's needs. Now, at Steps 3 and 4, he applies the theoretical approach he has selected. He begins making theoretical inferences to interpret and explain the processes or roots underlying Annie Wilkes's concerns as they are seen in Steps 1 and 2.

Step 3: Theoretical Inferences. At Step 3, concepts from the counselor's selected therapy, Cognitive Behavior Therapy, are applied to explain the experiences causing and the mechanisms maintaining Annie's severely problematic thoughts, feelings, and behaviors. The counselor tentatively matches the theme groups in Step 2 with this theoretical approach. In other words, the symptom constellations in Step 2, which were distilled from the symptoms in Step 1, now are combined using theory to show what are believed to be the underlying causes or psychological etiology of Annie Wilkes's current needs (Neukrug & Schwitzer, 2006; Schwitzer, 2006, 2007).

According to Cognitive Behavior Therapy (Beck, 1995, 2005; Ellis, 1994; Ellis & MacLaren, 2005), irrational thinking, faulty beliefs, or other forms of cognitive errors lead individuals to engage in problematic behaviors and to experience negative moods and attitudes. As can be seen in Figure 12.1, when the counselor applied these Cognitive Behavior Therapy concepts, he explained at Step 3 that the various issues noted in Step 1 (manic symptoms, psychotic thoughts and behaviors, negative parenting, antisocial behaviors.), which can be understood to be themes of (a) dealing with Bipolar Disorder, (b) dealing with psychotic thoughts and behaviors, and (c) dealing with childhood emotional trauma

(Step 2), are rooted in or caused by several cognitive distortions and faulty core beliefs ("I could not stand to be like my mother and therefore do not have Bipolar Disorder"; "Manic Episodes give me special powers to save children and others and I must use these powers," "I have learned life is hopeless for some children, so I can save them by death") and by inaccurate, problem behavioral responses (continuing to experience Bipolar Disorder, continuing to act on psychotic, antisocial thoughts). These are detailed on Figure 12.1.

Step 4: Narrowed Inferences. At Step 4, the clinician's selected theory continues to be used to address still-deeper issues when they exist (Schwitzer, 2006, 2007). At this step, "still-deeper, more encompassing, or more central, causal themes" are formed (Neukrug & Schwitzer, 2006, p. 207). Continuing to apply Cognitive Behavior Therapy concepts at Step 4, Ms. Wilkes's counselor presented two deepest, most-fundamental cognitive distortions of events that he believed to be most explanatory and causal regarding Annie's history and present functioning: the distortions that (a) "I have lived through awful experiences, know what a terrible world it is for some children and other people, and I alone can save them" and (b) "There is no reason I should change because I know what I am doing and what the world needs from me." When all four steps are completed, the client information in Step 1 leads to logical-intuitive groupings on the basis of common denominators in Step 2, the groupings then are explained using theory at Step 3, and then, finally, at Step 4, further deeper explanations are made. From start to finish, the thoughts, feelings, behaviors, and physiological features in the topmost portions are connected on down the pyramid into deepest dynamics.

The completed pyramid now is used to plan treatment, through which the counselor expects to work with Annie Wilkes to confront her cognitive distortions, faulty core beliefs, negative behavioral consequences, and deepest distortion of events.

TREATMENT PLANNING

At this point, Annie Wilkes's clinician at the Overlook Psychotherapy Center has collected all available information about the problems that have been of concern to her and the psychiatric team that performed her assessment. Based upon this information, the counselor developed a five-axis *DSM-IV-TR* diagnosis and then, using the "inverted pyramid" (Neukrug & Schwitzer, 2006; Schwitzer, 1996, 1997), formulated a working clinical *explanation* of Annie Wilkes's difficulties and their etiology that we called the *case conceptualization*. This, in turn, guides us to the next critical step in our clinical work, called the *treatment plan,* the primary purpose of which is to map out a logical and goal-oriented strategy for making positive changes in the client's life. In essence, the treatment plan is a road map *"for reducing or eliminating disruptive symptoms that are impeding the client's ability to reach positive mental health outcomes"* (Neukrug & Schwitzer, 2006, p. 225). As such, it is the cornerstone of our work with not only Ms. Wilkes, but with all clients who present with disturbing and disruptive symptoms and/or personality patterns (Jongsma & Peterson, 2006; Jongsma, Peterson, & McInnis, 2003a, 2003b; Seligman, 1993, 1998, 2004).

A comprehensive treatment plan must integrate all of the information from the biopsychosocial interview, diagnosis, and case conceptualization into a coherent plan of action. This *plan* comprises four main components, which include (1) a behavioral definition of the problem(s), (2) the selection of achievable goals, (3) the determination of treatment modes, and (4) the documentation of how change will be measured. The *behavioral definition of the problem(s)* consolidates the results of the case conceptualization into a concise hierarchical list of problems and concerns that will be the focus of treatment. The *selection of achievable goals* refers to assessing and prioritizing the client's concerns into a *hierarchy of urgency* that also takes into account the client's motivation for change, level of dysfunction, and real-world influences on his or her problems. The *determination of treatment modes* refers to selection of the specific interventions, which are matched to the uniqueness of the client and to his or

Figure 12.1   Annie Wilkes's Inverted Pyramid Case Conceptualization Summary: Cognitive
Behavior Therapy

1. IDENTIFY AND LIST CLIENT CONCERNS

Manic episodes
Erratic mood
Diminished sleep, sleep disturbances
Excessive energy
Highly charged to accomplish goals
  of nursing and helping infants
Diagnosed and prescribed for Bipolar
  Disorder
Periods of "crashing"
Psychotic thoughts during mania
Confuses murder with saving children's
  lives
Sees child patients as helpless and
  needing saving

Child history of harming animals
Child history of fire-setting
History of mother with Bipolar Disorder
History of parents with alcohol abuse
History of parental fighting & violence
History of removal to foster care
Problem alcohol use
Troubled work history
Fired on occasions
Prosecuted for murder

2. ORGANIZE CONCERNS INTO LOGICAL THEMATIC GROUPINGS

1. Dealing with routine effects of Bipolar Disorder
2. Dealing with the psychotic effects of Bipolar Disorder
3. Dealing with the learned experiences of a traumatic
   household background and foster care

**3. THEORETICAL INFERENCES: ATTACH THEMATIC
GROUPINGS TO INFERRED AREAS OF DIFFICULTY**

Cognitive Distortions and Faulty Core Beliefs

1. I could not possibly stand to live if I was similar to my mother
   and I will never be the kind of person my parents were;
   therefore, I cannot and do not have Bipolar Disorder like
   she did (or have an alcohol problem like she did)
2. When I have my bouts, they give me extraordinary abilities
   to save children and help others; therefore I must act on
   the ideas and plans I have during my bouts
3. I know from my upbringing that some children have no hope,
   and during my bouts I am able to help them out of their misery
   (by killing them)

Negative Behavioral Consequences

1. Continuing to experience untreated manic episodes and Bipolar Disorder
2. Acting on impulses to murder child hospital patients and
   other antisocial acts such as kidnapping

4. NARROWED INFERENCES: SUICIDALITY AND DEEPER DIFFICULTIES

Deepest Faulty Core Belief

1. I have lived through awful experiences and know
   what a terrible world it is for some children and
   other people, and I alone can save them
2. There is no reason I should change because
   I know what I am doing and what the world needs from me

her goals and clearly tied to a particular theoretical orientation (Neukrug & Schwitzer, 2006). Finally, the clinician must establish how change will be measured, based upon a number of factors, including client records and self-report of change, in-session observations by the clinician, clinician ratings, results of standardized evaluations such as the Beck Depression Inventory-II (Beck, Steer, & Brown, 1996), pre-post treatment comparisons, and reports by other treating professionals.

The four-step method discussed above can be seen in Figure 6.1 (p. 109) and is outlined below for the case of Annie Wilkes, followed by her specific treatment plan.

Step 1: Behavioral Definition of Problems. The first step in treatment planning is to carefully review the case conceptualization, paying particular attention to the results of Step 2 (Thematic Groupings), Step 3 (Theoretical Inferences), and Step 4 (Narrowed Inferences). The identified clinical themes reflect the core areas of concern and distress for the client, while the theoretical and narrowed inferences offer clinical speculation as to their origins. In the case of Annie Wilkes, there are three primary areas of concern. The first, "dealing with the routine effects of Bipolar Disorder," refers to her erratic mood, diminished sleep, excessive energy, periods of depression, and problematic alcohol use. The second, "dealing with the psychotic effects of Bipolar Disorder," refers to her grandiose thoughts during mania, and confusion between capturing and/or killing people with helping them. The third, "dealing with the learned experiences of a traumatic household and foster care," and refers to the basis for her antisocial behaviors. These symptoms and personality patterns are consistent with the diagnosis of Bipolar Disorder, Most Recent Episode Manic, Severe With Mood Congruent Psychotic Features and Antisocial Personality Disorder (APA, 2000a; Critchfield & Smith-Benjamin, 2006; Jones, 2004; Livesley, 2007; Scott & Gutierrez, 2004).

Step 2: Identify and Articulate Goals for Change. The second step is the selection of achievable goals, which is based upon a number of factors

including the most pressing or urgent behavioral, emotional, and interpersonal concerns and symptoms as identified by the client and clinician, the willingness and ability of the client to work on those particular goals, and the realistic (real-world) achievability of those goals (Neukrug & Schwitzer, 2006). At this stage of treatment planning, it is important to recognize that not all of the client's problems can be addressed at once, so we focus initially on those that cause the greatest distress and impairment. New goals can be created as old ones are achieved. In the case of Annie Wilkes, the goals are divided into three prominent clusters. The first, "dealing with the routine effects of Bipolar Disorder," requires that we assist her in maintaining stability sufficiently so she can participate in therapy, stabilizing her mood, eating, sleeping and activity levels, and reducing her alcohol use. The second, "dealing with the psychotic effects of her Bipolar Disorder," requires that we eliminate her psychotic symptoms, moderate her grandiose thoughts and balance them with realistic self-appraisal, and assist her to recognize the difference between helping and hurting others. The last, "dealing with the learned experiences of a traumatic household and foster care," requires that we help her to recognize the relationship between early family violence and her antisocial behavior and to reconcile feelings of loss and abandonment related to her childhood foster placement.

Step 3: Describe Therapeutic Interventions. This is perhaps the most critical step in the treatment planning process because the clinician must now integrate information from a number of sources, including the case conceptualization, the delineation of the client's problems and goals, and the treatment literature, paying particular attention to *empirically supported treatment* (EST) and *evidence-based practice* (EBP). In essence, the clinician must align the treatment approach with scientific evidence from the fields of counseling and psychotherapy. Wampold (2001) identifies two types of evidence-based counseling research: studies that demonstrate "absolute efficacy," that is, the fact that counseling and psychotherapy work, and those that demonstrate "relative efficacy," that is, the fact that certain theoretical/technical approaches work best for certain clients with particular problems (Psychoanalysis, Gestalt Therapy, Cognitive Behavior Therapy, Brief Solution-Focused Therapy, Cognitive Therapy, Dialectical Behavior Therapy, Person-Centered Therapy, Expressive/Creative Therapies, Interpersonal Therapy, and Feminist Therapy); and when delivered through specific treatment modalities (individual, group, and family counseling). In the case of Annie Wilkes, we have decided to use Cognitive Behavior Therapy because of its demonstrated effectiveness with clients experiencing Bipolar Disorder accompanied by Antisocial Personality Features (Critchfield & Smith-Benjamin, 2006; Jones, 2004; Livesley, 2007; Looper & Kirmayer, 2002; Scott & Gutierrez, 2004). The approach relies on a variety of cognitive techniques (reframing, challenging irrational thoughts, and cognitive restructuring) and behavioral techniques (reinforcement for and shaping of adaptive behavior, extinction of maladaptive behaviors, systematic desensitization, exposure with response prevention (Ball et al., 2006; Frank et al., 2005; Milkowitz, 2008). Further, the use of psychoeducation (Colom et al., 2003) has been found to be effective in helping clients gain a deeper understanding of Bipolar Disorder and developing resources within the family and community for coping with it. Finally, medication is considered to be a critical facet of treatment for Bipolar Disorder (Arana, Rosenbaum, & Hyman, 2000). Specific techniques for Ms. Wilkes will include correction of faulty cognitions, assistance in medication management, reconciliation of internal family-of-origin conflicts, and both individual and group support for bipolar awareness.

Step 4: Provide Outcome Measures of Change. This last step in treatment planning requires that we specify how change will be measured and indicate the extent to which progress has been made toward realizing these goals (Neukrug & Schwitzer, 2006). The counselor has considerable flexibility in this phase and may choose from a number of objective domains (psychological tests and measures of self-esteem, depression, psychosis, interpersonal relationship, anxiety, etc.), quasi-objective measures (the *DSM-IV-TR's* Axis V GAF scale; pre-post clinician, client, and psychiatric ratings), and subjective ratings (client self-report, clinician's in-session observations). In Annie Wilkes's case, we have implemented a number of these, including regular attendance in counseling and medication management sessions, increase and stabilization of her GAF, clinical observations, and client self-report of stabilized mood and improved reality contact, and expressed understanding of the impact of early traumatic experiences.

The completed treatment plan is now developed through which the counselor and Annie Wilkes will begin their shared work to modify and hopefully decrease her prominent symptomatology, build coping skills, improve the quality of her relationships, and move in the direction of overall positive change. Annie Wilkes's treatment plan follows and is summarized in Table 12.1.

TREATMENT PLAN

Client: Annie Wilkes

Service Provider: Overlook Psychotherapy Center—Individual Male Counselor

BEHAVIORAL DEFINITION OF PROBLEMS:

1. Dealing with routine effects of Bipolar Disorder—Erratic mood, diminished sleep, excessive energy with periods of crashing, periods of depression, problem alcohol use

2. Dealing with the psychotic effects of Bipolar Disorder—Psychotic grandiose thoughts during mania, confuses capturing and/or killing with helping

3. Dealing with the learned experiences of a traumatic household background and foster care—Antisocial beliefs and behaviors

GOALS FOR CHANGE:

1. Dealing with routine effects of Bipolar Disorder

   • Maintain stability of symptoms sufficient to participate in counseling
   • Stabilization of mood
   • Stabilization of eating and sleeping patterns and activity level
   • Reduced alcohol use

2. Dealing with the psychotic effects of Bipolar Disorder

   • Elimination of psychotic symptoms related to Bipolar Disorder
   • Moderate grandiose thoughts and balance them with realistic self-appraisal
   • Recognition of the difference between helping and hurting others

3. Dealing with the learned experiences of a traumatic household background and foster care

   • Recognize the role of early family violence and marital disruption in shaping distorted perception of self, others, and reality
   • Reconcile feelings of loss and abandonment related to foster placement

THERAPEUTIC INTERVENTIONS:

An intermediate- to long-term course of individual counseling (6 months to a year) focusing on Cognitive Behavioral strategies, psychotropic medication, and psychoeducational support

1. Dealing with routine effects of Bipolar Disorder

   • Identify and correct faulty cognitions that give rise to unrealistic self-appraisal as well as to depression
   • Use behavioral strategies including relaxation and imagery to regulate her stress, arousal, and energy level
   • Develop a schedule that provides for routine sleep and healthy eating
   • Provide direct feedback to client about appearance, hygiene, and energy level, and reinforce self-monitoring in these areas
   • Using positive reinforcement and shaping, assist client to evaluate her thoughts and behaviors positively
   • Assist client in identifying emotional, behavioral, and interpersonal triggers for maladaptive alcohol use
   • Refer for psychiatric evaluation to determine the need for medication
   • Refer to psychoeducational support group for Bipolar Disorder symptom awareness and management

(Continued)

(Continued)

2. Dealing with the psychotic effects of Bipolar Disorder

- Assist client in identifying emotional, behavioral, and interpersonal triggers for psychotic symptoms
- Use cognitive strategies to help client differentiate reality from fantasy and the role of arousal and cognitive distortion in precipitating psychotic symptoms
- Refer for evaluation to determine the need for medication
- Address compliance issues experienced by clients with Bipolar Disorder
- Make plans for hospitalization in the event of relapse

3. Dealing with the learned experiences of a traumatic household background and foster care

- Assist client to verbalize sadness and anger over early maltreatment and abandonment
- Disabuse client through cognitive restructuring and reframing of the belief that because she was harmed as a child that she must harm others
- Help client to understand that her negative self-evaluation stems from early traumatic family experiences

OUTCOME MEASURES OF CHANGE:

Compliance with counseling and psychiatric treatment, stabilization of mood, elimination of psychotic symptoms, and awareness of the role of early life experiences in her current life and symptoms as measured by:

- Compliance in treatment indicated by regular attendance in counseling and effective use of medication
- No psychiatric hospitalization for a 6-month period
- Gradual increase in clinician's rating of client's GAF to the mild range (>70)
- Observations by the counselor and psychiatrist as well as client's self-report of improved and sustained self-care along with elimination of psychotic symptoms
- Clinician's observations of stabilized mood, healthy self-statements, and decreased irrational thinking
- Reduced frequency of stress-related alcohol abuse as reflected in client's record keeping and random blood-alcohol-level testing
- Expressed understanding of early relational trauma
- Regular attendance in bipolar psychoeducational group

Table 12.1   Annie Wilkes's Treatment Plan Summary: Cognitive Behavior Therapy

Goals for Change	Therapeutic Interventions	Outcome Measures of Change
Dealing with routine effects of Bipolar Disorder	Dealing with routine effects of Bipolar Disorder	Compliance with counseling and psychiatric treatment, stabilization of mood, elimination of psychotic symptoms, and awareness of the role of early life experiences in her current life and symptoms as measured by:
Maintain stability of symptoms sufficient to participate in counseling	Identify and correct faulty cognitions that give rise to unrealistic self-appraisal as well as to depression	
Stabilization of mood	Use behavioral strategies including relaxation and imagery to regulate her stress, arousal, and energy level	Compliance in treatment indicated by regular attendance in counseling and effective use of medication
Stabilization of eating and sleeping patterns and activity level	Develop a schedule that provides for routine sleep and healthy eating	
Reduced alcohol use	Provide direct feedback to client about appearance, hygiene, and energy level, and reinforce self-monitoring in these areas	No psychiatric hospitalization for a 6-month period
Dealing with the psychotic effects of Bipolar Disorder	Using positive reinforcement and shaping, assist client to evaluate her thoughts and behaviors positively	Gradual increase in clinician's rating of client's GAF to the mild range (>70)
Elimination of psychotic symptoms related to Bipolar Disorder	Assist client in identifying emotional, behavioral, and interpersonal triggers for maladaptive alcohol use	Observations by the counselor and psychiatrist as well as client's self-report of improved and sustained self-care along with elimination of psychotic symptoms
Moderate grandiose thoughts and balance them with realistic self-appraisal	Refer for psychiatric evaluation to determine the need for medication	
Recognition of the difference between helping and hurting others	Refer to psychoeducational support group for Bipolar Disorder symptom awareness and management	Clinician's observations of stabilized mood, healthy self-statements, and decreased irrational thinking
Dealing with the learned experiences of a traumatic household background and foster care	Dealing with the psychotic effects of Bipolar Disorder	Reduced frequency of stress-related alcohol abuse as reflected in client's record keeping and random blood-alcohol-level testing
Recognize the role of early family violence and marital disruption in shaping distorted perception of self, others, and reality	Assist client in identifying emotional, behavioral, and interpersonal triggers for psychotic symptoms	
Reconcile feelings of loss and abandonment related to foster placement	Use cognitive strategies to help client differentiate reality from fantasy and the role of arousal and cognitive distortion in precipitating psychotic symptoms	Expressed understanding of early relational trauma
	Refer for evaluation to determine the need for medication	Regular attendance in bipolar psychoeducational group
	Address compliance issues experienced by clients with Bipolar Disorder	

(Continued)

Table 12.1 (Continued)

Goals for Change	Therapeutic Interventions	Outcome Measures of Change
	Make plans for hospitalization in the event of relapse	
	<u>Dealing with the learned experiences of a traumatic household background and foster care</u>	
	Assist client to verbalize sadness and anger over early maltreatment and abandonment	
	Disabuse client through cognitive restructuring and reframing of the belief that because she was harmed as a child that she must harm others	
	Help client to understand that her negative self-evaluation stems from early traumatic family experiences	

CASE 12.2 *THE COLOR PURPLE'S* MISS CELIE

INTRODUCING THE CHARACTER

Celie is the central character in Alice Walker's 1983 Pulitzer Prize–winning novel, *The Color Purple,* which was made into an Academy Award–winning movie in 1985, directed by Stephen Spielberg, and later adapted into a Broadway musical. Set in the rural American south, *The Color Purple* is a story that centers on a group of African American characters who, although unrelated by blood, share the legacy of oppression, race hatred, ignorance . . . and hope. As the tale unfolds, the characters—including the disenfranchised Shug, the oppressed and depressed Albert, the angry and subversive Ms. Sophia, and the naïve and innocent Celie—each must come to terms with, and ultimately overcome, the oppressions in their lives. Some of these oppressions include alcoholism, racial injustice, religious disaffection, personal enslavement, and the overt effects of being an African American person living when and where these characters spent their

lifetimes. Spanning several decades, the story is about racism, subjugation, and powerlessness over forces seemingly beyond one's control, and in the end, freedom, liberation, faith, and love. The following basic case summary and diagnostic impressions describe the negative reactions to traumatic life events and ongoing moderate problems with mood that are problems Celie possibly experienced.

Meet the Client

You can assess the client in action by viewing clips of Miss Celie's video material at the following websites:

- http://www.youtube.com/watch?v=ZsoHqApn_4E Miss Celie stands up
- http://www.youtube.com/watch?v=8uxvzizaweo Celie and Nettie united at last
- http://www.youtube.com/watch?v=dM60tZnG3i8 Nettie and Celie separated

Basic Case Summary

Identifying Information. Celie Booker, who prefers to be called Miss Celie, is a 51-year-old African American woman who lives on a plantation with her sister, Nettie, and her children, Adam and Olivia. Occupationally, Miss Celie co-owns a small seamstress shop with her lifelong friend, Ms. Sophia. It may be relevant to note that Ms. Sophia recently was released from a 5-year prison sentence for assaulting a white woman. Regarding relationship status, Miss Celie was married for 30 years to Albert Booker, whom she described as violent, dependent on alcohol, and physically abusive throughout their marriage. Miss Celie was appropriate and engaged throughout the interview; however, she expressed ambivalence about the need for, or potential benefits of, counseling. She voiced her concern that her church pastor might be a better source of support but was willing to participate in the interview.

Presenting Concern. Celie was brought to the counseling office by her sister, who had become increasingly concerned about what she described as "the darkness" Celie was experiencing. By "darkness," Nettie was referring to the nightmares, "fits" of nerves, and melancholy that had come over her sister of late, and that "was clouding her." It is estimated that Celie may have been experiencing symptoms suggesting Posttraumatic Stress Disorder (PTSD) in reaction to past physical abuse, and chronic symptoms of Dysthymic Disorder.

Background, Family Information, and Relevant History. Miss Celie was born on a farm outside of Mobile, Alabama, one of two children to unmarried partners, Mae and Eugene Washington. Mae Washington had seven other children by four men before Eugene but had not raised any of them, and these half-siblings were not known to Celie. Shortly after Celie's birth, her mother met another man, who was physically, emotionally, and sexually abusive to her and the girls. Miss Celie grew up treated more like a farmhand than as a daughter and was impregnated by her "stepfather" when she was 13. The child of that union as well as a second child were each taken away from her at birth, and in both instances, Celie was told that the child had died. The client recalled beginning to experience periods of depressed mood sometime during these years.

Miss Celie describes that when she was 17, she was "promised" to an adult widowed neighbor, Albert Booker, who, she says, was in actuality attracted to Celie's sister, who refused him. By Miss Celie's report, he, like Celie's stepfather, physically and emotionally abused her and treated her like a servant. Miss Celie says that while she became briefly elated when Nettie came to live with her and Albert, Miss Celie's hopes were immediately "dashed" when, on rebuking his sexual advances, Nettie was sent away by Albert. Miss Celie described this event as "heartbreaking." Shortly after, she appears to have begun experiencing another extended period of mild to moderate depression that lasted for nearly a decade and was characterized by long periods of silence, periods of declining to eat, and refusal to attend church.

As she described it, it was only after a visit by Shug Avery, whom Miss Celie referred to as "a fiery daughter of a Baptist minister," that Miss Celie says she began to gradually show an interest in life. Miss Celie recalls that her friendship with Shug "changed my world." She characterized Shug as a strong support, a self-confident role model, and as an occasional sexual partner. Miss Celie presented Shug's influence as catalyzing her to leave the "abuse and oppression" of her marriage, and in turn, to live on her own. She opened a small seamstress service with her friend, Ms. Sophia, and was sought out for her skills, particularly in making beautiful wedding dresses. When further queried by the counselor, Miss Celie volunteered that although successful at her business, she also had been saddened by the painful reality that her marriage to Albert had taken the best years of her life.

Miss Celie reported that she had hoped to someday reconnect with Nettie, her "long lost sister," who by that time had been out of her life for almost four decades. Miss Celie recalled that when she was 48 years old, while cleaning Albert's room, she found a package of letters that had been sent to her from her "beloved sister." As she described it, mustering the courage to confront Albert, Celie was told that her sister and the two children she thought were dead were living in Africa. She said that "in a showing of great compassion and guilt," Albert paid for her sister and children, now grown, to come to the United States. Subsequently, a year ago, on the day of her 50th birthday, Miss Celie, who had inherited her biological father's farm, was finally reunited with Nettie, her long lost children Adam and Olivia, and their spouses and children.

Problem and Counseling History. Prior to her visit to the clinic, Miss Celie had never received professional counseling services. She had participated in faith-based spiritual counseling on several occasions at her local church. She was accompanied by her sister, Nettie, and her two children, Adam and Olivia, who had grown increasingly concerned for their mother who, while overjoyed at their recent reunion, had recently voiced concerns that they found to be frightening. One stormy night several months after the reunion, Miss Celie had awoken from a dream screaming and pulling at her hair. The next morning she confided to Nettie that she had been experiencing horrific nightmares for the last several years, a feeling that "My body was numb" as well as intrusive recollections of episodes of physical and sexual abuse by Albert and "the other men he used to bring home with him at night." She was definitely afraid of loud noises, experienced episodes of agitation, a racing

heart, and vomiting that she called "the jitters." Although Miss Celie began the interview in a very reserved, almost numbed fashion, she became increasingly tearful and agitated as she reluctantly related the painful details of what was, up to that point, her most deeply private and tortured inner experiences.

In addition to these concerns, Miss Celie said she had been consulting her minister "on and off for years and years" for assistance with feelings of depressed mood. She describing feeling depressed much of the time ("as often as not"), but "not so badly that it gets in my way." Further, by her description, her mood seems reactive to everyday events, such as improving when seeing her adult children or completing successful sewing projects. She added that as many days as not she feels "slow" or fatigued, during which times it can be difficult for her to concentrate. Based on Miss Celie's report she appears to have been experiencing at least some dysthymic symptoms consistently since adolescence.

Miss Celie reported that she has had "only a couple of visits to the doctor" throughout her life.

Goals for Counseling and Course of Therapy to Date. Miss Celie has been seen for one extended intake interview to date. She appears to present anxiety symptoms of PTSD and mood symptoms of Dysthymic Disorder. Goals are to continue assessment in subsequent sessions to confirm initial diagnostic impressions; attempt to engage Miss Celie in the counseling relationship; and develop a conceptualization and plan that potentially applies Africentric and other counseling models. The client also has agreed to a referral to the Walker Regional Women's Center for a medical examination.

Diagnostic Impressions

Axis I.   309.1 Posttraumatic Stress Disorder, Chronic, With Delayed Onset

300.4 Dysthymic Disorder, Early Onset

Axis II.   V71.09 No Diagnosis on Axis II

Axis III.   None

Axis IV.   Problems with primary support group—History of sexual and physical abuse in family of origin, history of physical and emotional abuse in marital relationship

Problems related to the social environment—Childhood years spent in slavery, problems of discrimination, and racism in adulthood

Problems with access to health care—History of inadequate health care services

Axis V.   GAF = 53 (current)

GAF = 60 (highest level past year)

DISCUSSION OF DIAGNOSTIC IMPRESSIONS

Miss Celie arrived at the counseling center at the urging of her sister, who was worried about two domains of her functioning: her reactions to past traumatic events and her mood.

The *DSM-IV-TR's* Anxiety Disorders section includes all of the diagnosable disorders that feature increased arousal, excessive worry, or other signs of anxiety that cause distress or impairment, including panic (including Acute Stress Disorder and PTSD, both of which, by definition, occur only in the aftermath of, or as a result of, a traumatic life event). Likewise, the *DSM-IV-TR's* Mood Disorders section includes all of the diagnosable disorders that feature a disturbance in mood. The Mood Disorders include Depressive Disorders (in which the client experiences unipolar depression), Bipolar Disorders (in which the client experiences manic, hypomanic, or mixed episodes), and mood disorders that are due to substance use or a medical condition. The Anxiety Disorders and Mood Disorders probably comprise the client concerns most commonly seen by counseling professionals. Before moving on to a discussion of differential diagnoses for Miss Celie, it is important for counselors to be aware that diagnostic labels and the expectations they create may communicate gender bias. This may be particularly so in the case of certain personality disorders that reinforce traditional stereotyped perceptions of men and women (Antisocial Personality Disorder

for men and Dependent Personality Disorder for women), and anxiety and eating disorders, which are disproportionately assigned to women (Eriksen & Kress, 2008).

First examined were Celie's reactions to trauma. This case described what we portrayed as Celie's clinically significant negative reactions to her exposure to the traumatic experience of being physically and sexually abused by her mother's romantic partner, and later, physically abused by her husband and sexually abused by her husband and some of his male friends. She experienced repeated events characterized by threat to her physical integrity (she was sexually assaulted), threatened and actual physical injury (she was physically abused), and subjected to threat serious physical damage. Her reactions are assumed to have included intense fear and helplessness. These characteristics meet the *DSM-IV-TR* definition of a traumatic event.

Since the assault, she has been reexperiencing the event through persistent nightmares and intrusive daytime recollections of the abusive events with her husband. She reported feeling as though she were "numb" and detached, and until the interview has avoided conversations about her traumatic events. She had signs of anxiety, including being easily startled, feeling agitated, feeling her heart race, and being nauseous. According to the case timeline, Celie's symptoms had been present for many years. These factors suggest a diagnosis of PTSD. Because symptoms have persisted more than 3 months, the specifier, Chronic, is listed. Because the symptoms began more than 6 months after the events ended, the additional specifier, With Delayed Onset, is used.

Differential diagnoses might include Acute Stress Disorder and Adjustment Disorder. However, Acute Stress Disorder allows for a maximum duration of symptoms of 1 month, whereas PTSD fits when symptoms have lasted beyond 4 weeks. Whereas Adjustment Disorders are negative reactions to any sort of life stressors, in this case, Celie had experienced exposure to an extreme stressor meeting the diagnostic definition of trauma, and her reactions conform to the specific constellation of symptoms characteristic of PTSD and Acute Stress Disorder, which go beyond the general criteria set for Adjustment Disorder.

Next examined were Celie's problems with mood. She reported having experienced low mood for many years. She described "as often as not" feeling depressed but "not so bad that it gets in my way." Her mood was reactive to happy events like seeing her children. She also reported fatigue and difficulty concentrating. She estimated that these symptoms had been present persistently since adolescence. Taken together, Celie reported a long-term experience of moderately depressed mood and related symptoms without meeting the criteria for a Major Depressive Disorder. In this case, with no evidence that her mood disturbance is due to the direct consequences of a general medication condition such as hypothyroidism, or to substance use such as alcohol, the diagnosis is Dysthymia.

A differential diagnosis that might be considered is whether her mood symptoms are an aspect of the PTSD she is experiencing. This is important partly because there is evidence that in the past, mental health professionals have sometimes tended to overdiagnosis the presentations of African American clients with more severe symptoms of mental disorders (Strakowski, McElroy, Keck, & West, 1996). However, in Celie's case, although PTSD includes symptoms of numbed detachment, this disorder addresses features of anxiety, whereas Celie's mood symptoms

fully meet the criteria for Dysthymia. Therefore, Dysthymia is used in addition to PTSD.

To finish the diagnosis, Celie's critical psychosocial stresses are emphasized on Axis IV, and on Axis V her functioning is represented by GAF scores ranging from a recent period of moderate symptoms, and recently, the slightly more noticeable moderate difficulties in social and other areas of functioning that led to her counseling visit. The information on these axes is consistent with the information on Axis I.

CASE CONCEPTUALIZATION

During Celie Booker's first meeting at the clinic, her assigned counselor collected as much information as possible about the symptoms and situations leading Celie's sister to suggest a counseling referral. Her counselor collected a thorough history, listened to Celie's client report, made her own counselor observations, and collected other data. Based on the intake, Miss Celie's counselor developed diagnostic impressions, describing her concerns as falling into the categories of PTSD and Dysthymic Disorder. She also identified critical psychosocial factors. A case conceptualization next was developed. Whereas the purpose of diagnostic impressions is to *describe* the client's concerns, the goal of case conceptualization is to better *understand* and clinically *explain* the person's experiences (Neukrug & Schwitzer, 2006). It helps the counselor understand the etiology leading to, and the factors sustaining, Miss Celie's posttraumatic and dysthymic concerns. In turn, case conceptualization sets the stage for treatment planning. Treatment planning then provides a road map that plots out how the counselor and client expect to move from presenting concerns to positive outcomes (Seligman, 1993, p. 157)—helping Miss Celie improve her mood and reduce her posttraumatic and additional depressive symptoms.

When forming a case conceptualization, the clinician applies a purist counseling theory, an integration of two or more theories, an eclectic mix of theories, or a solution-focused combination of tactics, to his or her understanding of the client. In this case, Celie Booker's counselor based her conceptualization on psychotherapeutic integration of two theories (Corey, 2009). Psychotherapists very commonly integrate more than one theoretical approach in order to form a conceptualization and treatment plan that will be as efficient and effective as possible for meeting the client's needs (Dattilo & Norcross, 2006; Norcross & Beutler, 2008). In other words, counselors using the psychotherapeutic integration method attempt to flexibly tailor their clinical efforts to "the unique needs and contexts of the individual client" (Norcross & Beutler, 2008, p. 485). Like other counselors using integration, Celie Booker's clinician chose this method because she had not found one individual theory that was comprehensive enough, by itself, to address all of the "complexities," "range of client types," and "specific problems" seen among her everyday caseload (Corey, 2009, p. 450). Further, Celie Booker's counselor was aware of literature suggesting that an integration of approaches sometimes is particularly responsive to the needs of clients from ethnically diverse backgrounds (Corey, 2009; Ivey, Ivey, D'Andrea, & Simek-Morgan, 2005).

Specifically, Miss Celie's counselor selected an integration of (a) Schema-Focused Cognitive Behavior Therapy and (b) Feminist Therapy. She selected this approach based on Miss Celie's presentation of mood concerns and posttraumatic anxiety symptoms, along with a history of very negative psychosocial stresses and social-political environment problems—and her knowledge of current outcome research and suggested best practices with clients experiencing these types of concerns (Critchfield & Smith-Benjamin, 2006; Fotchmann & Gelenberg, 2005; Hollon, Thase, & Markowitz, 2002; Livesley, 2007; Philpot, Brooks, Lusterman, & Nutt, 1997; Remer, 2008; Westen & Morrison, 2001). According to the research and the Feminist Therapy literature, cognitive therapy focusing on family schema—as well as Feminist Therapy focusing on sociopolitical and cultural context and empowerment—may be indicated for women with a combination of concerns such as Miss Celie's. Miss Celie's

counselor is comfortable theoretically integrating these approaches.

The counselor used the Inverted Pyramid Method of case conceptualization because this method is especially designed to help clinicians more easily form their conceptual pictures of their clients' needs (Neukrug & Schwitzer, 2006; Schwitzer, 1996, 1997). The method has four steps: Problem Identification, Thematic Groupings, Theoretical Inferences, and Narrowed Inferences. The counselor's clinical thinking can be seen in Figure 12.2.

Step 1: Problem Identification. The first step is Problem Identification. Aspects of the presenting problem (thoughts, feelings, behaviors, physiological features), additional areas of concern besides the presenting concern, family and developmental history, in-session observations, clinical inquiries (medical problems, medications, past counseling, substance use, suicidality), and psychological assessments (problem checklists, personality inventories, mental status exam, specific clinical measures) all may contribute information at Step 1. The counselor "casts a wide net" in order to build Step 1 as exhaustively as possible (Neukrug & Schwitzer, 2006, p. 202). As can be seen in Figure 12.2, the counselor identified all Miss Celie's current and long-standing presenting problems (anxiety and posttraumatic symptoms plus symptoms of depression), the abusive experiences of her childhood and adulthood, and important social and environmental and other factors.

Step 2: Thematic Groupings. The second step is Thematic Groupings. The clinician organizes all of the exhaustive client information found in Step 1 into just a few intuitive-logical clinical groups, categories, or themes, on the basis of sensible common denominators (Neukrug & Schwitzer, 2006). Four different ways of forming the Step 2 theme groups can be used: Descriptive-Diagnosis Approach, Clinical Targets Approach, Areas of Dysfunction Approach, and Intrapsychic Approach. As can be seen in Figure 12.2, Miss Celie's counselor selected the Intrapsychic

Approach. This approach sorts together all of the Step 1 information about the "client's adjustment, development, distress, or dysfunction" in order "to show clinical patterns in the ways life events are associated with the person's personal experience and identity" (Neukrug & Schwitzer, 2006, p. 205).

Interestingly, the counselor grouped together all of the factors in Step 1 into just two themes capturing the two intrapsychic patterns she believes Miss Celie has been dealing with since early in her life. Specifically, she grouped: all of the Step 1 data pertaining to abuse and trauma into the theme, "a pattern of anxiety symptoms and posttraumatic symptoms associated with seeing, and being resigned to, being physically and sexually abused as her assigned role in life"; and all of the Step 1 data pertaining to oppressive situations and depressive symptoms into the theme, "a pattern of almost lifelong depressive symptoms associated with seeing, and being resigned to, childhood slavery, racism, and gender discrimination as her assigned role in life." In this case example, the counselor used the Intrapsychic Approach to group much diverse information together to show how external life experiences have been associated with Celie's experience of self.

So far, at Steps 1 and 2, the counselor has used her intake evaluation skills and clinical judgment to begin meaningfully understanding Miss Celie's situation. Now, at Steps 3 and 4, she applies an integration of the two theoretical approaches she has selected. She begins making theoretical inferences to interpret and explain the processes underlying Miss Celie's problematic dynamics as they are seen in Steps 1 and 2.

Step 3: Theoretical Inferences. At Step 3, concepts from the counselor's theoretical integration of two approaches—Schema-Focused Cognitive Therapy and Feminist Therapy—are applied to explain the experiences causing, and the mechanisms maintaining, Celie Booker's problematic thoughts, feelings, and behaviors. The counselor tentatively matches the theme groups in Step 2

with this theoretical approach. In other words, the symptom constellations in Step 2, which were distilled from the symptoms in Step 1, now are combined using theory to show what are believed to be the underlying causes or psychological etiology of Celie Booker's current needs (Neukrug & Schwitzer, 2006; Schwitzer, 2006, 2007).

A combination of approaches was used. First, generally speaking, according to Cognitive Behavior Therapy (Beck, 1995, 2005; Ellis, 1994; Ellis & MacLaren, 2005), irrational thinking, faulty beliefs, or other forms of cognitive errors lead individuals to engage in problematic behaviors and to experience negative moods and attitudes. More specifically, when the cognitive behavioral approach, Schema-Focused Cognitive Therapy, is used, there is an emphasis on identifying jointly held core beliefs that emerge in families (Dattilo, 2001, 2005, 2006). According to the approach, these jointly held core beliefs—or family schema—often have a strong influence on individual family members' thoughts, feelings, and behaviors. In the case of individuals experiencing depression and low self-esteem, schema learned in one's family of origin is believed to cause attitudes and feelings of self-devaluing, weakness, inadequacy, or inability to fill major life roles (Beck, 1995, 2005; Dattilo, 2001, 2005, 2006). As can be seen in the figure, Miss Celie's counselor presented two such distorted core beliefs: (a) "As a child, it was my family role to be available for sexual abuse and a target for physical abuse by my mother's boyfriend"; and (b) "As an adult woman, it was my role to be available for sexual abuse by my husband and his friends, and a target for his physical abuse."

Second, Feminist Therapy was applied. This second approach was thought to complement the schema already identified as a source of Celie's posttraumatic anxiety symptoms by further addressing her dysthymic symptoms. According to Feminist Therapy, symptoms are understood primarily to be coping mechanisms and survival strategies rather than psychopathology (Worell

& Johnson, 1997). According to the theory, psychological distress is reformulated and redefined by an understanding that personal experiences also intimately tied to political experiences; a recognition of the role of oppressive factors on women's functioning; and a focus on restoring egalitarian relationships and the individual's self- and political empowerment (Enns, 2004; Eriksen & Kress, 2005; Remer, 2008). As can be seen in Figure 12.2, when the counselor applied these Feminist Therapy concepts, she additionally explained at Step 3 that the various Step 1 issues, which can be understood in Step 2 to be patterns of difficulties from abusive and oppressive life events, were rooted in the following: Celie's severely negatively gender-role (and race-) related experiences, and severely unequal access to power, have negatively affected her psychological well-being.

Step 4: Narrowed Inferences. At Step 4, the clinician's selected theory continues to be used to address still-deeper issues when they exist (Schwitzer, 2006, 2007). At this step, "still-deeper, more encompassing, or more central, causal themes" are formed (Neukrug & Schwitzer, 2006, p. 207). Miss Celie's counselor continued to use psychotherapeutic integration of two approaches.

First, continuing to apply Schema-Focused Cognitive Therapy concepts at Step 4, Miss Celie's counselor presented a single, deepest, most-fundamental faulty family schema that she believed to be most explanatory and causal regarding Celie's combination of presenting problems: the shared family core belief that "It is just my place to live with the awful abuses I must endure and I must just live with the consequences." Second, continuing to apply Feminist Therapy, the counselor presented a single, most deeply rooted feminist psychology inference: Celie blames herself and endures her role rather than recognizing, integrating, and acting on the social-political factors responsible for her negative well-being. These two narrowed inferences together form the basis for understanding the

etiology and maintenance of Celie Booker's combination of difficulties.

When all four steps are completed, the client information in Step 1 leads to logical-intuitive groupings on the basis of common denominators in Step 2, the groupings then are explained using theory at Step 3, and then, finally, at Step 4, further deeper explanations are made. From start to finish, the thoughts, feelings, behaviors, and physiological features in the topmost portions are connected on down the pyramid into deepest dynamics.

TREATMENT PLANNING

At this point, Miss Celie's clinician at the Walker Regional Women's Center has collected all available information about the problems that have been of concern to her and her family. Based upon this information, the counselor developed a five-axis *DSM-IV-TR* diagnosis and then, using the "inverted pyramid" (Neukrug & Schwitzer, 2006; Schwitzer, 1996, 1997), formulated a working clinical *explanation* of Miss Celie's difficulties and their etiology that we called the *case conceptualization*. This, in turn, guides us to the next critical step in our clinical work, called the *treatment plan,* the primary purpose of which is to map out a logical and goal-oriented strategy for making positive changes in the client's life. In essence, the treatment plan is a road map "for reducing or eliminating disruptive symptoms that are impeding the client's ability to reach positive mental health outcomes" (Neukrug & Schwitzer, 2006, p. 225). As such, it is the cornerstone of our work with not only Miss Celie, but with all clients who present with disturbing and disruptive symptoms and/or personality patterns (Jongsma & Peterson, 2006; Jongsma et al., 2003a, 2003b; Seligman, 1993, 1998, 2004).

A comprehensive treatment plan must integrate all of the information from the biopsychosocial interview, diagnosis, and case conceptualization into a coherent plan of action. This

Figure 12.2 Miss Celie's Inverted Pyramid Case Conceptualization Summary: Psychotherapeutic Integration of Schema-Focused Cognitive Therapy and Feminist Therapy

1. IDENTIFY AND LIST CLIENT CONCERNS

Physical abuse by stepfather
Sexual abuse by stepfather
Physical abuse by husband
Sexual abuse by husband
Sexual abuse by husband's friends
Nightmares
Easily agitated
Racing heart
Nausea
Childhood spent in slavery
Experienced racism, discrimination
Experienced gender-based inequality
and abuses

Chronic low mood often since adolescence
Chronic fatigue often since adolescence
Chronic poor concentration often since
adolescence
Medical condition leading to depressive
symptoms ruled out
"Numb" detachment
Avoids conversations about abuses
Denies "anything out of the ordinary"
Lack of access to adequate health and
social care

2. ORGANIZE CONCERNS INTO LOGICAL THEMATIC GROUPINGS

1. A pattern of anxiety symptoms and post-traumatic symptoms associated with seeing, and being resigned to, being physically and sexually abused as her assigned role in life
2. A pattern of almost lifelong depressive symptoms associated with seeing, and being resigned to, childhood slavery, racism, and gender discrimination as her assigned role in life

3. THEORETICAL INFERENCES: ATTACH THEMATIC GROUPINGS TO INFERRED AREAS OF DIFFICULTY

Psychotherapeutic Integration

Schema-Focused Cognitive Theory

Distorted core beliefs:

1. "As a child, it was my family role to be available for sexual abuse and a target for physical abuse by my mother's boyfriend"
2. "As an adult woman, it was my role to be available for sexual abuse by my husband and his friends, and a target for his physical abuse"

Feminist Therapy

Celie's severely negative gender-role (and race-) related experience, and severely unequal access to power, have negatively affected her psychological well-being

4. NARROWED INFERENCES: SUICIDALITY AND DEEPER DIFFICULTIES

Psychotherapeutic Integration

Schema-Focused Cognitive Theory

Fundamental faulty family schema:

"It is just my place to live with the awful abuses I must endure and I must just live with the consequences"

Feminist Therapy

Celie blames self and endures her role rather than recognizing, integrating, and acting on the social political factors responsible for her negative well-being *plan* comprises four main components, which include (1) a behavioral definition of the problem(s), (2) the selection of achievable goals, (3) the determination of treatment modes, and (4) the documentation of how change will be measured. The *behavioral definition of the problem(s)* consolidates the results of the case conceptualization into a concise hierarchical list of problems and concerns that will be the focus of treatment. The *selection of achievable goals* refers to assessing and prioritizing the client's concerns into a *hierarchy of urgency* that also takes into account the client's motivation for change, level of dysfunction, and real-world influences on his or her problems. The *determination of treatment modes* refers to selection of the specific interventions, which are matched to the uniqueness of the client and to his or her goals and clearly tied to a particular theoretical orientation (Neukrug & Schwitzer, 2006). Finally, the clinician must establish how change will be measured, based upon a number of factors, including client records and self-report of change, in-session observations by the clinician, clinician ratings, results of standardized evaluations such as the Beck Anxiety Inventory (Beck & Steer, 1990) or a family functioning questionnaire, pre-post treatment comparisons, and reports by other treating professionals.

The four-step method discussed above can be seen in Figure 6.1 (p. 109) and is outlined below for the case of Miss Celie, followed by her specific treatment plan.

Step 1: Behavioral Definition of Problems. The first step in treatment planning is to carefully review the case conceptualization, paying particular attention to the results of Step 2 (Thematic Groupings), Step 3 (Theoretical Inferences), and Step 4 (Narrowed Inferences). The identified clinical themes reflect the core areas of concern and distress for the client, while the theoretical and narrowed inferences offer clinical speculation as to their origins. In the case of Miss Celie, there are two primary areas of concern. The first, "a pattern of anxiety and posttraumatic symptoms," refers to her nightmares, her numb detachment, avoidance of conversations about abuses suffered, denial of "anything out of the ordinary, and anxiety-based signs of physiological arousal including ready agitation, nausea, and a racing heart." The second, "a pattern of almost lifelong depressive symptoms," refers to her chronic low mood, fatigue, and poor concentration often since adolescence. These symptoms and stresses are consistent with the diagnosis of PTSD, Chronic, with Delayed Onset and Dysthymic Disorder, Early Onset (APA, 2000a; Bradley et al., 2005; Bryant et al., 2008; Depression Guideline Panel, 1993; Dobson, 1993; Foa & Keane, 2000; Hollon, Thase, & Markowitz, 2002).

Step 2: Identify and Articulate Goals for Change. The second step is the selection of achievable goals, which is based upon a number of factors, including the most pressing or urgent behavioral, emotional, and interpersonal concerns and symptoms as identified by the client and clinician, the willingness and ability of the client to work on those particular goals, and the realistic (real-world) achievability of those goals (Neukrug & Schwitzer, 2006). At this stage of treatment planning, it is important to recognize that not all of the client's problems can be addressed at once, so we focus initially on those that cause the greatest distress and impairment. New goals can be created as old ones are achieved. In the case of Miss Celie, the goals are divided into two prominent areas. The first, "a pattern of anxiety and posttraumatic stress symptoms," requires that we help Miss Celie to understand the societally based gender, racial, and socioeconomic conditions that gave rise to her maltreatment, relieve the cognitive, emotional, and behavioral symptoms of posttraumatic stress, verbalize an understanding of how these symptoms developed, and develop and implement effective coping skills and behaviors that will promote healing. We will also work with Miss Celie to challenge the self-destructive core beliefs that have contributed to her pathological world- and self-view, and, finally, create a plan for maintaining therapeutic gains. The second, "a pattern of almost lifelong depressive symptoms," requires that we help Miss Celie to understand the societally based gender, racial, and socioeconomic conditions that gave rise to her external and internal oppression, alleviate her depressive symptoms, and strengthen her sense of self and overall competence to make free choices in her life.

Step 3: Describe Therapeutic Interventions. This is perhaps the most critical step in the treatment planning process because the clinician must now integrate information from a number of sources, including the case conceptualization, the delineation of the client's problems and goals, and the treatment literature, paying particular attention to *empirically supported treatment* (EST) and *evidence-based practice* (EBP). In essence, the clinician must align his or her treatment approach with scientific evidence from the fields of counseling and psychotherapy. Wampold (2001) identifies two types of evidence-based counseling research: studies that demonstrate "absolute efficacy," that is, the fact that counseling and psychotherapy work, and those that demonstrate "relative efficacy," that is, the fact that certain theoretical/technical approaches work best for certain clients with particular problems (Psychoanalysis, Gestalt Therapy, Cognitive Behavior Therapy, Brief Solution-Focused Therapy, Cognitive Therapy, Dialectical Behavior Therapy, Person-Centered Therapy, Expressive/Creative Therapies, Interpersonal Therapy, and Feminist Therapy); and when delivered through specific treatment modalities (individual, group, and family counseling).

In the case of Miss Celie, we have decided to use a two-pronged or integrated approach to therapy comprised of Schema-focused Cognitive Therapy and Feminist Therapy. Schema-Focused Cognitive Therapy (Dattilo, 2001, 2005, 2006; Young, Klosko, & Weishart, 2003) is a variant of cognitive therapy (Beck, 1997) and is based on the premise that people form schemas, or mental representations, perceptions and expectations about themselves, relationships, and their roles within them, based upon early (and often traumatic) life experiences, and in particular their family-of-origin

abuses and disruptions. The therapist's goal is to help clients recognize, understand, and modify these schema. It has been found effective in helping clients to gain self-understanding, improve relational functioning, diminish symptoms related to anxiety and depression, and to develop mature and flexible role expectations and behaviors (Hoffart, Verslund, & Sexton, 2002; Young, 1990; Young et al., 2003). Specific techniques for Miss Celie that are drawn from this approach will include exploration of her particular schema and the way that they perpetuate symptoms of anxiety and posttraumatic stress, providing support and empathy for expression of painful feelings and negative self-beliefs stemming from relationship with parents and oppressors, challenging self- and relational attributions that undermine development of a positive self-image, participation in imaginal and in vivo exposure with response prevention to elements of traumatic events, and group support.

The counselor will also use Feminist Therapy (Enns, 2004; Eriksen & Kress, 2005; Evans, Kincade, Marbley, & Seem, 2005; Remer, 2008; Worell & Johnson, 1997), which uses an eclectic array of cognitive, behavioral, and interpersonal techniques designed to help clients understand the societal bases for the misuse of power and oppression, and in so doing, assist them to overcome the influence of these abuses. In the process, clients deal with conflicting feelings between traditional and newfound values, integrate messages of strength, power, and competence into their identity, and develop a positive and life-affirming perception of themselves and others (Ballou, Hill, & West, 2008; Neukrug, 2011). Specific techniques drawn from this approach will include exploring the basis for her depressive symptoms in the societal oppression of women and her personal experiences in slavery; contracting on the topics and pace of counseling to ensure an egalitarian relationship; supportive encouragement in the expression of pain and self-hatred; focusing on wellness, inner resources, and strength to offset the effects of pathologizing; challenge ruminative; and distorted thinking; change her distorted sense of responsibility for trauma; developing assertive communication and self-advocacy skills; stress-management techniques, including relaxation training, psychoeducation, guided imagery, meditation, and contemplative techniques; and referral to relevant community resources for health and education.

Step 4: Provide Outcome Measures of Change. This last step in treatment planning requires that we specify how change will be measured and indicate the extent to which progress has been made toward realizing these goals (Neukrug & Schwitzer, 2006). The counselor has considerable flexibility in this phase and may choose from a number of objective domains (psychological tests and measures of self-esteem, depression, psychosis, interpersonal relationship, anxiety, etc.), quasi-objective measures (the *DSM-IV-TR's* Axis V GAF scale; pre-post clinician, client and psychiatric ratings), and subjective ratings (client self-report, clinician's in-session observations). In Miss Celie's case,

we have implemented a number of these, including pre-post measures on the Beck Depression Inventory-II (Beck et al., 1996), and Beck Anxiety Inventory (Beck & Steer, 1990), post measures of GAF functioning in the mild range (>70), client self-reported awareness of and ability to challenge the tenets of her self-negating cognitive schema, clinician-observed replacement of maladaptive cognitive schema with adaptive, life-affirming and personal power-based beliefs about herself and relationships, and client-reported elimination of negative self-talk.

The completed treatment plan is now developed through which the counselor and Miss Celie will begin their shared work of modifying her cognitive schema and reducing her symptoms of depression, anxiety, and posttraumatic stress within the context of a supportive, collaborative, and empowering therapeutic relationship. The treatment plan appears below and is summarized in Table 12.2.

TREATMENT PLAN

Client: Celie Booker

Service Provider: Walker Regional Women's Center

BEHAVIORAL DEFINITION OF PROBLEMS:

1. A pattern of anxiety and posttraumatic symptoms associated with seeing, and being resigned to being physically and sexually abused as her assigned role in life—Nightmares, numb detachment, avoidance of conversations about abuses suffered, denial of "anything out of the ordinary," and anxiety-based signs of physiological arousal, including ready agitation, nausea, and a racing heart

2. A pattern of almost lifelong depressive symptoms associated with seeing, and being resigned to, childhood slavery, racism, and gender discrimination as her assigned role in life—Chronic low mood, fatigue, and poor concentration often since adolescence

(Continued)

(Continued)

GOALS FOR CHANGE:

1. A pattern of anxiety and posttraumatic symptoms associated with seeing, and being resigned to being physically and sexually abused as her assigned role in life

   - Understand the societally based gender, racial, and socioeconomic conditions that gave rise to her maltreatment
   - Understand how her traumatic history molded maladaptive schemas that undermined her self-esteem, worldview, and capacity to relate effectively
   - Relieve the cognitive, emotional, behavioral, and physiological symptoms of posttraumatic stress
   - Examine life experiences that confirm and refute the thoughts, feelings, and behaviors that flow from maladaptive schema
   - Develop and implement effective coping skills in order to lead a fulfilling life
   - Implement behaviors that promote healing, evolving acceptance of past events, and responsible living
   - Create a plan for maintaining therapeutic gains

2. A pattern of almost lifelong depressive symptoms associated with seeing, and being resigned to, childhood slavery, racism, and gender discrimination as her assigned role in life

   - Understand the societally based gender, racial, and socioeconomic conditions that contributed to past external and ongoing internal oppression
   - Alleviate her depressive symptoms
   - Strengthen her sense of self and overall competence to make free choices in her life
   - Develop a plan for independent living, including vocational growth and development

THERAPEUTIC INTERVENTIONS:

A moderate- to long-term course (9–12 months) of integrated Cognitive Behavior and Feminist Therapy supplemented with group support

1. A pattern of anxiety and posttraumatic symptoms associated with seeing, and being resigned to being physically and sexually abused as her assigned role in life

   - Psychoeducation about the nature of family-based cognitive schema
   - Exploration of her particular schema and the way that they perpetuate symptoms of anxiety and posttraumatic stress
   - Identifying schema-based triggers for poor self-image, passive-dependent relational style, and her subservient role
   - Providing support and empathy for expression of painful feelings and negative self-beliefs stemming from relationship with parents and oppressors

- Challenging self and relational attributions that undermine development of a positive self-image
- Participate in imaginal and in vivo exposure with response prevention to elements of traumatic events
- Practice thought-stopping for unwanted and intrusive recollections
- Modify irrational thoughts about the trauma and her perceived role
- Learn skills of eye movement desensitization and reprocessing (EMDR) to reduce emotional and physiological reactivity to trauma recollections
- Participation in trauma-focused group therapy, including relaxation training
- Discuss and implement relapse strategies for PTSD symptoms

2. A pattern of almost lifelong depressive symptoms associated with seeing, and being resigned to, childhood slavery, racism, and gender discrimination as her assigned role in life

- Exploring the basis for her depressive symptoms in societal oppression of women and her personal experiences in slavery
- Contracting on the topics and pace of counseling to ensure an egalitarian relationship
- Supportive encouragement in the expression of pain and self-hatred, focusing on wellness, inner resources, and strength to offset the effects of pathologizing
- Challenge ruminative and distorted thinking to change distorted sense of responsibility for trauma
- Developing assertive communication and self-advocacy skills
- Stress management techniques including relaxation training, psychoeducation, guided imagery, meditation, and contemplative techniques
- Referral to relevant community resources for health and education

OUTCOME MEASURES OF CHANGE:

The development of healthy, positive, and self-affirming attitudes toward herself centered on empowerment, personal agency, and strength accompanied by elimination of depressive and post-traumatic stress symptoms as measured by:

- Pre-post measures on the Beck Depression Inventory
- Pre-post measures on the Beck Anxiety Inventory
- Post-only measures of GAF functioning in the mild range (>70)
- Client self-reported awareness of and ability to challenge the tenets of her self-negating cognitive schema
- Clinician-observed replacement of maladaptive cognitive schema with adaptive, life-affirming, and personal power-based beliefs about herself and relationships
- Client-reported elimination of negative self-talk and negative interpretations of experiences
- Clinician observation of statements and behavior reflecting self-assertion
- Client self-report of engagement in life and self-affirming activities within and outside of the home

Table 12.2 Miss Celie's Treatment Plan Summary: Psychotherapeutic Integration of Schema-Focused Cognitive Therapy and Feminist Therapy

Goals for Change	Therapeutic Interventions	Outcome Measures of Change
A pattern of anxiety and posttraumatic symptoms associated with seeing, and being resigned to being physically and sexually abused as her assigned role in life	A pattern of anxiety and posttraumatic symptoms associated with seeing, and being resigned to being physically and sexually abused as her assigned role in life	The development of healthy, positive, and self-affirming attitudes toward herself centered on empowerment, personal agency, and strength accompanied by elimination of depressive and posttraumatic stress symptoms as measured by:
Understand the societally based gender, racial, and socioeconomic conditions that gave rise to her maltreatment	Psychoeducation about the nature of family-based cognitive schema	
	Exploration of her particular schema and the way that they perpetuate symptoms of anxiety and posttraumatic stress	Pre-post measures on the Beck Depression Inventory
Understand how her traumatic history molded maladaptive schemas that undermined her self-esteem, worldview, and capacity to relate effectively	Identifying schema-based triggers for poor self-image, passive-dependent relational style, and her subservient role	Pre-post measures on the Beck Anxiety Inventory

Post-only measures of GAF functioning in the mild range (>70) |
| Relieve the cognitive, emotional, behavioral, and physiological symptoms of posttraumatic stress | Providing support and empathy for expression of painful feelings and negative self-beliefs stemming from relationship with parents and oppressors | Client self-reported awareness of and ability to challenge the tenets of her self-negating cognitive schema |
| Examine life experiences that confirm and refute the thoughts, feelings, and behaviors that flow from maladaptive schema | Challenging self- and relational attributions that undermine development of a positive self-image

Participate in imaginal and in vivo exposure with response prevention to elements of traumatic events | Clinician-observed replacement of maladaptive cognitive schema with adaptive, life-affirming, and personal power-based beliefs about herself and relationships |
| Develop and implement effective coping skills in order to lead a fulfilling life | Practice thought-stopping for unwanted and intrusive recollections

Modify irrational thoughts about the trauma and her perceived role | Client-reported elimination of negative self-talk and negative interpretations of experiences |
| Implement behaviors that promote healing, evolving acceptance of past events, and responsible living | Learn skills of EMDR to reduce emotional and physiological reactivity to trauma recollections | Clinician observation of statements and behavior reflecting self-assertion |
| Create a plan for maintaining therapeutic gains | Participation in trauma-focused group therapy, including relaxation training

Discuss and implement relapse strategies for PTSD symptoms | Client self-report of engagement in life and self-affirming activities within and outside of the home |
| A pattern of almost lifelong depressive symptoms associated with seeing, and being resigned to, childhood slavery, racism, and gender discrimination as her assigned role in life | A pattern of almost lifelong depressive symptoms associated with seeing, and being resigned to, childhood slavery, racism, and gender discrimination as her assigned role in life | |

Goals for Change	Therapeutic Interventions	Outcome Measures of Change
Understand the societally based gender, racial, and socioeconomic conditions that contributed to past external and ongoing internal oppression Alleviate her depressive symptoms Strengthen her sense of self and overall competence to make free choices in her life Develop a plan for independent living, including vocational growth and development	Exploring the basis for her depressive symptoms in societal oppression of women and her personal experiences in slavery Contracting on the topics and pace of counseling to ensure an egalitarian relationship Supportive encouragement in the expression of pain and self-hatred, focusing on wellness, inner resources, and strength to offset the effects of pathologizing Challenge ruminative and distorted thinking to change distorted sense of responsibility for trauma Developing assertive communication and self-advocacy skills Stress-management techniques, including relaxation training, psychoeducation, guided imagery, meditation, and contemplative techniques Referral to relevant community resources for health and education	

CASE 12.3   *ONE FLEW OVER THE CUCKOO'S NEST'S* CHIEF BROMDEN

INTRODUCING THE CHARACTER

In Ken Kesey's 1962 book, *One Flew Over the Cuckoo's Nest,* the Native American character Chief Bromden narrates a story about life in a state psychiatric facility. The book was later made into an Academy Award–winning movie of the same title starring Will Sampson as the Chief and Jack Nicholson as protagonist Randle Patrick McMurphy (Zaentz, Douglas, & Forman, 1975). Actor Will Sampson was a significant choice for the role because he, himself, is a Muscogee-Creek Indian. Interestingly, there are differences between the book's and movie's storylines and portrayals of Chief Bromden. In the book, the Chief narrates the

story, which chronicles the psychiatric misadventures of R. P. McMurphy, a fellow patient with antisocial personality features who feigns mental illness in order to avoid going to prison for statutory rape. In the movie, on the other hand, the Chief is an imposing 6-foot 7-inch, 350-pound, mountain of a man who feigns mutism and has elected to remain silent since being hospitalized. The title phrase, "one flew over the cuckoo's nest," is a line from a children's rhyme Chief Bromden's grandmother sang to him as a child; "flying over the cuckoo's nest" means to go too far over the line, as McMurphy and other characters seem to do as the plot unfolds, and of course, the "cuckoo's nest" is a slang term for a psychiatric hospital.

Over the course of the story, McMurphy helps the Chief regain his self-respect and liberates him from his self-imposed silence; meanwhile, McMurphy, himself, unsuccessfully attempts to topple the oppressive power structure of the psychiatric facility, which is headed by clinical director, Nurse Ratched. Following a long tradition of negative popular culture portrayals of mental health professionals, Ratched's character is satirically presented in stereotype as a tyrannical, demeaning, punitive, and emasculating institutional psychiatric nurse. In fact, Ratched is so threatening that when Chief Bromden feigns being "deaf and dumb" in the movie version, it is as a defense, in order to become somewhat invisible, like a fly on the wall, and thereby avoid the troubles and harassment that other patients experience at the hands of Nurse Ratched, her henchmen, and society's various persecutors.

As the story nears its conclusion, McMurphy attempts one last, especially egregious but unsuccessful, assault on the power structure of the facility, rallying the patients together in revolt against the ward's system. After he led the failed patient uprising, Nurse Ratched arranges for McMurphy to be treated with a lobotomy procedure, leaving him in a vegetative state. McMurphy's downfall, however, rallies Chief's Bromden's inner resources and empowers the Chief to escape from the institution and its (stereotypically) horrid conditions. The story is about injustice, abuse of power, as well as the social and racial politics that have combined to imprison and disenfranchise both McMurphy and Bromden. The following basic case summary and diagnostic impressions present our construction of Chief Bromden's mental health concerns at a time when we imagine him to have been recently discharged from inpatient psychiatric care; we focus on the complex symptoms of a long-standing schizophrenic disorder and, secondarily, alcohol abuse we think he may have experienced.

Meet the Client

You can assess the client in action by viewing clips of Chief Bromden's video material at the following websites:

- http://www.youtube.com/watch?v=AG1 QPYCfaBQ The Chief speaks
- http://www.youtube.com/watch?v=nr Q9evXIle4 The Chief flies over the cuckoo's nest

BASIC CASE SUMMARY

Identifying Information. "Chief" Bromden is a 37-year-old Native American male who identifies himself as a Columbia Indian of the Pacific Northwest. He was recently discharged from an Oregon state psychiatric hospital, where he resided for 15 years. Since his discharge, he has been living in government subsidized housing and attending the day treatment program at the Oregon Bridge Center. Bromden prefers the sobriquet "Chief." Chief Bromden's appearance at the Center was appropriate and consistent with regional Native cultural norms.

Presenting Concern. During the first week of his daytime stay at the Oregon Bridge Center, Chief Bromden was interviewed by the director of intake services. Written medical and psychiatric historical notes also were available. The client sat quietly and passively as his file was reviewed, and he offered very simple and direct answers about his 15-year stay at the psychiatric hospital and his memory of the life events leading to his hospitalization. He volunteered that he was attending the Bridge Program as a condition of discharge and his goal was to manage his long-standing mental health problems so that he could remain living independently. Chief Bromden presents a history of increasingly prominent symptoms of a schizophrenic disorder, first suggested in childhood and adolescence and fully emerging in young adulthood and adulthood.

He also voluntarily raised concerns about his use of alcohol to manage his symptoms. He said he had recently lost his best friend, R. P. McMurphy, was despondent and had twice visited a bar on the outskirts of town in order to "get my head right." However, he chose not to drink, and instead walked the streets for hours before being picked up by the police and escorted home. He said that he was "afraid that if I pick up the bottle again I will have to surrender my spirit that I have only recently reacquired." Chief Bromden appears to have experienced Alcohol Abuse at times during his life cycle.

Background, Family, and Relevant History. Chief Bromden was born and raised on Indian tribal lands surrounding the Columbia River in the Pacific Northwest region of the United States. His father was a Native American tribal chief, Tee Ah Millatoona, and his mother was an Anglo school teacher, Mary Louise Bromden. Bromden's most prominent memories of childhood and adolescence are predominantly negative ones. He recalls being exposed at an early age to his father's difficulties and what Bromden called "humiliations" attempting to work with the U.S. government on behalf of his tribal people. Bromden recalled this as diminishing his father as an idealized male role model. Chief Bromden similarly recalls perceiving his Anglo mother as being "emasculating" and "belittling" toward his father and his father's culture. Chief Bromden recalls that throughout childhood, he felt emotionally abused at having to take his mother's "white" last name rather than his father's. Further, he recalls that his mother "berated my father to submit" by selling his tribal lands to enable the construction of hydroelectric dams on the Columbia River. Positive highlights of his childhood and adolescence primarily revolved around playing high school football, which he said allowed him to travel and see cities and areas other than the one in which he grew up.

Problem and Counseling History. During the childhood and adolescent time period described above, Chief Bromden appears to have experienced an early hallucination, viewing his mother as growing taller and taller until he perceived her to be "twice as tall as my father." He remembers feeling angry and remorseful about his father's use of alcohol and believed his father had "shrunk" from alcohol abuse and emasculation by Chief's mother and the white establishment. Likewise, he appears to have experienced an early delusion of being "invisible to white men." Following childhood and adolescence, Chief Bromden was enlisted in the U.S. Army and fought in World War II. This period provided structure and purposefulness for the client. It also appears to have been a time period during which his mental health concerns more fully emerged. Over this young adult time period and into adulthood, he appears to have begun to experience prominent, resilient, well-defined delusions and hallucinations. His primary delusion was a firm belief in an entity he referred to as the "Combine," which he described as a mechanized matrix or industrial complex. According to his delusion, the "Combine" machine is "huge," efficient, and well-organized, and its purpose is to control human thought and behavior. For example, it can insert fear or other emotions into individuals. Further, it is staffed by smoothly operating workmen. Along similar lines, his primary hallucinations were auditory ones of hearing the Combine in operation: gears turning, machines chugging, and a "rhythm" like a "thundering pulse." He sometimes confused his delusion and hallucinations pertaining to the Combine with hydroelectric dams.

Following discharge from the Army as a result of his continued symptoms and use of alcohol, Chief Bromden was occasionally incarcerated in local jails and subsequently remanded to hospitalized psychiatric care. During this period, his delusions and hallucinations continued as described above. He also experienced visual hallucinations of a "fog machine" operated by the Combine being used to cloud the air inside the psychiatric ward and the delusion that the Combine arranged for the death of a fellow patient. In addition, he developed a new delusional narrative in which he perpetrates a "mercy killing" on a fellow patient who recently has undergone a lobotomy procedure and then violently escapes from the hospital ward.

Although some symptoms persist, over the course of his hospitalization Chief Bromden experienced a reduction in delusions and hallucinations. At the time of his discharge, he reported no longer seeing the fog or having the fog machine delusion; by comparison, he reports currently "seeing the world and seeing myself more clearly." He also reported in the current interview that he understood his narrative about his hospital uprising and escape to have been a delusion (but added: "But it's all true even if it didn't happen").

Goals for Counseling and Course of Therapy to Date. Successful mitigation of symptoms via antipsychotic medication and milieu therapy during 15 years of hospitalized treatment recently resulted in the patient's discharge into independent living on the conditions that he reside in government-subsidized housing for community psychiatry patients and attend daily treatment at a bridge program. The primary goal is to develop a plan for supportive and life-skills counseling consistent with the following diagnostic impressions:

Diagnostic Impressions

Axis I.   295.30 Schizophrenia, Paranoid Type, Episodic With Interepisode Residual Symptoms

305.00 Alcohol Abuse

Axis II.   71.09 No Diagnosis on Axis II

Axis III.   None

Axis IV.   Problem related to social environment—Ethnic discrimination

Other psychosocial and environmental problems—History of exposure to war (WWII), history of extended psychiatric hospitalization

Problem related to primary support group—Childhood history of parental discord

Axis V.   GAF = 45 (at admission)

GAF = 61 (at discharge)

DISCUSSION OF DIAGNOSTIC IMPRESSIONS

Chief Bromden came to the Oregon Bridge Center day treatment program following discharge from inpatient hospitalization to address symptoms of Schizophrenia. Secondarily, Chief presented problems with alcohol use.

The *DSM-IV-TR* section "Schizophrenic and Other Psychotic Disorders" contains a variety of mental disorders featuring delusions, prominent hallucinations, disorganized speech, disorganized behavior, or catatonic behavior. Included in this section are schizophrenic disorders (Schizophrenia, Schizophreniform Disorder, and Schizoaffective Disorder), Delusional Disorder (Erotomanic, Grandiose, Jealous, Persecutory,

Somatic, and Mixed), and several other psychotic disorders (Brief Psychotic Disorder, Shared Psychotic Disorder, and psychotic disorders that are due to substance use or a medical problem).

Chief Bromden presented a long-standing history characterized by the complex features of Schizophrenia. During adolescence, the Chief experienced periods during which he had visual hallucinations (seeing his mother grow extraordinarily tall and his father shrink) and delusions (being invisible to white men) without other prominent symptoms. Providing these periods each lasted less than 6 months, during childhood and early adolescence, he probably was experiencing Schizophreniform Disorder.

During young adulthood and adulthood, Chief began experiencing persistent delusions (belief in the thought- and behavior-controlling "Combine" machine; belief in the story of his escape from the "Cuckoo's Nest"), auditory hallucinations (hearing the Combine rhythmically chug), and visual hallucinations (of a fog-making machine). His social functioning was impaired, he drank alcohol with problematic consequences, and his behavior led to being jailed on occasions. Taken together, Chief experienced a pattern of characteristic psychotic symptoms (delusions and hallucinations), with social dysfunction, lasting beyond 6 months. Further, there is no evidence of mood symptoms (suggesting a diagnosis of Schizoaffective Disorder or Mood Disorder With Psychotic Features) or that his symptoms were the direct consequence of a general medical condition or substance dependence, or any history of Autistic Disorder or another childhood Pervasive Developmental Disorder. Therefore, the diagnosis is Schizophrenia.

He most prominently experienced preoccupation is with his delusion about the Combine and related hallucinations. By comparison, he did not exhibit other characteristic symptoms, such as disorganized speech or behavior or inappropriate affect. Therefore, Paranoid Type is used. After his initial episode, he experienced a long pattern during which there were periods of intense delusions

and hallucinations, and in between these intense periods, other periods during which the hallucinations subsided and intensity of the delusions greatly reduced but did not completely disappear. Therefore, the longitudinal course specifier used is Episodic with Interepisode Residual Symptoms.

Schizophrenia is a challenging diagnosis. Several differential diagnoses might be considered. There must be no evidence that the client's or patient's symptoms are the direct consequence of a general medical condition (e.g., Psychotic Disorder Due to a General Medical Disorder or Delirium Due to a General Medical Condition) or substance use (e.g., Substance-Induced Psychotic Disorder or Substance-Induced Delirium). Criteria regarding characteristic schizophrenic symptoms, psychosocial dysfunction, duration, and exclusionary considerations all must be considered. One suggested resource for new clinicians is Noll's *The Encyclopedia of Schizophrenia and Other Psychotic Disorders* (2007). Based on our clinical evidence, Chief Bromden's history best matched the complex criteria for Schizoaffective Disorder.

Further, differential diagnosis requires effectively understanding the client's concerns. Accurately identifying and describing the counseling presentations of Native American clients may require the counselor's special attention (Garrett, 1999). Native cultural norms regarding extraordinary auditory and visual experiences, narrative presentation, use of silence and space, issues of social isolation, and other cultural considerations sometimes must be differentiated when making a diagnosis (Garrett, 1999; Garrett & Pichette, 2000).

Secondarily, Chief Bromden also reported a history of problematic alcohol use. The Substance-Related Disorders of the *DSM-IV-TR* comprise all of the Substance Use Disorders (Dependence and Abuse) and Substance Induced Disorders (Intoxication, Withdrawal, and substance-induced disruptions in mood, sleep, and sexual function) related to the use of 11 classes of drugs (including alcohol), medications, and toxins.

Chief reported a history of drinking alcohol to the point of intoxication, leading to his occasional arrest. He continued his drinking despite his awareness of this ongoing problematic consequence. Therefore, the diagnosis is Substance Abuse and, more specifically, Alcohol Abuse. Alcohol Dependence might be a reasonable differential consideration; however, Chief's use pattern meets the criteria for the less advanced diagnosis, abuse, rather than the more advanced diagnosis, dependence. Another differential consideration is whether Chief Bromden was engaged in nonproblematic social or recreational drinking, which would not require a diagnosis; however, his use met the criteria for a maladaptive pattern of substance-related behavior resulting in negative life consequences (Inaba & Cohen, 2000)—namely, recurrent use leading to recurrent substance-related legal problems—and therefore warranted a diagnosis indicating clinical significance. Chief Bromden reports having better current control over his drinking behavior; if symptoms diminish, in the future this diagnosis might no longer be applicable.

To round out the diagnosis, Chief's critical psychosocial stresses are emphasized on Axis IV, and on Axis V his functioning is represented by GAF scores ranging from serious symptoms and serious impairment at the time of hospital admission, in comparison with mild symptoms causing some difficulties as the time of discharge. The information on these axes is consistent with the information on Axis I.

CASE CONCEPTUALIZATION

During Chief Bromden's first week at the Oregon Bridge Center, the intake services director obtained current and historical information about the symptoms and consequences leading, at this point, to Chief's inpatient discharge and admission to the day program. Included among the intake materials were a thorough history, past medical and psychological records, interviews, and observations. Based on the intake process, the intake services director developed diagnostic impressions, confirming previous diagnoses describing Chief Bromden's symptoms as a

schizophrenic disorder, along with alcohol abuse. Next, a case conceptualization was developed. Whereas the purpose of diagnostic impressions is to *describe* the client's concerns, the goal of case conceptualization is to better *understand* and clinically *explain* the person's experiences (Neukrug & Schwitzer, 2006). It helps the clinician understand the etiology and process of the schizophrenia and related symptoms the Chief was experiencing. Case conceptualization sets the stage for treatment planning. Treatment planning then provides a road map that plots out how the therapy team at the day center and the client expect to move from presenting concerns to positive outcomes (Seligman, 1993, p. 157)—helping Chief Bromden continue controlling the symptoms of Schizophrenia, maintain daily functioning, and continue reduced reliance on alcohol.

When forming a case conceptualization, the clinician applies a purist counseling theory, an integration of two or more theories, an eclectic mix of theories, or a solution-focused combination of tactics, to his or her understanding of the client. In this case, the intake director based his conceptualization on psychotherapeutic integration of two theories (Corey, 2009). Psychotherapists very commonly integrate more than one theoretical approach in order to form a conceptualization and treatment plan that will be as efficient and effective as possible for meeting the client's needs (Dattilo & Norcross, 2006; Norcross & Beutler, 2008). In other words, counselors using the psychotherapeutic integration method attempt to flexibly tailor their clinical efforts to "the unique needs and contexts of the individual client" (Norcross & Beutler, 2008, p. 485). Like other counselors using integration, Chief's clinician chose this method because he had not found one individual theory that was comprehensive enough, by itself, to address all of the "complexities," "range of client types," and "specific problems" seen among his everyday caseload (Corey, 2009, p. 450).

Specifically, the director of intake services selected an integration of (a) Cognitive Behavior Therapy and (b) Cognitive Remediation Therapy.

He selected this approach based on Chief Bromden's chronic, long-standing experience of Schizophrenia and related symptoms, and his own knowledge of current outcome research with clients experiencing these types of concerns (McGurk, Twamley, Spitzer, McHugo, & Mueser, 2007; Pfammatter, Junghan, & Brenner, 2006; Tarrier & Bobes, 2000). According to the research, Cognitive Behavior Therapy is one treatment approach indicated when assisting clients to address their psychotic and other schizophrenic symptoms and the distress these symptoms cause (Tarrier & Bobes, 2000; Tarrier et al., 2001; Turkington, Kingdon, & Weiden, 2006), whereas an integrated approach emphasizing Cognitive Remediation Therapy is indicated to strengthen their cognitive abilities and reduce the losses in neurocognitive functioning they often experience (Wykes & Reeder, 2005; Wykes et al., 2003).

The counselor used the Inverted Pyramid Method of case conceptualization because this method is especially designed to help clinicians more easily form their conceptual pictures of their clients' needs (Neukrug & Schwitzer, 2006; Schwitzer, 1996, 1997). The method has four steps: Problem Identification, Thematic Groupings, Theoretical Inferences, and Narrowed Inferences. The counselor's clinical thinking can be seen in Figure 12.3.

Step 1: Problem Identification. The first step is Problem Identification. Aspects of the presenting problem (thoughts, feelings, behaviors, physiological features), additional areas of concern besides the presenting concern, family and developmental history, in-session observations, clinical inquiries (medical problems, medications, past counseling, substance use, suicidality), and psychological assessments (problem checklists, personality inventories, mental status exam, specific clinical measures) all may contribute information at Step 1. The counselor "casts a wide net" in order to build Step 1 as exhaustively as possible (Neukrug & Schwitzer, 2006, p. 202). As can be seen in Figure 12.3, the intake director identified not only Chief Bromden's prominent history of schizophrenic

symptoms (delusions, hallucinations, and negative symptom consequences) and problems resulting from alcohol use, but also positive past experiences (high school football, military service), parental and family dynamics, and sociocultural context—all of which were important to describing Chief Bromden's clinical situation.

Step 2: Thematic Groupings. The second step is Thematic Groupings. The clinician organizes all of the exhaustive client information found in Step 1 into just a few intuitive-logical clinical groups, categories, or themes, on the basis of sensible common denominators (Neukrug & Schwitzer, 2006). Four different ways of forming the Step 2 theme groups can be used: Descriptive-Diagnosis Approach, Clinical Targets Approach, Areas of Dysfunction Approach, and Intrapsychic Approach. As can be seen in the figure, the intake director selected the Descriptive-Diagnosis Approach. This approach sorts together all of the various Step 1 information about the client's adjustment, development, distress, or dysfunction "to show larger clinical problems as reflected through a diagnosis" (Neukrug & Schwitzer, 2006, p. 205).

The director made a straightforward grouping of all of Chief's various affective, cognitive, and physiological symptoms of Schizophrenia—plus the family and cultural contexts that seemed to influence the nature and content of his delusional narratives and hallucinations; he noted all of these together under "Schizophrenia." Likewise, he grouped Chief's problematic alcohol use and its consequences under "History of Alcohol Abuse." The counselor's conceptual work at Step 2 gave him a way to think about Chief's functioning and concerns more insightfully.

So far, at Steps 1 and 2, the director of intake services has used his clinical assessment skills and his clinical judgment to begin critically understanding Chief Bromden's needs. Now, at Steps 3 and 4, he applies the theoretical approach he has selected. He begins making theoretical inferences to explain the factors leading to Chief's issues as they are seen in Steps 1 and 2.

Step 3: Theoretical Inferences. At Step 3, concepts from the counselor's theoretical integration of two approaches—Cognitive Behavior Therapy and Cognitive Remediation—are applied to the experiences causing, and the mechanisms maintaining, Chief Bromden's functioning. The counselor tentatively matches the theme groups in Step 2 with this theoretical approach. In other words, the symptom constellations in Step 2, which were distilled from the symptoms in Step 1, now are combined using theory to show what are believed to be the underlying processes or psychological mechanisms of Chief Bromden's current needs (Neukrug & Schwitzer, 2006; Schwitzer, 2006, 2007).

First, Cognitive Behavior Therapy was applied primarily to Chief Bromden's needs regarding his prominent schizophrenic symptomology. According to Cognitive Behavior Therapy (Beck, 1995, 2005; Ellis, 1994; Ellis & MacLaren, 2005), irrational thinking, faulty beliefs, or other forms of cognitive errors lead individuals to engage in problematic behaviors and experience their behavioral consequences. As can be seen in Figure 12.3, when the intake director applied these Cognitive Behavior Therapy concepts to Chief Bromden's Schizophrenia, he explained at Step 3 that the various issues noted in Step 1, which can be understood in Step 2 to be a theme of recurrent Schizophrenia with contextual influences, lead to inferences that the client must (Bustillo, Lauriello, Horan, & Keith, 2001; Pfammatter et al., 2006; Rector & Beck, 2002): (a) learn to distinguish hallucinations from actual visional and auditory events; (b) learn to distinguish delusional narratives from actual reality; and (c) reinforce the importance of taking medications, complying with treatment, and coping with obstacles.

Second, Cognitive Remediation Therapy was applied primarily to Chief Bromden's needs regarding declines or deficits in neurocognitive functioning, which sometimes results from long-standing Schizophrenia and prolonged treatment (Wykes & Reeder, 2005). As also can be seen in Figure 12.3, when the director applied these concepts, he additionally inferred at Step 3: Now that the client's psychotic symptoms have subsided, he may continue to experience neurocognitive deficits that can interfere with his coping (Wykes et al., 2003; Wykes & Reeder, 2005).

Step 4: Narrowed Inferences. At Step 4, the clinician's selected theory continues to be used to address still-deeper issues when they exist (Schwitzer, 2006, 2007). At this step, "still-deeper, more encompassing, or more central, causal themes" are formed (Neukrug & Schwitzer, 2006, p. 207). Chief Bromden's counselor continued to use psychotherapeutic integration of two approaches.

First, continuing to apply Cognitive Behavior Therapy concepts at Step 4, the director of intake services presented a single, deepest theoretical inference that he believed to be most fundamental for Chief Bromden from a cognitive behavioral perspective: Despite the biological basis of the client's symptoms, he can use cognitive-behavioral practices to manage their effects and reduce their consequences. Second, continuing to apply Cognitive Remediation, the director presented a single, deepest theoretical inference that he believed to be most fundamental for Chief Bromden from a cognitive rehabilitation perspective: Despite the neurocognitive deficits resulting from the client's Schizophrenic Disorder, with extensive, focused practice he can regain better attending, reasoning, and memory skills. These two narrowed inferences, together, form the basis for understanding the Chief's current counseling situation.

When all four steps are completed, the client information in Step 1 leads to logical-intuitive groupings on the basis of common denominators in Step 2, the groupings then are explained using theory at Step 3, and then, finally, at Step 4, further deeper explanations are made. From start to finish, the thoughts, feelings, behaviors, and physiological features in the topmost portions are connected on down the pyramid into deepest dynamics.

Figure 12.3 Chief Bromden's Inverted Pyramid Case Conceptualization Summary: Psychotherapeutic Integration of Cognitive Behavior Therapy and Cognitive Remediation Therapy

1. IDENTIFY AND LIST CLIENT CONCERNS

History of diagnosis of Schizophrenia
History of inpatient hospitalization
Early visual hallucination of towering mother
Prominent delusions of Combine
Auditory hallucinations of Combine gears
Visual hallucinations of Combine fog machine
Delusion of Combine killing inpatient
Delusion of narrative of mercy killing and escape
Currently without prominent symptoms
Currently recognizes escape narrative as delusion
Currently sober and compliant with treatment

Positive high school football & travel experience
Positive army enlistment experience
History of alcohol use leading to jail
History of jail plus symptoms leading to hospitalization
Native American upbringing
Multicultural parents (Anglo mother, Native father)
Recalls father primarily as humiliated in tribal actions with U.S. government
Recalls father primarily humiliated and belittled by mother
Recalls with regret father's selling of tribal land for hydro dams

2. ORGANIZE CONCERNS INTO LOGICAL THEMATIC GROUPINGS

1. Schizophrenia, Paranoid Type, Episodic With Interepisodic Symptoms (with influences of family and cultural context)
2. History of Alcohol Abuse (resulting in jail and other negative consequences)

3. THEORETICAL INFERENCES: ATTACH THEMATIC GROUPINGS TO INFERRED AREAS OF DIFFICULTY

Psychotherapeutic Integration

Cognitive Behavior Therapy

1. Client must learn to distinguish hallucinations from actual visional and auditory events
2. Client must learn to distinguish delusional narratives from actual reality
3. Client must reinforce importance of taking medications, complying with treatment, and coping with obstacles

Cognitive Remediation Therapy

Now that the client's psychotic symptoms have subsided, he may continue to experience neurocognitive deficits that can interfere with his coping

4. NARROWED INFERENCES: SUICIDALITY AND DEEPER DIFFICULTIES

Psychotherapeutic Integration

Cognitive Behavior Therapy

Despite the biological basis of the client's symptoms, he can use cognitive behavioral practices to manage their effects and reduce their consequences

Cognitive Remediation Therapy

Despite the neurocognitive deficits resulting from the client's schizophrenic disorder, with extensive, focused practice he can regain better attending, reasoning, and memory skills

TREATMENT PLANNING

At this point, Chief Bromden's clinician at the Oregon Bridge Center has collected all available information about the problems that have been of concern to him and the psychiatric team that performed the assessment. Based upon this information, the counselor developed a five-axis *DSM-IV-TR* diagnosis and then, using the "inverted pyramid" (Neukrug & Schwitzer, 2006; Schwitzer, 1996, 1997), formulated a working clinical *explanation* of Chief Bromden's difficulties and their etiology that we called the *case conceptualization.* This, in turn, guides us to the next critical step in our clinical work, called the *treatment plan,* the primary purpose of which is to map out a logical and goal-oriented strategy for making positive changes in the client's life. In essence, the treatment plan is a road map "for reducing or eliminating disruptive symptoms that are impeding the client's ability to reach positive mental health outcomes" (Neukrug & Schwitzer, 2006, p. 225). As such, it is the cornerstone of our work with not only Chief Bromden, but with all clients who present with disturbing and disruptive symptoms and patterns (Jongsma & Peterson, 2006; Jongsma et al., 2003a, 2003b; Seligman, 1993, 1998, 2004).

A comprehensive treatment plan must integrate all of the information from the biopsychosocial interview, diagnosis, and case conceptualization into a coherent plan of action. This *plan* comprises four main components, which include (1) a behavioral definition of the problem(s), (2) the selection of achievable goals, (3) the determination of treatment modes, and (4) the documentation of how change will be measured. The *behavioral definition of the problem(s)* consolidates the results of the case conceptualization into a concise hierarchical list of problems and concerns that will be the focus of treatment. The *selection of achievable goals* refers to assessing and prioritizing the client's concerns into a *hierarchy of urgency* that also takes into account the client's motivation for change, level of dysfunction, and real-world influences on his or her

problems. The *determination of treatment modes* refers to selection of the specific interventions, which are matched to the uniqueness of the client and to his or her goals and clearly tied to a particular theoretical orientation (Neukrug & Schwitzer, 2006). Finally, the clinician must establish how change will be measured, based upon a number of factors, including client records and self-report of change, in-session observations by the clinician, clinician ratings, results of standardized evaluations such as the Beck Depression Inventory (Beck & Steer, 1990) or a family functioning questionnaire, pre-post treatment comparisons, and reports by other treating professionals.

The four-step method discussed above can be seen in Figure 6.1 (p. 109) and is outlined below for the case of Chief Bromden, followed by his specific treatment plan.

Step 1: Behavioral Definition of Problems. The first step in treatment planning is to carefully review the case conceptualization, paying particular attention to the results of Step 2 (Thematic Groupings), Step 3 (Theoretical Inferences), and Step 4 (Narrowed Inferences). The identified clinical themes reflect the core areas of concern and distress for the client, while the theoretical and narrowed inferences offer clinical speculation as to their origins. In the case of Chief Bromden, there are two primary areas of concern. The first, "Schizophrenia, Paranoid Type, Episodic With Inter-episode Residual Symptoms," refers to his history of diagnosis of Schizophrenia and inpatient hospitalizations, early visual hallucination of a towering mother, prominent delusions and hallucinations of the "Combine," delusions of mercy killing and escape, and currently being without prominent symptoms. The second, "Alcohol Abuse," refers to his history of episodes of excessive alcohol use and incarcerations. Many of Chief Bromden's symptoms, particularly his alcoholism, can be contextualized within the sociopolitical oppression of American Indians (Diller, 2007). These symptoms and stresses are consistent with the diagnosis of Schizophrenia, Paranoid

Type, Episodic With Inter-episodic Residual Symptoms; and Alcohol Abuse (APA, 2000a).

Step 2: Identify and Articulate Goals for Change. The second step is the selection of achievable goals, which is based upon a number of factors, including the most pressing or urgent behavioral, emotional, and interpersonal concerns and symptoms as identified by the client and clinician, the willingness and ability of the client to work on those particular goals, and the realistic (real-world) achievability of those goals (Neukrug & Schwitzer, 2006). At this stage of treatment planning, it is important to recognize that not all of the client's problems can be addressed at once, so we focus initially on those that cause the greatest distress and impairment. New goals can be created as old ones are achieved. In the case of Chief Bromden, the goals are divided into two prominent areas. The first, "Schizophrenia, Paranoid Type, Episodic With Inter-episode Residual Symptoms" requires that we help Chief Bromden to control (or eliminate) his active psychotic symptoms through medication compliance, distinguish between hallucinations/delusions and reality, improve his social skills and problem-solving, remediate neurocognitive deficits, including working memory, executive functioning, attention, and processing speed and increase his goal-directed behaviors. The second, "Alcohol Abuse," requires that we help Chief Bromden to recognize the relationship between alcohol abuse and sociopolitical oppression of the American Indian, recognize the relationship between alcohol use and psychotic symptomatology, identify social, behavioral, emotional, physiological, and cognitive triggers for alcohol use, develop effective coping strategies to eliminate reliance upon alcohol, and to establish a sustained recovery from the maladaptive use of alcohol.

Step 3: Describe Therapeutic Interventions. This is perhaps the most critical step in the treatment planning process because the clinician must now integrate information from a number of sources, including the case conceptualization, the delineation of the client's problems and goals, and the

treatment literature, paying particular attention to *empirically supported treatment* (EST) and *evidence-based practice* (EBP). In essence, the clinician must align his or her treatment approach with scientific evidence from the fields of counseling and psychotherapy. Wampold (2001) identifies two types of evidence-based counseling research: studies that demonstrate "absolute efficacy," that is, the fact that counseling and psychotherapy work, and those that demonstrate "relative efficacy," that is, the fact that certain theoretical/technical approaches work best for certain clients with particular problems (Psychoanalysis, Gestalt Therapy, Cognitive Behavior Therapy, Brief Solution-Focused Therapy, Cognitive Therapy, Dialectical Behavior Therapy, Person-Centered Therapy, Expressive/Creative Therapies, Interpersonal Therapy, and Feminist Therapy); and when delivered through specific treatment modalities (individual, group, and family counseling).

In the case of Chief Bromden, we have decided to use a two-pronged "integrated" approach comprised of Cognitive Behavior Therapy and Cognitive Remediation Therapy. Cognitive Behavior Therapy (Beck, 1995, 2005; Ellis, 1994; Ellis & MacLaren, 2005) has been found to be highly effective in counseling and psychotherapy with adults who experience the symptoms of Schizophrenia (McGurk et al., 2007; Pfammatter et al., 2006) and Alcohol Abuse (Longabaugh & Morgenstern, 1999). The approach relies on a variety of cognitive techniques (reframing, challenging irrational thoughts, and cognitive restructuring) and behavioral techniques (reinforcement for and shaping of adaptive behavior, extinction of maladaptive behaviors, systematic desensitization, and exposure with response prevention) (Ball et al., 2006; Frank et al., 2005; Milkowitz, 2008). Specific techniques drawn from this approach will include identification of and desensitization (imaginal and in vivo) to triggers of behavioral, emotional, and physiological stress that precipitate psychotic reaction; identification and refutation of irrational (and delusional) thoughts about the "Combine" and conspiracies; cognitive restructuring and reframing of thoughts related to oppression and conspiracies; and in vivo shaping and reinforcement of appropriate social behavior.

The second component of treatment will be Cognitive Remediation Therapy, which employs an array of tasks designed to address and improve the client's cognitive functioning in areas that contribute to the positive and negative symptoms of Schizophrenia and other psychotic disorders (Wykes & Reeder, 2005; Wykes et al., 2003). Techniques drawn from this model will include verbal and computerized exercises designed and proven to strengthen many of the cognitive skills that are deficient in Schizophrenia, including executive control (reasoning and problem-solving), verbal and visual working memory, social cognition, and speed of processing.

Step 4: Provide Outcome Measures of Change. This last step in treatment planning requires that we specify how change will be measured and indicate the extent to which progress has been made toward realizing these goals (Neukrug & Schwitzer, 2006). The counselor has considerable flexibility in this phase and may choose from a number of objective domains (psychological tests and measures of self-esteem, depression, psychosis,

interpersonal relationship, anxiety, etc.), quasi-objective measures (the *DSM-IV-TR's* Axis V GAF scale; pre-post clinician, client, and psychiatric ratings), and subjective ratings (client self-report, clinician's in-session observations). In Chief Bromden's case, we have implemented a number of these, including client self-reported alcohol abstinence, a pre-post improved measure on the Alcohol Use Inventory (Horn, Wanberg, & Foster, 1990), a 3-month post measure of GAF functioning in the mild to moderate range (60–70), and a 6–12 month measure of functioning in the mild range (>70), client self-report of absence of psychotic symptoms, counselor observation and client self-report of improved social functioning, medical evidence of no psychiatric hospitalization for 6 months, and rehabilitation center report of improved functioning on measured areas of cognitive functioning.

The completed treatment plan is now developed through which the counselor and Chief Bromden will work together to reduce the impact of his Schizophrenic symptoms, to assist him with his alcohol abuse, and to improve his overall functioning. Chief Bromden's treatment plan is as follows and is summarized in Table 12.3.

TREATMENT PLAN

Client: Chief Bromden

Service Provider: Oregon Bridge Center

BEHAVIORAL DEFINITION OF PROBLEMS:

1. Schizophrenia, Paranoid Type, Episodic With Inter-episode Residual Symptoms—History of diagnosis of Schizophrenia and inpatient hospitalizations, early visual hallucination of a towering mother, prominent delusions and hallucinations of the "Combine," delusions of mercy killing and escape, and currently being without prominent symptoms

2. History of Alcohol Abuse—Repeated episodes of alcohol abuse leading to jail (currently in remission)

GOALS FOR CHANGE:

1. Schizophrenia, Paranoid Type, Episodic With Inter-episode Residual Symptoms

- Control (or eliminate) his active psychotic symptoms through medication compliance
- Distinguish between hallucinations/delusions and reality
- Improve social skills and problem solving
- Remediate neurocognitive deficits (working memory, executive functioning, attention and processing speed)
- Increase his goal-directed behaviors

2. History of Alcohol Abuse

- Recognize the relationship between alcohol abuse and sociopolitical oppression of the American Indian
- Recognize the relationship between alcohol use and psychotic symptomatology
- Identify social, behavioral, emotional, physiological, and cognitive triggers for alcohol use
- Develop effective coping strategies to eliminate reliance upon alcohol
- Establish a sustained recovery from the maladaptive use of alcohol

THERAPEUTIC INTERVENTIONS:

A moderate-term course of individual Cognitive Behavior and Cognitive Remediation Therapy (6–9 months)

1. Schizophrenia, Paranoid Type, Episodic With Inter-episode Residual Symptoms

- Psychoeducational group counseling around social skills, medication compliance, and positive symptom management
- Identification of and desensitization (imaginal and in vivo) to triggers of behavioral, emotional, and physiological stress that precipitate psychotic reaction
- Identification and refutation of irrational (and delusional) thoughts about the "Combine" and conspiracies
- Cognitive restructuring and reframing of thoughts related to oppression and conspiracies
- In vivo shaping and in vivo reinforcement of appropriate social behavior
- Cognitive tasks (verbal and computerized) to strengthen executive control (reasoning and problem-solving, verbal and visual working memory, social cognition and speed of processing)

2. History of Alcohol Abuse

- Discuss feelings of oppression and their relationship to drinking
- Do a cost-benefit analysis of drinking and sobriety
- Develop a list of behaviors, attitudes, and feelings involved with use and relapse
- Identify and refute thoughts that precipitate the perceived need to drink
- Identify bodily and physiological states that lead to drinking
- Practice stress-management techniques, including breathing, progressive muscle relaxation, and meditation and plan for use in daily life
- Develop and establish rituals that enhance sobriety
- Attendance in alcohol support group
- Co-create a relapse contract and long-term plan for abstinence

(Continued)

(Continued)

OUTCOME MEASURES OF CHANGE:

The immediate reduction, and eventual elimination of, psychotic symptomatology, awareness of the role of racial oppression in his life, alcohol abstinence, and long-term adaptive functioning as measured by:

- 3-month post measures of GAF functioning in the mild to moderate range (60–70)
- 6–12 month measure of functioning in the mild range (>70)
- Client self-reported alcohol abstinence
- Pre-post improved measure on the Alcohol Use Inventory
- Client self-report of absence of psychotic symptoms
- Counselor observation and client self-report of improved social functioning
- Medical evidence of no psychiatric hospitalization for 6 months
- Rehabilitation center report of improved functioning on measured areas of cognitive functioning

Table 12.3   Chief Bromden's Treatment Plan Summary: Psychotherapeutic Integration of Cognitive Behavior Therapy and Cognitive Remediation

Goals for Change	Therapeutic Interventions	Outcome Measures of Change
Schizophrenia, Paranoid Type, Episodic With Interepisode Residual Symptoms	Schizophrenia, Paranoid Type, Episodic With Interepisode Residual Symptoms	The immediate reduction and eventual elimination of psychotic symptomatology, awareness of the role of racial oppression in his life, alcohol abstinence, and long-term adaptive functioning as measured by:
Control (or eliminate) his active psychotic symptoms through medication compliance	Psychoeducational group counseling around social kills, medication compliance, and positive symptom management	
Distinguish between hallucinations/delusions and reality	Identification of and desensitization (imaginal and in vivo) to triggers of behavioral, emotional, and physiological stress that precipitates psychotic reaction	3-month post measures of GAF functioning in the mild to moderate range (60–70)
Improve social skills and problem solving	Identification and refutation of irrational (and delusional) thoughts about the "Combine" and conspiracies	6–12 month measure of functioning in the mild range (>70)
Remediate neurocognitive deficits (working memory, executive functioning, attention and processing speed)	Cognitive restructuring and reframing of thoughts related to oppression and conspiracies	Client self-reported alcohol abstinence
Increase his goal-directed behaviors	In vivo shaping and in vivo reinforcement of appropriate social behavior	Pre-post improved measure on the Alcohol Use Inventory

Goals for Change	Therapeutic Interventions	Outcome Measures of Change
History of Alcohol Abuse Recognize the relationship between alcohol abuse and sociopolitical oppression of the American Indian Recognize the relationship between alcohol use and psychotic symptomatology Identify social, behavioral, emotional, physiological, and cognitive triggers for alcohol use Develop effective coping strategies to eliminate reliance upon alcohol Establish a sustained recovery from the maladaptive use of alcohol	Cognitive tasks (verbal and computerized) to strengthen executive control (reasoning and problem solving, verbal and visual working memory, social cognition, and speed of processing History of Alcohol Abuse Discuss feelings of oppression and their relationship to drinking Do a cost-benefit analysis of drinking and sobriety Develop a list of behaviors, attitudes, and feelings involved with use and relapse Identify and refute thoughts that precipitate the perceived need to drink Identify bodily and physiological states that lead to drinking Practice stress-management techniques, including breathing, progressive muscle relaxation, and meditation and plan for use in daily life Develop and establish rituals that enhance sobriety Attendance in alcohol support group Co-create a relapse contract and long-term plan for abstinence	Client self-report of absence of psychotic symptoms Counselor observation and client self-report of improved social functioning Medical evidence of no psychiatric hospitalization for 6 months Rehabilitation center report of improved functioning on measured areas of cognitive functioning

CASE 12.4 *SPIDER-MAN'S* PETER PARKER

INTRODUCING THE CHARACTER

Peter Parker, who transforms into the fantasy hero Spider-Man, is the creation of Marvel Comics writer and editor, Stan Lee, and artist and cowriter, Steve Ditko. Peter Parker first appeared in the August 1962 issue of *Amazing Fantasy #15.* Since the character's creation, Peter Parker, also known as Spider-Man, has appeared as a television cartoon character; in graphic novels; in newspaper comic strips; and most recently in a series of movies starring actor Tobey Maguire, including *Spider-Man* (Avad &

Raimi, 2002), *Spider-Man 2* (Avad & Raimi, 2004), and *Spider-Man 3* (Avad & Raimi, 2007).

Peter, an orphan being raised by his paternal uncle, Ben, along with his wife, May, was introduced to the comic world as an angst-ridden teen and high school student who while facile in science and academics was extremely shy, self-conscious, and uncomfortable with girls, particularly with Mary Jane Watson, his neighbor and love interest. Although early Spider-Man stories pitted the hero against fantasy ne'er-do-wells such as Green Goblin, Dr. Octopus, and Venom, later story lines focused on more reality-based issues such as drug abuse and terrorism.

Peter's critical transformation into a super hero occurs during a high school field trip to a science museum. There, he is bitten by a radioactive spider, which transforms him into a web-casting, wall-climbing, lightening fast, super-strong, and sensorially acute alter-persona soon after known to the comic book world as Spider-Man. Up to that point in comic book history, teenagers had been relegated to the secondary role of sidekick (such as Batman's Robin and Captain America's Bucky). Spider-Man soon became one of the most popular comic book superheroes—wrestling with crime and criminals by night and the challenges of adolescence during the day. In the basic case summary and diagnostic impressions that follow, we present Peter Parker's experiences as illustrations of a moderate, recurrent depressive mood disorder, coexisting with a change in personality due to a medical problem.

Meet the Client

You can assess the client in action by viewing clips of Peter Parker's video material at the following websites:

- http://www.youtube.com/watch?v=dg83 d4VziLk Origin of a superhero
- http://www.youtube.com/watch?v= Hm4BxQen6SM Awakening with powers
- http://www.youtube.com/watch?v= IuOkwCcMjEc Death of Uncle Ben
- http://www.youtube.com/watch?v=N-PYuGYkdyM Mary Jane Watson

---

BASIC CASE SUMMARY

Identifying Information. Peter Parker is a 17-year-old white male adolescent who currently is a senior in Midtown High School. He lives at home with his Aunt May, who recently lost her husband, Parker's Uncle Ben, to gun violence. Parker was referred by his aunt at the urging of his Midtown High School school counselor who has noticed

visible changes in Peter's behavior and mood. His aunt also reports seeing clear behavioral and mood changes at home. Although ambivalent about participating in counseling, Peter was polite and compliant during the interview.

Presenting Concern. The school counselor referred Peter Parker due to changes she noticed in his mood, beginning about 4 months ago, shortly after the death of Peter's uncle. Peter was nearby when his uncle was killed. His uncle was a victim of a carjacking and murder. Peter believes he could have heroically saved his uncle and blames himself for his uncle's death. Correspondingly, Peter was self-reproaching in the interview and described himself as worthless. He says he has had trouble staying asleep at night and regularly is awakened by nightmares centering on violence and death. He volunteered that he is unsure whether he feels "depressed" as suggested by his aunt and school counselor, but did admit that he has been feeling "angry and irritated" "almost constantly" since his uncle's murder. When queried, he said he also is having difficulty taking pleasure in his school work, "even science, which I used to really love," or enjoying his school newspaper photography, which formerly was one of his special interest highlights. Both his aunt and counselor report that although he continues to perform well academically and is engaged successfully in extracurricular activities as a photographer for the school newspaper, he has begun to struggle to concentrate on his work, is having trouble meeting deadlines, and has missed several homework assignments. He also seems to no longer spend time in the evenings with friends in the neighborhood.

His aunt raised a second concern in addition to Peter's reaction to the loss of his uncle. She described changes in his behavior and reactions that she has noticed since prior to the shooting, "going back to his field trip last fall at the science museum." She said that since he returned from the field trip, his behavior has become increasingly unpredictable. She said that persistently since the museum visit his mood quickly changes from calm to angry to remorseful; sometimes he becomes pushy and aggressive, and even seems able to "climb the walls" and "bounce from place to place"; he is increasingly suspicious and worried about being attacked or "found out" by others; and in the evenings he impulsively puts on a costume and goes into downtown streets "looking for trouble." His aunt reports all of these are easily noticeable, dramatic changes from his behavior and reactions prior to the field trip.

Background, Family Information, and Relevant History. Peter is a high school senior at Midtown High School in Forest Hills, New York, where he had been living with his paternal uncle and aunt, Ben and May Parker, and now lives with just his aunt. He was adopted by his aunt and uncle at the time of his parents' deaths early in his life. Initially believing that his parents Richard and Mary died in a plane crash when he was 6 years old, he later discovered that they were killed in the line of duty as U.S. Special Forces Operatives.

As a child, Peter was seen in individual play therapy soon after his relocation to his aunt and uncle's home. At that time, he was experiencing night terrors, enuresis, and breathing difficulties that were later attributed to panic attacks. Although the symptoms subsided within 9 months and he made a good adjustment in his new school, Peter continued to experience mild symptoms of anxiety and generalized but manageable fears during childhood.

Peter said the Parkers raised him in a "traditional Protestant household," in which he was taught the importance of honesty, hard work, kindness, and loyalty. Peter says he has a small circle of friends, most of whom share his academic and scientific interests and who he says are generally regarded by others as "nerds." Peter said that while he "has always been shy with girls," Peter feels very close with his neighbor, Mary Jane Watson, who lives in an abusive household and whom he would like to be able to protect.

Turning to very recent history, Peter was queried specifically about his recent museum field trip event, after which his aunt noticed persistent personality changes. Peter was reticent to respond, but did admit that during the trip to the science museum, he was bitten by an unusual spider. It is Peter's belief that the bite has slowly transformed him into a person with great strength, speed, and sensory acuity. He said after the bite, he became more able to "just act on impulses."

In fact, he reported that in order to try to capitalize upon these sudden gifts, he entered a local wrestling match, which he easily won. However, he says he was "cheated out" of his prize money. When a thief soon afterward robbed the wrestling promoter who had "cheated" him out of his winnings, Peter said he was so uncontrollably angry at the promoter that he chose to allow the thief to escape rather than "using my new super abilities to capture him." Peter believes it was the very same thief who went on to carjack and kill his beloved Uncle Ben.

As the client described it, over the course of the next several months, which has coincided with his final months in high school, Peter has worked diligently to hone his newfound "skills" and apparently views himself as a vigilante who can redeem himself for his uncle's death by fighting the street criminals he seems to fear. He says he has kept his dual identity a secret, even from those closest to him, and as a result, has become increasingly socially isolated, "misunderstood," and lonely, spending most of his time "in the darkness and shadows" as well as in the company of other "outcasts" and criminals.

Problem and Counseling History. In our counseling meeting, Peter presented as a conventional appearing teenager. He seemed somewhat suspicious of his environment and could be described as exhibiting a piercing glance through which he seemed to take in everything around him. He expressed himself in a rather mechanical fashion and spoke from an intellectual as opposed to an emotional way. He frequently choked back tears when describing the death of his uncle and the loss of his parents, but was equally if not more concerned about losing control of his feelings. Although articulate and seemingly self-aware, he was self-effacing.

Peter described ongoing difficulties in relationships with girls whom he worried perceived him to be a bookworm and a nerd. Nevertheless, he attested to a love of science and was thinking about a career in crime fighting. He alluded to the nightmares he had as a child as well as to feelings of sadness over not having known or being able to remember much about his parents. When asked about the recent death of his uncle Ben, Peter was unable to hold back a torrent of tears that he quickly stifled and replaced with intense anger. He noticed that these mood swings have been more frequent of late and that while he does not drink or use drugs, he has been engaging in what might be considered reckless, dangerous, and thrill-seeking behavior that has put him in direct contact with criminals. He realized the potential harm this behavior might cause him, but believes that it is "my mission to save people . . . I couldn't help my Uncle Ben."

Goals for Counseling and Course of Therapy to Date. To date Peter has had one counseling session and also was referred for one medical examination by his primary care physician. Referral information from his school counselor and results of his initial counseling session appear in this report. Consistent with Peter's description of receiving a spider bite, chemical screen and neurological testing as part of his medical examination were positive for a spider bite with radioactive venom affecting his frontal lobes and other nervous system sites, resulting in a syndrome characterized by heightened impulsivity, inhibition, and other personality changes. Recommendation is for ongoing psychotherapy to address depressive symptoms and personality effects of radioactive spider bite syndrome.

Diagnostic Impressions

Axis I. 296.22 Major Depressive Disorder, Single Episode, Moderate

310.1 Personality Change Due to Radioactive Spider Bite Syndrome, Combined Type

Axis II. V71.09 No Diagnosis on Axis II

Axis III. Radioactive Spider Bite Syndrome

Axis IV. Problems with primary support group—Recent death of uncle, death of parents at age 6

Other psychosocial and environmental problems—Exposure to street crime

Axis V. GAF = 60 (current)

GAF = 80 (highest level past year)

DISCUSSION OF DIAGNOSTIC IMPRESSIONS

Peter Parker was urged to attend counseling by his aunt and his school counselor, both of whom had noticed changes in Peter's mood, and personality, in recent months.

All of the diagnoses contained in the *DSM-IV-TR's* Mood Disorders section feature a disturbance in mood. The Mood Disorders include Depressive Disorders (in which the client experiences unipolar depression), Bipolar Disorders (in which the client experiences manic, hypomanic, or mixed episodes), and mood disorders that are due to substance use or a medical condition. All of the diagnoses contained in the section, Mental Disorders Due to a General Medical Condition, feature psychological and behavioral symptoms that are the directly due to the physiological consequences of medical problem. One of the conditions appearing in this section is Personality Change Due to a General Medical Condition. Changes in personality that are the direct result of a medical condition can include emotional lability, disinhibition, aggressiveness, apathy, and/or paranoia.

The psychotherapist first evaluated Peter Parker's mood concerns. Peter described his mood as angry and irritable, although he was unsure whether he felt depressed. He described feelings of self-reproach and worthlessness; reported having difficulty maintaining sleep and having nightmares; said he has little interest in, and finds little pleasure in, the photography and schoolwork that formerly he enjoyed; and is having trouble concentrating. He has experienced these symptoms for more than 2 weeks, and they are interfering with his ability to function at school and elsewhere. Peter's presentation meets the criteria of a Major Depressive Episode. Mood Episodes are the building blocks for making a Mood Disorder diagnosis.

Peter has experienced no Manic or Hypomanic Episodes; in turn, the diagnosis is Major Depressive Disorder and not a Bipolar Disorder. The current episode is the first that he has experienced, so, the course is specified as Single Episode. Finally, his current episode is described: He experiences meet multiple criteria for a Major Depressive Episode. He is experiencing distress along with more than minor impairment in occupational functioning. Conversely, his symptoms are not substantially beyond those needed for the diagnosis and are not causing severe problems with work or social functioning. The best fit among the severity specifiers is Moderate.

One differential diagnosis that might be considered because Peter's mood change is in reaction to a life event is Adjustment Disorder With Depressed Mood. Whereas Adjustment Disorders With Depressed Mood are negative affective reactions to life stressors in the absence of another diagnosable Axis I disorder, in this case, Peter's symptoms conform to the specific criteria for a Major Depressive Episode, which go beyond the general criteria set for Adjustment Disorder.

Another differential consideration is Acute Stress Disorder or Posttraumatic Stress Disorder (PTSD), since Peter has some symptoms of anxiety such as difficulty with sleep and concentration. However, his symptoms primarily are in the area of mood rather than anxiety and meet the criteria for a Major Depressive Disorder. It is notable that Peter's mood is angry and irritable, rather than depressed; this is consistent with presentations of depression sometimes seen in children and adolescents (APA, 2000a, p. 356).

The psychotherapist next evaluated Peter Parker's changes in personality and behavior. Peter's aunt reported that in contrast to his behavior prior to his science museum field trip, his behavior had become unpredictable, his mood quickly changed from anger to remorse, he was uncharacteristically "pushy" and aggressive, was suspicious and worried, and engaged in impulsive acts like wandering downtown streets at night seeking "trouble" and wearing unusual costumes. These symptoms might be characteristic of a Personality Disorder. Peter did report that he remembered getting a spider bite during his museum visit, and his therapist referred him for a physical exam and toxicology screening along with the counseling intake. Lab test results from the exam revealed biochemical evidence of Radioactive Spider Bite Syndrome, which produces changes in personality. In such cases the diagnosis is a Mental Disorder Due to a General Medical Condition, more specifically: Personality Change Due to Radioactive Spider Bite Syndrome, Combined Type. Combined Type is used because Peter was experiencing a combination of features, including mood lability, poor impulse control, aggressiveness, and paranoid ideation.

One differential consideration is whether these personality changes were severe symptoms associated with Major Depressive Disorder. However, because the therapist expertly referred Peter Parker for a physical exam, evidence was found indicating that personality changes were, instead, the direct consequence of a medical problem. (Damage to the frontal lobe and hemispheric strokes are more common examples of gمتةmedical conditions that can cause personality change than is Radioactive Spider Bite Syndrome, for which Peter Parker is the only known patient).

To complete the diagnosis, the medical condition associated with the diagnosis listed on Axis I must be listed on Axis III, Peter's relevant stressors are emphasized on Axis IV, and on Axis V his functioning is represented by GAF scores ranging from the presence of good functioning with only expectable reactions to life stressors within the past year, to the current, moderately serious symptoms affecting several aspects of his functioning, which led to his referral. The information on all five axes is consistent.

CASE CONCEPTUALIZATION

When Peter Parker came for his first counseling appointment, his assigned counselor collected thorough information about the symptoms and situations leading to his referral. She collected information about his current symptoms and presentation, recent situational factors and other events. Based on her thorough intake evaluation, the counselor developed diagnostic impressions, describing Peter's presenting concerns by a single episode of Major Depressive Disorder, and Personality Change Due to General Medical Condition, which was a radioactive spider bite. A case conceptualization next was developed. Whereas the purpose of diagnostic impressions is to *describe* the client's concerns, the goal of case conceptualization is to better *understand* and clinically *explain* the person's experiences (Neukrug & Schwitzer, 2006). It helps the counselor understand the etiology leading to Peter's depressive disorder and personality change, and the factors maintaining these concerns. In turn, case conceptualization sets the stage for treatment planning. Treatment planning then provides a road map that plots out how the counselor and client expect to move from presenting concerns to positive outcomes (Seligman, 1993, p. 157)—helping Peter improve his low mood and related symptoms, and reducing the problematic aspects of his change in personality.

When forming a case conceptualization, the clinician applies a purist counseling theory, an integration of two or more theories, an eclectic mix of theories, or a solution-focused combination of tactics, to his or her understanding of the client. In this case, Peter Parker's counselor based her conceptualization on psychotherapeutic integration of two theories (Corey, 2009). Psychotherapists very commonly integrate more than one theoretical approach in order to form a conceptualization and treatment plan that will be as efficient and effective as possible for meeting the client's needs (Dattilo & Norcross, 2006; Norcross & Beutler, 2008). In other words, counselors using the psychotherapeutic integration method attempt to flexibly tailor their clinical efforts to "the unique needs and contexts of the individual client" (Norcross & Beutler, 2008, p. 485). Like other counselors using integration, Peter's clinician chose this method because she had not found one individual theory that was comprehensive enough, by itself, to address all of the "complexities," "range of client types," and "specific problems" seen among her everyday caseload (Corey, 2009, p. 450).

Specifically, Peter Parker's counselor selected an integration of (a) Cognitive Behavior Therapy and (b) Reality Therapy. She selected this approach based on Peter's presentation of intrapersonal mood concerns along with interpersonal personality problems, her knowledge of current outcome research, and suggested best practices with clients experiencing these types of concerns (Critchfield & Smith-Benjamin, 2006; Glasser, 1998, 2001, 2003; Fotchmann & Gelenberg, 2005; Hollon, Thase, & Markowitz, 2002; Westen & Morrison, 2001). According to the research, Cognitive Behavior Therapy is one treatment approach indicated when assisting clients with depressive disorders (Fotchmann & Gelenberg, 2005; Hollon et al., 2002; Westen & Morrison, 2001), whereas an integrated approach emphasizing Reality Therapy can be useful when addressing behavioral and interpersonal choices such as those confronting Peter Parker following his recent experiences (Wubbolding, 2000, 2007). Peter's counselor is comfortable theoretically integrating these approaches.

The counselor used the Inverted Pyramid Method of case conceptualization because this method is especially designed to help clinicians more easily form their conceptual pictures of their clients' needs (Neukrug & Schwitzer, 2006; Schwitzer, 1996, 1997). The method has four steps: Problem Identification, Thematic Groupings, Theoretical Inferences, and Narrowed Inferences. The counselor's clinical thinking can be seen in Figure 12.4.

Step 1: Problem Identification. The first step is Problem Identification. Aspects of the presenting problem (thoughts, feelings, behaviors, physiological features), additional areas of concern besides the presenting concern, family and developmental history, in-session observations, clinical inquiries (medical problems, medications, past counseling, substance use, suicidality), and psychological assessments (problem checklists, personality inventories, mental status exam, specific clinical measures) all may contribute information at Step 1. The counselor "casts a wide net" in order to build Step 1 as exhaustively as possible (Neukrug & Schwitzer, 2006, p. 202). As can be seen in Figure 12.4, the counselor identified Peter Parker's various primary concerns (angry mood and all of the other symptoms of major depression; all of the symptoms of personality change); important recent events and situations (loss of uncle, etc.); important medical and clinical concerns (spider bite, Radioactive Spider Bite Syndrome); and related issues, thoughts, feelings, and behaviors (guilt, self-reproach, etc.). She attempted to go beyond just the current, noticeable symptoms leading to Peter's referral, in order to be descriptive as she could.

Step 2: Thematic Groupings. The second step is Thematic Groupings. The clinician organizes all of the exhaustive client information found in Step 1 into just a few intuitive-logical clinical groups, categories, or themes, on the basis of sensible common denominators (Neukrug & Schwitzer, 2006). Four different ways of forming the Step 2 theme groups can be used: Descriptive-Diagnosis Approach, Clinical Targets Approach, Areas of Dysfunction Approach, and Intrapsychic Approach. As can be seen in the figure, Peter's counselor selected the Intrapsychic Approach. This approach sorts together all of the Step 1 information about the "client's adjustment, development, distress, or dysfunction" in order "to show clinical patterns in the ways life events are associated with the person's personal experience and identity" (Neukrug & Schwitzer, 2006, p. 205).

Peter's counselor formed two interesting symptom constellations to capture the two intrapsychic patterns and resulting behaviors she attributed to Peter. She grouped together his symptoms of depression, loss of his uncle, guilt, and self-reproach about responsibility for his uncle's death, and so on into Theme 1: Symptoms of depression due to guilt and self-reproach about causing or not preventing uncle's death. She grouped together his unpredictable personality features and risky vigilant behaviors into Theme 2: Indicators of choosing risky, erratic vigilant behaviors capitalizing on spider bite–induced changes in personality and abilities to repair guilt and self-reproach. In this case example, the counselor used the Intrapsychic Approach to group together various information about changes in thinking, mood, behavior, and physiology in order to show how external life experiences have been associated with dimensions of Peter's experience of self.

So far, at Steps 1 and 2, the counselor has used her clinical assessment skills and her clinical judgment to begin meaningfully understanding Peter Parker's needs. Now, at Steps 3 and 4, she applies the theoretical approach she has selected. She begins making theoretical inferences to interpret and explain the processes or roots underlying Peter's concerns as they are seen in Steps 1 and 2.

Step 3: Theoretical Inferences. At Step 3, concepts from the counselor's theoretical integration of two approaches—Cognitive Behavior Therapy and Reality Therapy—are applied to explain the experiences causing, and the mechanisms maintaining, Peter Parker's problematic changes in mood and behavior. The counselor tentatively matches the theme groups in Step 2 with this theoretical approach. In other words, the symptom constellations in Step 2, which were distilled from the symptoms in Step 1, now are combined using theory to show what are believed to be the underlying causes or psychological etiology of Peter Parker's current needs (Neukrug & Schwitzer, 2006; Schwitzer, 2006, 2007).

First, Cognitive Behavior Therapy was applied primarily to Peter's depressive needs. According to Cognitive Behavior Therapy (Beck, 1995, 2005; Ellis, 1994; Ellis & MacLaren, 2005), irrational thinking, faulty beliefs, or other forms of cognitive errors lead individuals to engage in problematic behaviors and to experience negative moods and attitudes. As can be seen in Figure 12.4, when the counselor applied these Cognitive Behavior Therapy concepts, she explained at Step 3 that the various issues noted in Step 1 (mood and other adolescent symptoms of depression), which can be understood in Step 2 to be a theme of loss and guilt, are rooted in or caused by Peter's irrational belief, "It is my fault my uncle is dead, and therefore I do not deserve to be happy or to move on with my life."

Second, Reality Therapy was applied. This second approach was thought to complement the irrational belief as a source of Peter's depressive symptoms by further addressing his recent problematic changes. According to Reality Therapy, individuals choose actions in attempts to satisfy their needs—more importantly, relationship needs. Therefore, according to the theory, the counseling focus is on what actions and behaviors clients are choosing and evaluating the degree to which present actions are leading to need satisfaction or other desired consequences (Glasser, 1998, 2001, 2003). The Reality Therapy conceptualization addresses the individual's present-day wants pertaining to the type of person he or she wishes to be, desires for family, whether and how the person intends to change his or her life, and similar questions about the choices the individual is making and is willing to make for the future (Wubbolding, 2000, 2007).

As can be seen in the figure, when the counselor applied these Reality Therapy concepts, she additionally explained at Step 3 that the various Step 1 issues, which can be organized in Step 2 to be indicators of choosing erratic vigilante behaviors to repair guilt, could be understood as follows: Peter's current behaviors are leading to risky, harmful possible consequences, and these behaviors are poor need-satisfying choices.

Step 4: Narrowed Inferences. At Step 4, the clinician's selected theory continues to be used to address still-deeper issues when they exist (Schwitzer, 2006, 2007). At this step, "still-deeper, more encompassing, or more central, causal themes" are formed (Neukrug & Schwitzer, 2006, p. 207). Peter Parker's counselor continued to use psychotherapeutic integration of two approaches.

First, continuing to apply Cognitive Behavior Therapy concepts at Step 4, Peter's counselor presented a single, most-fundamental faulty belief that she believed to be most explanatory and causal regarding Peter's primary reasons for referral: the deepest irrational self-statement that "I must redeem myself for my uncle's death by vigilantism; otherwise I don't deserve to exist." Second, continuing to apply Reality Therapy, the counselor presented a single, most deeply rooted Reality Therapy inference: Peter is focused on past events rather than making good choices now and learning to make good choices for the future. These two narrowed inferences, together, form the basis for understanding the etiology and maintenance of Peter's difficulties.

When all four steps are completed, the client information in Step 1 leads to logical-intuitive groupings on the basis of common denominators in Step 2, the groupings then are explained using theory at Step 3, and then, finally, at Step 4, further deeper explanations are made. From start to finish, the thoughts, feelings, behaviors, and physiological features in the topmost portions are connected on down the pyramid into deepest dynamics.

Figure 12.4 Peter Parker's Inverted Pyramid Case Conceptualization Summary: Psychotherapeutic Integration of Cognitive Behavior Therapy and Reality Therapy

1. IDENTIFY AND LIST CLIENT CONCERNS

Angry

Irritable

Feelings of worthlessness

Poor sleep

Nightmares

Diminished school performance

Loss of interest in school and
   photography

Witnessed uncle's death by gun violence

Self-reproaching and guilty

Feels uncle's death is his fault

Believes he could have saved uncle

Personality and behavior changes

Recent Radioactive Spider Bite Syndrome

Acts unpredictably

Acts pushy and aggressively

Acts impulsively/poor impulse control

Suspicious and worried

Wearing unusual costumes

Adopted clandestine alter-identity

Engages in risky, dangerous vigilantism

2. ORGANIZE CONCERNS INTO LOGICAL THEMATIC GROUPINGS

1. Symptoms of depression due to guilt and self-reproach about causing or not preventing uncle's death
2. Indicators of choosing risky, erratic vigilante behaviors capitalizing on spider bite-induced changes in personality and abilities to repair guilt and self-reproach

3. THEORETICAL INFERENCES: ATTACH THEMATIC GROUPINGS TO INFERRED AREAS OF DIFFICULTY

Psychotherapeutic Integration

Cognitive Behavior Therapy

Irrational belief:

"It is my fault my uncle is dead and therefore I do not deserve to be happy or to move on with the rest of my life"

Reality Therapy

Current behaviors are leading to risky, harmful possible consequences and these behaviors are poor need-satisfying choices

4. NARROWED INFERENCES: SUICIDALITY AND DEEPER DIFFICULTIES

Psychotherapeutic Integration

Cognitive Behavior Therapy

Deepest faulty belief:

"I must redeem myself for my uncle's death by vigilantism; otherwise I don't deserve to exist

Reality Therapy

Peter is focused on past events rather than making good choices now and learning how to make good choices for the future

TREATMENT PLANNING

At this point, Peter's clinician at the Midtown High School Counseling Center has collected all available information about the problems that have been of concern to him. Based upon this information, the counselor developed a five-axis *DSM-IV-TR* diagnosis and then, using the "inverted pyramid" (Neukrug & Schwitzer, 2006; Schwitzer, 1996, 1997), formulated a working clinical *explanation* of Peter's difficulties and their etiology that we called the *case conceptualization.* This, in turn, guides us to the next critical step in our clinical work, called the *treatment plan,* the primary purpose of which is to map out a logical and goal-oriented strategy for making positive changes in the client's life. In essence, the treatment plan is a road map "for reducing or eliminating disruptive symptoms that are impeding the client's ability to reach positive mental health outcomes" (Neukrug & Schwitzer, 2006, p. 225). As such, it is the cornerstone of our work with not only Peter, but with all clients who present with disturbing and disruptive symptoms and/or personality patterns (Jongsma & Peterson, 2006; Jongsma et al., 2003a, 2003b; Seligman, 1993, 1998, 2004).

A comprehensive treatment plan must integrate all of the information from the biopsychosocial interview, diagnosis, and case conceptualization into a coherent plan of action. This *plan* comprises four main components, which include (1) a behavioral definition of the problem(s), (2) the selection of achievable goals, (3) the determination of treatment modes, and (4) the documentation of how change will be measured. The *behavioral definition of the problem(s)* consolidates the results of the case conceptualization into a concise hierarchical list of problems and concerns that will be the focus of treatment. The *selection of achievable goals* refers to assessing and prioritizing the client's concerns into a *hierarchy of urgency* that also takes into account the client's motivation for change, level of dysfunction, and real-world influences on his or her problems. The *determination of treatment modes*

refers to selection of the specific interventions, which are matched to the uniqueness of the client and to his or her goals and clearly tied to a particular theoretical orientation (Neukrug & Schwitzer, 2006). Finally, the clinician must establish how change will be measured, based upon a number of factors, including client records and self-report of change, in-session observations by the clinician, clinician ratings, results of standardized evaluations such as the Beck Depression Inventory-II (Beck, 1996) or a family functioning questionnaire, pre-post treatment comparisons, and reports by other treating professionals.

The four-step method discussed above can be seen in Figure 6.1 (p. 109) and is outlined below for the case of Peter, followed by her specific treatment plan.

Step 1: Behavioral Definition of Problems. The first step in treatment planning is to carefully review the case conceptualization, paying particular attention to the results of Step 2 (Thematic Groupings), Step 3 (Theoretical Inferences), and Step 4 (Narrowed Inferences). The identified clinical themes reflect the core areas of concern and distress for the client, while the theoretical and narrowed inferences offer clinical speculation as to their origins. In the case of Peter, there are two primary areas of concern. The first, "symptoms of depression due to guilt and self-reproach about causing or not preventing his uncle's death," refers to his feelings that his uncle's death was his fault, feelings of guilt and self-reproach, anger, irritability, feelings of worthlessness, poor sleep with nightmares, diminished school performance, and loss of interest in school and photography. The second, "indicators of choosing risky, erratic vigilante behaviors capitalizing on spider bite–induced changes in personality and abilities to repair guilt and self-reproach refers to headaches, poor sleep, and fatigue," refers to personality and behavior changes following a recent radioactive spider bite, unpredictable, pushy, and aggressive behavior, impulsivity, suspiciousness, and worry. These symptoms and stresses are consistent with the diagnosis of Major Depressive Disorder, Single Episode, Moderate; and Personality Change Due to Radioactive Spider Bite Syndrome, Combined Type (Andrews, Slade, Sunderland, & Anderson, 2007; APA, 2000a; Chuang, 2009; Dobson, 1989; Hollon, Thase, & Markowitz, 2002).

Step 2: Identify and Articulate Goals for Change. The second step is the selection of achievable goals, which is based upon a number of factors, including the most pressing or urgent behavioral, emotional, and interpersonal concerns and symptoms as identified by the client and clinician, the willingness and ability of the client to work on those particular goals, and the realistic (real-world) achievability of those goals (Neukrug & Schwitzer, 2006). At this stage of treatment planning, it is important to recognize that not all of the client's problems can be addressed at once, so we focus initially on those that cause the greatest distress and impairment. New goals can be created as old ones are achieved. In the case of Peter, the goals are divided into two prominent clusters. The first, "symptoms of depression due to guilt and self reproach about causing or not preventing uncle's death," requires that we help Peter to alleviate his depressed mood and return to previous levels of functioning, appropriately grieve his loss, identify the relationship between his depression, guilt, and the loss of his uncle, identify his irrational guilt-based thoughts, develop healthy cognitive patterns and beliefs, learn and implement relapse prevention strategies, and to develop a positive reconnection with memories of his uncle. The second, "indicators of choosing risky, erratic, vigilante behaviors capitalizing on spider bite-induced changes in personality," requires that we assist Peter to medically stabilize his condition through compliance with physical treatment, live life to the fullest by learning physical and psychological coping strategies, reduce fear and anxiety associated with the medical condition, accept the physical changes and monitor their impact on his daily functioning, and accept the role of psychological/stress factors in the exacerbation of his condition.

Step 3: Describe Therapeutic Interventions. This is perhaps the most critical step in the treatment planning process because the clinician must now integrate information from a number of sources, including the case conceptualization, the delineation of the client's problems and goals, and the treatment literature, paying particular attention to *empirically supported treatment* (EST) and *evidence-based practice* (EBP). In essence, the clinician must align his or her treatment approach with scientific evidence from the fields of counseling and psychotherapy. Wampold (2001) identifies two types of evidence-based counseling research: studies that demonstrate "absolute efficacy," that is, the fact that counseling and psychotherapy work, and those that demonstrate "relative efficacy," that is, the fact that certain theoretical/technical approaches work best for certain clients with particular problems (Psychoanalysis, Gestalt Therapy, Cognitive Behavior Therapy, Brief Solution-Focused Therapy, Cognitive Therapy, Dialectical Behavior Therapy, Person-Centered Therapy, Expressive/Creative Therapies, Interpersonal Therapy, and Feminist Therapy); and when delivered through specific treatment modalities (individual, group, and family counseling).

In the case of Peter, we have decided to use a two-pronged integrated approach to therapy comprised of Cognitive Behavior Therapy and Reality Therapy. Cognitive Behavior Therapy (Beck, 1995, 2005; Ellis, 1994; Ellis & MacLaren, 2005) has been found to be highly effective in counseling and psychotherapy with adults (and adolescents) who experience the symptoms of Major Depressive Disorder related to loss (Fiorini & Mullen, 2006; Neimeyer, 2000; Servaty-Seib, 2004). The approach relies on a variety of cognitive techniques (reframing, challenging irrational thoughts, and cognitive restructuring) and behavioral techniques (reinforcement for and shaping of adaptive behavior, extinction of maladaptive behaviors, systematic desensitization, and exposure with response prevention) (Ball et al., 2006; Frank et al., 2005; Milkowitz, 2008). Peter's loss-based depression will be addressed through a combination of individual techniques that include identifying and understanding the stages of grief; verbalizing circumstances of loss and identifying related irrational thoughts and feelings; exploring feelings of anger, sadness, and guilt related to loss, and reframing in a non-guilt-inducing manner; imaginal desensitization around the experience of his uncle's death; developing and engaging in healthy mourning rituals; and scheduling activities that have a high likelihood for stress relief and relaxation.

We have also decided to use Reality Therapy (Glasser, 1998, 2001, 2003) due to its emphasis on client's recognition of the role of choices in their life, how those choices affect their happiness (and unhappiness), and how they can make healthier and life-affirming choices. The WDEP system (Wubbolding et al., 2004; Wubbolding & Brickell, 1998; Wubbolding & Colleagues, 1998) provides the structure for intervention by helping clients to identify their wants (W) and their direction (D), to evaluate the efficacy of their current direction and its outcome (E), and to plan accordingly (P). Given Peter's general life competencies and past successful adjustment both at home and at school, Reality Therapy's emphasis on strengthening the client's internal locus of control as well fostering insight and change through the therapeutic relationship will assist him to reclaim responsibility in and for his life, as well as to effectively problem-solve. This particular form of counseling/psychotherapy has proven effective in treating a wide range of problems, including anxiety, depression, anger management, and relationship issues (Radtke, Sapp, & Farrell, 1997; Wubbolding, 2000; Wubbolding & Brickell, 1999). Specific techniques for Peter will include recognizing the medical basis for his changed personality functioning; taking responsibility for the thoughts, feelings, and behaviors that resulted from this condition; using physiological, behavioral, and emotional monitoring to minimize the need to engage in risky and harmful behaviors; recognizing the possible adverse consequences of these behaviors to both himself and others; practicing statements of responsibility and choice; and joining a support group for medical conditions that lead to personality change.

Step 4: Provide Outcome Measures of Change. This last step in treatment planning requires that we specify how change will be measured and indicate the extent to which progress has been made toward realizing these goals (Neukrug & Schwitzer, 2006). The counselor has considerable flexibility in this phase and may choose from a number of objective domains (psychological tests and measures of self-esteem, depression, psychosis, interpersonal relationship, anxiety, etc.), quasi-objective measures (the *DSM-IV-TR's* Axis V GAF scale; pre-post clinician, client, and psychiatric ratings), and subjective ratings (client self-report, clinician's in-session observations). In Peter's case, we have implemented a number of these, including improved pre-post measures on the Beck Depression Inventory-II (Beck, Steer, & Brown,1996), Beck Anxiety Inventory (Beck & Steer,1990), and Clinical Anger Scale (Snell, Gum, Shuck, Mosely, & HIte, 1995); spouse and client report of improvement in overall life, family and work satisfaction, aunt's report of Peter's improvement in mood, activity level, and outlook, and the development of adaptive responses to stress.

The completed treatment plan is now developed through which the counselor and Peter will be able to use the techniques of Cognitive Behavior Therapy and Reality Therapy to reduce Peter's stressful feelings, and eliminate his disruptive physiological, emotional, cognitive and behavioral symptoms. Peter Parker's treatment plan appears below, and a summary can be found in Table 12.4.

TREATMENT PLAN

Client: Peter Parker

Service Provider: Midtown High School Counseling Center

BEHAVIORAL DEFINITION OF PROBLEMS:

1. Symptoms of depression due to guilt and self-reproach for causing or not preventing uncle's death—Feeling that his uncle's death was his fault, self-reproach and guilt, anger, irritability, feelings of worthlessness, poor sleep with nightmares, diminished school performance, and loss of interest in school and photography

2. Indicators of choosing risky, erratic vigilante behaviors capitalizing on spider bite–induced changes in personality and abilities to repair guilt and self-reproach—Personality and behavior changes following a recent radioactive spider bite; unpredictable, pushy, and aggressive behavior, impulsivity, suspiciousness, and worry

GOALS FOR CHANGE:

1. Symptoms of depression due to guilt and self-reproach for causing or not preventing uncle's death

   - Alleviate depressed mood and return to previous levels of functioning
   - Appropriately grieve his loss
   - Identify the relationship between his depression, guilt, and the loss of his uncle
   - Identify his irrational guilt-based thoughts
   - Develop healthy cognitive patterns and beliefs
   - Develop a health mourning ritual
   - Learn and implement relapse prevention strategies

2. Indicators of choosing risky, erratic vigilante behaviors capitalizing on spider bite–induced changes in personality and abilities to repair guilt and self-reproach

   - Medically stabilize his condition through compliance with physical treatment
   - Reduce fear and anxiety associated with the medical condition
   - Accept the physical changes and monitor their impact on his daily functioning
   - Accept the role of psychological/stress factors in the exacerbation of his condition
   - Live life to the fullest by learning physical and psychological coping strategies

(Continued)

(Continued)

THERAPEUTIC INTERVENTIONS:

A short- to moderate-term course of individual Cognitive Behavior and Reality Therapy centered counseling (3–6 months)

1. Symptoms of depression due to guilt and self-reproach for causing or not preventing uncle's death

   - Identify and understand the stages of grief
   - Verbalize circumstances of loss- and identify-related irrational thoughts and feelings
   - Explore feelings of anger, sadness, and guilt related to loss and reframe in a non-guilt-inducing manner
   - Imaginal desensitization around the experience of his uncle's death
   - Identify positive characteristics of lost loved one
   - Schedule activities that have a high likelihood of stress relief
   - Develop and implement program for regular exercise and relaxation strategies

2. Indicators of choosing risky, erratic vigilante behaviors capitalizing on spider bite–induced changes in personality and abilities to repair guilt and self-reproach

   - Recognizing the medical basis for his changed personality functioning
   - Taking responsibility for the thoughts, feelings, and behaviors that resulted from this condition
   - Using physiological, behavioral, and emotional monitoring to minimize the need to engage in risky and harmful behaviors
   - Discussing the adverse consequences of these behaviors to both himself and others
   - Practicing statements of responsibility and choice for his thoughts and actions
   - Joining a support group for medical conditions that lead to personality change

OUTCOME MEASURES OF CHANGE:

The resolution of guilt-driven grief, elimination of depression, and responsible management of his medical condition and its consequences as measured by:

   - Stabilization of clinician's rating of client's GAF to the mild range (>70)
   - Improved pre-post scores on Beck Depression Inventory-II
   - Client self-report of improved overall mood, with reduced and tolerable guilt
   - Client's report of acceptance of and responsible choices in managing medical his condition
   - Clinician observation of client's decreased stress level
   - Incident-free police record for a period of 1 year

Table 12.4   Peter Parker's Treatment Plan Summary: Psychotherapeutic Integration of Cognitive Behavior Therapy and Reality Therapy

Goals for Change	Therapeutic Interventions	Outcome Measures of Change
Symptoms of depression due to guilt and self-reproach for causing or not preventing uncle's death	Symptoms of depression due to guilt and self-reproach for causing or not preventing uncle's death	The resolution of guilt-driven grief, elimination of depression, and responsible management of his medical condition and its consequences as measured by:
Alleviate depressed mood and return to previous levels of functioning	Identify and understand the stages of grief	Stabilization of clinician's rating of client's GAF to the mild range (>70)
Appropriately grieve his loss	Verbalize circumstances of loss and identify related irrational thoughts and feelings	Improved pre-post scores on Beck Depression Inventory II
Identify the relationship between his depression, guilt, and the loss of his uncle	Explore feelings of anger, sadness, and guilt related to loss and reframe in a non-guilt-inducing manner	Client self-report of improved overall mood, with reduced and tolerable guilt
Identify his irrational guilt-based thoughts	Imaginal desensitization around the experience of his uncle's death	Client's report of acceptance of and responsible choices in managing medical his condition
Develop healthy cognitive patterns and beliefs	Identify positive characteristics of lost loved one	Clinician observation of client's decreased stress level
Develop a healthy mourning ritual	Schedule activities that have a high likelihood for stress relief	Incident-free police record for a period of 1 year
Learn and implement relapse prevention strategies	Develop and implement program for regular exercise and relaxation strategies	
Indicators of choosing risky, erratic vigilante behaviors capitalizing on spider bite-induced changes in personality and abilities to repair guilt and self-reproach	Indicators of choosing risky, erratic vigilante behaviors capitalizing on spider bite-induced changes in personality and abilities to repair guilt and self-reproach	
Medically stabilize his condition through compliance with physical treatment	Recognizing the medical basis for his changed personality functioning	
Reduce fear and anxiety associated with the medical condition	Taking responsibility for the thoughts, feelings, and behaviors that resulted from this condition	
Accept the physical changes and monitor their impact on his daily functioning	Using physiological, behavioral, and emotional monitoring to minimize the need to engage in risky and harmful behaviors	
Accept the role of psychological/stress factors in the exacerbation of his condition	Discussing the adverse consequences of these behaviors to both himself and others	
Live life to the fullest by learning physical and psychological coping strategies	Practicing statements of responsibility and choice for his thoughts and action	
	Joining a support group for medical conditions that lead to personality change	

CASE 12.5 *WINNIE THE POOH'S* CHRISTOPHER ROBIN

INTRODUCING THE CHARACTER

Christopher Robin is the central figure in the fictional works of British author A. A. Milne, which include *When We Were Very Young* (1924), *Winnie the Pooh* (1926), *Now We Are Six* (1927), and *The House at Pooh Corner* (1928). The fanciful stories feature 6-year-old Christopher Robin and his stuffed toys Winnie the Pooh (a bear), Eeyore (a donkey), Tigger (a tiger), and mother and son Kanga and Roo, as well as the woodland creatures Owl and Rabbit. Since their publication, the books featuring Christopher Robin and his friends in the Hundred Acre Wood, most prominently Winnie the Pooh, have been made into a number of animated films. The most famous of these movies are *The Many Adventures of Winnie the Pooh* (Lounsbery & Reitherman, 1977) and *Winnie the Pooh and the Blustery Day* (Reitherman, 1968), both created by the Walt Disney Company.

Although never introduced to the reader or audience as imaginary characters, it is clear that all of Christopher Robin's friends are his beloved stuffed animals brought to life through his vivid imagination. Each one personifies a unique quality, including Winnie's loving innocence, Owl's wisdom, Rabbit's cynicism, Piglet's fearfulness, Tigger's love for life, Eeyore's sadness, and Kanga's and Roo's compassion. Although the adventures of Christopher Robin and his friends clearly are flights of imagination, the lessons learned have provided generations of children and grown-ups with bits of wisdom that somehow, yet invariably, get lost along the way to adulthood. As we imagine him, Christopher Robin may be experiencing the impairments in human social interaction, and restricted interests and activities, that together are characteristic of Asperger's Disorder. Details follow in the basic case summary and diagnostic impressions below.

Meet the Client

You can assess the client in action by viewing clips of Christopher Robin's video material at the following website:

- http://www.youtube.com/watch?v=6W8 p5KG7eMA Christopher and Winnie

---

BASIC CASE SUMMARY

Identifying Information. Christopher Robin is a 6-year-old boy who has been at the Hundred Acre Day School for Boys for just over 3 months. He resides in London with his parents. Although Christopher has done adequately in his studies thus far, he prefers creative and solitary activities, including drawing, play acting, and free play on the school's spacious athletic fields. He appears to be an active and appropriately energetic boy. However, he was remarkably withdrawn and reluctant to engage the counselor during his intake meeting. Although ample toys, games, and distractions were available to Christopher in the play therapy room during the interview, he exclusively held, talked to, and played with the stuffed bear (he named Winnie), stuffed pig (he named Piglet), and stuffed rabbit (he named Rabbit) that he brought with him to the session.

Presenting Problem. Christopher arrived for an evaluation session on referral from the school counselor and with his parents' permission. Initiating the referral were his teachers', classroom assistants', counselors', and parents' concerns about his lack of interest in engaging with his classmates and peers, his lack of initiative seeking out any objects or themes of play beyond his stuffed animal collection, and his failure to make eye contact or meaningfully pay attention to and respond to his teachers at school.

Likewise, his parents report that at home he plays exclusively with his stuffed animals, declines any solicitations by his father to try soccer or other sports or outdoor activities, rejects encouragement by his mother to play board games or video games, and does not socially interact at all with their weekly housecleaner, or with adults or children who are neighbors.

The Day School's headmistress, Eloise Rathbone, has become concerned that Christopher may not be "ready for school" or may have needs beyond the school's resources. Like his teachers, she is concerned because he has had some difficulty adjusting to the social demands of leaving home every day to attend school; during the day he mainly spends his time with isolative behavior, spends excessive time in imaginary play with his stuffed animals, and shows a heightened level of distractibility during his classes. However, Ms. Rathbone does describe Christopher as an otherwise "very pleasant child."

Background, Family Information, and Relevant History. Christopher was born in the socioeconomically affluent London suburb of Blustershire, the only child of Alexander and Annaleise Robin. His parents, who are well-established and loyal patrons of the arts throughout London, report that they have hoped throughout 16 years of marriage to have a child and finally were successful with the birth of Christopher. Christopher's father described himself as a prolific and somewhat driven and reclusive author of children's books who spends most of his days cloistered in his study and, by his description, has been only rarely available to the family. Christopher's mother, Annaleise, reports that she has been extensively involved in the Labour Party in England and is often out of the house during days, evenings, or weekends. A part-time nanny, Olive Rockwell, provides additional child care when Christopher's parents are unavailable. His parents describe Ms. Rockwell as "very caring" but "a bit domineering." They say they have encouraged her to occupy Christopher's time with "playful distractions."

Christopher was described by his parents as "a rather sickly child with a host of respiratory and digestive ailments" that precluded physical activity. Therefore, much of his early childhood was spent indoors in the company of either the nanny or one or two "chosen" playmates, but mostly with his "precious stuffed animals." In a separate interview, Ms. Rockwell noted that Christopher "could virtually spend hours engaged in fanciful adventures with this ragamuffin band." Not only did Christopher play with his stuffed friends, he would draw pictures of them, fashion clothing out of paper to protect them from the elements, and would at times attempt to take them into the bath with him. Christopher's connection with his "stuffed friends" became

more problematic when at 5-1/2 years of age he began kindergarten at the Blustershire School for the Gifted and Creative.

According to his kindergarten teacher at Blustershire, Christopher was a very pleasant, creative, and easygoing child who had difficulty making friends but who "easily won the hearts of teachers." He was a child who cried easily when his stuffed toys were taken away during other class activities and who withdrew from others. During times when he was separated from his animals, he would sit alone in a corner and draw, suck his thumb, have conversations with absent imaginary friends, and occasionally rock back and forth. Although Christopher successfully met the academic criteria for passage into the first grade, his parents and teachers were concerned that due to his lack of social interest and his overly restricted interests in his toys, he would need a smaller classroom environment for first grade than could be provided by Blustershire. As a result, he was transferred to the Hundred Acre Day School for Boys.

Problem and Counseling History. Christopher was referred to the school guidance center by the school counselor and headmistress out of concern that his growing preoccupation with his imaginary friends and socially isolative behavior might be suggestive of incipient psychological disorder. Due to his known behavior, the school counselor asked ahead of time that Christopher bring one or two of his favorite stuffed animals with him.

Christopher presented as a slender, yet healthy-looking child with fair skin, blue eyes, and blond hair, who sported a stuffed animal under each arm. He introduced one as his favorite, Winnie, a bear, and the other as Winnie's best friend, Tigger, a threadbare tiger. Christopher sat throughout the interview engaged primarily in play with his toys. However, when asked by the counselor, he shared adventures that he has had with Winnie, Tigger, and his other friends. Given the opportunities, he drew pictures of his imaginary Hundred Acre Wood and pleasantly chatted about his favorite, Winnie the Pooh, but made little eye contact with the counselor. When asked about his being at the school, Christopher said that "I like it well enough, but I miss my room at home." Christopher became particularly animated only when discussing his most recent adventure with his friends.

Goals for Counseling and Course of Therapy to Date. As a result of the initial meeting with the school counselor, it was recommended that Christopher be referred for a play assessment and the development of a plan for play therapy and other developmentally appropriate treatment with the school's psychological consultant, Dr. Gleewell,

a certified child counselor specializing in creative expression. Dr. Gleewell would use a variety of expressive materials, including a sandtray, puppets, arts and crafts, as well as metaphoric storytelling in order to determine any possible underlying psychological issues that might be contributing to Christopher's behavior; and to intervene with treatment. The primary goal of additional evaluation and treatment is to promote the client's ability to remain enrolled at and be successful at the Day School. Specific objectives will be determined.

Diagnostic Impressions

Axis I. 299.80 Asperger's Disorder

Axis II. 71.09 No Diagnosis on Axis II

Axis III. Early childhood respiratory and digestive problems

Axis IV. Educational problem—Problems adjusting to educational environment

Axis V. GAF = 53 (current)

GAF = 59 (highest prior to attending school)

DISCUSSION OF DIAGNOSTIC IMPRESSIONS

Christopher Robin was referred to the school guidance center because the school staff had become worried about his social isolation and inordinate preoccupation with his imaginary friends. According to reports by his teachers and parents, Christopher's primary engagement was with his Hundred Acre Wood stuffed animals. They described his focus on his animals as an almost all-encompassing preoccupation. In fact, when separated from his toys of interest, he had imaginary conversations with them, sat alone and drew pictures of them, and rocked. His teachers and parents also reported that outside of his interest in his toys, Christopher exhibited almost no interest in playing with or otherwise engaging his classmates, neighborhood children, or other peers;

and he made very little eye contact with them or with adults such as his teachers and housekeeper. In fact, he paid very little attention to others.

The Disorders Usually First Diagnosed in Infancy, Childhood, or Adolescence is a wide-reaching section of the *DSM-IV-TR* and is organized into many groupings of disorders that all share the feature of occurring early in the life cycle. Autistic Disorder and Asperger's Disorder both appear in the grouping titled "Pervasive Developmental Disorders." Increasingly, being able to identity, evaluate, diagnose, and provide treatment and support for students with these disorders are important clinical skills for counseling professionals who work with children, adolescents, young adults, and adults in school, college and university, and community settings (Adreon & Durocher, 2007; Van Bergeijk, Klin, & Volkmar, 2008).

In our imagined case, Christopher Robin presented impaired development in social interaction and restricted interests and activities. Although he preferred to be isolated, Christopher had no significant delay in language development. Similarly, no other developmental delays in cognition or other age-appropriate skills were noted outside of his lack of social interaction and lack of interest in the world around him. In such cases of restricted, stereotypical, consuming interests, and impaired social interactions in the absence of delays in language or other cognitive development, the diagnosis is Asperger's Disorder.

Regarding differential diagnoses, Autistic Disorder might be considered. Like all of the Pervasive Developmental Disorders, both Asperger's and Autistic Disorders are characterized by problems with social interactions. However, Autistic Disorder requires delay or impairment in early language development not found with Asperger's Disorder. Further, when making the diagnosis of Asperger's Disorder, Rett's Disorder and Childhood Disintegrative Disorder both must be ruled out; the essential feature of these two disorders is developmental deficits (Rett's Disorder) or regression in functioning (Childhood Disintegrative Disorder) following an early period of normal development. Both can be ruled out in Christopher's case.

To wrap up the diagnosis, Christopher's physical health problems are listed on Axis III, his school stress is emphasized on Axis IV, and on Axis V his functioning is represented by GAF scores ranging from the presence of moderate symptoms before beginning school, to the current, moderately serious symptoms affecting school and other functioning, which led to his referral. The information on these axes is consistent with the Axis I diagnosis describing Christopher's patterns of behavior.

CASE CONCEPTUALIZATION

When Christopher Robin came to counseling, first he participated in an evaluation session.

The intake counselor collected as much information as possible about the problematic situations in class and outside of class that led to Christopher's referral by his teachers, parents, and other adults at school. The counselor first used evaluation information to develop diagnostic impressions. Christopher's concerns were described by Asperger's Disorder. Next, the counselor developed a case conceptualization. Whereas the purpose of diagnostic impressions is to *describe* the client's concerns, the goal of case conceptualization is to better *understand* and clinically *explain* the person's experiences (Neukrug & Schwitzer, 2006). It helps the counselor understand the etiology leading to Christopher's presenting concerns and the factors maintaining these behaviors. In turn, case conceptualization sets the stage for treatment planning. Treatment planning then provides a road map that plots out how the counselor and client expect to move from presenting concerns to positive outcomes (Seligman, 1993, p. 157)—helping Christopher increase his abilities to socialize more appropriately and engage in "real-world" activities and interests.

When forming a case conceptualization, the clinician applies a purist counseling theory, an integration of two or more theories, an eclectic mix of theories, or a solution-focused combination of tactics, to his or her understanding of the client. In this case, Christopher's counselor based her conceptualization on a purist theory applicable to the behavioral needs of child clients, the Expressive Creative Arts Approach to play therapy and counseling with children. She selected this approach based on her knowledge of current outcome research and the best practice literature pertaining to child clients dealing with the Autism spectrum and especially communication problems like Asperger's Disorder (Gladding, 2005; Kazdin & Weisz, 2003; Mowder, Rubinson, & Yasik, 2009; Vernon & Clemente, 2005). The Expressive Creative Arts Approach is consistent with this counselor's professional therapeutic viewpoint about clinical work with child and early adolescent clients.

The counselor used the Inverted Pyramid Method of case conceptualization because this method is especially designed to help clinicians more easily form their conceptual pictures of their clients' needs (Neukrug & Schwitzer, 2006; Schwitzer, 1996, 1997). The method has four steps: Problem Identification, Thematic Groupings, Theoretical Inferences, and Narrowed Inferences. The counselor's clinical thinking can be seen in Figure 12.5.

Step 1: Problem Identification. The first step is Problem Identification. Aspects of the presenting problem (thoughts, feelings, behaviors, physiological features), additional areas of concern besides the presenting concern, family and developmental history, in-session observations, clinical inquiries (medical problems, medications, past counseling, substance use, suicidality), and psychological assessments (problem checklists, personality inventories, mental status exam, specific clinical measures) all may contribute information at Step 1. The counselor "casts a wide net" in order to build Step 1 as exhaustively as possible (Neukrug & Schwitzer, 2006, p. 202). As can be seen in Figure 12.5, the counselor thoroughly noted not just all of Christopher's verbal expressive concerns, social isolation, and aspects of his preoccupation with his imaginary animals, and so on—but also, as much important information as she could find regarding his developmental experiences and inner experience. She attempted to go beyond just listing the main behaviors causing the referral and to be as complete as she could.

Step 2: Thematic Groupings. The second step is Thematic Groupings. The clinician organizes all of the exhaustive client information found in Step 1 into just a few intuitive-logical clinical groups, categories, or themes, on the basis of sensible common denominators (Neukrug & Schwitzer, 2006). Four different ways of forming the Step 2 theme groups can be used: Descriptive-Diagnosis Approach, Clinical Targets Approach, Areas of Dysfunction Approach, and Intrapsychic Approach. As can be seen in the figure,

Christopher's counselor selected the Areas of Dysfunction Approach. This approach sorts together all of the Step 1 information into "areas of dysfunction according to important life situations, life themes, or life roles and skills" (Neukrug & Schwitzer, 2006, p. 205).

The counselor grouped together (a) his obstacles to verbal expression, social isolation, withdrawal, and so on, into the theme, "withdrawal, lack of engagement, lack of verbal communication" as well as (b) his preoccupied behaviors with his animal toys, focus on his imaginary friends' lives, separation symptoms, and so on, into the theme, "all-encompassing preoccupation with lives of stuffed animals." She evaluated these two areas to be related but separate themes. Her conceptual work at Step 2 gave the counselor a way to begin understanding and organizing Christopher's areas of functioning of concern more clearly and meaningfully.

So far, at Steps 1 and 2, the counselor has used her clinical assessment skills and her clinical judgment to begin meaningfully understanding Christopher's needs. Now, at Steps 3 and 4, she applies the theoretical approach she has selected. She begins making theoretical inferences to interpret and explain the processes or roots underlying Christopher's concerns as they are seen in Steps 1 and 2.

Step 3: Theoretical Inferences. At Step 3, concepts from the counselor's selected theory, Expressive Creative Arts Therapy, are applied to explain the aspects of Christopher's problematic behaviors. The counselor tentatively matches the theme groups in Step 2 with this theoretical approach. In other words, the symptom constellations in Step 2, which were distilled from the symptoms in Step 1, now are combined using theory to show what is believed to be the underlying etiology of Christopher's current needs (Neukrug & Schwitzer, 2006; Schwitzer, 2006, 2007).

The Expressive Creative Arts Therapy approach is based on the assumption that verbal approaches to engagement and relationship with some children is limited and ineffective, especially with children who—based on their developmental predispositions, earlier experiences, or other neurological and psychosocial factors—are reluctant to communicate through traditional verbal means (Gladding, 2005; Okun, 2007; Vernon & Clemente, 2005). According to the model, children with such difficulties verbally communicating have not yet developed sufficient skills and coping mechanisms, and therefore may benefit from art-oriented or other creative expression-oriented methods of engaging and sharing their needs and inner lives (Gladding, 1995, 2005; Lev-Wiesel & Daphna-Tekoha, 2000).

As can be seen in the figure, when the counselor applied these Expressive Creative Arts Therapy constructs, she made one theoretical inference at Step 3 to explain the issues identified in Step 1, leading to the themes at Step 2: Christopher has failed, so far, to develop abilities, skills, and mechanisms that facilitate verbal communication. This is presented in Figure 12.5.

Step 4: Narrowed Inferences. At Step 4, the clinician's selected theory continues to be used to address still-deeper issues when they exist (Schwitzer, 2006, 2007). At this step, "still-deeper, more encompassing, or more central, causal themes" are formed (Neukrug & Schwitzer, 2006, p. 207). Continuing to apply Creative Expressive Arts Therapy concepts at Step 4, Christopher's counselor presented a single, most-fundamental construct that she believed to be most explanatory Christopher's needs. This was a deeper inference that Christopher does have a rich, active inner language that he can learn to express to others with exposure to creative expressive methods. When all four steps are completed, the client information in Step 1 leads to logical-intuitive groupings on the basis of common denominators in Step 2, the groupings then are explained using theory at Step 3, and then, finally, at Step 4, further deeper explanations are made. From start to finish, the thoughts, feelings, behaviors,

and physiological features in the topmost portions are connected on down the pyramid into deepest dynamics.

The completed pyramid now is used to plan the treatment and techniques that will be employed in work with Christopher Robin as we have portrayed him in this case.

TREATMENT PLANNING

At this point, Christopher's clinician at the Hundred Acre Day School Counseling Center has collected all available information about the problems that have been of concern to his family and school. Based upon this information, the counselor developed a five-axis *DSM-IV-TR* diagnosis and then, using the "inverted pyramid" (Neukrug & Schwitzer, 2006; Schwitzer, 1996, 1997), formulated a working clinical *explanation* of Christopher's difficulties and their etiology that we called the *case conceptualization*. This, in turn, guides us to the next critical step in our clinical work, called the *treatment plan,* the primary purpose of which is to map out a logical and goal-oriented strategy for making positive changes in the client's life. In essence, the treatment plan is a road map "for reducing or eliminating disruptive symptoms that are impeding the client's ability to reach positive mental health outcomes" (Neukrug & Schwitzer, 2006, p. 225). As such, it is the cornerstone of our work with not only Christopher, but with all clients who present with disturbing and disruptive symptoms and patterns (Jongsma & Peterson, 2006; Jongsma, Peterson, & McInnis, 2003a, 2003b; Seligman, 1993, 1998, 2004).

A comprehensive treatment plan must integrate all of the information from the biopsychosocial interview, diagnosis, and case conceptualization into a coherent plan of action. This *plan* comprises four main components, which include (1) a behavioral definition of the problem(s), (2) the selection of achievable goals, (3) the determination of treatment modes, and (4) the documentation of how change will be measured. The *behavioral*

Figure 12.5   Christopher Robin's Inverted Pyramid Case Conceptualization Summary: Expressive Creative Arts Play Therapy

1. IDENTIFY AND LIST CLIENT CONCERNS

Born into high SES family
High-achieving parents
Child care by "caring but domineering" nanny
Nanny encouraged distractions through play
Physical ailments during early childhood
Prior to age 5-½ years, almost exclusive play at home with stuffed animals
Drew pictures, made costumes, etc., for animals
Fails to effectively communicate verbally

At age 5-½ years, kindergarten
Withdrawn, sits in corner, sucks thumb when separated from stuffed animals
Occasionally sit and rock without toys
Imaginary conversations
Social isolation from kindergarten forward
Withdrawn, reluctant to interact
Fails to play sports or games with father
Current social isolation at school & current low interest in play/peers
All-encompassing focus on stuffed animals
All-encompassing preoccupation with lives of imaginary friends
Anguish when separated from toys

2. ORGANIZE CONCERNS INTO LOGICAL THEMATIC GROUPINGS

1. Withdrawal, lack of engagement, lack of verbal communication
2. All-encompassing preoccupation with lives of stuffed animals

3. THEORETICAL INFERENCES: ATTACH THEMATIC GROUPINGS TO INFERRED AREAS OF DIFFICULTY

Expressive Creative Arts Therapy Inference
Christopher has failed, so far, to develop abilities, skills, and mechanisms that facilitate verbal communication

4. NARROWED INFERENCES: SUICIDALITY AND DEEPER DIFFICULTIES

Deeper Expressive Creative Arts Therapy Inference
Christopher does have a rich active inner language, which he can learn to express to others with exposure to creative expressive methods

definition of the problem(s) consolidates the results of the case conceptualization into a concise hierarchical list of problems and concerns that will be the focus of treatment. The *selection of achievable goals* refers to assessing and prioritizing the client's concerns into a *hierarchy of urgency* that also takes into account the client's motivation for change, level of dysfunction, and real-world influences on his or her problems. The *determination of treatment modes* refers to selection of the specific interventions, which are matched to the uniqueness of the client and to his or her goals and clearly tied to a particular theoretical orientation (Neukrug & Schwitzer, 2006). Finally, the clinician must establish how change will be measured, based upon a number of factors, including client records and self-report of change, in-session observations by the clinician, clinician ratings, results of standardized evaluations such as the Conners 3 (Conners, 2008) or a family functioning questionnaire, pre-post treatment comparisons, and reports by other treating professionals.

The four-step method discussed above can be seen in Figure 6.1 (p. 109) and is outlined below for the case of Christopher followed by his specific treatment plan.

Step 1: Behavioral Definition of Problems. The first step in treatment planning is to carefully review the case conceptualization, paying particular attention to the results of Step 2 (Thematic Groupings), Step 3 (Theoretical Inferences), and Step 4 (Narrowed Inferences). The identified clinical themes reflect the core areas of concern and distress for the client, while the theoretical and narrowed inferences offer clinical speculation as to their origins. In the case of Christopher, there are two primary areas of concern. The first, "withdrawal, lack of engagement and verbal communication," refers to isolative behavior at home and at school, reluctance to interact, failure to play sports and games with father, low interest in play with peers, and occasional sitting and rocking without toys. The second, "all encompassing preoccupation with the lives of his stuffed animals," refers to almost exclusive play at home and

conversations with stuffed animals, drawing pictures of and making costumes for stuffed animals, and all-encompassing focus on stuffed animals and their imaginary lives. These symptoms and stresses are consistent with the diagnosis of Asperger's Disorder (APA, 2000a; Hersen & Ammerman, 2000; Kundert & Trimarchi, 2006; Meyer, Mundy, van Hecke, & Durocher, 2006; Parritz & Troy, 2011).

Step 2: Identify and Articulate Goals for Change. The second step is the selection of achievable goals, which is based upon a number of factors including the most pressing or urgent behavioral, emotional, and interpersonal concerns and symptoms as identified by the client and clinician, the willingness and ability of the client to work on those particular goals, and the realistic (real-world) achievability of those goals (Neukrug & Schwitzer, 2006). At this stage of treatment planning, it is important to recognize that not all of the client's problems can be addressed at once, so we focus initially on those that cause the greatest distress and impairment. New goals can be created as old ones are achieved. In the case of Christopher, the goals are divided into two prominent areas. The first, "withdrawal, lack of engagement and verbal communication," requires that we help Christopher to strengthen his basic (external) expressive language skills and the ability to communicate simply with others, to increase the frequency of positive interactions with parents and peers, to strengthen the basic emotional bond with his parents, to engage in reciprocal and cooperative interactions with others on a regular basis, and to help his parents, teachers, and peers to develop a level of understanding and acceptance of Christopher's capabilities and to set realistic expectations for his behavior. The second, "solitary, repetitive, stereotypical, and purposeless behaviors and play," requires that we help Christopher to reduce the amount of time that he engages in play with stuffed animals, shape and reinforce play with other toys and materials, increase the frequency of play with parents and peers, and to attain the highest, most realistic level of overall functioning.

Step 3: Describe Therapeutic Interventions. This is perhaps the most critical step in the treatment planning process because the clinician must now integrate information from a number of sources, including the case conceptualization, the delineation of the client's problems and goals, and the treatment literature, paying particular attention to *empirically supported treatment* (EST) and *evidence-based practice* (EBP). In essence, the clinician must align his or her treatment approach with scientific evidence from the fields of counseling and psychotherapy. Wampold (2001) identifies two types of evidence-based counseling research: studies that demonstrate "absolute efficacy," that is, the fact that counseling and psychotherapy work, and those that demonstrate "relative efficacy," that is, the fact that certain theoretical/technical approaches work best for certain clients with particular problems (Psychoanalysis, Gestalt Therapy, Cognitive Behavior Therapy, Brief Solution-Focused Therapy, Cognitive Therapy, Dialectical Behavior Therapy, Person-Centered Therapy, Expressive/Creative Therapies, Interpersonal Therapy, and Feminist Therapy; and when delivered through specific treatment modalities (individual, group, and family counseling).

In the case of Christopher, we have decided to use an eclectic play-based/expressive-artistic intervention based upon child-centered and cognitive behavioral play therapy as well as Social Stories and Lego Therapy. It is important to note that "specific interventions proposed for clinical disturbances . . . have included individual psychotherapy for the child and/or caregiver, parent training with emphasis on developmental expectations and sensitive responsiveness, family therapy or caregiver/child dyadic therapy" (Zeanah & Boris, 2005, p. 365). Child-Centered Play Therapy (CCPT) is a humanistic and nondirective approach to child counseling that derives from the work of Carl Rogers (Rogers, 1951, 1961) and Virginia Axline (1947). It is based upon the premise that children have an inherent capacity for self-understanding, self-expression, positive relationships, and mental health, which can be nurtured and facilitated under the therapeutic conditions of attuned empathy congruence and unconditional positive regard. In the nonjudgmental and nonhurried playspace that provides the child access to toys, materials, and activities for the full expression of thoughts, feelings, and behaviors, he or she can work through conflicts, gain self-acceptance, and effective coping skills for living in the world (Landreth, 2002; Moustakas, 1959; Nordling, Cochran, & Cochran, 2010). It has been effectively applied to a wide range of child behavior and emotional problems, including the symptoms of Asperger's Disorder (Baggerly, Ray, & Bratton, 2010; VanFleet, Sywulak, Caporaso, Sniscak, & Guerney, 2010). Specific techniques that will be drawn from this approach will include utilizing unconditional positive regard, acceptance, attuned empathy, focused tracking, and selective limit-setting with Christopher as he engages with the different materials and activities in the playroom (arts-and-crafts, puppets, dollhouse, drawing, storytelling, role-playing).

Cognitive Behavior Play Therapy was originally devised as a means of applying the empirically proven methods of cognitive and behavior therapy to working with children, particularly in the playroom (Knell, 1993, 1994). This approach relies on a variety of cognitive techniques (reframing, challenging irrational thoughts, and cognitive restructuring) and behavioral techniques (reinforcement for and shaping of adaptive behavior, extinction of maladaptive behaviors, systematic desensitization, exposure with response prevention). However, the cognitive behavioral play therapist also uses artistic and expressive playroom materials, such as board games, puppets, dolls, drawings, storytelling, and the sandtray to achieve these ends. An example would be engaging a child through the use of puppets in a conversation about feelings and relating with others while verbalizing possible thoughts that impair social relatedness. This technique has been effectively applied to a variety of childhood emotional and behavioral problems, including symptoms of Asperger's Disorder (Drewes, 2009). Specific techniques drawn from this approach will include using puppets and role play in a group play format to address Christopher's social disinterest, shaping social behavior through sandtray miniature play, and creating cartoon strip stories around the themes of withdrawal and positive engagement.

More recently, creative techniques, that is, those that employ art, music, dance, drama, and play, have been used to enhance sensory integration, social skills, communication, and symbolic thinking. Social Stories (Gray & Garand, 1983) is one such methodology that relies upon the use of picture stories to teach social problem-solving skills and it has been found to be useful in working with children with Autism Spectrum Disorders (Kokina & Kern, 2010). Another play-based intervention that has been found to be both useful and effective with these children is Lego therapy (LeGoff, 2004), which uses Legos to teach social skills. Lego toys are naturally attractive and sensorily appealing, and as such can capture the attention of children with Autism Spectrum disorders for long periods. The play therapist works with children individually or in groups to build Lego-based social scenarios through which clients can interact. In Christopher's case, we will use elements of both Social Stories and Lego therapy to enhance his social and communication skills.

Finally, and in working directly with Christopher's parents, we will provide psycho-educational support so that they may understand the manifestations of Asperger's Disorder and refer them to an autism support group and encourage them to join the Autism Society of London to expand their knowledge and support.

Step 4: Provide Outcome Measures of Change. This last step in treatment planning requires that we specify how change will be measured and indicate the extent to which progress has been made toward realizing these goals (Neukrug & Schwitzer, 2006). The counselor has considerable flexibility in this phase and may choose from a number of objective domains (psychological tests and measures of self-esteem, depression, psychosis, interpersonal relationship, anxiety, etc.), quasi-objective measures (the *DSM-IV-TR's* Axis V GAF scale; pre-post clinician, client and psychiatric ratings), and subjective ratings (client self-report, clinician's in-session observations). In Christopher's case, we have implemented a number of these, including clinician- and parent-reported improvement in verbal communication, social interaction and creative/expressive play; teacher-reported increased frequency of decreased isolative play and increased interactive play; and clinician- and parent-reported improvement in verbal communication, social interaction, and creative/expressive play, with materials and objects in addition to stuffed animals.

The completed treatment plan is now developed through which the counselor, Christopher, and his parents and teachers will begin their shared work of improving his social communication skills, reducing the amount of time playing with his stuffed animals, increasing the amount of social play, and connecting his parents with Autism spectrum support. The treatment plan is described below and is summarized in Table 12.5.

TREATMENT PLAN

Client: Christopher Robin

Service Provider: Hundred Acre Day School Counseling Center

BEHAVIORAL DEFINITION OF PROBLEMS:

1. Withdrawal, lack of engagement and verbal communication—Isolative behavior at home and at school, reluctance to interact, failure to play sports and games with father, low interest in play with peers, and occasional sitting and rocking without toys

(Continued)

(Continued)

2. All-encompassing preoccupation with lives of stuffed animals—Almost exclusive play at home and conversations with stuffed animals, drawing pictures of and making costumes for stuffed animals, and all-encompassing focus on stuffed animals and their imaginary lives

GOALS FOR CHANGE:

1. Withdrawal, lack of engagement and verbal communication

- Strengthen basic expressive language skills
- Strengthen ability to communicate simply with others
- Strengthen the basic emotional bond with his parents
- Increase the frequency of positive interactions with parents and peers
- Engage in reciprocal and cooperative interactions with others on a regular basis
- Help his parents, teachers, and peers to develop a level of understanding and acceptance of capabilities and set realistic expectations for behavior

2. All-encompassing preoccupation with lives of stuffed animals

- Reduce the amount of time engaging in play with stuffed animals
- Shape and reinforce play with other toys and materials
- Increase the frequency of play with parents and peers
- Attain the highest, most realistic level of overall functioning

THERAPEUTIC INTERVENTIONS:

An ongoing course of eclectic play-based/expressive-artistic intervention targeting psychological and social/interpersonal deficiencies supplemented with psychoeducation and group support for parents and teachers

1. Targeting psychological factors (solitary play with stuffed animals)

- Using unconditional positive regard, acceptance, attuned empathy, focused tracking, and selective limit-setting in the therapeutic playroom with different materials and activities (arts-and-crafts, puppets, dollhouse, drawing, storytelling, role-playing)
- Use effective contingency management to decrease repetitive and preoccupied play with stuffed animals
- Extinguish repetitive stuffed-animal play by reinforcing engagement with a broader array of play materials and activities
- Use Social Stories in individual counseling to stimulate social interest
- Use Legos in group counseling to build social interest and interaction

2. Targeting social interactions and communication

- Using unconditional positive regard, acceptance, attuned empathy, focused tracking, and selective limit-setting in the therapeutic playroom with other children using different materials and activities (arts-and-crafts, puppets, dollhouse, drawing, storytelling, role-playing)
- Employ frequent use of praise and positive reinforcement to increase verbalizations and social communication
- Use a token economy at home and in the school to build interactive play and social communication skills

- Implement a response-shaping program to facilitate his communicative language and social interaction skills
- Use Social Stories in individual counseling to stimulate social interest
- Use Legos in group counseling to build social interest and interaction

3. Targeting parenting

- Referral to an Autism support group
- Encouragement to join the Autism Society of London to expand knowledge and support base
- Psychoeducational support

OUTCOME MEASURES OF CHANGE:

Decreased preoccupation with stuffed-animal play, increased play with other objects and materials, and increased social interaction as measured by:

- Clinician- and parent-reported improvement in verbal communication, social interaction, and creative/expressive play
- Teacher-reported increased frequency of decreased isolative play and increased interactive play
- Clinician-observed play with materials and objects in addition to stuffed animals

Table 12.5 Christopher Robin's Treatment Plan Summary: Expressive Creative Arts Play Therapy

Goals for Change	Therapeutic Interventions	Outcome Measures of Change
Withdrawal, lack of engagement and verbal communication Strengthen basic expressive language skills Strengthen ability to communicate simply with others Strengthen the basic emotional bond with his parents Increase the frequency of positive interactions with parents and peers Engage in reciprocal and cooperative interactions with others on a regular basis	*Targeting psychological factors (solitary play with stuffed animals)* Using unconditional positive regard, acceptance, attuned empathy, focused tracking, and selective limit-setting in the therapeutic playroom with different materials and activities (arts-and-crafts, puppets, dollhouse, drawing, storytelling, role-playing) Use effective contingency management to decrease repetitive and preoccupied play with stuffed animals Extinguish repetitive stuffed-animal play by reinforcing engagement with a broader array of play materials and activities Use Social Stories in individual counseling to stimulate social interest	Decreased preoccupation with stuffed-animal play, increased play with other objects and materials, and increased social interaction as measured by: Clinician- and parent-reported improvement in verbal communication, social interaction, and creative/expressive play Teacher-reported increased frequency of decreased isolative play and increased interactive play Clinician-observed play with materials and objects in addition to stuffed animals

(Continued)

Table 12.5 (Continued)

Goals for Change	Therapeutic Interventions	Outcome Measures of Change
Help his parents, teachers, and peers to develop a level of understanding and acceptance of capabilities and set realistic expectations for behavior All-encompassing preoccupation with lives of stuffed animals Reduce the amount of time engaging in play with stuffed animals Shape and reinforce play with other toys and materials Increase the frequency of play with parents and peers Attain the highest, most realistic level of overall functioning	Use Legos in group counseling to build social interest and interaction Targeting social interactions and communication Using unconditional positive regard, acceptance, attuned empathy, focused tracking, and selective limit-setting in the therapeutic playroom with different materials and activities (arts-and-crafts, puppets, dollhouse, drawing, storytelling, role-playing) Employ frequent use of praise and positive reinforcement to increase verbalizations and social communication Use a token economy at home and in the school to build interactive play and social communication skills Implement a response-shaping program to facilitate his communicative language and social interaction skills Use Social Stories in individual counseling to stimulate interest Use Legos in group counseling to build social interest and interaction Targeting parenting Referral to an Autism support group Encouragement to join the Autism Society to expand knowledge and support base Psychoeducational support	

FOLLOW-UP: DIAGNOSIS, CASE CONCEPTUALIZATION, AND TREATMENT PLANNING THEMES—CHAPTER SUMMARY

This chapter presented an intricate clinical caseload composed of: three adults, Annie Wilkes, Miss Celie, and Chief Bromden; an adolescent, Peter Parker; and a child, Christopher Robin. The caseload had a gender balance of two female clients and three males. Among the caseload's diversity were four American clients: Of these, Miss Celie is African American (and from a postreconstruction historical time context), Chief Bromden is a Native American (he is a Columbia

Indian), and both Annie Wilkes and Peter Parker are white. Finishing the group is Christopher Robin, an international client in London. Upper-middle, middle, working-class, and low-socioeconomic statuses were represented by this group of clients. We believe all of these clients identified themselves as heterosexual.

Among this chapter's clients, Miss Celie and Peter Parker were urged to attend counseling by family members, and Christopher was referred to outpatient counseling by his school counselor with his parents' support. By comparison, Chief Bromden entered mandated day treatment at the Oregon Bridge Center following his discharge from psychiatric hospitalization, and Annie Wilkes initially came to counseling at the Overlook Psychotherapy Center seeking professional consultation with a legal courtroom matter but was referred on to a psychiatric center for evaluation.

Among the concerns presented by our clients in the chapter's caseload, Annie Wilkes sought consultation for concerns characterized diagnostically as Bipolar Disorder with severe mood-congruent psychotic features as well as Antisocial Personality Disorder; Miss Celie presented the delayed onset of PTSD along with a background of Dysthymic Disorder; Chief Bromden brought with him a history of episodes of the paranoid type of Schizophrenia as well as Alcohol Abuse; Peter Parker was dealing with both a single episode of moderate Major Depressive Disorder, and Personality Change Due to a General Medical Condition (namely, Radioactive Spider Bite Syndrome); and the youngest client, Christopher Robin, presented Asperger's Disorder.

Looking at the counseling theories represented, the adults' counselors formed case conceptualizations and then treatment plans based on Cognitive Behavior Therapy and three psychotherapeutic integrations: Schema-Focused Cognitive Therapy with Feminist Therapy, Cognitive Behavior Therapy With Cognitive Remediation, and Cognitive Behavior Therapy With Reality Therapy. Christopher Robin's child counselor used a multidimensional mix of Expressive Creative Arts Play Therapy.

In their treatment plans, these clients' counselors expressed hopes that their clients would achieve such outcomes as compliance with counseling, stabilization of mood, and elimination of psychotic symptoms (Annie Wilkes); development of self-affirming attitudes and elimination of depressive and posttraumatic symptoms (Miss Celie); reduction of psychotic symptoms, resolving of racial oppression effects, alcohol abstinence, and adaptive functioning (Chief Bromden); resolution of guilt and grief, and management of medical condition consequences (Peter Parker); and decreased stuffed-animal preoccupation, increased play with other items, and increased social interactions (Christopher Robin).

STUDY QUESTIONS AND LEARNING ACTIVITIES

Based on your understanding of this chapter's cases, consider and respond to these Study Questions and Learning Activities:

1. This caseload is an intricate one.

   a. If you were assigned this group of clients, what would be your initial reactions to their individual characteristics and differences? Working with both adults and children? Their reasons for referral?

   b. What would you identify as your greatest strengths for assisting these five clients? Your areas of greatest need for growth?

2. In their Basic Case Summaries, this chapter's counselors focused on their clients' earlier developmental and family experiences, presenting concerns, assessment of current distress, and areas and life roles in which they were experiencing difficulties, client strengths, and hopes for change. There was an emphasis on Annie Wilkes's problematic parental and developmental history plus the patterns, severity, and consequences of her own symptoms over her lifetime; origins of Miss Celie's mood and trauma concerns in traumatic early family and childhood experiences, marital and adult experiences, and

influences of social and racial context; both the psychosocial and medical origins of Peter Parker's difficulties; and thoroughly understanding the patterns and severity of Christopher Robin's needs as well as important family dynamics.

a. Keeping in mind that the initial counseling meeting, screening session, or intake interview usually requires the counselor to balance rapport and trust-building, on one hand, and assessment and information-gathering, on the other hand, what would you identify as your greatest strengths when engaging these five clients in the counseling process, and gathering the clinical information needed to conceptualize and plan for their counseling process? Your areas of greatest need for growth?

b. Looking at the five Basic Case Summaries, how does this type of clinical writing differ from your everyday thinking and conversation about people? What are your levels of comfort, skill, and experience with this type of professional writing? What steps can you take to further develop or improve these skills?

c. What suggestions would you have for one of more of the counselors in this chapter regarding missing, overlooked, or underemphasized—or overemphasized—information gathered and reported in the Basic Case Summaries? What would you like to have known more about? What methods could be used—clinical interview questions, observations, psychological measures, or other means—to find the additional information you would seek?

3. This chapter illustrated *DSM-IV-TR* diagnoses found in the following sections: Disorders Usually First Diagnosed in Infancy, Childhood, or Adolescence; Mental Disorders Due to a General Medical Condition; Substance-Related Disorders; Schizophrenia and Other Psychotic Disorders; Mood Disorders; Anxiety Disorders; and Personality Disorders—plus Other Conditions That May Be a Focus of Clinical Attention.

a. How familiar are you with these sections of the *DSM-IV-TR?* What is your comfort level using the *DSM-IV-TR* to explore these sets of concerns? Which of these groups of

disorders are likely to be most important to you in the practicum, internship, residency, or professional practice settings in which you hope to work?

b. What are your attitudes, reactions, or thoughts concerning diagnosis of childhood disorders? Concerning the diagnosis of behavioral consequences of problematic substance use? Concerning diagnosing lifelong patterns characterized as personality disorders? How can you further explore or develop your professional attitudes about diagnosis of these types of concerns?

c. What will be your next steps in gaining greater comfort and skills at diagnosis of the pervasive developmental disorders of childhood? Mental disorders due to medical problems? Alcohol use disorders? Schizophrenia? The depressive and bipolar mood disorders? Anxiety Disorders? Personality disorders?

d. What are your attitudes, reactions, or thoughts concerning use of Axis IV to record psychosocial and environmental stressors (such as Miss Celie's history of physical and sexual abuse) and Axis V to record general medical problems (such as Peter Parker's spider bite)? What will be your next steps in gaining greater comfort and skills with these axes?

e. Among this group of clients, Axis V Global Assessment of Functioning (GAF) scores ranged from 40 (Annie Wilkes's impairment) to 61 (Chief Bromden's present-day mild symptoms). What are your attitudes, reactions, or thoughts concerning use of Axis V GAF scores to estimate the client's overall level of functioning? Do you agree with the counselors' estimates found in this chapter? What will be your next steps in gaining greater comfort and skills estimating Axis V GAF scores?

4. This chapter's cases included two examples of case conceptualization and treatment planning using purist counselor theories (one adult approach and one child play-therapy model) and three examples of psychotherapeutic integration.

a. What is your level of familiarity with the various adult, and one play-therapy, counseling theories illustrated in this chapter:

Cognitive Behavior Therapy and Schema-Focused Cognitive Therapy? Feminist Therapy? Reality Therapy? Cognitive Remediation? For children, Expressive Creative Arts Play Therapy? What do you believe are their relative strengths and weaknesses? For which individuals do they seem to be a good match? For what types of client concerns do they seem to be potentially effective? What do the evidence and discussions found in the current literature say about this?

b. Which of these theories seem to be a good fit with your own attitudes and skills? Which interest you the most?

c. To learn more, review the resources and references cited in the chapter, interview a practicing counselor who uses these theories in his or her everyday work, seek clinical supervision from a supervisor experienced with the approach, enroll in a special topics class, or look for continuing education workshops and conference presentations covering these approaches.

d. What are your thoughts, reactions, and comfort level integrating multiple psychotherapeutic approaches to address the needs of your clients? Which theories are you most likely, or least likely, to consider integrating into your approach? How will you decide when, with whom, and in what ways, to integrate multiple approaches? To consider and learn more about integrating approaches such as Schema-Focused Cognitive Behavior Therapy with Feminist Therapy, Cognitive Behavior Therapy With Reality Therapy, or Cognitive Behavior Therapy with Cognitive Remediation, interview a practicing counselor who uses an integration of these theories in his or her everyday work, seek clinical supervision from a supervisor experienced with psychotherapeutic integration of these theories, or seek other professional consultations and learning opportunities.

5. The case conceptualizations found in this chapter began with casting a wide net for client concerns and dynamics, next formed intuitive-logical groupings to begin better understanding the clients' presentations, and then applied counseling theories to make clinical inferences about the clients' situations.

a. How does this type of professional clinical thinking differ from your everyday thinking, conversation, and analysis about people? What are your levels of comfort, skill, and experience with this type of clinical thinking? What steps can you take to further develop or improve your conceptualizing skills?

b. What are your thoughts, reactions, and critique of the ways these counselors grouped together: Annie Wilkes's dealing with routine Bipolar Disorder effects, dealing with psychotic Bipolar Disorder effects, and dealing with learned experiences from a traumatic background? Miss Celie's patterns of anxiety and posttraumatic symptoms, and almost lifelong depressive symptoms? Chief Bromden's Schizophrenia with family and cultural contextual influences, and Alcohol Abuse with negative consequences? Peter Parker's symptoms of depression due to guilt; and risky, erratic behavioral choices? Christopher Robin's withdrawal, and stuffed-animal preoccupation? Do you agree with each of these thematic groupings? How might you have organized these differently, more usefully, or more effectively?

c. What are your thoughts and reactions pertaining to the ways the counselors applied the various theoretical approaches in order to explain, make inferences about, and prepare for treatment planning with these clients? What were your reactions to the counselors' presentations of: Annie Wilkes's cognitive distortions and faulty core beliefs (Cognitive Behavior Therapy)? Miss Celie's distorted core beliefs and fundamental faulty family schema (Schema-Focused Cognitive Therapy) and enduring severely negative gender-role and race-related experiences (Feminist Therapy)? Chief Bromden's need to learn behavioral practices to cope with biologically based symptoms (Cognitive Behavior Therapy) and need to improve neurocognitive deficits (Cognitive Remediation Therapy)? Peter Parker's irrational and faulty beliefs (Cognitive Behavior Therapy) and poor need-satisfying choices (Reality Therapy)? Christopher Robin's failure to as yet develop expressions of his rich inner language (Expressive Creative Arts Play Therapy)? Do you agree with the ways the counselors used the various theories with these clients? How might you have applied the theories differently, more usefully, or more effectively?

6. A fully developed treatment plan was presented for each of the individuals comprising this chapter's caseload. The treatment plans provide goals for change, interventions, and outcome measures.

   a. How does this type of clinical writing, thinking, and preparation for the professional counseling process differ from your everyday approach to engaging in helpful relationships with people? What are your levels of comfort, skill, and experience with this type of professional writing, thinking, and preparation? What steps can you take to further develop or improve your treatment planning skills for the types of practicum, internship, residency, or work settings that are of most interest to you?

   b. This chapter's treatment plans first list goals for change for each "client" character, next apply the selected counseling theory to clearly state the interventions and approaches to be used, and finally identify ways to measure the expected changes. What are your thoughts, reactions, and critique of the ways this chapter's counselors prepared Annie Wilkes's, Miss Celie's, Chief Bromden's, Peter Parker's, and Christopher Robin's treatment plans? What interests you most about these plans? What raises questions for you?

   c. What are your thoughts and reactions pertaining to: the cognitive behavioral techniques (Annie Wilkes), schema-focused cognitive and feminist therapeutic approaches

(Miss Celie), cognitive behavioral and cognitive remediation activities (Chief Bromden), Cognitive Behavior and Reality Therapy methods (Peter Parker), and Expressive Creative Arts Play Therapy game-plan outlined as interventions? With which are you most familiar? Least familiar? Unfamiliar? Which will you select to learn more about through further reading, clinical supervision, or other professional development? Alternatively, which do not seem to be close fits with your own preferred approach?

   d. These clients' counselors used counselor observation, client report, change scores on psychological measures and the GAF, behavioral reports, and other means to measure outcomes. As you review the outcome measures found on Annie's, Celie's, Chief's, Peter's, and Christopher's treatment plans, consider these questions: Do the measures seem realistic and accomplishable? Are they concrete and specific enough to indicate change? Are they sensitive to the needs of the client? Which of these measures will become a regular part of your own repertoire, which might you decline to use, and what additional measures might you add to your own list? What new skills and competencies might you need to develop in order to effectively report on your own clients' outcomes?

7. Now, working independently, with a partner, or in a small group, select your own "client" from among the pop culture world of Characters in Literature and Comics. Develop your own narrative about the client's arrival at counseling. Then, prepare a fully completed Basic Case Summary, Diagnostic Impressions, Case Conceptualization, and Treatment Plan!

PART IV

EPILOGUE AND MEDIA RESOURCES

13

EPILOGUE

FINAL CONSIDERATIONS ABOUT OUR POPULAR CULTURE CASELOAD

The purpose of this textbook was to provide extensive and detailed coverage of three critical professional counseling skills: mental health diagnosis, case conceptualization, and treatment planning. The content of the text emphasized the interconnections between these three skills and highlighted how they are used together, in an integrated fashion, in everyday practice. We believe the approaches we used in the book are equally valid and can be equally valuable for all types of practitioners across the multiple disciplines providing services for clients in today's world of professional counseling and mental health care.

As you are well aware by now, we used popular culture to augment the text's content and to make the learning more lively, vivid, and well illustrated. We hope you have enjoyed our use of popular culture and found it to be a good way to increase learning. We also recognize that you might have a few questions about some of our character choices, client portrayals, and popular culture case scenarios. Therefore, in our Epilogue, we offer several caveats and disclaimers to help you understand how we developed the cases.

Choosing and Portraying Our Popular Culture Clients

One question that might be raised has to do with how and why we chose the characters we did from among the unlimited world of popular culture. Why did Claire appear in our book rather than any of the other *Breakfast Club* characters? Why did Elphaba join our caseload rather than another *Wizard of Oz* character? We certainly are aware of many, many alternative characters who would have made interesting and instructive clients. For instance, in his book *Reel Psychiatry: Movie Portrayals of Psychiatric Conditions,* Robinson (2003) provided an exhaustive description of hundreds of movie characters presenting diagnosable mental disorders. Similarly, other educators have focused on very contemporary characters we did not include here; for example, Fisher (2010) has analyzed the use of hip-hop lyrics, and characters and themes from *The Boondocks* cartoon appearing on The Cartoon Network's Adult Swim. In our case, we selected the various characters we did in order to build a caseload of 30 clients from a wide collection of media who could represent all of the classes of diagnosable psychological disorders, plus other conditions that can be a focus of counseling, found in the *Diagnostic and Statistical Manual of Mental Disorders, Fourth Edition, Text Revision..* In order to offer the most guidance for students and trainees, and their faculty and clinical supervisors, we needed to portray the full range of today's client presentations. We also tried to include characters with whom most of our readers would be at least somewhat familiar. If you did not find your favorite characters, populations, or media represented, we hope you will go on to develop your own cases based on your own clinical thinking!

Undoubtedly, readers noticed, too, that some of our clients were portrayed in surprising ways. Here again, keep in mind that our task was to devise a 30-client caseload that could reflect the extremely wide array of client presentations, etiologies, sustaining factors, and psychological and interpersonal experiences clinicians may see in professional practice. To accomplish this task, we needed to creatively construct (or reconstruct) some of our clients' life experiences. In our view, Edward Cullen, Jamal, Juno, Claire, Cleveland Brown, Smithers, Jack Bauer, sitcom character George Lopez, Chief Bromden, and Peter Parker all appear very close to their popular culture media portrayals—for these individuals, we only constructed the presenting concerns and needs that led them to become clients. However, to make the clinical points we intended, we needed to more heavily develop the hypothetical background experiences, stresses, or life challenges faced by Gretel, Naruto, Elphaba, Sophia, Jack McFarland, Fred the Baker, Maria, the Geico Caveman, Annie Wilkes, and Miss Celie—although we did this while preserving their traditional media portrayals.

Further, in order to transform some of our characters into useful client examples, we began with basic portrayals, but then reconstructed or reinvented them; these character-to-client transformations occurred most notably with: Miss Piggy (who was never portrayed on television as growing up in New Orleans' French Quarter), Mario (who never before has been presented with substance and personality disorders), Snoopy (who became a human boy with canine Snoopy's basic patterns), Jessie (who become a human girl with *Toy Story* Jessie's basic patterns), Belle (whom we reinvented as an international client in a European nation), Billie Jean (in which case we used Michael Jackson's portrayal as a starting place for inventing a fuller life history), Eleanor Rigby (for whom we used The Beatles' portrayal as a starting place for inventing a fuller life history), and Christopher Robin (whose basic patterns we exaggerated to create our case example).

Naturally, even for characters who did not undergo significant transformation, there can be discussion and debate about the diagnosis, dynamics, or needs we presented. For example, in our book, we prepared Annie Wilkes's presentation to fit the diagnoses of Bipolar Disorder and Antisocial Personality Disorder. By comparison, in his work, Shannon (2011) has made the case that Annie Wilkes might more likely be experiencing Borderline Personality Disorder. Once again, our creative constructions of some characters' lives, and transformations of others, allowed us to provide all of the examples and illustrations we needed for this book. Where you have other ideas about your favorite characters, we hope you will reanalyze based on your own clinical thinking!

Selecting and Presenting Therapeutic Approaches

As with choosing the characters, in this text we attempted to select and present a very wide range of counseling approaches—specifically, we aimed to provide illustrations using most of the main theories addressed in counseling and psychotherapy education and training today, offer demonstrations of the many ways in which the theories are often psychotherapeutically integrated in contemporary practice, and give examples of solution-focused and eclectic methods. We tried to be very careful to let readers know the basis for the selection of the therapeutic approach in each of our cases.

As we discussed in the text, most clinicians rely on a combination of evidence-based and best practice information, together with their own clinical expertise, to decide on treatment.

For nearly all of our cases, we provide widely accepted references and resources supporting the evidence-based selection of treatment. In a few cases, however, we mostly relied on the (fictional) counselor's clinical expertise. Primarily these included the cases of: Juno, Smithers, and Fred the Baker (all using person-centered counseling), Claire (applying a contemporary psychodynamic model), Tinkerbell and Billie Jean (for both of whom solution-focused counseling was selected), and Belle (employing Cognitive Behavior Therapy). Still other cases offered a balanced blend of evidence-based practice choices and decisions informed by clinical expertise; primarily these were: Jack McFarland, Eleanor Rigby, and Miss Celie. Jongsma and Peterson (2006) used a similar approach in which they clearly indicated which of the treatments they suggested were based on the available evidence (using an asterisk), and which of the treatments they suggested were best practices selected on the basis of clinical expertise. Since you may have ideas of your own, we believe reconsidering some of the approaches we used to form the case conceptualizations and treatment plans would be another effective use of your clinical thinking!

NEXT STEPS

Becoming competent with diagnosis, case conceptualization, and treatment planning is a critical part of the transition from natural helper to counseling professional. Hopefully, learning through use of this textbook has been an excellent start. As a next step, we suggest you study a wide range of original texts dealing with many different specific theoretical models and therapeutic approaches. It will come as no surprise that we next recommend "practice, practice, practice"! More specifically, when it is not feasible or ethically advisable to practice your clinical thinking skills with actual clients, we recommend forming cases based on popular culture—just as we did in this book—to continue your skill development. You can use pop culture clients to "practice" with individuals from populations to whom you do not have access, or those with presenting concerns and needs you do not have an immediate chance to see in real settings. Of course, this is just the bridge to true practice with real-life clients; we believe you will need to evaluate and apply your skills to real-life cases in classroom settings, practicum and internship sites, licensure and residence experiences, and ongoing workshops and professional development programs throughout your career—appropriately using faculty, clinical supervisors, and consultation with other professionals to support your ability to be effective with clients and challenge your continued growth. We hope, in the words of *Star Trek*'s Captain Jean-Luc Picard, that you will make it so!

14

GETTING TO KNOW THE CLIENTS THROUGH INTERNET SOURCES, PUBLISHED LITERATURE, AND FILM

GETTING TO KNOW OUR THIRTY CLIENTS

The clinical cases that we explored in this book were taken from the fictional world of popular culture. However, even the most unusual and seemingly extreme portrayals of fictional characters often are drawn from or based on, at one level or another, the stories of real-life people. It was our hope that by bringing some of these already-familiar characters to life for you in a clinical context, we could create a learning experience that would be intellectually rigorous, but also engaging and enjoyable.

In the body of the book, we provided you with a wealth of clinical information with which to develop and strengthen your diagnostic, case conceptualization, and treatment planning skills. In this appendix, we offer additional resources through which you can deepen your understanding of the fascinating characters we have presented. They are organized according to the chapters of the book in which they appear, under their respective headings.

CHAPTER 7: CHILDREN'S CHARACTERS AND VIDEO GAME CHARACTERS

Case 7.1 Miss Piggy

Internet Sources

> http://en.wikipedia.org/wiki/Miss_Piggy
>
> http://muppet.wikia.com/wiki/Miss_Piggy

Video Clips

> http://www.youtube.com/watch?v=hCNKgg RYW2I Miss Piggy on *The View*
>
> http://www.youtube.com/watch?v=Beuek MbXCIw Miss Piggy and Kermit
>
> http://www.youtube.com/watch?v=b7HYY KEbfLk Miss Piggy singing "I Will Survive"
>
> http://www.spike.com/video/miss-piggy-pizza-hut/2691925 Miss Piggy dishes it for Pizza Hut
>
> http://www.youtube.com/watch?v=XhbF5u9y MkU Miss Piggy meets Joan Rivers

Film

Henson, J., Lazer, D., Grade, L., & Starger, M. (Producers), & Frawley, J. (Director). (1979). *The Muppet movie* [Motion Picture]. Argentina: Henson Associates.

Case 7.2 Mario Alito

Internet Sources

http://en.wikipedia.org/wiki/Mario

http://mario.nintendo.com

http://en.wikipedia.org/wiki/List_of_Mario_games_by_year

Video Clips

http://www.youtube.com/watch?v=82TSWzOsPYc Mario hard at work

http://www.youtube.com/watch?v=iO10_IbDUBU Mario, the intergalactic star

Case 7.3 Gretel

Internet Source

http://en.wikipedia.org/wiki/Hansel_and_Gretel

Video Clips

http://www.youtube.com/watch?v=KxkIGXVwZTM Hansel and Gretel

http://www.youtube.com/watch?v=n7ZMFLyZ4BU Mickey and Minnie as Hansel and Gretel

http://www.youtube.com/watch?v=wqfOb8Yrqr0 Hansel and Gretel

Case 7.4 Naruto

Internet Sources

http://naruto.viz.com

http://en.wikipedia.org/wiki/Naruto

http://www.cartoonnetwork.com/tv_shows/naruto

Video Clips

http://www.hulu.com/watch/35645/naruto-enter-naruto-uzumaki#s-p12-n1-so-i0 Naruto's origin story

http://www.hulu.com/watch/35628/naruto-sasuke-and-sakura-friends-or-foes#s-p11-n1-so-i0 Naruto and friends

http://www.hulu.com/watch/35657/naruto-the-land-where-a-hero-once-lived#s-p10-n1-so-i0 A hero's journey

http://www.hulu.com/watch/60872/naruto-the-closed-door#s-p11-so-i0 The Closed Door

Case 7.5 Snoopy

Internet Source

http://en.wikipedia.org/wiki/Snoopy

Video Clips

http://www.youtube.com/watch?v=gKxXAwBRuVo Snoopy in a bad mood

http://www.youtube.com/watch?v=rNremK0cBEg Snoopy vs. the Red Barron

http://www.youtube.com/watch?v=hUQX2B67KL4 Snoopy loves dancing

http://www.youtube.com/watch?v=pq9hBEvFNlM Snoopy kisses Lucy

http://www.youtube.com/watch?v=iyIxW-ouwAg Snoopy and Charlie Brown

CHAPTER 8: TROUBLED YOUTH IN FILM AND ON STAGE

Case 8.1 Edward Cullen

Internet Sources

http://thecullensliveforever.webs.com/edwardsbio.htm

http://www.examiner.com/x-4908-Twilight-Examiner~y2009m4d2-Twilight-series-spawns-religion-Edward-Cullen-is-real-members-should-read-the-books-like-a-Bible

http://www.imdb.com/character/ch0058224/bio

http://www.robertpattinsonsite.com/twilight-movie.php

Video Clips

http://www.youtube.com/watch?v=bfYtIQG-xNQ Edward saves Bella and first reveals himself

http://www.youtube.com/watch?v=6VUUdy 7Eh18 Edward turned into a vampire

http://www.youtube.com/watch?v=Vc1UqeHhjeo Edward and Bella first conversation

Film

Godfrey, W. (Producer), & Hardwicke, K. (Director). (2008). *Twilight* [Motion Picture]. United States: Summit Entertainment.

Slade, D. (Director). (2010). *Eclipse* [Motion Picture]. United States: Summitt Entertainment.

Weitz, C. (Director). (2009). *New moon* [Motion Picture]. United States: Summitt Entertainment.

Literature

Meyer, S. (2008). *The Twilight saga collection.* New York, NY: Little, Brown Young Readers.

Case 8.2 Jamal Malik

Internet Sources

http://www.imdb.com/title/tt1010048/

http://en.wikipedia.org/wiki/Slumdog_millionaire

Video Clips

http://www.youtube.com/watch?v=Ak70A EHw1as Malik on *Who Wants To be a Millionaire*

http://www.youtube.com/watch?v=AIzbwV7on6Q Movie trailer

http://www.youtube.com/watch?v=__HQGvSqZ5I Growing up on the streets

Literature

Swarup, V. (2008). *Slumdog millionaire.* Canada: HarperCollins.

Film

Boyle, D., & Tandan, L. (Directors). (2008). *Slumdog millionaire* [Motion Picture]. United States: Caleador films.

Case 8.3 Juno MacGuff

Internet Sources

http://en.wikipedia.org/wiki/Juno_%28film%29

http://www.foxsearchlight.com/juno

Video Clips

http://www.fancast.com/movies/Juno/139277/ 715137535/Pregnancy-Test/videos Pregnancy test

http://www.fancast.com/movies/Juno/139277/ 607007915/-Juno-%3A-Discussing-Pregnancy/ videos Discussing adoption with her stepfather

http://www.fancast.com/movies/Juno/139277/ 607007527/-Juno-%3A-Hallway-Confrontation/ videos Hallway confrontation with Bleeker

Film

Reitman, J. (Director). (2007). *Juno* [Motion Picture]. United States: Fox Searchlight Pictures.

Case 8.4 Claire Standish

Internet Source

http://en.wikipedia.org/wiki/Breakfast_Club

Video Clips

http://www.youtube.com/watch?v=dkX8J-FKndE Movie trailer

http://www.youtube.com/watch?v=mgdUBSD wL9g Claire steps out of her comfort zone

http://www.youtube.com/watch?v=jsZkkqLDFmg videos Bender (the criminal) mocks Claire

Film

Hughes, J. (Director). (1985). *The breakfast club* [Motion Picture]. United States: A & M Films.

Case 8.5 Elphaba Thropp

Internet Sources

http://en.wikipedia.org/wiki/Wicked:_The_Life_ and_Times_of_the_Wicked_Witch_of_the_West

http://en.wikipedia.org/wiki/Wicked_(musical)

http://en.wikipedia.org/wiki/Elphaba_Thropp#Characteristics

Video Clips

http://www.youtube.com/watch?v=7P4QvtyZhoo Introduction to musical

http://www.youtube.com/watch?v=F4PCKL2vvhs&feature=PlayList&p=DF92D0BF970495A4&index=15 Elphaba

http://www.youtube.com/watch?v=3A2Q47Y8XHM&feature=PlayList&p=DF92D0BF970495A4&index=13 *Wicked* discussed on the View

Literature

Baum, L. F. (1900). *The wonderful wizard of oz.* Chicago, IL: George M. Hill Company.

Maguire, G. (2007). *Wicked: The life and times of the Wicked Witch of the West.* New York, NY: Harper.

Maguire, G. (2008). *Son of a witch: Volume two in the wicked years.* New York, NY: Harper.

Maguire, G. (2009). *A lion among men: Volume three in the wicked years.* New York, NY: Harper.

CHAPTER 9: ANIMATED CHARACTERS

Case 9.1 Cleveland Brown

Internet Sources

http://en.wikipedia.org/wiki/The_Cleveland_Show

http://www.fox.com/cleveland

Video Clips

http://www.youtube.com/watch?v=sT-sNBKpDEo *The Cleveland Show* trailer

http://www.youtube.com/watch?v=HHXZ-UMLY60 Welcome to Stoolbend

http://www.imdb.com/title/tt1195935/video gallery/content_type-Full%20Episode This link provides access to full episodes of *The Cleveland Show*

Case 9.2 Jessie

Internet Sources

http://en.wikipedia.org/wiki/Toy_Story_2

http://en.wikipedia.org/wiki/Jessie_(Toy_Story)

http://pixar.wikia.com/Jessie

Video Clip

http://www.youtube.com/watch?v=px0j1EHF8Y0 Jessie tells the story of her abandonment

Film

Plotkin, H., & Jackson, K. R. (Producers), & Lasseter, J. (Directors). (1999). *Toy story 2* [Motion Picture]. United States: Pixar Animation Studios.

Unkrich, L. (Director). (2010). *Toy story 3* [Motion Picture]. United States: Pixar Animation and Walt Disney Studios.

Case 9.3 Tinkerbell

Internet Sources

http://members.tripod.com/~tinkerbell_14/tinker bell.html

http://disney.go.com/fairies/#/characters/tinkerbell?int_cmp=fai_fran_tink_charaport_thumb_Intl

http://en.wikipedia.org/wiki/Tinkerbell

Video Clips

http://www.youtube.com/watch?v=A4XuWT7n-aw&feature=related Internal struggle with various emotions

http://www.youtube.com/watch?v=Y3k8nto5SgI&feature=related Shows her jealous nature

http://www.youtube.com/watch?v=WtEv3ktX30I&feature=related Her creative, mischievous side

Literature

Barrie, J. M. (1911). *Peter and Wendy.* New York, NY: Scribner.

Film

Geronimi, C., & Jackson, W. (Directors). (1953). *Peter Pan* [Motion Picture]. United States: RKO Radio Pictures.

Hogan, P. J. (Director). (2003). *Peter Pan.* [Motion Picture]. United States: Universal Pictures.

Case 9.4 Waylon Smithers

Internet Sources

http://en.wikipedia.org/wiki/Waylon_Smithers

http://www.thesimpsons.com/#/characters

http://simpsons.wikia.com/wiki/Waylon_Smithers

Video Clips

http://www.youtube.com/watch?v=QW6DTVK4aCk Smithers loves Mr. Burns

http://www.dailymotion.com/video/x7mjqk_the-simpsons-homers-brain_shortfilms Smithers and Burns perform brain surgery

http://www.dailymotion.com/video/x7mjf0_the-simpsons-homer-gets-hired_shortfilms Smithers and Burns hire Homer

Case 9.5 Belle Beastly

Video Clips

http://www.youtube.com/watch?v=DGSqt2fD4Xo Movie trailer

http://www.youtube.com/watch?v=oeoPtz0F2Ck Getting ready for Belle

http://www.youtube.com/watch?v=RaVZB6mdJtY&feature=related Belle's provincial life

Film

Trousdale, G., & Wise, K. (Directors). (1991). *Beauty and the beast* [Motion Picture]. United States: Walt Disney Pictures.

CHAPTER 10: ADULTS IN TELEVISION SITCOMS AND DRAMAS

Case 10.1 Jack Bauer

Internet Sources

http://24.wikia.com/wiki/Jack_Bauer

http://en.wikipedia.org/wiki/Jack_bauer

http://www.imdb.com/character/ch0009881/bio

http://www.tv.com/24/show/3866/summary.html

Video Clips

http://www.hulu.com/watch/994/24-kim-tells-jack-about-chase Kim Bauer tells her father about her boyfriend, Chase

http://www.youtube.com/watch?v=5CJ8OIDIrj0 A day in the life of Jack Bauer

http://www.youtube.com/watch?v=kBzwPvaBYWE Jack at work

Case 10.2 Sophia Petrillo

Internet Sources

http://en.wikipedia.org/wiki/Golden_Girls

http://en.wikipedia.org/wiki/Sophia_Petrillo

Video Clips

http://www.youtube.com/watch?v=GpalAkrZa4Q A day in the life of Sophia

http://www.youtube.com/watch?v=a4XJszcVt5Q Sophia wants to enter the convent

http://www.youtube.com/watch?v=FXLcSRoGB38 Sophia stands up

Case 10.3 George Lopez

Internet Source

http://en.wikipedia.org/wiki/George_Lopez_Show

Video Clips

http://www.youtube.com/watch?v=g30LQBLIbZ8 George drives the Batmobile http://www.youtube.com/watch?v=NjMom_EaQJ0 Trick or treat me right

http://www.youtube.com/watch?v=Nkf48tD3teM George and father-in-law, Vic

Case 10.4 Lieutenant Commander Data

Internet Sources

http://en.wikipedia.org/wiki/Data_%28Star_Trek%29

http://en.wikipedia.org/wiki/Star_Trek_The_Next_Generation

Video Clips

http://www.youtube.com/watch?v=DLIU5tC3LAs Data feels laughter

http://www.youtube.com/watch?v=XeyplUvxztE A tribute to Data

http://www.youtube.com/watch?v=GYp2dx652ho Is Datas human?

Film

Carson, D. (Director). (1994). *Star trek: Generations* [Motion Picture]. United States: Paramount Pictures.

Frakes, J. (Director). (1996). *Star trek: First contact* [Motion Picture]. United States: Paramount Pictures.

Case 10.5 Jack McFarland

Internet Sources

http://en.wikipedia.org/wiki/Will_and_grace

http://en.wikipedia.org/wiki/Jack_McFarland

Video Clips

http://www.youtube.com/watch?v=mARNVXhVy3U Nurse jack

http://www.youtube.com/watch?v=U0jV5XU-jrI Jack, the tap dancing fool

http://www.youtube.com/watch?v=ESsovl8ow00 Will asks Jack for advice

http://www.youtube.com/watch?v=5IiTyiWZggM Will meets Jack

CHAPTER 11: CHARACTERS IN MUSIC, MUSICALS, AND ADVERTISING

Case 11.1 Fred the Baker

Internet Sources

http://edition.cnn.com/2005/SHOWBIZ/TV/12/28/obit.vale/index.html

http://en.wikipedia.org/wiki/Dunkin_Donuts

http://en.wikipedia.org/wiki/Fred_the_baker

Video Clips

http://www.youtube.com/watch?v=83mJQXiG8Bw A Dunkin' Donuts Christmas

http://www.youtube.com/watch?v=gwfrBbNo5Jg Time to make the donuts

http://www.youtube.com/watch?v=5_mfiw_lD9s&p=028D0C49D86F0BAB&playnext=1&index=48 Fun in the kitchen with Fred

Case 11.2 Maria

Internet Sources

http://www.westsidestory.com/

http://en.wikipedia.org/wiki/West_side_story

Video Clips

http://www.youtube.com/watch?v=4oxfOncYiag *A Boy Like That*

http://www.youtube.com/watch?v=5_QffCZs-bg *Tonight*

http://www.youtube.com/watch?v=Ye7PIyIcCro *I Feel Pretty*

Film

Wise, R. (Producer), & Robbins, J. (Director). (1961). *West Side story* [Motion Picture]. United States: Mirisch.

Case 11.3 Billie Jean

Internet Source

http://en.wikipedia.org/wiki/Billie_jean

Video Clips

http://www.youtube.com/watch?v=Zi_XLOB
Do_Y Billie Jean by Michael Jackson

http://www.youtube.com/watch?v=Y8KjO1BsGb0
Michael Jackson performing Billie Jean

Case 11.4 Eleanor Rigby

Internet Sources

http://en.wikipedia.org/wiki/Eleanor_Rigby

http://www.stpeters-woolton.org.uk/index.php/
beatles-information/the-beatles.html

Video Clips

http://www.youtube.com/watch?v=IFeMhdXIqWc

http://www.youtube.com/watch?v=Ht-qVldmP00

Film

Dunning, G. (Director). (1968). *Yellow submarine*
[Motion Picture]. United Kingdom: Apple Corps.

Case 11.5 Geico Caveman

Internet Source

http://en.wikipedia.org/wiki/GEICO_Cavemen

Video Clips

http://www.youtube.com/watch?v=m9Dognr3BII
Cavemen chat

http://www.youtube.com/watch?v=3Mg_JIceCvk
Caveman and friends bowling

http://www.youtube.com/watch?v=sPPfYKbO-1M
Caveman plays tennis with Billie Jean King

http://www.youtube.com/watch?v=iomlEcaeZgQ
Therapy for the Caveman

http://www.youtube.com/watch?v=3F3qzfTCDG4
The Caveman protests

CHAPTER 12: CHARACTERS IN LITERATURE AND COMICS

Case 12.1 Annie Wilkes

Internet Sources

http://en.wikipedia.org/wiki/Misery_%28novel%29

http://en.wikipedia.org/wiki/Annie_Wilkes

Video Clips

http://www.youtube.com/watch?v=i5OlolbLXvw
Annie hurts Paul for lying

http://www.youtube.com/watch?v=64RdMFheer4
Annie from all sides

Literature

King, S. (1987). *Misery.* New York, NY: Viking.

Film

Reiner, R. (Director). (1990). *Misery* [Motion
Picture]. United States: Castle Rock Entertainment.

Case 12.2 Miss Celie

Internet Source

http://en.wikipedia.org/wiki/The_Color_Purple

Video Clips

http://www.youtube.com/watch?v=ZsoHqApn_4E
Miss Celie stands up

http://www.youtube.com/watch?v=8uxvzizaweo
Celie and Nettie united at last

http://www.youtube.com/watch?v=dM60tZnG3i8
Nettie and Celie separated

Film

Spielberg, S. (Director). (1985). *The color purple*
[Motion Picture]. United States: Amblin Entertainment.

Literature

Walker, A. (1982). *The color purple.* New York,
NY: Harcourt Brace Jovanovich.

Case 12.3 Chief Bromden

Internet Source

http://en.wikipedia.org/wiki/Chief_Bromden#Main_characters

Video Clips

http://www.youtube.com/watch?v=AG1QPYCfaBQ The Chief speaks

Film

Zaentz, S., & Douglas, M. (Producers), & Forman, M. (Director). (1975). *One flew over the cuckoo's nest* [Motion Picture]. United States: United Artists.

Literature

Kesey, K. (1962). *One flew over the cuckoo's nest*. New York, NY: Viking Press.

Case 12.4 Peter Parker

Internet Sources

http://marvel.com/universe/Spider-Man_%28Peter_Parker%29

http://en.wikipedia.org/wiki/Peter_parker

http://en.wikipedia.org/wiki/Fictional_history_of_Spider-Man#College_life

http://www.spiderfan.org/characters/himself/index.html

http://www.marveldirectory.com/individuals/s/spiderman.htm

http://www.superherostuff.com/Biographies/SpideyBio.html

Video Clips

http://www.youtube.com/watch?v=dg83d4VziLk Origin of a superhero

http://www.youtube.com/watch?v=Hm4BxQen6SM Awakening with powers

http://www.youtube.com/watch?v=luOkwCcMjEc Death of Uncle Ben

http://www.youtube.com/watch?v=N-PYuGYkdyM Mary Jane Watson

Film

Avad, A. (Producer), & Raimi, S. (Director). (2002). *Spider-Man* [Motion Picture]. United States: Columbia Pictures.

Avad, A. (Producer), & Raimi, S. (Director). (2004). *Spider-Man 2* [Motion Picture]. United States: Columbia Pictures.

Avad, A. (Producer), & Raimi, S. (Director). (2007). *Spider-Man 3* [Motion Picture]. United States: Columbia Pictures.

Case 12.5 Christopher Robin

Internet Sources

http://en.wikipedia.org/wiki/Christopher_Robin

http://www.just-pooh.com/christopher.html

Video Clip

http://www.youtube.com/watch?v=6W8p5KG7eMA Christopher and Winnie

Literature

Milne, A. A. (1924). *When we were very young.* London: Methuen.

Milne, A. A. (1926). *Winnie-the-pooh.* London: Methuen.

Milne, A. A. (1927). *Now we are six.* London: Methuen.

Milne, A. A. (1928). *The house at pooh corner.* London: Methuen.

Film

Lounsbery, J., & Reitherman, W. (Directors). (1977). *The many adventures of Winnie the Pooh* [Motion Picture]. United States: Walt Disney Productions.

Reitherman, W. (Producer), & Reitherman, W., & Lounsbery, J. (Directors). (1977). *The many adventures of Winnie the Pooh* [Motion Picture]. United States: Walt Disney Productions.

Reitherman, W. (Director). (1968). *Winnie the Pooh and the blustery day* [Motion Picture]. United States: Walt Disney Productions.

REFERENCES

Abel, S. (1995). The rabbit in drag: Camp and gender construction in the America animated cartoon. *Journal of Popular Culture, 29*(3), 183–202.

Abidin, R. R. (1997). Parenting Stress Index: A measure of the parent-child system. In C. P. Zalaquett & R. Woods (Eds.), *Evaluating stress: A book of resources* (pp. 277–291). Lanham, MD: Scarecrow Press.

Ackley, D. C. (1997). *Breaking free of managed care: A step-by-step guide to regaining control of your practice.* New York, NY: Guildford Press.

Adler, A. A. (1964). The structure of neurosis. In H. L. Ansbacher & R. R. Ansbacher (Eds.), *Superiority and social interest: A collection of later writings* (pp. 83–95). Evanston IL: Northwestern University Press. (Original work published 1933)

Adreon, D., & Durocher, J. S. (2007). Evaluating the college transition needs of individuals with high-functioning autism spectrum disorders. *Intervention in School and Clinic, 42,* 271–279.

Alexander, D. (2003). A Marijuana Screening Inventory (experimental version): Description and preliminary psychometric properties. *The American Journal of Drug and Alcohol Abuse, 29*(3), 619–646.

American Association for Geriatric Psychiatry. (2006). AAGP position statement: Principles of care for patients with dementia resulting from Alzheimer disease. *American Journal of Geriatric Psychiatry, 14,* 561–572. Retrieved from http://www.aagponline.org/prof/position_caredmnalz.asp

American Counseling Association. (2009). *The ACA encyclopedia of counseling.* Alexandria, VA: American Counseling Association.

American Psychiatric Association. (2000a). *Diagnostic and statistical manual of mental disorders* (4th ed., Text Rev.). Washington, DC: Author.

American Psychiatric Association. (2000b). Practice guidelines for the treatment of patients with major depressive disorder (Rev.). *American Journal of Psychiatry,* 157 (Suppl 4).

Amos, P. A. (2004). New considerations in the prevention of aversives, restraint, and seclusion: Incorporating the role of relationships into an ecological perspective. *Research and Practice for Persons With Severe Disabilities, 29,* 263–272.

Andrews, G., Slade, T., Sunderland, M., & Anderson, T. (2007). Issues for *DSM-V:* Simplifying *DSM-V* to enhance utility: The case of major depressive disorder. *The American Journal of Psychiatry, 164*(12), 1784–1785.

Anonymous. (2004). Guidelines for psychological practice with older adults. *American Psychologist, 59*(4), 236–260.

Anonymous. (2005). An adventure into Snoezelen therapy. *Nursing Homes, 54*(10), 64–74.

Anonymous. (2006). AAGP position statement: Practice guidelines of care for patients with dementia resulting from Alzheimer's disease. *American Journal of Geriatric Psychiatry, 14*(7), 561–572.

Anonymous. (2007). Practice guidelines for the treatment of patients with Alzheimer's disease and other dementias. *The American Journal Psychiatry, 164*(12), 4–39.

Anton, R. F., O'Malley, S. S., Ciraulo, D. A., Cisler R. A., Couper, D., Donovan, D. M., Gastfriend, D. R. et al. (2006). Combined pharmacotherapies and behavioral interventions for alcohol dependence: The COMBINE study: A randomized controlled trial. *Journal of the American Medical Association, 295*(17), 2003–2017.

Arana, G. W., & Rosenbaum, J. F., & Hyman, S. E. (2000). *Handbook of psychiatric drug therapy.* Philadelphia, PA: Lippincott Williams & Wilkins.

Ariel, S. (2005). Family play therapy. In C. E. Schaefer, J. McCormick, & A. Ohnogi (Eds.), *International handbook of play therapy: Advances in assessment, theory, research and practice* (pp. 3–22). Northvale, NJ: Jason Aronson.

Arkowitz, H., & Miller, W. R. (2008). Learning, applying and extending motivational interviewing. In H. Arkowitz, H. A. Westra, W. R. Miller, & S. Rollnick (Eds.), *Motivational interviewing in the treatment of psychological problems* (pp. 1–25). New York, NY: Guilford Press.

Arnold, L. E., Abikoff, H. B., Cantwell, D. P., Conners, C. K., Elliott, G., Greenhill, L. L., & Colleagues. (1997). National Institute of Mental Health collaborative multimodal treatment study of children with ADHD (the MTA). *Archives of General Psychiatry, 54*(9), 865–870.

Arthur, N. (2004). *Counseling international students: Clients from around the world.* New York, NY: Kluwer Academic/Plenum.

Ashcraft, C. (2003). Adolescent ambiguities in A*merican Pie:* Popular culture as a resource for sex education. *Youth & Society, 35*(1), 37–70.

Auld, F., & Hyman, M. (1991). *Resolution of inner conflict: An introduction to psychoanalytic therapy.* Washington, DC: American Psychological Association.

Avad, A. (Producer), & Raimi, S. (Director). (2002). *Spider-Man* [Motion Picture]. United States: Columbia Pictures.

Avad, A. (Producer), & Raimi, S. (Director). (2004). *Spider-Man 2* [Motion Picture]. United States: Columbia Pictures.

Avad, A. (Producer), & Raimi, S. (Director). (2007). *Spider-Man 3* [Motion Picture]. United States: Columbia Pictures.

Axline, V. (1947). *Play therapy.* New York, NY: Ballantine.

Ayalon, L., Gunn, A., Feliciano, L., & Arean, P. A. (2006). Effectiveness of nonpharmacological interventions for the management of neuropsychiatric symptoms in patients with dementia: A systematic review. *Archives of Internal Medicine, 166,* 2182–2188.

Bachar, E. (1998). The contributions of self-psychology to the treatment of anorexia and bulimia. *American Journal of Psychotherapy, 52*(2), 147–165.

Baer, J. S., & Peterson, P. L. (2002). Motivational interviewing with adolescents and young adults. In W. R. Miller & Rollnick, S. (Eds.), *Motivational interviewing: Preparing people for change* (2nd ed., pp. 320–332). New York, NY: Guilford Press.

Baggerly, J., Ray, D., & Bratton, S. (2010). *Child-centered play therapy research: The evidence base for effective practice.* New York, NY: Wiley.

Baker, R., & Siryk, B. (1984). Measuring adjustment to college. *Journal of Counseling Psychology, 31,* 179–189.

Ball, J. R., Mitchell, P. B., Corry, J. C., Skillecorn, A., Smith, M., & Malhi, G. S. (2006). A randomized controlled trial of cognitive therapy for bipolar disorders. *Journal of Clinical Psychiatry, 67,* 277–286.

Ballou, M., Hill, M., & West, C. (2008). *Feminist therapy theory and practice: A contemporary perspective.* New York, NY: Springer.

Barkley, R. A. (2006). *Attention-deficit hyperactivity disorder: A handbook for diagnosis and treatment.* New York, NY: Guilford.

Barrie, J. M. (1911). *Peter and Wendy.* New York, NY: Scribner.

Basch, M. F. (1980). *Doing psychotherapy.* New York, NY: Basic Books.

Baum, L. F. (1900). *The wonderful Wizard of Oz.* Chicago, IL: George M. Hill.

Beck, A. T. (1997). The past and future of cognitive therapy. *Journal of Psychotherapy Practice and Research, 6,* 276–284.

Beck, A. T., & Steer, R. A. (1990). *Beck Anxiety Inventory manual.* San Antonio, TX: Psychological Corporation.

Beck, A. T., Steer, R. A., & Brown G. K. (1996). *BDI-II, Beck Depression Inventory: Manual* (2nd ed.). Boston, MA: Harcourt Brace.

Beck, J. (1995). *Cognitive therapy: Basics and beyond.* New York, NY: Guilford Press.

Beck, J. (2005). *Cognitive therapy for challenging problems.* New York, NY: Guilford Press.

Beesdo, K., Bittner, A., Pine, D., Stein, M., Hoffler, M., Lieb, R., & Wittchen, H. (2007). Incidence of social anxiety disorder and the consistent risk for secondary depression in the first three decades of life. *Archives of General Psychiatry, 64*(8), 903–912.

Bell, J. (1992). In search of a discourse on aging: The elderly on television. *The Gerontologist, 32*(3), 305–311.

Bernal, G., & Saez-Santiago, E. (2006). Culturally-centered psychosocial interventions. *Journal of Community Psychology, 34*(2), 121–132.

Bernard, J. M., & Goodyear, R. K. (2004). *Fundamentals of clinical supervision* (4th ed.). New York, NY: Pearson.

Beres, L. (2002). Negotiating images: Popular culture, imagination, and hope in clinical social work practice. *Affilia, 17*(4), 429–447.

Berg, I. K. (1994). *Family based services: A solution-focused approach.* New York, NY: Norton.

Berry, J. W. (2003). Conceptual approaches to acculturation. In K. M. Chun, P. B. Organista, & G. Marin (Eds.), *Acculturation: Advances in theory, measurement, and applied research* (pp. 17–38). Washington, DC: American Psychological Association.

Bertolino, B., & O'Hanlon, B. (2002). *Collaborative, competency-based counseling and therapy.* Boston, MA: Allen & Bacon.

Best, S., & Kellner, D. (1999). Rap, black rage, and racial difference. *Enculturation, 2*(2), n.p.

Behavioral Health Network (BHN). (2005). *Provider manual.* Retrieved from http://www.bhn.com

Binks, C., Fenton, M., McCarthy, L., Lee, T., Adams, C. E., & Duggan, C. (2009). Psychological therapies for people with borderline personality disorder. *The Cochrane Collaboration, 1,* 1–22.

Bieschke, K., Perez, R., & DeBord, K. (Eds.). (2007). *Handbook of counseling and psychotherapy with lesbian, gay, bisexual and transgendered clients.* Washington, DC: American Psychological Association.

Bohart, A. C., & Greenberg, L. S. (Eds.). (1997). *Empathy reconsidered: New directions in psychotherapy.* Washington, DC: American Psychological Association.

Boyle, D., & Tandan, L. (Directors). (2008). *Slumdog millionaire* [Motion Picture]. United States: Caleador Films.

Bradley, R., Greene, J., Russ, E., Dutra, L., & Westen, D. (2005). A multidimensional meta-analysis of psychotherapy for PTSD. *American Journal of Psychiatry, 162,* 214–227.

Broadley, B. T. (1999). The actualizing tendency. *The Person-Centered Journal, 4,* 18–30.

Brody, V. (1999). *The dialogue of touch: Developmental play therapy.* Northvale, NJ: Jason Aronson.

Brooks, A., McCarthy, K., Ondaatje, E., & Zakaras, L. (2004). *Gift of the muse: Reframing the debate about the benefits of the arts.* Santa Monica, CA: Rand.

Brooks, K. (2006). Comfortably numb: Young people, drugs, and the seductions of popular culture. *Youth Studies Australia, 25,* 9–16.

Browne, R. (1984). Popular culture as the new humanities. *Journal of Popular Culture, 17*(4), 1–8.

Brunello, N., Davidson, J. R., Deahl, M., Kessler, R. C., Mendlewica, J., Racagni, G., Shalev, A. Y., & Zohar, J. (2001). Post-traumatic stress disorder: Diagnosis, and epidemiology, comorbidity and social consequences, biology and treatment. *Neuropsychobiology, 43*(3), 150–162.

Bryant, R., Mastrodomenico, J., Felmingham, K., Hopwood, S., Kenny, L., Kandris, E., Cahill, C., & Creamer, M. (2008). Treatment of acute stress disorder. *Archives of General Psychiatry, 65*(6), 659–667.

Budman, S., & Gurman, A. (1983). *Theory and practice of brief therapy.* New York, NY: Guilford Press.

Budney, A. J., Hughes, J. R., Moore, B. A., & Vandrey, R. (2004). Review of the validity and significance of cannabis withdrawal syndrome. *American Journal of Psychiatry, 161,* 1967–1977.

Bugental, J. F. T. (1990). Existential-humanistic psychotherapy. In J. K. Zeig & W. M. Munion (Eds.), *What is psychotherapy? Contemporary perspectives* (pp. 189–193). San Francisco, CA: Jossey-Bass.

Burlingame, G. M., & Fuhriman, A. (1987). Conceptualizing short-term treatment: A comparative review. *The Counseling Psychologist, 15,* 557–595.

Bustillo, J. R., Lauriello, J., Horan, W. P., & Keith, S. J. (2001). The psychological treatment of schizophrenia: An update. *American Journal of Psychiatry, 158,* 163–175.

Butler, R. N. (2001). The life review. *Journal of Geriatric Psychiatry, 35*(1), 7–10.

Butters, J. W., & Cash, T. F. (1987). Cognitive-behavioral treatment of women's body image dissatisfaction. *Journal of Consulting and Clinical Psychology, 55,* 889–897.

Cain, D. J. (2008). Person-centered therapy. In J. Frew & M. D. Spiegler (Eds.), *Contemporary psychotherapies for a diverse world* (pp. 177–227). Boston, MA: Lahaska Press.

Campbell, J. (1968). *The hero with a thousand faces.* Princeton, NJ: Princeton University Press.

Campbell, J., & Moyers, B. (1991). *The power of myth.* New York, NY: Anchor Books.

Carkhuff, R. (2000). *The art of helping in the 21st century* (8th ed.). New York, NY: Holt, Rinehart & Winston.

Carlson, J. D., & Englar-Carlson, M. (2008). Adlerian therapy. In J. Frew & M. D. Speigler (Eds.), *Contemporary psychotherapies for a diverse world* (pp. 93–140). Boston, MA: Lahaska Press.

Carlson, J., Watts, R. E., & Maniacci, M. (2006). *Adlerian therapy: Theory and practice.* Washington, DC: American Psychological Association.

Carroll, K., Ball, S. A., Nich, S. C., Martino, S., Frankforter, T. L., Farentinos, C., Kunkel, L., Mikulich-Gilbertson, S. K., Morgenstern, J., Obert, J. L., Polcin, D., Snead, N., & Woody, G. E. (2006). Motivational interviewing to improve treatment engagement and outcome in individuals seeking treatment for substance abuse: A multisite effectiveness study. *Drug and Alcohol Dependence, 81*(3), 301–312.

Casey, P., Dorwick, C., & Wilkinson, G. (2001). Adjustment disorders: Fault line in the psychiatric glossary. *The British Journal of Psychiatry, 179,* 479–481.

Cash, T. F., Phillips, K. A., Santos, M. T., & Hrabosky, J. I. (2004). Measuring "negative body image": Validation of the Body Image Disturbance Questionnaire in a non-clinical population. *Body Image: An International Journal of Research, 1,* 363–372.

Carson, D. (Director). (1994). *Star trek: Generations* [Motion Picture]. United States: Paramount Pictures.

Chambless, D. L., Baker, M. J., Baucom, D., Beutler, L. E., Calhoun, K. S., Crits-Christoph, P., et al. (1998). Update on empirically validated therapies: II. *The Clinical Psychologist, 51*(1), 3–16.

Chacko, A., Pellam, W. E., Jr., Gnagy, E. M., Greiner, A., Vallano, G., Bukstein, O., & Rancurello, M. (2005). Stimulant medication effects in a summer treatment program among young children with attention-deficit/hyperactivity disorder. *Journal of the American Academy of Child & Adolescent Psychiatry, 44,* 249–257.

Chewning, B., & Sleath, B. (1996). Medication decision-making and management: A client-centered approach. *Social Science & Medicine, 42*(3), 389–398.

Chuang, L. (2009). *Mental disorders secondary to general medical conditions.* Retrieved from http://emedicine.medscape.com/article/294131-overview

Cohen-Mansfield, J. (1991). *Instruction manual for the Cohen-Mansfield Agitation Inventory.* Rockville, MD: The Research Institute of the Hebrew Home of Greater Washington.

Coleman, B., & Sebesta, J. (Eds). (2008). *Women in American musical theater.* Jefferson, NC: McFarland.

Colom, F., Vieta, E., Martinez-Aran, A., et al. (2003). A randomized trial on the efficacy of group psychoeducation in the prophylaxis of recurrences in bipolar patients whose disease is in remission. *Archives of General Psychiatry, 60,* 402–407.

Conners, C. K. (2008). *Attention deficit hyperactivity disorder: The latest assessment and treatment strategies* (3rd ed.). Sudbury, MA: Jones & Bartlett Learning.

Conners, C. K. (2008). *Conners 3rd edition: Manual.* North Tanawanda, NY: Multi Health Systems.

Cooper, J. O., Heron, T. E., & Heward, W. L. (1987). *Applied behavior analysis.* Englewood Cliffs, NJ: Prentice Hall.

Corcoran, J., & Stephenson, M. (2000). The effectiveness of solution-focused therapy with child behavior problems: A preliminary report. *Families in Society, 81,* 468–474.

Corey, G. (2009). *Theory and practice of counseling and psychotherapy* (8th ed.). Belmont, CA: Brooks/Cole Cengage Learning.

Corsini, R. J. (2008). *Introduction.* In R. J. Corsini & D. Wedding (Eds.), *Current psychotherapies* (8th ed., pp. 1–14). Belmont, CA: Brooks/Cole.

Crain, W. (1992). *Theories of development: Concepts and applications* (3rd ed.). Englewood Cliffs, NJ: Prentice Hall.

Critchfield, K., & Smith-Benjamin, L. (2006). Principles for psychosocial treatment of personality disorder: Summary of the APA Division 12 Task Force/NASPR Review. *Journal of Clinical Psychology, 62*(6), 661–674.

Crits-Christoph, P., Siqueland, L., Blaine, J., Frank, A., Luborsky, L., Onken, L. S., et al. (1999). Psychosocial treatments for cocaine dependence: National Institute on Drug Abuse Collaborative Cocaine Treatment Study. *Archives of General Psychiatry, 56,* 493–502.

Danesi, M. (2008). *Popular culture: Introductory perspectives.* New Lanham, MD: Rowman & Littlefield.

Dattilo, F. M. (2001). Cognitive-behavior family therapy: Contemporary myths and misconceptions. *Contemporary Family Therapy, 23*(1), 3–18.

Dattilo, F. M. (2005). Restructuring family schemas: A cognitive-behavioral perspective. *Journal of Marital and Family Therapy, 31*(1), 15–30.

Dattilo, F. M. (2006). Cognitive-behavioral family therapy: A coming of age story. In R. L. Leahy (Ed.), *Contemporary cognitive therapy: Theory, research, and practice* (pp. 389–405). New York, NY: Guilford Press.

Dattilo, F. M., & Norcross, J. C. (2006). Psychotherapy integration and the emergence of instinctual territoriality. *Archives of Psychiatry and Psychotherapy, 8*(1), 5–6.

Davanloo, H. (2005). Intensive short-term dynamic psychotherapy. In H. Kaplan & B. Sadock (Eds.), *Comprehensive textbook of psychiatry* (8th ed.,

Vol. 2, pp. 2628–2652). Philadelphia, PA: Lippincott Williams & Wilkins.

De Jong, P., & Berg, I. K. (2002). *Interviewing for solutions* (2nd ed.). Pacific Grove, CA: Brooks/Cole.

Delong, H., & Pollack, M. H. (2008). Update on the assessment, diagnosis, and treatment of individuals with social anxiety disorder. *Focus, 6*, 431–437.

de Shazer, S. (1988). *Clues: Investigating solutions in brief therapy.* New York, NY: Norton.

de Shazer, S. (1991). *Putting difference to work.* New York, NY: Norton.

de Shazer, S., Dolan, Y. M. (with Korman, H., Trepper, T., McCullom, E., & Berg, I. K). (2007). *More than miracles: The state of the art of solution-focused brief therapy.* New York, NY: Haworth Press.

des Portes, V., Hagerman, V., & Hendren, R. L., (2003). Pharmacotherapy. In S. Ozonoff, S. J. Rogers, & R. L. Hendren (Eds.), *Autism spectrum disorders: A research review for practitioners* (pp. 168–186). Washington, DC: American Psychiatric Publishing.

Depression Guideline Panel. (1993). *Depression in primary care: Vol. 2. Treatment of major depression.* Clinical Practice Guideline No. 5, AHCPR Publication No. 93–0551. Rockville, MD: U.S. Department of Health and Human Services, Public Health Service, Agency for Health Care Policy and Research.

Diefenbach, D. L. (1997). The portrayal of mental illness on prime-time television. *Journal of Community Psychology, 25,* 289–302.

Diller, J. (2007). *Cultural diversity: A primer for the human services.* Belmont, CA: Brooks/Cole.

Dinkmeyer, D., & Sperry, L. (2000). *Counseling and psychotherapy: An integrated, individual psychology approach.* Columbus, OH: Merrill.

Dobson, K. S. (1989). A meta-analysis of the efficacy of cognitive therapy for depression. *Journal of Consulting and Clinical Psychology, 57,* 414–419.

Drewes, A. (2009). *Blending play therapy with cognitive-behavior therapy: Evidence-based and other effective treatments and techniques.* Hoboken, NJ: Wiley.

Drum, D. J., & Lawler, A. C. (1988). *Developmental interventions: Theories, principles, and practice.* Columbia, OH: Merrill.

Duffey, T. H. (2005). A musical chronology and the emerging life song. *Journal of Creativity in Mental Health, 1*(1), 141–147.

Dumont, F. (1993). Inferential heuristics in clinical problem formation: Selective review of their strengths and weaknesses. *Professional Psychology: Research and Practice, 24,* 196–205.

DuPaul, G. J., & Stoner, G. (2003). *AD/HD in the schools: Assessment and intervention strategies* (2nd ed.). New York, NY: Guilford Press.

DuPaul, G. J., & Weyandt, L. L. (2006). School-based intervention for children with attention deficit hyperactivity disorder: Effects on academic, social, and behavioral functioning. *International Journal of Disability, Development and Education, 53,* 161–176.

Eales, J., Keating, N., & Damsma, A. (2001). Seniors' experiences of client-centered residential care. *Aging & Society, 21,* 179–196.

Eells, T. D. (Ed.). (1997). *Handbook of psychotherapy case formulation.* New York, NY: Guilford Press.

Eikeseth, S., Smith, T., Jahr, E., & Eldevik, S. (2002). Intensive behavioral treatment at school for 4 to 7 year-old children with autism. *Behavior Modification, 2691,* 49–68.

Elkins, D. H. (1995). Psychotherapy and spirituality: Toward a theory of the soul. *Journal of Humanistic Psychology, 35,* 78–99.

Ellis, A. (1994). *Reason and emotion in psychotherapy* (Rev.). New York, NY: Kensington.

Ellis, A. (2004). *Rational emotive behavior therapy.* Amherst, NY: Prometheus Books.

Ellis, A., & MacLaren, C. (2005). *Rational emotive therapy: A therapist's guide* (2nd ed.). Atascadero, CA: Impact Publishers.

Eells, T. D. (Ed.). (1997). *Handbook of psychotherapy case formulation.* New York, NY: Guilford Press.

Enns, C. Z. (2004). *Feminist theories and feminist psychotherapies: Origins, themes, and diversity* (2nd ed.). New York, NY: Haworth Press.

Eriksen, K., & Kress, V. E. (2005). *Beyond the DSM story: Ethical quandaries, challenges, and best practices.* Thousand Oaks, CA: Sage.

Eriksen, K., & Kress, V. (2008). Gender and diagnosis: Struggles and suggestions for counselors. *Journal of Counseling and Development: JCD, 86*(2), 152–162.

Erikson, E. (1950). *Childhood and society.* New York, NY: Norton.

Evans, K., Kincade, E., Marbley, A., & Seem, S. (2005). Feminism and feminist therapy: Lessons from the past and hopes for the future. *Journal of Counseling and Development: JCD, 83*(3), 269–277.

Evans, N. J., Forney, D. S., & Guido-DiBrito, F. (1998). *Student development in college: Theory, research, and practice.* San Francisco, CA: Jossey-Bass.

Evans, N., & Levine, H. (1990). Perspectives on sexual orientation. In L. Moore (Ed.), *Evolving theoretical perspectives on students: New directions for student services* (pp. 49–58). San Francisco, CA: Jossey-Bass.

Eyberg, S. M., Nelson, M. N., & Boggs, S. (2008). Evidence-based psychosocial treatments for children and adolescents with disruptive behavior disorders. *Journal of Clinical Child and Adolescent Psychology, 37*(1), 215–237.

Farvid, P., & Braun, V. (2006). "Most of us guys are raring to go anytime, anyplace, anywhere": Male and female sexuality in Cleo and Cosmo. *Sex Roles, 55*(5–6), 295–310.

Federman, R., & Thomson, J. A., Jr. (2010). *Facing bipolar: The young adult's guide to dealing with bipolar disorder.* Oakland, CA: New Harbinger.

Feigenbaum, J. (2007). Dialectical behavior therapy: An increasing evidence base. *Journal of Mental Health, 16*(1), 51–68.

Fiorini, J., & Mullen, J. (2006). *Counseling children and adolescents through grief and loss.* Champaign, IL: Research Press.

Fisher, E. (2010 April). *MLK vs. Jay-Z: Rhetorical thoughts, strategies, & rhythms of Dr. Martin Luther King Jr. and hip-hop music.* Presentation at the Annual Hip Hop Conference of Cal U, California, PA.

Fishwick, M. (2002). *Popular culture in a new age.* Binghampton, NY: Haworth Press.

Flessner, C. A., Conolea, C. A., Woods, D. W., Franklin, M. E., & Keuthen, N. J. (2008). Styles of pulling in trichotillomania: Exploring differences in symptom severity, phenomenology, and functional impact. *Behavioral Research Therapy, 46,* 345–357.

Flessner, C. A., Woods, D. W., Franklin, M. E., Keuthen, N. J., Piacentini, J., Cashin, S. E., & Colleagues. (2007). The Milwaukee Inventory for Styles of Trichotillomania—Child version (MIST-C): The development of an instrument for the assessment of "focused" and "automatic" hair pulling in children and adolescents. *Behavior Modification, 31,* 896–918.

Flores, L., Ojeda, L., Yu-Ping, H., Gee, D., & Lee, S. (2006). The relation of acculturation, problem-solving appraisal, and career decision-making self-efficacy to Mexican American high school students' educational goals. *Journal of Counseling Psychology, 53*(20), 260–266.

Floyd, F. J., Haynes, S. N., Doll, E. R., Winemiller, D., Lemsky, C., Burgy, T. M., Werle, M., & Heilman, N. (1992). Assessing retirement satisfaction and perceptions of retirement experiences. *Psychology and Aging, 7*(4), 609–621.

Foa, E. B., & Keane, T. M. (Eds.). (2000). *Effective treatments for PTSD: Practice guidelines from the International Society of Traumatic Stress studies.* New York, NY: Guilford Press.

Fochtmann, L., & Gelenberg, A. (2005). *Guideline watch: Practice guidelines for the treatment of patients with major depressive disorder.* Arlington, VA: American Psychiatric Association.

Fontaine, J., & Hammond, N. (1996). Counseling issues with gay and lesbian adolescents. *Adolescence, 31,* 817–830.

Fouts, G., Callan, M., & Piasentin, K. (2006). Demonizing in children's television cartoons and Disney animated films. *Child Psychiatry and Human Development, 37,* 15–23.

Frakes, J. (Director). (1996). *Star Trek: First contact* [Motion Picture]. United States: Paramount Pictures.

Frances, A., First, M. B., & Pincus, H. N. (1995). *DSM-IV guidebook: The essential companion to the* Diagnostic and Statistical Manual of Mental Disorders. Washington, DC: American Psychiatric Association.

Frank, E., Kupfer, D. J., Thase, M. E., Mallinger, A. G., Swartz, H. A., & Eagiolini, A. M. (2005). Two-year outcomes for interpersonal and social rhythm therapy in individuals with bipolar I disorder. *Archives of General Psychiatry, 62,* 996–1004.

Frankel, F., Cantwell, D. P., Myatt, R., & Feinberg, D. T. (1999). Do stimulants improve self-esteem in children with ADHD and peer problems? *Journal of Child and Adolescent Psychopharmacology, 9,* 185–194.

Frankl, V. E. (1968). *Psychotherapy and existentialism.* New York, NY: Simon & Schuster.

Frawley. J. (Director). (1979). *The Muppet movie* [Motion Picture]. Argentina: Henson Associates.

Gaffney, S. (2006a). Gestalt therapy with groups: A developmental perspective. *Gestalt Journal of Australia & New Zealand, 2*(2), 6–28.

Gaffney, S. (2006b). Gestalt with groups: A cross cultural perspective. *Gestalt Review, 10*(3), 205–219.

Gardstrom, S. C. (1999). Music exposure and criminal behavior: Perceptions of juvenile offenders. *Journal of Music Therapy, 36,* 207–221.

Garrett, M. T. (1999). Understanding the "medicine" of Native American traditional values: An integrative review. *Counseling and Values, 43,* 84–98.

Garrett, M. T., & Pichette, E. F. (2000). Red as an apple: Native American acculturation and counseling with or without reservation. *Journal of Counseling and Development: JCD, 78,* 3–13.

Garner, D., Olmstead, M., & Polivy, J. (1983). Development and validation of a multidimensional eating disorder inventory for anorexia and bulimia. *International Journal of Eating Disorders, 2*(2), 15–34.

Geronimi, C., & Jackson, W. (Directors). (1953). *Peter Pan* [Motion Picture]. United States: RKO Radio Pictures.

Gil, E. (1984). *Play in family therapy.* New York, NY: Guilford Press.

Gilliam, J. (2006). *The Gilliam Autism Rating Scale* (2nd ed.). Austin, TX: PRO-ED.

Gingerich, W. J., & Eisengart, S. (2000). Solution-focused brief therapy: A review of the outcome research. *Family Process, 39*(4), 477–498.

Gladding, S. (1995). Creativity in counseling. *Counseling and Human Development, 28,* 1–12.

Gladding, S. (2005). *Counseling as art: The creative arts in counseling* (3rd ed.). Alexandria, VA: American Counseling Association.

Glasser, W. (1998). *Choice theory: A new psychology of personal freedom.* New York, NY: HarperCollins.

Glasser, W. (2001). *Counseling with choice theory: The new reality therapy.* New York, NY: HarperCollins.

Glasser, W. (2003). *Warning: Psychiatry can be hazardous to your health.* New York, NY: HarperCollins.

Glidewell, J. C., & Livert, D. E. (1992). Confidence in the practice of clinical psychology. *Professional Psychology: Research and Practice, 23,* 362–368.

Godfrey, W. (Producer), & Hardwicke, C. (Director). (2008). *Twilight* [Motion Picture]. United States: Summit Entertainment.

Goldenberg, J., Kosloff, S., & Greenberg, J. (2006). Existential underpinnings of approach and avoidance of the physical body. *Motivation and Emotion, 30,* 127–134.

Goldman, W., McCulloch, M., & Cuffel, B. (2003). A four-year study of enhancing outpatient psychotherapy in managed care. *Psychiatric Services, 54,* 41–49.

Gordon, T. (2000). *Parent effectiveness training: The proven program for raising responsible children.* New York, NY: Three Rivers Press.

Gordek, H., & Folsom, R. (2005). *National survey on drug use and health* (prepared for The Substance Abuse and Mental Health Service Administration–SAMHSA). Retrieved from http://oas.samhsa .gov/nsduh/2k5MRB/2k5SamplingError.pdf

Grabe, H. J., Volzke, H., Ludemann, J., Wolff, B., Schwahn, C., John, U., Meng, W., & Freyberger, H. J. (2005). Mental and physical complaints in thyroid disorders in the general population. *Acta Psychiatrica Scandinavica, 112*(July), 286–293.

Grant, B., Dawson, D., Stinton, F., Chou, P., Dufour, M., & Pickering, R. (2006). The 12-month prevalence and trends in *DSM-IV* alcohol abuse and dependence. United States, 1991–1992 and 2001–2002. *Alcohol Research and Health, 29*(2), 79–91.

Graves, B. (1999). Television and prejudice reduction: "When does television as a vicarious experience make a difference?" *Journal of Social Issues, 55*(4), 707–725.

Gray, C., & Garand, D. (1983). Social stories: Improving responses of students with autism with accurate social information. *Focus on Autism and Other Developmental Disabilities, 8*(April), 1–10.

Greene, G. J., Kondrat, D. C., Lee, M. Y., Clement, J., Siebert, H., Mentzer, R. A., & Pinnell, S. R. (2006). A solution-focused approach to case management and recovery with consumers who have a severe mental disability. *Families in Society, 87*(3), 339–350.

Greenspan, S. I., & Wieder, S. (2006). *Autism: Using the Floortime approach to help children relate, communicate, and think.* Cambridge, MA: Da Capo Press/Perseus Book Group.

Griffith, B. A., & Griggs, J. C. (2001). Religious identity status as a model to understand, assess, and interact with client spirituality. *Counseling and Values, 46,* 14–25.

Guarnaccia, P. J., DeLaCancela, V., & Carrillo, E. (1989). The multiple meanings of ataques de nervios in the Latino community. *Medical Anthropology, 11,* 47–62.

Gutterman, J. T. (2006). *Solution-focused counseling.* Alexandria, VA: American Counseling Association.

Haight, B., & Gibson, F. (Eds.). (2005). *Burnsides working with older adults: Group processes and techniques.* Boston, MA: Jones and Bartlett.

Hall, M., & Sutton, J. M., Jr. (2004). *Clinical supervision: A handbook for practitioners.* Boston, MA: Pearson Education.

Hanna, F. J., & Puhakka, K. (1991). When psychotherapy works: Pinpointing an element of change. *Psychotherapy, 28,* 598–607.

Hanna, F. J., & Ritchie, M. H. (1995). Seeking the active ingredients of psychotherapeutic change: Within and outside the context of therapy. *Professional Psychotherapy: Research and Practice, 26,* 176–183.

Harrison, P. L., & Oakland, T. (2000). *Adaptive behavior assessment system.* San Antonio, TX: The Psychological Corporation.

Hart, K.-P. (2000). Representing gay men on American television. *Journal of Men's Studies, 9*(1), 597–607.

Hartmann, D. P. (1984). Assessment strategies. In D. H. Barlow & M. Hersen (Eds.), *Single case environmental designs* (pp. 107–129). New York, NY: Pergamon Press.

Hays, D. G., McLeod, A. L., & Prosek, E. A. (2010). A mixed methodological analysis of the role of culture in the clinical decision-making process. *Journal of Counseling and Development: JCD, 88,* 114–121.

Hembree-Kigin, T. L., & McNeil, C. (1995). *Parent child interaction therapy.* New York, NY: Plenum Press.

Henggeler, S. W., Schoenwald, S. K., Borduin, C. M., Rowland, M. D., & Cunningham, P. B. (1998). *Multisytemic treatment of antisocial behavior in children and adolescents.* New York, NY: Guilford Press.

Henry, W. P. (1998). Science, politics, and the politics of science: The use and misuse of empirically validated treatments. *Psychotherapy Research, 8,* 126–140.

Heppner, P. P., Kivlighan, D. M., Jr., & Wampold, B. E. (1999). *Research design in counseling and psychotherapy* (2nd ed.). Pacific Grove, CA: Brooks/Cole.

Herek, G. M. (1995). Psychological heterosexualism in the United States. In A. D'Augelli & C. Patterson (Eds.), *Lesbian, gay, and bisexual identities over the lifespan: Psychological perspectives* (pp. 321–346). New York, NY: Oxford University Press.

Herron, W. G., Javier, R. A., Primavera, L. H., & Schultz, C. L. (1994). The cost of psychotherapy. *Professional Psychology: Research and Practice, 25,* 106–110.

Hersen, M., & Ammerman, R. (2000). *Advanced abnormal child psychology.* Mahwah, NJ: Lawrence Erlbaum.

Higgins, S. T., Budney, A. J., Bickel, W. K., Hughes, J. R., Foerg, F., & Badger, G. (1993). Achieving cocaine abstinence with a behavioral approach. *American Journal of Psychiatry, 150,* 763–769.

Higgins, S. T., & Silverman, K. (1999). *Motivating behavior change among illicit drug abusers: Research on contingency management interventions.* Washington, DC: American Psychological Association.

Hinkle, J. S. (1994). The *DSM-IV:* Prognosis and implications for mental health counselors. *Journal of Mental Health Counseling, 16,* 33–36.

Hoffart, A., Verslund, S., & Sexton, H. (2002). Self-understanding, empathy, guided discovery, and schema belief in schema-focused cognitive therapy of personality problems: A process-outcome study. *Cognitive Therapy and Research, 2692,* 199–219.

Hogan, P. J. (Director). (2003). *Peter Pan* [Motion Picture]. United States: Universal Pictures.

Hollon, S., Thase, M., & Markowitz, J. (2002). Treatment and prevention of depression. *Psychological Science in the Public Interest, 3*(2), 39–77.

Holmberg, C. B. (1998). *Sexualities and popular culture.* London: Sage.

Hopson, L., & Kim, J. (2004). A solution-focused approach to crisis intervention with adolescents. *Journal of Evidenced-Based Social Work, 1*(2–3), 93–110.

Horn, J. L., Wanberg, K. W., & Foster, F. M. (1990). *Guide to the Alcohol Use Inventory (AUI).* Minneapolis, MN: National Computer Systems.

Hosie, T. W., & Erik, R. R. (1993). ACA reading program: Attention deficit disorder. *American Counseling Association Guidepost, 35,* 15–18.

Howlin, P., Magiati, I., & Charman, T. (2009). Systematic review of early intensive behavioral interventions for children with autism. *Journal of Intellectual and Developmental Disabilities, 114*(1), 23–41.

Hughes, J. (Producer & Director). (1985). *The breakfast club* [Motion Picture]. United States: A & M Films.

Hyler, S. (1988). DSM III at the cinema: Madness in the movies. *Comprehensive Psychiatry, 29,* 195–206.

Hyler, S. E., Gabbard, G. O., & Schneider, I. (1991). Homicidal maniacs and narcissistic parasites: Stigmatization of mentally ill persons in the movies. *Hospital and Community Psychiatry, 42,* 1044–1048.

Inaba, D. S., & Cohen, W. E. (2000). *Uppers, downers, all-arounders: Physical and mental effects of psychoactive drugs* (5th ed.). Ashland, OR: CNS.

Indick, W. (2004). Classical heroes in modern movies: Mythological patterns of the superhero. *Journal of Media Psychology, 9,* 1–13.

Ivey, A. E., Ivey, M. B., D'Andrea, M., & Simek-Morgan, L. (2005). *Theories of counseling and psychotherapy: A multicultural perspective.* Boston, MA: Allyn & Bacon/Longman.

Jaffe, J. H., Rawson, R. A., & Ling, W. (2005). Cocaine-related disorders. In B. J. Sadock & V. Sadock (Eds.), *Kaplan & Sadock's comprehensive textbook of psychiatry* (pp. 1220–1238). Philadelphia, PA: Williams & Wilkins.

Jernberg, A. (1979). *Theraplay: A new treatment using structured play for problem children and their families.* San Francisco, CA: Jossey-Bass.

Jernberg, A., & Booth, P. (1999). *Theraplay: Helping parents and children build better relationships through attachment-based play* (2nd ed.). San Francisco, CA: Jossey-Bass.

Jernberg, A., & Jernberg, E. (1993). Family Theraplay for the family tyrant. In T. Kottman & C. Schaefer (Eds.), *Play therapy in action: A casebook for practitioners* (pp. 45–96). Northvale, NJ: Jason Aronson.

Jernberg, A., Booth, P., Koller, T., & Allert, A. (1991). *Manual for the administration and the clinical interpretation of the Marshak interaction method (MIM): Pre-school and school-aged* (Rev.). Chicago, IL: Theraplay Institute.

Johnson, S. (2006). *Everything bad is good for you: How today's popular culture is actually making us smarter.* New York, NY: Penguin.

Jones, J. B. (2003). *Our musicals, ourselves: A social history of the American musical theatre.* Hanover, NH: Brandeis University Press.

Jones, S. (2004). Psychotherapy of bipolar disorder: A review. *Journal of Affective Disorders, 80,* 101–114.

Jongsma, A., & Peterson. (2006). *The complete adult psychotherapy treatment planner.* New York, NY: Wiley.

Jongsma, A., Peterson, L. M., & McInnis, W. (2003a). *The adolescent psychotherapy treatment planner.* New York, NY: Wiley.

Jongsma, A., Peterson, L. M., & McInnis, W. (2003b). *The child psychotherapy treatment planner.* New York, NY: Wiley.

Kaczmarek, M., & Backlund, B. (1991). Disenfranchised grief: The loss of an adolescent romantic relationship. *Adolescence, 26,* 102, 253–259.

Kaiser Family Foundation. (2001). *Talking with kids about tough issues: A national survey of parents and kids.* Retrieved from http://www.kff.org/Kaiserpolls/3017-index.cfm

Kazdin A. E. (1995). *Conduct disorders in childhood and adolescence* (2nd ed.). Thousand Oaks, CA: Sage.

Kazdin, A. E., Weisz, J. (Eds.). (2003). *Evidence-based psychotherapies for children and adolescents.* New York, NY: Guilford Press.

Keel, P. K., Heatherton, T. F., Dorer, D., Joiner, T. E., & Zalta, A. K. (2006). Point prevalence of bulimia nervosa in 1982, 1992, and 2002. *Psychological Medicine, 36,* 119–127.

Kesey, K. (1962). *One flew over the cuckoo's nest.* New York, NY: Viking Press.

Keshen, A. (2006). A new look at existential psychotherapy. *American Journal of Psychotherapy, 60*(3), 285–298.

Kessler, R. C., McGonagle, K. A., Zhao, S., Nelson, C. B., Hughes, M., Eshleman, S., Wittchen, H. U., & Kendler, K. S. (1994). Lifetime and 12-month prevalence of *DSM-III-R* psychiatric disorders in the United States. *Archives of General Psychiatry, 51*(1), 8–19.

Kessler, R. C., Sonnega, A., Brommet, E., Hughes, M., & Nelson, C. B. (1995). Post-traumatic stress disorder in the National Comorbidity Survey. *Archives of General Psychiatry, 52*(12), 1048–1060.

King, B. H., Hodapp, R. M., & Dykens, E. M. (2005). Mental retardation. In B. J. Sadock & V. Sadock (Eds.), *Kaplan & Sadock's comprehensive textbook of psychiatry* (pp. 3076–3106). Philadelphia, PA: Williams & Wilkins.

King, S. (1987). *Misery.* New York, NY: Viking Press.

Kleinke, C. L. (1994). *Common principles of psychotherapy.* Pacific Grove, CA: Brooks/Cole.

Klerman, G. L., & Weissman, M. M. (1993). *New applications of interpersonal psychotherapy.* Washington, DC: American Psychiatric Press.

Knell, S. (1993). *Cognitive-behavioral play therapy.* Northvale, NJ: Jason Aronson.

Knell, S. (1994). Cognitive-behavioral play therapy. In K. O'Conner & C. Schafer (Eds.), *Handbook of play therapy: Vol 2. Advances and innovations* (pp.111–142). New York, NY: Wiley.

Kohut, H. (1971). *The analysis of the self.* New York, NY: International Universities Press.

Kohut, H. (1977). *The restoration of the self.* New York, NY: International Universities Press.

Kohut, H. (1984). *How does analysis cure?* New York, NY: International Universities Press.

Kokina, A., & Kern, L. (2010). Social Story™, Interventions for students with autism spectrum disorders: A meta-analysis. *Journal of Autism and Developmental Disorders, 40*(7), 812–826.

Koller, T., & Booth, P. (1997). Fostering attachment through family Theraplay. In K. O'Connor & L. M. Braverman (Eds.), *Play therapy theory and practice: A comparative presentation* (pp. 204–233). New York, NY: Wiley.

Konner, J., & Perlmutter, A. (Producers). (1988). *Joseph Campbell and the power of myth* [DVD]. United States: Public Broadcasting Service.

Krabbandam, L., & Aleman, A. (2003). Cognitive rehabilitation in schizophrenia: A quantitative analysis of controlled studies. *Psychopharmacology, 169,* 376–382.

Kundert, D. K., & Trimarchi, C. I. (2006). Pervasive developmental disorders. In *Chronic health-related disorders in children: Collaborative medical and psychoeducational interventions* (pp. 213–235). Washington, DC: American Psychological Association.

Kunen, S., Niederhauser, R., Smith, P. O., Morris, J. A., & Marx, B. D. (2005). Race disparities in psychiatric rates in emergency departments. *Journal of Consulting & Clinical Psychology, 73,* 116–126.

LaBruzza, A. L., & Mendez-Villarrubia, J. M. (1994). *Using DSM-IV: A clinician's guide to psychiatric diagnosis.* Northvale, NJ: Jason Aronson.

Lacourse, E., Claes, M., & Villenueve, M. (2001). Heavy metal music and adolescent suicidal risk. *Journal of Youth & Adolescence, 30*(3), 321–332.

Lamb, S., & Brown, L. (2007). *Packaging girlhood: Rescuing our daughters from marketers' schemes.* New York, NY: St. Martin's Press.

Lamb, S., Brown, L., & Tappan, M. (2009). *Packaging boyhood: Saving our sons from superheroes, slackers and other media stereotypes.* New York, NY: St. Martin's Press.

Landreth, G. (1991). *Play therapy: The art of the relationship* (2nd ed.). New York, NY: Brunner-Routledge.

Landreth, G. (2002). *Play therapy: The art of the relationship.* Muncie, IN: Accelerated Development.

Landreth, G., & Sweeney, D. (1997). Child-centered play therapy. In K. O'Conner & L. M. Braverman (Eds.), *Play therapy and practice: A comparative presentation* (pp. 17–45). New York, NY: Wiley.

Lawrence, M., Condon, K., Jacobi, K., & Nicholson, E. (2006). Play therapy for girls displaying social aggression. In C. E. Schaefer & H. G. Kaduson (Eds.), *Contemporary play therapy* (pp. 212–237). New York, NY: Guilford Press.

Lazarus, A. A. (2005). Multimodal therapy. In J. C. Norcross & M. R. Goldfried (Eds.), *Handbook of psychotherapy integration* (2nd ed., pp. 105–120). New York, NY: Oxford University Press.

Lazarus, A. A. (2008). Multimodal therapy. In R. J. Corsini & D. Wedding (Eds.), *Current psychotherapies* (8th ed., pp. 368–401). Belmont, CA: Brooks/Cole.

Lazarus, A. A., Beutler, L. E., & Norcross, J. C. (1992). The future of technical eclecticism. *Psychotherapy, 29*(1), 11–20.

LeGoff, D. (2004). Use of Lego as a therapeutic medium for improving social competence. *Journal of Autism and Developmental Disorders, 34*(5), 557–571.

Leiblum, S. (Ed.). (2006). *Principles and practice of sex therapy.* New York, NY: Guilford Press.

Leiper, R., & Maltby, M. (2004). *The psychodynamic approach to therapeutic change.* Thousand Oaks, CA: Sage.

Leitch, M. L. (1998). Contextual issues in teen pregnancy and parenting: Refining our scope of inquiry. *Family Relations, 47*(2), 145–148.

Lemoire, S. J., & Chen, C. P. (2005). Applying person-centered counseling to sexual minority adolescents. *Journal of Counseling and Development: JCD, 83*(2), 146–154.

Leone, C., & D'Arienzo, J. (2000). Sensation-seeking and differentially arousing television commercials. *Journal of Social Psychology, 140*(6), 710–720.

Levinson, R. (1975). From Olive Oyl to Sweet Polly Purebred: Sex role stereotypes in televised cartoons. *Journal of Popular Culture, 9*(3), 561–572.

Lev-Wiesel, R., & Daphna-Tekoha, S. (2000). The self-revelation through color technique: Understanding clients' relationships with significant others through the use of color. *American Journal of Art Therapy, 39,* 35–41.

Lieberman, A. F., & Pawl, J. H. (1990). Disorders of attachment and secure-base behavior in the second year of life: Conceptual issues and clinical intervention. In M. T. Greenberg, A. Cichetti, & E. M. Cummings (Eds.), *Attachment in the preschool years: Theory, research and intervention* (pp. 375–398). Chicago, IL: University of Chicago Press.

Linehan, M. M. (1993a). *Cognitive-behavioral treatment of borderline personality disorder.* New York, NY: Guilford Press.

Linehan, M. M. (1993b). *Skills training manual for treating borderline personality disorder.* New York, NY: Guilford Press.

Linehan, M. M., Heard, H. L., & Armstrong, H. E. (1993). Naturalistic follow-up of a behavioral treatment for chronically parasuicidal borderline patients. *American Journal of Psychiatry, 50,* 971–974.

Lines, D. (2002). *Brief counseling in the schools.* London: Sage.

Livesley, W. (2007). An integrated approach to the treatment of personality disorder. *Journal of Mental Health, 16*(1), 131–148.

Livingston, G., Johnston, K., Katona, C., Paton, J., Lyketsos, C. G., & Old Age Task Force of the World Federation of Biological Psychiatry.

(2005). Systematic review of psychological approaches to the management of neuropsychiatric symptoms of dementia. *American Journal of Psychiatry, 162,* 1996–2021.

Loganbill, C., Hardy, E., & Delworth, U. (1982). Supervision: A conceptual model. *The Counseling Psychologist, 10,* 3–42.

Longabaugh, R., & Morgenstern, J. (1999). Cognitive-behavioral coping skills therapy for alcohol dependence: Current status and future directions. *Alcohol Research & Health, 2392,* 78–85.

Looper, K., & Kirmayer, L. (2002). Behavioral medicine approaches to somatoform disorders. *Journal of Consulting and Clinical Psychology, 70*(3), 810–827.

Lovaas, O. I., Ackerman, A., Alexander, D., Firestone, P., Perkins, M. B., & Colleagues. (1987). *Teaching developmentally disabled children: The ME book.* Austin, TX: Pro-Ed.

Lowenstein, L. (Ed.). (2008). *Assessment and treatment activities for children, adolescents and families: Practitioners share their most effective techniques.* Toronto, ON, Canada: Champion Press.

Lowenstein, L. (Ed.). (2010). *Assessment and treatment activities for children, adolescents and families: Vol. 2. Practitioners share their most effective techniques.* Toronto, ON, Canada: Champion Press.

Lowis, M., Edwards, A. C., & Burton, M. (2009). Coping with retirement: Well-being, health and religion. *The Journal of Psychology, 143*(4), 427–448.

Lykestos, C., Colenda, C., Beck, C., Blank, K., Doraiswamy, M., Kalunian, D., & Yaffe, D. (2006). Position statement of the American Association for Geriatric Psychiatry regarding principles of care for patients with dementia resulting from Alzheimer's disease. *American Journal of Geriatric Psychiatry, 14*(7), 561–572.

MacDonald, A. J. (1994). Brief therapy in adult psychiatry. *Journal of Family Therapy, 16,* 415–426.

Macdonald, D. (1998). A theory of mass culture. In J. Storey (Ed.), *Cultural theory and popular culture: A reader* (pp. 22–36). New York, NY: Prentice Hall.

Magee, W. J., Eaton, W. E., Wittchen, H., McGonagle, K. A., & Kessler, R. C. (1996). Agoraphobia, simple phobia, and social phobia in the National Comorbidity Survey. *Archives of General Psychiatry, 53*(2), 159–168.

Maguire, G. (2007). *Wicked: The life and times of the Wicked Witch of the West.* New York, NY: Harper.

Maguire, G. (2008). *Son of a witch.* New York, NY: Harper.

Maguire, G. (2009). *A lion among men.* New York, NY: Harper.

Mahalick, J. R. (1990). Systematic eclectic models. *The Counseling Psychologist, 18,* 655–679.

Mahoney, M. (1991). *The human change processes: The scientific foundations of psychotherapy.* New York, NY: Basic Books.

Marinucci, M. (2005). Television, generation X and third wave feminism: A contextual analysis of the Brady Bunch. *The Journal of Popular Culture, 38*(3), 505–524.

Markland, D., Ryan, R. M., Tobin, V. J., & Rollnick, S. (2005). Motivational interviewing and self-determination theory. *Journal of Social & Clinical Psychology, 24,* 811–831.

Martell, C. R. (2007). Behavioral therapy. In A. B. Rochlen (Ed.), *Applying counseling theories: An online case-based approach* (pp. 143–156). Upper Saddle River, NJ: Pearson Prentice Hall.

Martin, J., Slemon, A., Hiebert, B., Halberg, E., & Cummings, A. (1989). Conceptualizations of novice and experienced counselors. *Journal of Counseling Psychology, 36,* 395–400.

Matthys, W., & Lochman, J. (2010). *Oppositional defiant disorder and conduct disorder in childhood.* New York, NY: Wiley.

Mattingly, C. (2006). Pocahontas goes to the clinic: Popular culture as *lingua franca* in a cultural borderland. *American Anthropologist, 108*(3), 494–501.

May, R. (1988). *Psychoanalytic psychotherapy in a college context.* New York, NY: Praeger.

McAuliffe, G., & Associates. (2008). *Culturally alert counseling: A comprehensive introduction.* Thousand Oaks, CA: Sage.

McBride, D., & Glenapp, A. (2000). Using randomized designs to evaluate client-centered programs to prevent adolescent pregnancy. *Family Planning Perspectives, 32*(5), 227–235.

McCauley, C., Woods, K., Coolidge, C., & Kulick, W. (1983). More aggressive cartoons are funnier. *Journal of Personality and Social Psychology, 44*(4), 817–823.

McGurk, S., Twamley, E., Spitzer, D., McHugo, G., & Mueser, K. (2007). A meta-analysis of cognitive remediation in schizophrenia. *The American Journal of Psychiatry, 164*(12), 1791–1802.

McLeod, K. (2006). "We are the champions": Masculinities, sports and popular culture. *Popular Music and Society, 29*(5), 531–547.

McWilliams, N. (1994). *Psychoanalytic diagnosis: Understanding personality structure in the clinical process.* New York, NY: Guilford Press.

McWilliams, N. (1999). *Psychoanalytic case formulation*. New York, NY: Guilford Press.

Meehl, P. (1960). The cognitive activity of the clinician. *American Psychologist, 15,* 19–27.

Meier, S. T. (1999). Training the practitioner-scientist: Bridging case conceptualization, assessment, and intervention. *The Counseling Psychologist, 27,* 589–613.

Meier, S. T. (2003). *Bridging case conceptualization, assessment, and intervention.* Thousand Oaks, CA: Sage.

Meier, S. T., & Davis, S. R. (2005). *The elements of counseling* (5th ed.). Belmont, CA: Thompson Brooks/Cole.

Mendez-Villarrubia, J. M., & LaBruzza, A. (1994). Issues in the assessment of Puerto Rican and other Hispanic clients, including *Ataques de nervios* (Attacks of nerves). In A. L. LaBruzza & J. M. Mendez-Villarrubia (Eds.), *Using DSM-IV: A clinician's guide to psychiatric diagnosis* (pp. 141–196). Northvale, NJ: Jason Aronson.

Messer, S. B., & Warren, S. (1995). *Models of brief psychodynamic therapy: A comparative approach.* New York, NY: Guilford Press.

Meyer, J. A., Mundy, P. C., van Hecke, A. V., & Durocher, J. S. (2006). Social attribution processes and comorbid psychiatric symptoms in children with Asperger's syndrome. *Autism, 10,* 383–402.

Meyer, S. (2008). *The twilight saga collection.* New York, NY: Little, Brown Young Readers.

Meyer, S., & Schwitzer, A. M. (1999). Stages of identity development among college students with minority sexual orientations. *Journal of College Student Psychotherapy, 13,* 41–65.

Meyers, S. M., Plauche-Johnson, C., & Council on Children with Disabilities. (2007). Management of children with autism spectrum disorder. *Pediatrics, 120*(5), 1162–1182.

Milkowitz, D. J. (2008). Adjunctive psychotherapy for bipolar disorders: A developmental psychopathology view. *Development and Psychopathology, 16,* 667–678.

Miller, B., Benson, B., & Galbraith, K. (2000). Family relationships and adolescent pregnancy risk: A research synthesis. *Developmental Review, 21*(1), 1–38.

Miller, E. T., & Rollnick, S. (2002). *Motivational interviewing: Preparing people for change* (2nd ed.). New York, NY: Guilford Press.

Miller, P. H. (1993). *Theories of developmental psychology* (3rd ed.). New York, NY: Freeman.

Milne, A. A. (1924). *When we were very young.* London: Methuen.

Milne, A. A. (1926). *Winnie-the-Pooh.* London: Methuen.

Milne, A. A. (1927). *Now we are six.* London: Methuen.

Milne, A. A. (1928). *The house at Pooh Corner.* London: Methuen.

Miranda, A., Presentacion, M. J., Garcia, R., & Siegenthaler, R. (2009). Intervention with students with ADHD: Analysis of the effects of a multi-component and multi-contextualized program on academic and socio-emotional adjustment. *Advances in Learning and Behavioral Disabilities, 22,* 227–263.

Moni, K., & Jobling, A. (2008). A case for including popular culture in literacy education for young adults with Down syndrome. *Australian Journal of Language and Literacy, 31*(3), 260–277.

Moos, R. H., & Timko, C. (2008). Outcome research on 12-step and other self-help programs. In M. Galanter & H. D. Kleber (Eds.), *The American Psychiatric Publishing textbook of substance abuse treatment* (4th ed., pp. 511–521). Arlington, VA: American Psychiatric Publishing.

Morgan, S. P. (2005). Depression: Turning toward life. In C. K. Germer, R. D. Siegel, & P. R. Fulton (Eds.), *Mindfulness and psychotherapy* (pp. 130–151). New York, NY: Guilford Press.

Moustakas, C. E. (1959). *Psychotherapy with children.* New York, NY: Harper & Row.

Mowder, B., Rubinson, F., & Yasik, A. (Eds.). (2009). *Evidence-based practice in infant and early childhood psychology.* New York, NY: Wiley.

Munro, A. (1999). *Delusional disorder, paranoia and related illnesses.* New York, NY: Cambridge University Press.

Munson, C. E. (2001). *The mental health diagnostic desk reference: Visual guides and more for learning to use the* Diagnostic and Statistical Manual (DSM-IV-TR) (2nd ed.). Binghamton, NY: Haworth Press.

Murphy, M. J. (1996). The Wizard of Oz as cultural narrative and conceptual model for psychotherapy. *Psychotherapy, 33*(4), 531–538.

Nathan, P. E., & Gorman, J. M. (Eds.). (2002). *A guide to treatments that work.* New York, NY: Oxford University Press.

National Institute on Drug Abuse (NIDA). (2008). *NIDA InfoFacts: Treatment approaches for drug addiction.* Retrieved from http://www.nida.nih.gov/PDF/InfoFacts/Treatment08.pdf

Neighbors, H. W., Trierweiler, S. J., Ford, B. C., & Muroff, J. R. (2003). Racial differences in *DSM* diagnosis using a semi-structured instrument: The importance of clinical judgment in the diagnosis of African Americans. *Journal of Health & Social Behavior, 44,* 237–256.

Neimeyer, R. (2000). Grief therapy and research as essential tensions: Prescriptions for a progressive partnership. *Death Studies, 24,* 603–610.

Neukrug, E. S. (2001). *Skills and techniques for human service professionals: Counseling environment, helping skills, treatment issues.* Belmont, CA: Wadsworth.

Neukrug, E. S. (2002). *Skills and techniques for human service professionals: Counseling environment, helping skills, treatment issues.* Pacific Grove, CA: Brooks/Cole.

Neukrug, E. S. (2003). *The world of the counselor: An introduction to the counseling profession* (2nd ed.). Pacific Grove, CA: Brooks/Cole.

Neukrug, E. (2011). *Counseling theory and practice.* Belmont, CA: Brooks/Cole.

Neukrug, E. S., & Schwitzer, A. M. (2006). *Skills and tools for today's counselors and psychotherapists: From natural helping to professional helping.* Belmont, CA: Wadswoth/Thompson Brooks/Cole.

Newman, E., Weathers, F. W., Nader, K., Kaloupek, D. G., Pynoos, R. S., & Blake, D. D. (2004). *Clinician-administered PTSD Scale for Children and Adolescents (CAPS-CA).* Los Angeles, CA: Western Psychological Services.

Norcross, J. C., & Beutler, L. E. (2008). Integrative psychotherapies. In R. J. Corsini & D. Wedding (Eds.), *Current psychotherapies* (8th ed., pp. 481–511). Belmont, CA: Brooks/Cole.

Noll, R. (2007). *The encyclopedia of schizophrenia and other psychotic disorders (Facts on File Library of Health and Living).* Retrieved from http://www.fofweb.com/Subscription/Default.asp?BID=7

Nordling, W., Cochran, J., & Cochran, N. (2010). *A practical guide to developing therapeutic relationships with children.* New York, NY: Wiley.

Nye, R. D. (1992). *The legacy of B. F. Skinner: Concepts and perspectives, controversies and misunderstandings.* Pacific Grove, CA: Brooks/Cole.

Nystul, M. S. (1999). An interview with Paul Pederson. *Journal of Individual Psychology, 55,* 216–224.

Oberst, U. E., & Stewart, A. E. (2003). *Adlerian psychotherapy: An advanced approach to individual psychology.* New York, NY: Brunner-Routledge.

O'Farrell, T., & Fals-Stewart, W. (2003). Alcohol abuse. *Journal of Marital and Family Therapy, 29*(1), 121–146.

Okun, B. F. (2007). *Effective helping, interviewing, and counseling techniques* (7th ed.). Pacific Grove, CA: Brooks/Cole.

Olson, D. H., & Gorall, D. M. (2003). Circumplex model of marital and family systems. In F. Walsh (Ed.), *Normal family processes* (3rd ed., pp. 514–547). New York, NY: Guilford Press.

Ometo, A., & Kurtzman, H. (Eds.). (2006). *Sexual orientation and mental health: Examining identity and development in lesbian, gay and bisexual people.* Washington, DC: American Psychological Association.

Ott, B. (2003). "I'm Bart Simpson, who the hell are you?" A study in postmodern identity reconstruction. *The Journal of Popular Culture, 37*(1), 56–82.

Packwood-Freeman, C., & Merskin, D. (2006). Having it his way: The construction of masculinity in fast-food TV advertising. In L. Rubin (Ed.), *Food for thought: Essays on eating and culture* (pp. 277–293). Jefferson, NC: McFarland.

Paris, J. (2000). Childhood precursors of borderline personality disorder. *Psychiatric Clinics of North America, 23,* 77–88.

Parritz, R. H., & Troy, M. (2011). *Disorders of childhood: Development and psychopathology.* New York, NY: Wadsworth.

Patton, M. J., & Meara, N. M. (1992). *Psychoanalytic counseling: Ideas from psychoanalytic thought . . . translated for counselors.* New York, NY: Wiley.

Patton, M. J., & Robbins, S. B. (1982). Kohut's self-psychology as a model for college-student counseling. *Professional Psychology, 13,* 876–888.

Paul, G. L. (Ed.). (1988). *Assessment in residential treatment settings.* Champaign, IL: Research Press.

Pederson, P. B. (1991). Counseling international students. *The Counseling Psychologist, 19,* 10–58.

Pfammatter, M., Junghan, U. M., & Brenner, H. D. (2006). Efficacy of psychological therapy in schizophrenia: Conclusions from meta-analyses. *Schizophrenia Bulletin, 32*(S1), S64–80.

Phillips, K. A. (2005). *The broken mirror.* New York, NY: Oxford University Press.

Phillips, K. A., McElroy, S. L., Keck, P. E., Pope, H. G., & Hudson, J. I. (1993). Body dysmorphic disorder: 30 cases of imagined ugliness. *American Journal of Psychiatry, 181,* 699–702.

Philpot, C. L., Brooks, G. R., Lusterman, D. D., & Nutt, R. L. (1997). *Bridging separate gender worlds: Why men and women clash and how therapists can bring them together.* Washington, DC: American Psychological Association.

Plotkin, H., & Jackson, K. R. (Producers), & Lasseter, J. (Director). (1999). *Toy story 2* [Motion Picture]. United States: Pixar Animation Studios.

Polster, E., & Polster, M. (1999). *From the radical center: The heart of gestalt therapy.* Cleveland, OH: The Gestalt Institute of Cleveland Press.

Poyrazli, S., Kavanaugh, P. R., Baker, A., & Al-Timimi, N. (2004). Social support and demographic correlates of acculturative stress in international students. *Journal of College Counseling, 7,* 73–82.

Prochaska, J. O., Norcross, J. C., & DiClemente, C. C. (1994). *Changing for good.* New York, NY: Morrow.

Project MATCH Research Group. (1997). Matching alcoholism treatments to patient heterogeneity: Project MATCH post-treatment drinking outcomes. *Journal of Studies on Alcohol, 58,* 7–29.

Quimby, K. (2005). Will & Grace: Negotiating (gay) marriage on prime-time television. *Journal of Popular Culture, 38*(4), 713–731.

Radtke, L., Sapp, M., & Farrell, W. C. (1997). Reality therapy: A meta-analysis. *Journal of Reality Therapy, XVII*(1), 4–9.

Raskin, N. J., & Rogers, C. R. (2000). Person-centered therapy. In R. J. Corsini & D. Wedding (Eds.), *Current psychotherapies* (6th ed., pp. 133–167). Itasca, IL: Peacock.

Rector, N. A., & Beck, A. T. (2002). A clinical review of cognitive therapy for schizophrenia. *Current Psychiatry Report, 4,* 284–292.

Reich, L., & Kolbasovsky, A. (2006). *Mental health provider's guide to managed care: Industry insiders reveal how to successfully participate and profit in today's system.* New York, NY: Norton.

Reif, S. (2005). *How to reach and teach ADD/ADHD children.* San Francisco, CA: Jossey-Bass.

Reiner, R. (Director). (1990). *Misery* [Motion Picture]. United States: Castle Rock Entertainment.

Reitherman, W. (Director). (1968). *Winnie the Pooh and the blustery day* [Motion Picture]. United States: Walt Disney Productions.

Reitherman, W. (Producer), & Reitherman, W., & Lounsbery, J. (Directors). (1977). *The many adventures of Winnie the Pooh* [Motion Picture]. United States: Walt Disney Productions.

Reitman, J. (Director). (2007). *Juno* [Motion Picture]. United States: Fox Searchlight Pictures.

Remer, P. (2008). Feminist therapy. In J. Frew & M. D. Spiegler (Eds.), *Contemporary psychotherapies for a diverse world* (pp. 397–441). Boston, MA: Lahaska Press.

Reynolds, J. F., Mair, D. C., & Fischer, P. C. (1995). *Writing and reading mental health records: Issues and analyses* (2nd ed.). Mahwah, NJ: Erlbaum.

Robertie, K., Weidenbenner, R., Barrett, L., & Poole, R. (2008). Milieu multiplex: Using movies in the treatment of adolescents with sexual behavior problems. In L. Rubin (Ed.), *Popular culture in counseling, psychotherapy, and play-based interventions* (pp. 99–122). New York, NY: Springer.

Robbins, S. B. (1989). Role of contemporary psychoanalysis in counseling psychology. *Journal of Counseling Psychology, 36,* 267–278.

Robbins, S. B., & Zinni, V. R. (1988). Implementing a time-limited treatment model: Issues and solutions. *Professional Psychology: Research and Practice, 19,* 53–57.

Robinson, D. J. (2003). *Reel psychiatry: Movie portrayals of psychiatric conditions.* Port Huron, MI: Rapid Psychler Press.

Rogers, C. (1951). *Client-centered therapy: Its current practice, implications and theory.* London: Constable.

Rogers, C. R. (1961). *On becoming a person.* Boston, MA: Houghton Mifflin.

Rogers, C. R. (1977). *Carl Rogers on personal power: Inner strength and its revolutionary impact.* New York, NY: Delacorte Press.

Rogers, C. R. (1986). Rogers, Kohut, and Erickson: A personal perspective on some similarities and differences. In J. K. Zeig (Ed.), *The evolution of psychotherapy* (pp. 179–187). New York, NY: Brunner/Mazel.

Rogers, S. J. (1998). Neuropsychology of autism in young children and its implications for early intervention. *Mental Retardation and Developmental Disabilities Research Reviews, 4,* 104–112.

Rose, A. (1995). Metaphor with an attitude: The use of *The Mighty Morphin Power Rangers* television series as a therapeutic metaphor. *International Journal of Play Therapy, 4*(2), 59–72.

Rosen, J. C., Reiter, J., & Orosan, P. (1995). Cognitive-behavioral body-image therapy for body dysmorphic disorder. *Journal of Consulting and Clinical Psychology, 63,* 263–269.

Rosenberg, R., & Kosslyn, S. (2010). *Abnormal psychology.* New York, NY: Worth Publishers.

Rubin, L. (Ed.). (2006a). *Psychotropic drugs and popular culture: Essays on medicine, mental health and the media.* Jefferson, NC: McFarland.

Rubin, L. (Ed.). (2006b). *Using superheroes in counseling and play therapy.* New York, NY: Springer.

Rubin, L. (2008). Introduction. In L. Rubin (Ed.), *Popular culture in counseling, psychotherapy and play-based interventions (*pp. xxi–ivii). New York, NY: Springer.

Russell, J. M. (2007). Existential psychotherapy. In A. B. Rochlen (Ed.), *Applying counseling theories: An online case-based approach* (pp. 107–125). Upper Saddle River, NJ: Pearson Prentice Hall.

Saatcioglu, O., Erim, R., & Cakmak, D. (2006). Role of family in alcohol and substance abuse. *Psychiatry and Clinical Neurosciences, 60,* 125–132.

Saravanan, P., Visser, T., & Dayan, C. M. (2006). Psychological wellbeing correlates with free T4 but not free T3 levels in patients on thyroid hormone replacement. *Journal of Clinical Endocrinology & Metabolism, 91*(September), 3389–3393.

Savage, T., Harley, D., & Nowak, D. (2005). Applying social empowerment strategies as tools for self-advocacy in counseling lesbian and gay male clients. *Journal of Counseling and Development: JCD, 83*(2), 131–137.

Schaeffer, C. E., & Carey, L. (Eds.). (1994). *Family play therapy.* Northvale, NJ: Jason Aronson.

Schlossberg, N. K. (1995). *Counseling older adults in transition* (2nd ed.). New York, NY: Springer.

Schmaling, K. B., & Hernandez, D. V. (2005). Detection of depression among low-income Mexican Americans in primary care. *Journal of Health Care for the Poor and Underserved, 16,* 780–790.

Schwartz, R., & Feisthamel, K. (2009). Disproportionate diagnosis of mental disorders among African American versus European American clients: Implications for counseling theory, research and practice. *Journal of Counseling and Development: JCD, 87*(3), 295–301.

Schwitzer, A. M. (1996). Using the inverted pyramid heuristic in counselor education and supervision. *Counselor Education and Supervision, 35,* 258–267.

Schwitzer, A. M. (1997). The inverted pyramid framework applying self psychology constructs to conceptualizing college student psychotherapy. *Journal of College Student Psychotherapy, 11*(3), 29–47.

Schwitzer, A. M. (2005). Self-development, social support, and student help-seeking: Research summary and implications for college psychotherapists. *Journal of College Student Psychotherapy, 20*(2), 29–52.

Schwitzer, A. M., Boyce, D., Cody, P., Holman, A., & Stein, S. (2006). Clinical supervision and professional development using clients from literature, popular fiction and entertainment media. *Journal of Creativity and Mental Health, 1*(1), 57–80.

Schwitzer, A. M., & Everett, A. (1997). Reintroducing the *DSM-IV:* Responses to ten counselor reservations about diagnosis. *The Virginia Counselors Journal, 25,* 54–64.

Schwitzer, A. M., Hatfield, T., Jones, A. R., Duggan, M. H., Jurgens, J., & Winninger, A. (2008). Confirmation among college women: The eating disorders not otherwise specified diagnostic profile. *The Journal of American College Health, 56,* 607–615.

Schwitzer, A. M., MacDonald, K. E., & Dickinson, P. (2008). Using pop culture characters in clinical training and supervision. In L. Rubin (Ed.), *Popular culture in counseling, psychotherapy, and play-based interventions* (pp. 315–342). New York, NY: Springer.

Schwitzer, A. M., Rodriguez, L. E., Thomas, C., & Salimi, L. (2001). The eating disorder NOS diagnostic profile among college women. *Journal of American College Health, 49,* 157–166.

Scott, J., & Gutierrez, M. (2004). The current status of psychological treatments in bipolar disorders: A systematic review of relapse prevention. *Bipolar Disorders, 6,* 498–503.

Selfhout, M., Delsing, M., der Bogt, T., & Meeus, W. (2008.). Heavy metal usage and hip-hop style preferences and externalizing problem behavior. *Youth and Society, 39,* 435–452.

Seligman, L. (1993). Teaching treatment planning. *Counselor Education and Supervision, 33,* 287–297.

Seligman, L. (1996). *Diagnosis and treatment planning* (2nd ed.). New York, NY: Plenum Press.

Seligman, L. (1998). *Selecting effective treatments: A comprehensive systematic guide to treating mental disorders.* Upper Saddle River, NJ: Merrill/Prentice Hall

Seligman, L. (2004). *Diagnosis and treatment planning* (3rd ed.). New York, NY: Plenum Press.

Seligman, L., & Reichenberg, L. (2007). *Selecting effective treatments: A comprehensive systematic guide to treating mental disorders.* New York, NY: Wiley.

Seligman, M. E. P. (1990). *Learned optimism.* New York, NY: Pocket Books.

Servaty-Seib, H. L. (2004). Connections between counseling theories and current theories of grief and mourning. *Journal of Mental Health Counseling, 26*(2), 125–145.

Shannon, J. (2011, November). *Understanding personality disorders.* Seminar for Health Professionals, Institute for Brain Potential, Norfolk, VA.

Sharma, T., & Harvey, P. (Eds.). (2000). *Cognition in schizophrenia: Impairments, importance and treatment strategies.* Oxford, UK: Oxford University Press.

Shapiro, F. (Ed.). (2002). *EMDR as an integrative psychotherapy approach: Experts of diverse orientations explore the paradigm prism.* Washington, DC: American Psychological Association.

Shapiro, R. (2005). *EMDR solutions: Pathways to healing.* New York, NY: W. W. Norton.

Sicile-Kira, C., & Grandin, T. (2004). *Autism spectrum disorders: The complete guide to understanding autism, Asperger's syndrome, pervasive developmental disorder, and other ASDs.* New York, NY: Perigee Books.

Singer, D., & Singer, J. (2007). *Imagination and play in the electronic age.* London: Harvard University Press.

Slade, D. (Director). (2010). *Eclipse* [Motion Picture]. United States: Summit Entertainment

Snell, W. E., Jr., Gum, S., Shuck, R. L., Mosley, J. A., & Hite, T. L. (1995). The Clinical Anger Scale: Preliminary reliability and validity. *Journal of Clinical Psychology, 51,* 215–226.

Spector, A., Davies, S., Woods, B., & Orrell, M. (2000). Reality orientation for dementia: A systematic review of the evidence of effectiveness from randomized controlled trials. *The Gerontologist, 40,* 206–212.

Spielberg, S. (Director). (1985). *The color purple* [Motion Picture]. United States: Amblin Entertainment.

Spira, A. P., & Edelstein, B. A. (2006). Behavioral interventions for agitation in older adults with dementia: An evaluative review. *International Psychogeriatrics, 18,* 195–225.

Spitzer, R. L., Gibbon, M., Skodol, A., Williams, J. B., & First, M. B. (Eds.). (1994). *DSM-IV casebook: A learning companion to the* Diagnostic and Statistical Manual of Mental Disorders, Fourth Edition. Washington, DC: American Psychiatric Association.

Stanton, M. D., & Shadish, W. R. (1997). Outcome, attrition, and family-couples treatment for drug abuse: A meta-analysis and review of the controlled, comparative studies. *Psychological Bulletin, 122,* 170–191.

Steenbarger, B. N. (1994). Duration and outcome in psychotherapy: An integrative review. *Professional Psychology: Research and Practice, 25*(2), 111–119.

Stein, D. J., Christiansen, G. A., & Hollander, E. (Eds.). (1999). *Trichotillomania.* Washington, DC: American Psychiatric Press.

Stern, B., Barak,, B., & Gould, S. (1987). Sexual Identity Scale: A new self-assessment measure. *Sex Roles, 17*(9/10), 503–519.

Strain, J. J., Hammer, J. S., McKenzie, D. P., Blumenfeld, M., Muskin, P., Newstadt, G., Wallack, J., Wilner, A., & Schleifer, S. S. (1998). Adjustment disorder: A multisite study of its utilization and interventions in the consultation-liaison psychiatry setting. *General Hospital Psychiatry, 20*(3), 134–149.

Strakowski, S. M., McElroy, S. L., Keck, P. E., & West, S. A. (1996). Racial influences on diagnosis in psychotic mania. *Journal of Affective Disorders, 39,* 157–162.

Substance Abuse and Mental Health Services Organization, Office of Applied Studies. (2006). *Results from the 2005 National Survey on Drug Use and Health: National findings* (NSDUH Series H-30, DHHS Publication No. SMA 06-4194). Rockville, MD: Author.

Swan, K. (1995). *Saturday morning cartoons and children's perceptions of social reality* (Report No. PS 023908). San Francisco, CA: Paper Presented at the Annual Meeting of the American educational Research Association. (ERIC Document Reproduction Services No. ED 390579)

Swarup, V. (2008). *Slumdog millionaire.* Toronto, ON, Canada: Harper.

Sweeney, T. J. (1998). *Adlerian counseling: A practitioner's approach* (4th ed.). Philadelphia, PA: Accelerated Development.

Taffel, R. (2005). *Breaking through to teens: A new psychotherapy for the new adolescence.* New York, NY: Guilford Press.

Tarrier, N., & Bobes, J. (2000). The importance of psychosocial interventions and patient involvement in the treatment of schizophrenia. *International Journal of Psychiatry in Clinical Practice, 4,* S35-S51.

Tarrier, N., Kinney, C., McCarthy, E., Wittkowski, A., Yusupoff, L., Gledhill, A., Morris, J., & Humphreys, L. (2001). Are some types of psychotic symptoms more responsive to cognitive-behaviour therapy? *Behaviour & Cognitive Psychotherapy, 29,* 45–55.

Taylor, S. (1996). Meta-analysis of cognitive-behavioral treatments for social phobia. *Journal of Behavior Therapy and Experimental Psychiatry, 27*(1), 1–9.

Teyber, E. (1992). *Interpersonal process in psychotherapy: A guide for clinical training* (2nd ed.). Pacific Grove, CA: Brooks/Cole.

Teyber, E. (2000). *Interpersonal process in psychotherapy: A guide for clinical training* (4th ed.). Pacific Grove, CA: Brooks/Cole.

Thompson, T., & Zerbino, E. (1995). Gender roles in animated cartoons: Has the picture changed in 20 years? *Sex Roles, 32*(9/10), 651–673.

Thorne, B. (2002). Person-centered therapy. In W. Dryden (Ed.), *Handbook of individual therapy* (4th ed., pp. 131–157). London: Sage.

Tiggerman, M. (2005). Television and adolescent body image: The role of program content and viewing motivation. *Journal of Social and Clinical Psychology, 24*(3), 361–381.

Tippins, S., & Reiff, M. (2004). *ADHD: A complete and authoritative guide.* Elk Grove Village, IL: American Academy of Pediatrics.

Trierweiler, S. J., Muroff, J. R., Jackson, J. S., Neighbors, H. W., & Munday, C. (2005). Clinician race, situational attributions, and diagnoses of mood versus schizophrenia disorders. *Cultural Diversity & Ethnic Minority Psychology, 11,* 351–364.

Trousdale, G., & Wise, K. (Directors). (1991). *Beauty and the beast* [Motion Picture]. United States: Walt Disney Pictures.

Tsai, J. (2008). *Leading edge cognitive disorders research.* Happauge, NY: Nova.

Turkington, D., Kingdon, D., & Weiden, P. J. (2006). Cognitive behavior therapy for schizophrenia. *American Journal of Psychiatry, 163,* 365–373.

Unkrich, L. (Director). (2010). *Toy story 3* [Motion Picture]. United States: Pixar Animation and Walt Disney Studios.

Van IJzendoorn, M. H., Vereijken, C., Bakermans-Kranenburg, M. J., & Riksen-Walraven, M. (2004). Assessing attachment security with the Attachment Q Sort: Meta-analytic evidence for the validity of the Observer AQS. *Child Development, 75*(4), 1188–1213.

Van Bergeijk, E., Klin, A., & Volkmar, F. (2008). Supporting more able students on the autism spectrum: College and beyond. *Journal of Autism and Developmental Disorders, 38,* 1359–1370.

Van Deurzen, E. (1991). Ontological insecurity revisited. *Journal of the Society for Existential Analysis, 2,* 38–48.

Van Deurzen, E. (2002). *Existential counseling and psychotherapy in practice* (2nd ed.). London: Sage.

VanFleet, R., Sywulak, K. A., Caporaso, C., Sniscak, C. C., & Guerney, L. (2010). *Child-centered play therapy.* New York, NY: Guilford Press.

Vaughn, S. C. (1997). *The talking cure.* New York, NY: Henry Holt.

Vernon, A. (2009). Applications of rational-emotive behavior therapy with children and adolescents.

In A. Vernon (Ed.), *Counseling children & adolescents* (4th ed., pp. 173–202). Denver, CO: Love Publishing.

Vernon, A., & Clemente, R. (2005). *Assessment and intervention with children and adolescents: Developmental and multicultural considerations.* Alexandria, VA: American Counseling Association.

Vontress, C. E., Johnson, J. A., & Epp, L. R. (1999). *Cross-cultural counseling: A casebook.* Alexandria, VA: American Counseling Association.

Vuust, P., & Frith, C. (2008). Anticipation is the key to understanding music and the effects of music on emotion. *Behavioral and Brain Sciences, 31*(5), 599–600.

Walker, A. (1982). *The color purple.* New York, NY: Harcourt Brace Jovanovich.

Wampold, B. E. (2001). *The great psychotherapy debate: Models, methods, and findings.* Mahwah, NJ: Erlbaum.

Watts, R. E. (Ed.). (2003). *Adlerian, cognitive and constructivistic therapies: An integrative dialogue.* New York, NY: Springer.

Watts, R. E. (2007). Counseling conservative Christian couples: A spiritually sensitive perspective. In O. J. Morgan (Ed.), *Counseling and spirituality: Views from the profession* (pp. 165–186). Boston, MA: Lahaska/Houghton Mifflin.

Wedding, D. (2005). *Movies & mental illness: Using films to understand psychopathology.* Cambridge, MA: Hogrefe.

Weinberg, G. (1996). *The heart of psychotherapy.* New York, NY: St. Martin's Griffin.

Weissman, M. M., Markowitz, J. C., & Klerman, G. L. (2000). *Comprehensive guide to interpersonal psychotherapy.* New York, NY: Basic Books.

Weitz, C. (Director). (2009). *New moon* [Motion Picture]. United States: Summit Entertainment.

Wells, K. C., Pelham, W. E., Kotkon, R., Hoza, B., & Abikoff, H., & Colleagues (2000). Psychosocial treatment strategies in the MTA study: Rationale, methods, and critical issues in design and implementation. *Journal of Abnormal Child Psychology, 28*(6), 483–505.

Wenar, C. (1990). *Psychopathology from infancy through adolescence* (2nd ed.). New York, NY: Random House.

Westen, D., & Morrison, K. (2001). A multidimensional meta-analysis of treatments for depression, panic, and generalized anxiety disorder: An empirical examination of the status of empirically supported therapies. *Journal of Consulting and Clinical Psychology, 69*(6), 875–899.

White, M. (1989). Pseudo-encopresis: From avalanche to victory, from vicious to virtuous cycles. In *Selected papers* (pp. 115–124). Adelaide, Australia: Dulwich Centre Publications. Reprinted from *Family Systems Medicine, 2*[2], 1984).

White, M. (2007). *Maps of narrative practice.* New York, NY: W. W. Norton.

Wilson, C., Nairn, R., Coverdale, J., & Panapa, A. (2000). How mental illness is portrayed in children's television: A prospective study. *British Journal of Psychiatry, 176,* 440–443.

Winger, G., Woods, J., & Hoffman, F. (2004). *A handbook on drug and alcohol abuse: The biomedical aspects.* New York, NY: Oxford University Press.

Wise, R. (Producer), & Robbins, J. (Director). (1961). *West side story* [Motion Picture]. United States: Mirisch.

Wolpe, J. (1990). *The practice of behavior therapy* (4th ed.). New York, NY: Pergamon Press.

Woods, B. (2004). Reducing the impact of cognitive impairment in dementia. In A. D. Baddeley, M. D. Kopelman, & B. A. Wilson (Eds.), *Essential handbook of memory disorders for clinicians* (pp. 285–300). New York, NY: Wiley.

Woods, B., Spector, A., Jones, C., Orrell, M., & Davies, S. (1998). Reminiscence therapy for dementia. *Cochrane Database of Systematic Reviews, 3:* CD001120.

Woodside, M., & McClam, T. (1998). *Generalist case management: A method of human services delivery.* Pacific Grove, CA: Brooks/Cole.

Worell, J., & Johnson, N. G. (Eds.). (1997). *Shaping the future of feminist psychology: Education, research, and practice.* Washington, DC: American Psychological Association.

Wubbolding, R. E. (2000). *Reality therapy for the 21st century.* Philadelphia, PA: Brunner-Routledge.

Wubbolding, R. E. (2007). Reality therapy theory. In D. Capuzzi & D. R. Gross (Eds.), *Counseling and psychotherapy: Theories and interventions* (4th ed., pp. 289–312). Upper Saddle, NJ: Merrill Prentice Hall.

Wubbolding, R. E., & Brickell, J. (1998). *Counseling with reality therapy.* Oxon, UK: Winslow Press.

Wubbolding, R. E., Brickell, J., Imhof, L., In-Za Kim, R., Lojk, L., & Al-Rashidi, B. (2004). Reality therapy: A global perspective. *International Journal for the Advancement of Counseling, 26,* 219–228.

Wubbolding, R. E., & Colleagues. (1998). Multicultural awareness: Implications for reality therapy and choice theory. *International Journal of Reality Therapy, 17,* 4–6.

Wykes, T., Reeder, C., Williams, C., Corner, J., Rice, C., & Everett, B. (2003). Are the effects of cognitive remediation therapy (CRT) durable? Results from an exploratory trial in schizophrenia. *Schizophrenia Research, 61,* 163–174.

Wykes, T., & Reeder, C. (2005). *Cognitive remediation therapy for schizophrenia.* New York, NY: Routledge.

Yalom, I. D. (1980). *Existential psychotherapy.* New York, NY: Basic Books.

Yalom, I. D. (2003). *The gift of therapy: An open letter to a new generation of therapists and their patients.* New York, NY: HarperCollins (Perennial).

Young, J., Klosko, J., & Weishart, M. (2003). *Schema therapy: A practitioner's guide.* New York, NY: Guilford Press.

Young, J. E. (1990). *Cognitive therapy for personality disorders: A schema-focused approach.* Sarasota, FL: Professional Resource Exchange.

Young, T. (1993). Women as comic book superheroes: The weaker sex in the Marvel universe. *Journal of Human Behavior, 30*(2), 49–50.

Yudofsky, S., & Hales, R. (2007). *The American Psychiatric Publishing textbook of neuro-psychiatry and behavioral neuroscience.* Arlington, VA: American Psychiatric Publishing.

Zeanah, C. H., & Boris, N. W. (2005). Disturbances and disorders of attachment in early childhood. In C. H. Zeanah, Jr. (Ed.), *Handbook of infant mental health* (pp. 353–368). New York, NY: Guilford Press.

Zaentz, S., & Douglas, M. (Producers), & Forman, M. (Director). (1975). *One flew over the cuckoo's nest* [Motion Picture]. United States: United Artists.

Zero to Three Association. (2005). *Diagnostic classification of mental health and developmental disorders of infancy and early childhood.* Washington, DC: Zero to Three: National Center for Infants, Toddlers and Families.

INDEX

ABOUT THE AUTHORS

Alan M. "Woody" Schwitzer, PhD is a Licensed Psychologist and Professor of Counseling at Old Dominion University (ODU) in Norfolk, Virginia. Dr. Schwitzer completed his graduate degrees in Counseling Psychology at Virginia Commonwealth University and interned at The University of Texas at Austin Counseling and Mental Health Center. Prior to full-time faculty work, he was Assistant Director of the Tulane University Counseling and Testing Center and then Assistant Professor and Training Director of the James Madison University Counseling and Student Development Center. Dr. Schwitzer is past editor of the *Journal of College Counseling.* He has Chaired the Council of Journal of Editors of the American Counseling Association (ACA), and currently reviews articles for the *Journal of American College Health* and *Journal of College Student Development,* publications of the American College Health Association and American College Personnel Association. Dr. Schwitzer has published over 40 journal, magazine, and newspaper articles primarily examining college and university student adjustment, development, learning, and counseling. He also specializes in teaching diagnosis, case conceptualization, and treatment planning. His previous books include *Skills and Tools for Today's Counselors and Psychotherapists: From Natural Helping to Professional Counseling* and *Promoting Student Learning and Student Development at a Distance.* Among Dr. Schwitzer's recent awards are the Ralph M. Berdie Memorial Award for Research and Scholarship in the Field of College Student Affairs and the American College Counseling Association's Outstanding Contribution to Professional Knowledge Award. Woody lives near the Lafayette River with his wife, two dogs, and cat. He maintains a private practice focusing on consultation, training, and continuing education.

Lawrence "Larry" Rubin, PhD, LMHC, RPTS is a Professor of Counselor Education at St. Thomas University in Miami, Florida, where he directs the Mental Health Counseling Program and is a private practice psychologist, professional counselor, and play therapist. Dr. Rubin, past president of the Florida Association for Play Therapy, currently serves on the Board of Directors of the Association for Play Therapy. Dr. Rubin's research interests and publications lie at the intersection of psychology and popular culture. He is a prolific writer and editor. His book, *Psychotropic Drugs and Popular Culture: Medicine, Mental Health and the Media,* won the 2006 Ray and Pat Browne Award for Best Anthology. His other books include *Food for Thought: Essays on Eating and Culture, Popular Culture in Counseling, Psychotherapy and Play-based Intervention, Using Superheroes in Counseling and Play Therapy, Messages: Self-help Through Popular Culture, Mental Illness* *and Popular Media: Essays on the Representation of Psychiatric Disorders and Play-based Interventions for Children and Adolescents With Autism Spectrum Disorders.* Larry blogs about popular culture and psychology for *Psychology Today* magazine and is the Area Chair of the Division of Mental Health, Mental Illness and Popular Culture for the Popular Culture Association. He lives in Ft. Lauderdale with his wife, two children, and five pets.

The authors would be glad to hear from you! They can be reached at aschwitz@odu.edu and lrubin@stu.edu, respectively.

SAGE Research Methods Online

The essential tool for researchers

Sign up now at www.sagepub.com/srmo for more information.

An expert research tool

- An **expertly designed taxonomy** with more than 1,400 unique terms for social and behavioral science research methods
- **Visual and hierarchical search tools** to help you discover material and link to related methods

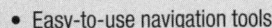

- Easy-to-use navigation tools
- Content organized by complexity
- Tools for citing, printing, and downloading content with ease
- Regularly updated content and features

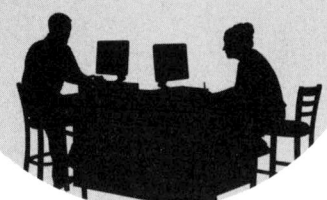

A wealth of essential content

- The most comprehensive picture of quantitative, qualitative, and mixed methods available today
- More than **100,000 pages of SAGE book and reference material** on research methods as well as editorially selected material from SAGE journals
- More than **600 books** available in their entirety online

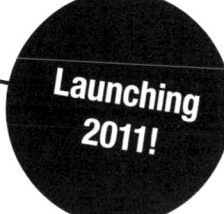

Launching 2011!

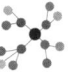 **$SAGE** research methods online

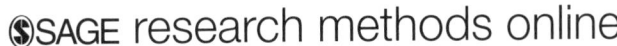